Sexually Transmitted Diseases

REPRODUCTIVE MEDICINE

A Series of Textbooks and Monographs

Volume 1 Practical Pediatric and Adolescent Gynecology, Sir John Dewhurst

Volume 2 Amniotic Fluid and Its Clinical Significance, edited by Merton Sandler

Volume 3 Clinical Sexuality, edited by Stephen F. Pariser, Stephen B. Levine, and Malcolm L. Gardner

Volume 4 Clinical and Diagnostic Procedures in Obstetrics and Gynecology. Part A: Obstetrics. Part B: Gynecology, edited by E. Malcolm Symonds and Frederick P. Zuspan

Volume 5 Continuous Transcutaneous Blood Gas Monitoring, edited by Renate Huch and Albert Huch

Volume 6 Fetal Physiology and Medicine, Second, Revised Edition, edited by Richard W. Beard and Peter W. Nathanielsz

Volume 7 Sexually Transmitted Diseases: A Clinical Syndrome Approach, edited by Vincent A. Spagna and Richard B. Prior

Other volumes in preparation

Sexually Transmitted Diseases
A Clinical Syndrome Approach

edited by
VINCENT A. SPAGNA
RICHARD B. PRIOR
The Ohio State University
College of Medicine
Columbus, Ohio

Marcel Dekker, Inc. New York and Basel

Library of Congress Cataloging in Publication Data

Main entry under title:

Sexually transmitted diseases.

(Reproductive medicine ; v. 7)
Includes bibliographies and index.
1. Venereal diseases--Diagnosis. 2. Diagnosis, Differential. 3. Syndromes. I. Spagna, Vincent A. II. Prior, Richard B.
[DNLM: 1. Venereal Diseases. W1 RE213P v. 7 / WC 140 S5185]
RC200.5.S49 1985 616.9'5 85-1602
ISBN 0-8247-7310-1

Marcel Dekker, Inc.
270 Madison Avenue, New York, New York 10016

Current printing (last digit):
10 9 8 7 6 5 4 3 2 1

PRINTED IN THE UNITED STATES OF AMERICA

To Aunt Fran
V. A. S.

To Tina, Pam, Chris, and Rick
R. B. P.

About the Series

Some time ago, the publishers, Marcel Dekker, Inc., interested us in developing a new concept in editing a series of books on *Reproductive Medicine*, which would span the Atlantic Ocean by the editors' representation in Europe and in the United States. In general, many of the books destined for production in this series that relate specifically to obstetrics and gynecology will have an author or editor in Europe and one in the United States. This concept of bringing contributors from the two continents together permits an academic discussion of similar and dissimilar points of view in relation to any given topic.

Marcel Dekker is particularly well placed to introduce such a concept. Their previous experience has involved the development and merging of European publishing experience into the United States scene. At present, Dekker's main office is in New York, with supplementary offices in Europe. Hence, the amalgamation of authors, under joint editorship, and the established experience for distribution of books, have made this experiment one that is particularly well adapted to these publishers. This is a new venture in medical publishing and one which will grow and develop with time.

E. Malcolm Symonds, M.D.
Frederick P. Zuspan, M.D.

Foreword

The rate of increase of gonorrhea in the early 1970s was described as "a national outrage" by the head of the Venereal Disease Control Branch at the Centers for Disease Control (CDC), and rightly so. The National Commission on Venereal Disease reported to the Assistant Secretary for Health that a pandemic of sexually transmitted diseases (STDs) was developing and made recommendations to reduce the number of cases. The American Medical Association and the American Academy of Family Physicians also called for cooperation at all levels in controlling the spread and the expensive consequences of STDs by urging "intensified public and professional education which will result in increased awareness, exact diagnosis, effective treatment, prompt reporting and proper epidemiological investigation of venereal disease."

Implementing these precepts continues to be timely, for neither physicians at CDC (and other public health physicians) nor their colleagues in clinical practice and academia foresaw the increasing numbers of STDs—there are now at least 25 distinct entities. Nor did they predict the vast involvement of people, largely between the ages of 15 and 35, who would suffer the consequences of the STD juggernaut.

Another unforeseeable factor in the spread of STDs was the variation and multiplication of sexual activities, leading to an imaginative "mix and match of mucous membranes" (as one epidemiologist put it). These activities seem to be limited only by the flexibility, stamina, and availability of willing partners. The youth of society seem to have been anesthetized to the possibilities of pain, loss of time and money, sterility, or even death in the case of the latest STD, the acquired immune deficiency syndrome. Today more people are transmitting more disease with "tender loving care" than at any other time in history.

Unprotected anonymous intercourse is a not uncommon practice, resulting in new disease manifestations in the same old places as well as old diseases occupying anatomical locations hitherto unaffected by STDs. A homosexual male, asked to describe bathhouse activities, replied, "Organs and orifices, orifices and organs." Careful histories reveal that heterosexuals also are employing insertion/reception techniques other than the time-honored genital/genital activity.

In editing *Sexually Transmitted Diseases: A Clinical Syndrome Approach*, Drs. Spagna and Prior recognized the numerous presenting symptoms and signs of today's STDs and grouped them according to a rational clinical methodology that should enhance the diagnostic and therapeutic abilities of clinicians of various specialties in dealing with the multiple manifestations of modern sexual gymnastics. The editors are also well aware of the hiatus within the medical education system in teaching about STDs ever since public and professional opinion welcomed penicillin as Ehrlich's "magic bullet" in the early 1950s, proclaimed syphilis and gonorrhea to be conquered, and almost completely [with the exception of the CDC and the American Social Health Association (ASHA)] abandoned the field, in both education and research. The subject of STDs is now slowly being restored to the curricula of medical schools, residency programs, and continuing medical education organizations.

Thanks to some dedicated people in both the CDC and the ASHA, along with some state and local health officers, concerned professional organizations, and legislators interested in a group of diseases long held to be an untouchable topic because of the nature of transmission, there is an increasing public and professional awareness and dedication to controlling these diseases, which wreak such havoc on our youth and thereby our future. Indeed, recent congressional action "intends that a strong well-defined research program be developed and believes that the National Institute of Allergy and Infectious Diseases [NIAID] must begin to take a far more aggressive and responsible posture in confronting this epidemic through basic and clinical investigation, as well as prevention research strategies." The Advisory Council of NIAID has responded by adopting recommendations calling for expansion of the current teaching and research programs in STDs.

The American Medical Association in June 1984 reaffirmed its interest in STD control by passing a resolution to "continue to urge increased efforts at all levels of the federation to bring sexually transmitted diseases under control through professional and public education, supportive efforts of the State Departments of Health, Centers for Disease Control, the National Institutes of Health, and other appropriate organizations." In 1983 the prestigious and authoritative AMA Council on Scientific Affairs noted that STDs continue to increase and to pose a hazard, estimating that one out of every four Americans between the ages of 15 and 55 is affected by one of the STDs. The American Social Health Association, a United Way agency located at 260 Sheridan Avenue, Palo Alto, CA 94306, distributes literature on STDs to multiple audiences, operates the VD National Hotline (800-227-8922), and sponsors the Venereal Diseases Research Fund and the Herpes Resource Center with its many local chapters.

Spagna and Prior insist on excellence in the management of STDs. This volume thoroughly explains the various syndromes and their accurate diagnosis through detailed histories, painstaking observation, and intelligent use of laboratory facilities in and out of the physician's office. The editors and authors are aware of the need for a responsible approach to the control of these many diseases and present their advice in a professionally and socially responsible manner, including a list of questions commonly asked by patients, with appropriate answers.

Although the physician's battle against disease and disability is never-ending, the consequences of STDs are unacceptable and will be decreased only by educating those at risk, those who treat, those who control resources, and those who teach, that loving one another also means that the transmission of disease by close human contact is unwise, unwarranted, and unloving. One hopes that future editions of this useful reference will include, along with inexpensive, rapid, effective diagnostic and therapeutic modalities, information that the numbers of STD cases—along with their tangible and intangible costs—are exhibiting a steady and meaningful decline.

Sam A. Nixon, M.D.

Director, Division of Continuing Education
The University of Texas
Health Science Center at Houston
Houston, Texas

Preface

Sexually transmitted diseases (STDs) are seen by a variety of health care providers, including specialists in family practice, obstetrics and gynecology, internal medicine, urology, and dermatology. These physicians see on a daily basis patients who have an STD as their chief complaint. Additionally, some physicians see patients who must be evaluated for STDs as part of their normal examination. These physicians include gynecologists and specialists in obstetrics and reproductive medicine since unsuspected and undetected STDs can cause serious complications in women and neonates. Traditionally, gonorrhea and syphilis are thought of as *the* "venereal diseases"; however, newer STDs have recently been recognized, and currently there are over 20 different types that are transmitted by sexual contact.

Sexually Transmitted Diseases is a concise, clinically oriented presentation of the various pathological conditions associated with the traditional and the newly recognized sexually transmitted infectious agents. The usual textbook approach to STDs has been the presentation of distinct and separate disease entities. While satisfying the organizational integrity of a comprehensive publication of medical disorders, it is difficult to extrapolate this information to actual clinical situations that present to the physician. The "syndrome" approach of *Sexually Transmitted Diseases* allows the clinician to construct an organized differential diagnosis around those pathological situations that are clinically apparent.

Sexually Transmitted Diseases is directed toward physicians, medical students, nurses, public health officials, and other paraprofessionals involved in the evaluation, management, and treatment of patients with STDs. A review of basic reproductive anatomy is presented, followed by an overview of the epidemiology of STDs. Then, the etiology, pathophysiology, clinical parameters, laboratory diagnosis, and proper management of the various disease entities are elaborated with guideline discussions of the commonly encountered clinical problems. Current treatment regimens recommended for a particular STD are incorporated into the appropriate chapter, and pertinent references are included at the end of each chapter. Color photographs are also included where necessary to show and compare important clinical conditions.

The clinical syndrome approach with emphasis on the differential diagnosis should be especially helpful to private practitioners who encounter STDs in their daily practices. Accordingly, we have included a separate chapter, specifically directed to these physicians, which deals with the outpatient approach to STDs and which coalesces much of the material presented in this book. Finally, we have included a chapter that contains 108 of the most frequently asked questions about "VD" from patients attending an STD clinic. Examples of short, straightforward answers are included. We hope that this chapter will give the health care provider some insight into the patient's perspective of STDs.

We wish to acknowledge Frederick P. Zuspan, who invited us to develop this book and who has enthusiastically supported our efforts. We also wish to thank the contributors for their participation and cooperation during this project.

Vincent A. Spagna
Richard B. Prior

Contents

Contributors

Ian M. Baird, M.B., Ch.B. Director, Infectious Diseases, Riverside Methodist Hospital, Columbus, Ohio

Richard C. Bump, M.D. Assistant Professor, Department of Obstetrics and Gynecology, The Ohio State University College of Medicine, Columbus, Ohio

James H. Caldwell, M.D. Professor, Division of Gastroenterology, Department of Medicine, The Ohio State University College of Medicine, Columbus, Ohio

Charles Camisa, M.D. Director, Division of Dermatology, and Assistant Professor, Department of Medicine, The Ohio State University College of Medicine, Columbus, Ohio

Blaise L. Congeni, M.D. Assistant Professor, Department of Pediatrics, Northeastern Ohio Universities College of Medicine, Rootstown, Ohio

James Q. Del Rosso, D.O. Clinical Instructor, Department of Dermatology, Southeastern College of Osteopathic Medicine, North Miami Beach, Florida

David A. Eschenbach, M.D. Professor, Department of Obstetrics and Gynecology, University of Washington, Seattle, Washington

Robert J. Fass, M.D. Professor, Division of Infectious Diseases, Department of Medicine, The Ohio State University College of Medicine, Columbus, Ohio

Thomas M. File, Jr., M.D. Associate Professor, Department of Medicine, Northeastern Ohio Universities College of Medicine, Rootstown, Ohio, and Chief, Infectious Disease Service, Akron City Hospital, Akron, Ohio

William G. Gardner, M.D. Associate Professor, Department of Medicine, Northeastern Ohio Universities College of Medicine, Rootstown, Ohio, and Director, Infectious Diseases, Akron General Medical Center, Akron, Ohio

Carol A. Kitchen, R.N. Registered Nurse, Venereal Disease Clinic, Columbus Health Department, Columbus, Ohio

Merry B. Krempasky, L.P.N. Licensed Practical Nurse, Venereal Disease Clinic, Columbus Health Department, Columbus, Ohio

David R. Lambert, M.D. Clinical Instructor, Division of Dermatology, Department of Medicine, The Ohio State University College of Medicine, Columbus, Ohio

Joseph G. Lossick, D.O., M.S. Epidemiologist, Division of Sexually Transmitted Diseases, Centers for Disease Control, Atlanta, Georgia, and Director, Sexually Transmitted Disease Research, Venereal Disease Clinic, Columbus Health Department, Columbus, Ohio

John A. Negulesco, Ph.D. Associate Professor, Department of Anatomy, The Ohio State University College of Medicine, Columbus, Ohio

Michael F. Para, M.D. Assistant Professor, Division of Infectious Diseases, Department of Medicine, The Ohio State University College of Medicine, Columbus, Ohio

Joseph F. Plouffe, M.D. Associate Professor, Division of Infectious Diseases, Department of Medicine, The Ohio State University College of Medicine, Columbus, Ohio

Richard B. Prior, Ph.D. Associate Professor, Division of Infectious Diseases, Department of Medicine, The Ohio State University College of Medicine, Columbus, Ohio

Vincent A. Spagna, M.D. Clinical Assistant Professor, Division of Infectious Diseases, Department of Medicine, The Ohio State University College of Medicine, Columbus, Ohio

Courtland Storck Clinical Associate, Venereal Disease Clinic, Columbus Health Department, Columbus, Ohio

James S. Tan, M.D. Chairman, Infectious Disease Subcouncil, Northeastern Ohio Universities College of Medicine, Rootstown, Ohio, and Chairman, Department of Medicine, Akron City Hospital, Akron, Ohio

Michael L. Tapper, M.D. Chief, Section of Infectious Diseases, Department of Medicine, Lenox Hill Hospital, New York, New York

Frank W. Yoder, M.D. Clinical Assistant Professor, Division of Dermatology, Department of Medicine, The Ohio State University College of Medicine, Columbus, Ohio

ONE

Basic Anatomy and Physiology

John A. Negulesco
The Ohio State University
College of Medicine
Columbus, Ohio

INTRODUCTION

The reproductive organs of the male and female are complicated anatomical structures frequently subjected to infections and/or abnormal growths due to the very nature of their narrow passages and secretory cells lining their lumina. Capable of rapid proliferation and often uncontrolled division, the parenchyma of the reproductive organs often leads to pathological functions when stimulated by physiological imbalances as well as external agents. The variety of injurious agents invading these areas cover the knowledge spectrum of a well-trained microbiologist by involving bacteria, flagellates, various groups of vermes, viruses, and most recently the acquired immune deficiency syndrome (AIDS).

A comprehensive and complete coverage of the reproductive organs is well beyond the scope of this chapter. We have attempted, however, to describe in a synoptic yet, hopefully, clear fashion the salient points in the anatomy of the male and female reproductive organs. Whenever necessary, the text is highlighted by original illustrations for a quick review and emphasis of the described area. It is our hope that the physician and student will use this chapter as a guide only and will eventually find the time to enjoy some of the classics in anatomy suggested at the end of the chapter in order to receive a complete knowledge of the relations of these organs and their intricate lymphatics, blood supply, and innervation.

REPRODUCTIVE ORGANS OF THE MALE

Major Genital Organs and Accessory Glandular Structures

There are five important genital organs in the anatomy of the male:

1. Testes and their internal adnexa
2. Ductus deferens
3. Seminal vesicles
4. Ejaculatory ducts
5. Penis

In addition, one must also consider two accessory glandular structures: the prostate and the bulbourethral glands.

The testes (Fig. 1) are paired compound tubular glands which produce the spermatozoa (reproductive cells of the male) and two major hormonal compounds: testosterone and some estrogen. The two organs develop under the kidneys within the extraperitoneal connective tissue of the upper lumbar region of the embryo. Body temperature plays an important factor in the regulation of spermatogenesis and the generation of viable sperm cells. Ideal physiological conditions necessitate a climate a few degrees below the physiological temperature of the human body (37°C). Thus one can appreciate why testes must take the time and require the necessary effort to leave the protected and soothingly warm environment of the peritoneal cavity, sometimes before birth, in order to descend to the colder climate of the scrotal pouch. The migration process takes 7 to 8 months; and, if unsuccessful, one or both testes may remain trapped within the peritoneal cavity, with resultant failure of development known as cryptorchidism. If the condition is not surgically corrected, the individual reaches adulthood lacking reproductive ability, since the core temperature of the body may inhibit or inactivate the process of spermatogenesis. Several historians maintain that at the height of the Roman Empire any male witness during a civil trial needed two intact testes, which had to be displayed to the judges, in order to testi-fy.

Under normal conditions the testis reaches the iliac fossa of the false or greater pelvis by the third intrauterine month, and by the fifth month it is already near the mouth of the internal or deep inguinal ring of the abdominal wall. Although the length of the inguinal canal (Fig. 1) in the fetus is relatively short (1.5 cm), it is believed that it takes the testis 2 or 3 months to descend through the abdominal weakness of the inguinal canal to reach the scrotum. The total migration of the

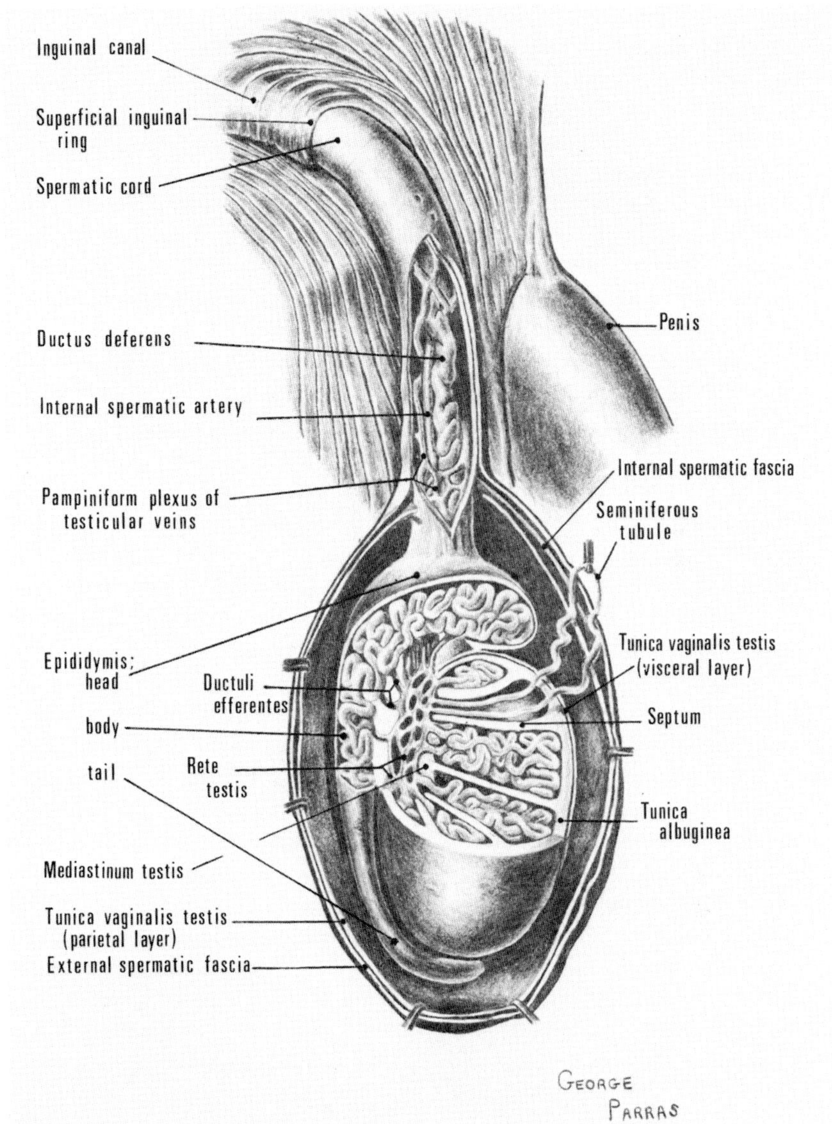

Fig. 1 Sagittal view of the testicle. (Illustration by George Parras, M.D.)

organ is completed by the eighth month of the gestation. A peritoneal protrusion, the processus vaginalis testis, precedes the testis during its descent through the inguinal region and mouth of the scrotum. Once the testis reaches its final destination within the scrotal pouch, the processus vaginalis adheres as a closed serous membrane or sac around and along the anterior and lateral sides of the organ to form or become known as the tunica vaginalis testis (Fig. 1). This latter addition often requires surgical intervention when its lining cells continue uninterruptedly their secretory activity or when its connection with the peritoneal cavity is not obliterated. Either condition results in a hydrocele, an abnormal accumulation of a large quantity of serous or peritoneal fluid within this circumtesticular structure.

The adult but not senile testis is about 4.5 cm long, 3 cm wide, and 2 cm thick and weighs between 9 to 15 g. The testes of an elephant, although much larger and weighing several kilograms, do not descend into the scrotal sac. The advantages are obvious and necessary should one consider a stampede through the wild African bush.

The entire testis is surrounded by a thick fibrous connective tissue coat, the tunica albuginea (Latin, "resembling egg white") (Fig. 1). At the posterior aspect of the organ, the white tunic enters the substance of the testis to form the mediastinum testis (Latin, "middle septum") (Fig. 1). This zone represents the point of entrance and exit for the numerous connectors of the organ: ducts, blood vessels, lymphatics, and some nervous fibers. The mediastinum testis also represents the area where partitions of fibrous connective tissue (septa) (Fig. 1) project toward the surface of the organ to divide it into multiple (as many as 400) compartments or lobules containing the seminiferous tubules (800 to 1600 per testis) (Fig. 1). Certain epithelial cells lining these tubules produce the spermatozoa (seminal lineage), while others, the Sertoli cells, like good nurses, support, protect, and feed the developping germinal cells. Each seminiferous tubule (70 to 80 cm long) extends from the cortex to the mediastinum testis, where it elongates to form a straight duct (plural tubuli recti) which connects to the tubular network of the rete testis (Fig. 1). This network of canals terminates at the superior end of the mediastinum testis into 12 to 20 efferent ducts (ductuli efferentes) (Fig. 1) which were patiently measured by the anatomical forefathers to be from 15 to 20 cm in length. The ductuli efferentes penetrate the white and fibrous testicular tunic (tunica albuginea) to drain into the single duct comprising the head of the epididymis (Greek, *epi* = on, *didymos* = twin; plural testes) (Fig. 1). The C-shaped and highly convoluted epididymis (7 m in length, 0.4 mm in diameter) is positioned along the posterior aspect of the testis, and it can be subdivided into a head (which rests upon the superior pole of the testis), a body (along the posterior border of the organ), and a tail (which attaches to the inferior pole of the testis). The tail of the epididymis continues with or becomes the (45 cm long) ductus (vas) deferens (NA, conveying away), which transports the spermatozoa from the testis to the prostatic urethra in conjunction with the ductuli efferentes and the epididymis. The course of the ductus deferens (Fig. 1) retraces the early descent of the testis through the inguinal canal and its subabdominal projections. The ductus deferens and the associated blood vessels and nerves which subserve it (deferential artery, vein, and branches of the inferior hypogastric plexus) or the testis (testicular artery, pampiniform plexus of veins, lymphatics, and autonomic fibers) are the constituents of the spermatic cord (Fig. 1). Although the ductus lies in the midst of the other constituents of the spermatic cord, it is readily palpable and recognizable during standard anatomical or vasectomy dissections owing to its heavier or more muscular feel when rolled between the index and large (pollex) fingers. After traversing the inguinal canal, the ductus deferens gains access to the cavity of the lesser or true pelvis via the mouth of the deep inguinal ring. Within the true pelvis, the ductus descends retroperitoneally and sequentially crosses the external iliac vessels, medial to the obturator nerve and vessels, to reach the posterior wall of the bladder (Fig. 2). At this site, the ductus deferens curves and descends over and medial to the ureter and seminal vesicle [the mnemonic used here remains "bridge (ductus) over the water (ureter)"] . The terminal portion of the ductus positioned just medial to the seminal vesicles enlarges significantly to form the ampulla of the organ (Fig. 2). Near or within the upper and posterior surface of the prostate the ductus deferens undergoes another luminar change and, by narrowing significantly, joins the minuscule duct of the seminal vesicles to form, on each side, the (2 cm long) ejaculatory duct (Fig. 2). The two ejaculatory ducts enter and cross the glandular substance of the prostate to drain into the prostatic urethra.

The two highly tortuous and lobulated seminal vesicles, slightly smaller than a person's small finger, are located against the fundus of the urinary bladder (Fig. 2). During each ejaculation, the alkaline contribution of the seminal vesicles (rich in globulin, vitamin C, and fructose) is added to the seminal fluid to nurse and enhance the motility of the spermatozoa.

The prostate, which is a tubuloalveolar gland, is considered to be an accessory genital organ of the male reproductive tract (Fig. 2). Measuring about 3 cm by 2 cm, the gland lies under the urinary bladder and is crossed in a superior-inferior fashion by the (3 to 4 cm long) prostatic urethra. The prostate has two lobes (left and right) which can be histologically subdivided into about 30 to 50 branched tubuloalveolar glands. These structures, in turn, drain via 20 to 30 prostatic ducts into the prostatic sinuses which are found on either side of the urethral crest within the prostatic urethra (Fig. 2). Commonly labeled with the misnomer "prostrate" by the novice student of anatomy, the organ can indeed force an individual to become prostrate when aggravated by infection, abscess, or carcinoma. The prostate can be examined by palpation, or it can be massaged by inserting a finger into the rectum. Prostatic massage is utilized to stimulate the secretion of prostatic fluid, rich in protein, lysozymes, and acid phosphatase, for laboratory analysis following collection at the end of the penile urethra.

Roughly the size of the nail of the small finger or compared by anatomists to peas, the bulbourethral glands (of Cowper) are sandwiched between the two

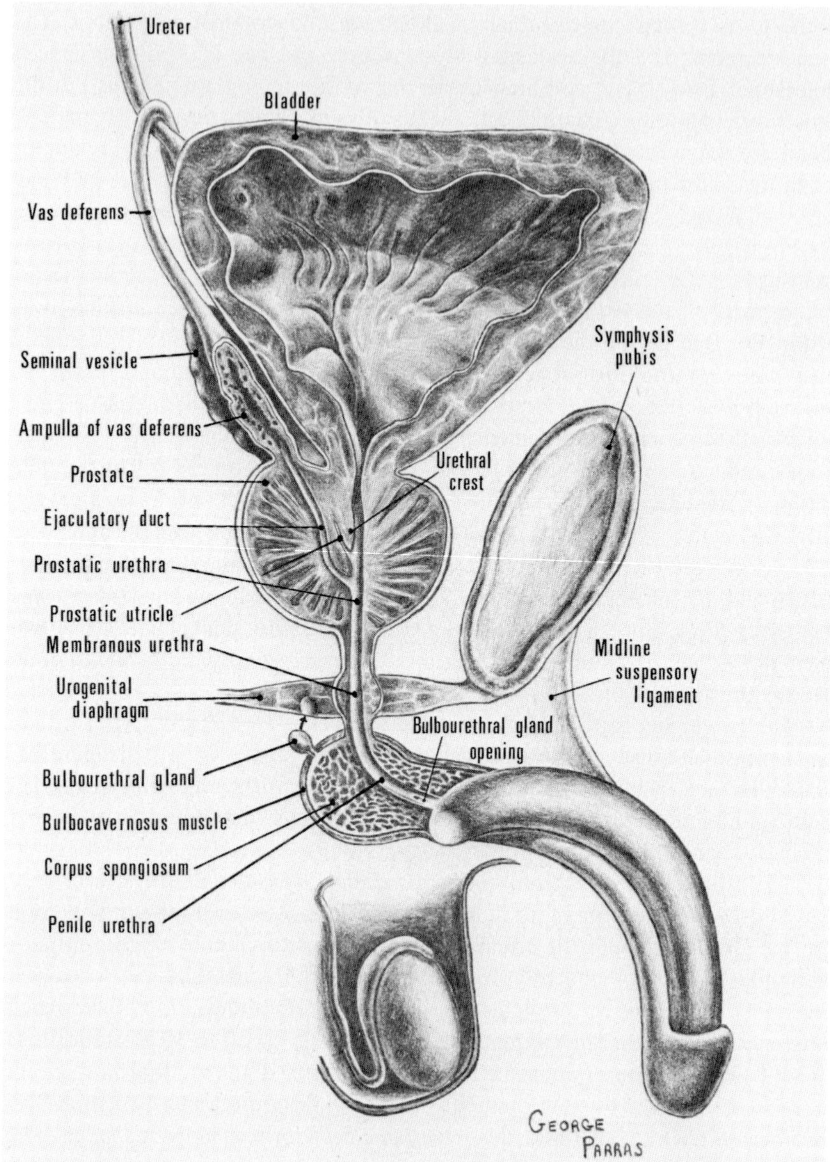

Fig. 2 Male internal reproductive organs. (Illustration by George Parras, M.D.)

layers of the urogenital diaphragm embedded within the muscular fibers of the sphincter urethrae muscle (Fig. 2). The fortunate amateur dissector occasionally discovers one or both tubuloalveolar glands posterolateral to the free or membranous portion of the urethra (Fig. 2). The mucoid secretion of the bulbourethral glands adds texture to the seminal fluid expelled during ejaculation.

The male copulatory organ, the penis, demonstrating variations in size and weight, is basically formed by the union of three bodies of erectile tissue. During the erect position, two of these bodies are arranged side by side on the dorsal aspect of the organ as the corpora cavernosa penis (singular, corpus cavernosum) while the third or unpaired mesial body lies underneath as the corpus spongiosum penis (cavernosum urethrae). The corpora cavernosa (Latin, *caverna* = grotto) recieve their name from their cross-sectional appearance in which they display the enlarged meshwork of intercommunicating venous cavities within their internal anatomy. These venous spaces are lined with endothelium continuous with that of the venous channels which drain them. The third portion of the urethra, the penile or spongy urethra, traverses the corpus spongiosum along its entire length from the bulb to its terminal expansion, the glans penis, where it connects to the ambient environment at the external urethral orifice (Fig. 3). The glans penis (Fig. 3) is formed by the terminal or dilated end of the corpus spongiosum as it surrounds the blunt end portion of the corpora cavernosa penis. The prominent posterior margin of the glans extends backward over the corpora cavernosa as the corona (Latin, "garland," "crown"). In the uncircumcised male the corona and the glans penis are covered by a free fold of skin called the prepuce (Latin, *preputium*), or foreskin (Fig. 3). The two corpora cavernosa penis are closely bound by a dense fibroelastic sheath called the tunica albuginea which unites at their midline as the septum penis. Another fascial plane, the fascia penis or Buck's fascia, surrounds the tunica albuginea (and its corpora cavernosa) and splits to enclose ventrally the single corpus spongiosum penis (Fig. 3). This deep fascial layer splits again to enclose the corresponding muscles which surround and subserve the bodies of erectile tissue (the bulbocavernosus muscle over the bulb of the corpus spongiosum and the two ischiocavernosus muscles over the crura of the corpora cavernosa penis). External to Buck's fascia (deep fascia of the penis) is a looser layer of fibrous tissue called the superficial fascia (Fig. 3) which contains and conveys the blood vessels (e.g., superficial dorsal vein of the penis). It should be pointed out that the major vessels of the penis (e.g., deep dorsal vein and its right and left deep dorsal arteries, their branches, the nerves, and venous tributaries) course between the tunica albuginea and Buck's fascia (deep fascia of the penis).

Contrary to common belief, the penis is not a skin-held appendage which intermittently becomes engorged with blood. Instead, the organ is firmly attached via its root to the osseous elements of the pelvis and to the pelvic diaphragm. On researching the inferior border of the pubic symphysis, the two corpora cavernosa split from each other to form the crura of the penis (Fig. 3). Each crus bends sharply inferiorly and laterally to attach to its corresponding inferior pubic ramus. An ischiocavernosus mucle sourrounds to protect and constrict, when necessary, each

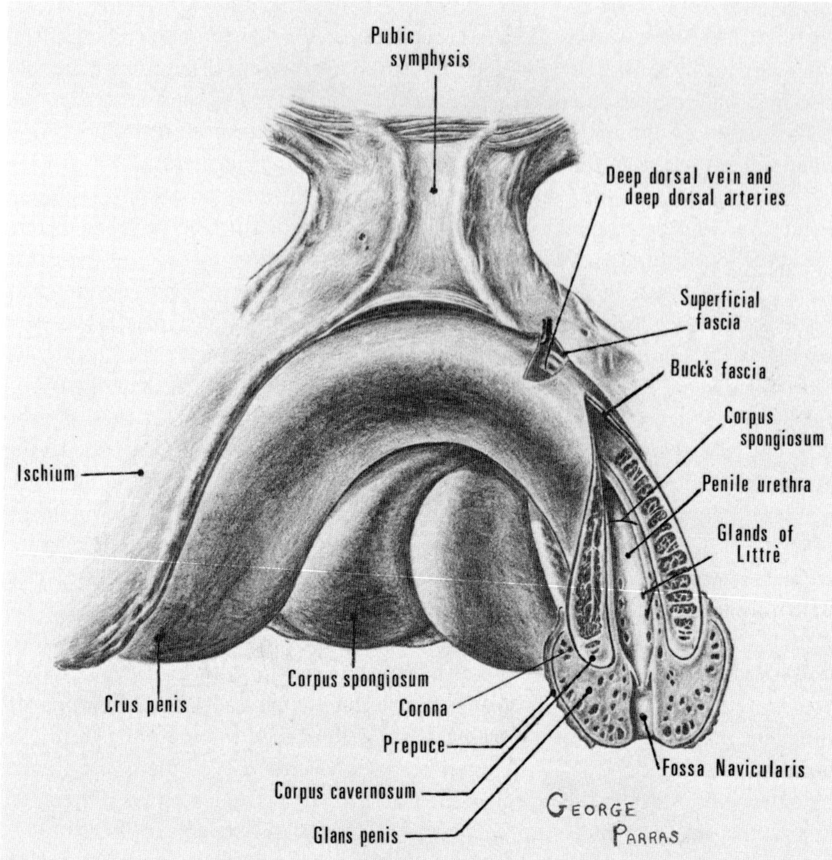

Fig. 3 Penis with sagittal view of internal structures. (Illustration by George Parras, M.D.)

crus along its entire bony attachment. Similarly, the inferioposterior or expanded portion of the corpus spongiosum (bulb of the penis) is overlaid by two symmetrical muscles (bulbocavernosus) united along the midline by a fibrous raphe. Through the fascial lining of this muscle, the bulb assumes a stable attachment to the central tendinous point of the perineum (perineal body). Because of its ability to squeeze out the last drop of urine from the penile urethra (which traverses the corpus spongiosum), the bulbocavernosus muscle (Fig. 2) becomes a significant structure when considering the prevalent cases of urinary incontinence as the individual gets older.

The dorsal aspect of the penis is also well anchored by a midline suspensory ligament which connects the fascia of the two cavernous bodies (just before their split into crura) to the symphysis pubis (Fig. 2). Secondary attachments are found on the two margins of the suspensory ligament where the left and right fundiform ligaments interconnect the fascia over the symphysis pubis with the cavernous and the scrotal fascia.

Male Urethra (Urethra Virilis or Masculina)

The main functions of the urethra are to convey urine from the bladder to the external environment and to allow the passage of sperm between the prostate and the tip of the penis during ejaculation (Fig. 2). The anatomy books describe the male urethra as a 15- to 20-cm passage line by transitional epithelium which can be subdivided into three functional parts (Fig. 2):

1. Prostatic (via prostate lined by transitional epithelium and about 2.5 to 4.5 cm long)
2. Membranous (via urogenital diaphragm lined by pseudostratified columnar epithelium and about 1 to 1.5 cm long)
3. Spongy (via bulb and body of corpus spongiosum lined by pseudostratified columnar epithelium and about 14 to 15 cm long)

It is fairly obvious that the urethra of a midget's penis is noticeably shorter than that of a basketball center.

The beginning of the urethral canal starts within the bladder neck as a semilunar orifice just anterior to the uvula of the bladder (Latin, *uva* = grape, NA a fleshy mass). The prostatic portion of the urethra is the most complex portion of the passage, showing several modifications.

The posterior wall of the tube shows a slight elevation called the urethral crest which may represent an extension of the uvula of the bladder. On either side of the crest, one may locate with the help of a hand lens, a groove called the prostatic sinus which contains about 25 minute openings of the ducts of the prostate gland (Fig. 2).

Roughly along its midlength, the urethral crest enlarges to form a microscopic eminence known as the seminal colliculus. The colliculus contains a blind central depression, the prostatic utricle (Latin, "leather bag"), which is thought to be the male homolog of the uterus and vagina (Fig. 2). Anterior to this structure a careful examination reveals the two (or more) openings of the ejaculatory ducts (Fig. 2). It is at this point in the male urogenital system that the reproductive passage (openings of ejaculatory ducts) connects with the urinary system (prostatic urethra and colliculus) for the conveyance of sperm via the remaining urethral canal during ejaculation (Fig. 2).

The membranous portion of the urethra receives its name from its passage through the two membranous layers surrounding the deep perineal pouch (containing sphincter urethrae and/or vaginae muscles, deep transverse perineus muscles, internal pudendal artery, artery of the bulb, and dorsal nerve of the penis or clitoris).

In a superior-inferior fashion, the urethra crosses the membranous layer of the pelvic fascia or the superior layer of the urogenital diaphragm, the deep pouch of the perineum via the sphincter urethrae (vaginae in the female) muscle, and the membranous perineal membrane or the inferior layer of the urogenital diaphragm.

The bulbourethral glands of the male are found on either side of the urethra within the muscular fasciculi of the sphincter urethrae muscle. The glands are actually sandwiched between the membranous layer of the pelvic fascia (above) and the perineal membrane(below). The ducts of these glands perforate the inferior fascial layer of the urogenital diaphragm (perineal membrane) in order to enter and drain into the bulbar portion of the spongy urethra (Fig. 2). Thus no glands open or drain into the lumen of the membranous urethra.

The third portion of the male urethra, the spongy (penile) part, enters and traverses in sequence the entire length of the bulb of the penis and its narrower anterior projection, the corpus spongiosum (Fig. 2). The transverse (5 to 6 mm wide) passage terminates at the tip of the glans penis in a vertical slit (external urethral orifice) through which it connects to the external environment (Fig. 3). In essence, it can be seen that the male urethra traverses through one gland (prostate) and both perineal pouches: the deep pouch as the membranous part of the urethra and the superficial pouch as the spongy urethra. Besides the openings of the bulbourethral glands into its bulbar portion, the spongy urethra receives the numerous openings of the small mucous urethral glands of Littre (Fig. 3). The majority of these glands drain into the proximal two-thirds of the spongy urethra, thus slightly behind the dilatation of this passage within the glans penis (fossa navicularis urethrae).

The entire urethral passage can be viewed and examined through an urethroscope. This instrument enables the physician to examine not only the colliculus seminalis (verumontanum), but also the finer structures such as the prostatic utricle and the openings of the ejaculatory ducts.

REPRODUCTIVE ORGANS OF THE FEMALE

External Genitalia

The female reproductive organs develop both within and ouside the body cavity. The external genitalia project outside the body surface within the urogenital triangle subdivision of the perineum, and the internal organs of reproduction rest under the protective covering of the peritoneal lining of the true or lesser pelvic cavity.

The external genitalia of the female consist of the mons pubis, the two labia majora, and the structures which lie between them (labia minora, clitoris, urethra, and vestibule of vagina). Collectively these structures are known as the vulva or pudendum femininum.

The labia majora (Fig. 4) are longitudinally prominent (bilateral) skin folds which protect the lateral margins of the urogenital cleft. Both anteriorly and posteriorly, the two labia fuse to form the corresponding labial commissures (Fig. 4).

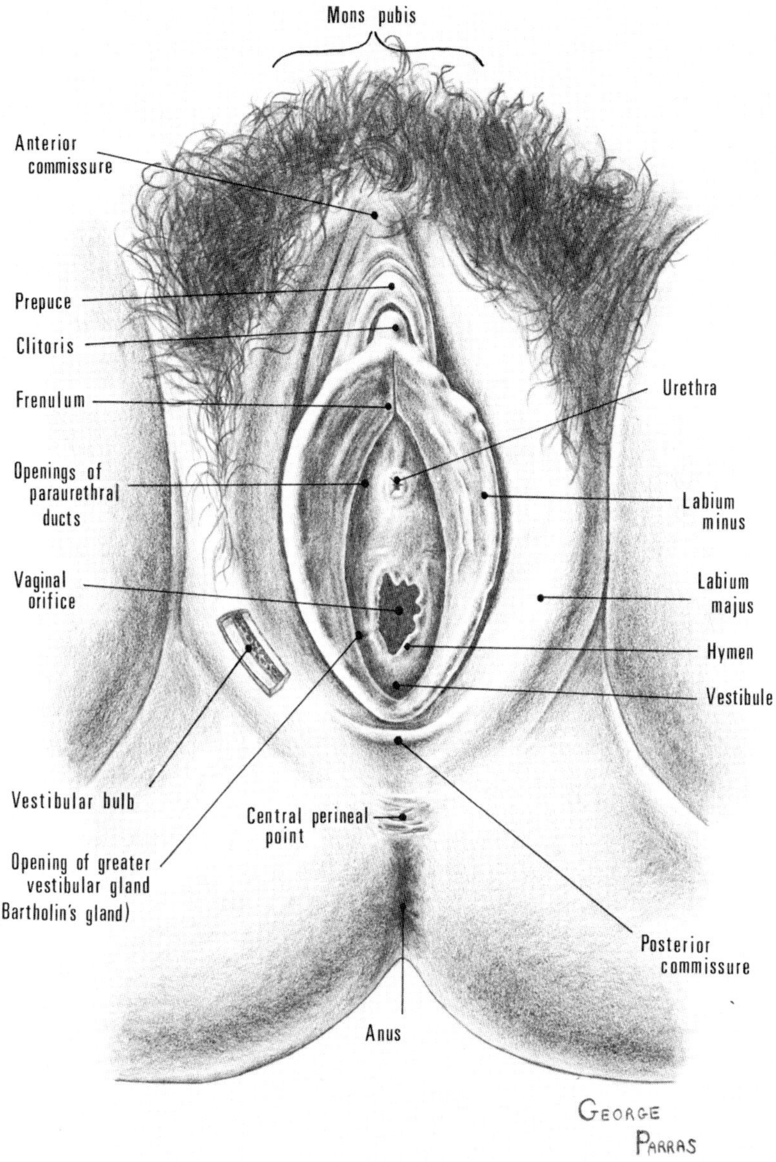

Fig. 4 External genitalia of the female. (Illustration by George Parras, M.D.)

The posterior commissure is formed by the tapering of the labia majora in front of the anus, while the more prominent anterior commissure continues superiorly as a fatty prominence called the mons pubis (Fig. 4). The midline of the two labia is lined with smooth skin, and it is provided with numerous openings of the large sebaceous glands it contains within.

Just internal or medial to the labia majora, there are two smaller cutaneous folds called the labia minora which guard the midline openings of the urethra and vagina (Fig. 4). The fat-free labia minora are covered with hairless skin which, like the majora, contains multiple openings of sebaceous glands. Above the two labia minora split to send their cutaneous contributions above the clitoris as the prepuce of the organ, while below it they form its frenulum (Latin, "bridle") (Fig. 4). Although considered as the morphological equivalent of the penis, the female clitoris is not traversed by the urethra. Instead, this latter structure descends and drains, independently, between clitoris and vagina.

The subclitoral cleft between the two labia minora is called the vestibule of the vagina. The vestibule, as the name suggests, is an entrance court which receives the openings of the urethra, the vagina, and the ducts of the greater vestibular glands.

The female urethra is a short structure (4 to 5 cm long) which connects the urinary bladder to the vaginal vestibule. The terminal portion of this organ is called the external urethral orifice, and its aperture is located just anterior to the vagina (Fig. 4). On close examination, numerous minute openings of the urethral mucous glands are found along the wall of the tube, while the minuscule openings of the paraurethral glands (Skene's glands) may be located on either side of the external urethral orifice (Fig. 4). These small openings are connected to the slender paraurethral ducts of Skene, which, along with urethral glands and lacunae, may be infected to harbor *Neisseria gonorrhoeae* and a multitude of other exotic microorganisms. The urethral glands are believed to be homologous to the male prostate.

The vaginal orifice is located posterior to the urethra and it is partly or sometimes completely closed, in the virginal state, by a thin membranous fold of tissue, the hymen. Following perforation of this imperfect annular fold several small, fleshy fragments persist around the vaginal opening, to old age, as hymenal caruncles. In the normal anatomic position and assuming that the urinary bladder is empty, the 8- to 9-cm long vaginal canal is almost parallel in position to the osseous elements comprising the caudal region of the sacrum (Fig. 5).

Although generously endowed with smooth muscles, the vagina should not be compared to a rubber garden hose. Under resting conditions its anterior (7 to 8 cm long) and posterior (8.5 to 9 cm long) walls are collapsed and actually touching along the midline. The upper part of the vagina receives the cervix of the uterus along the superior border of its anterior wall (Fig. 5). In the normal anatomic position, the vagina is directed upward and backward. The junction between the uterus and vagina, although continuous and circular in nature, is subdivided by anatomists into four uterovaginal spaces called fornices (Latin, "arches" or "vaults").

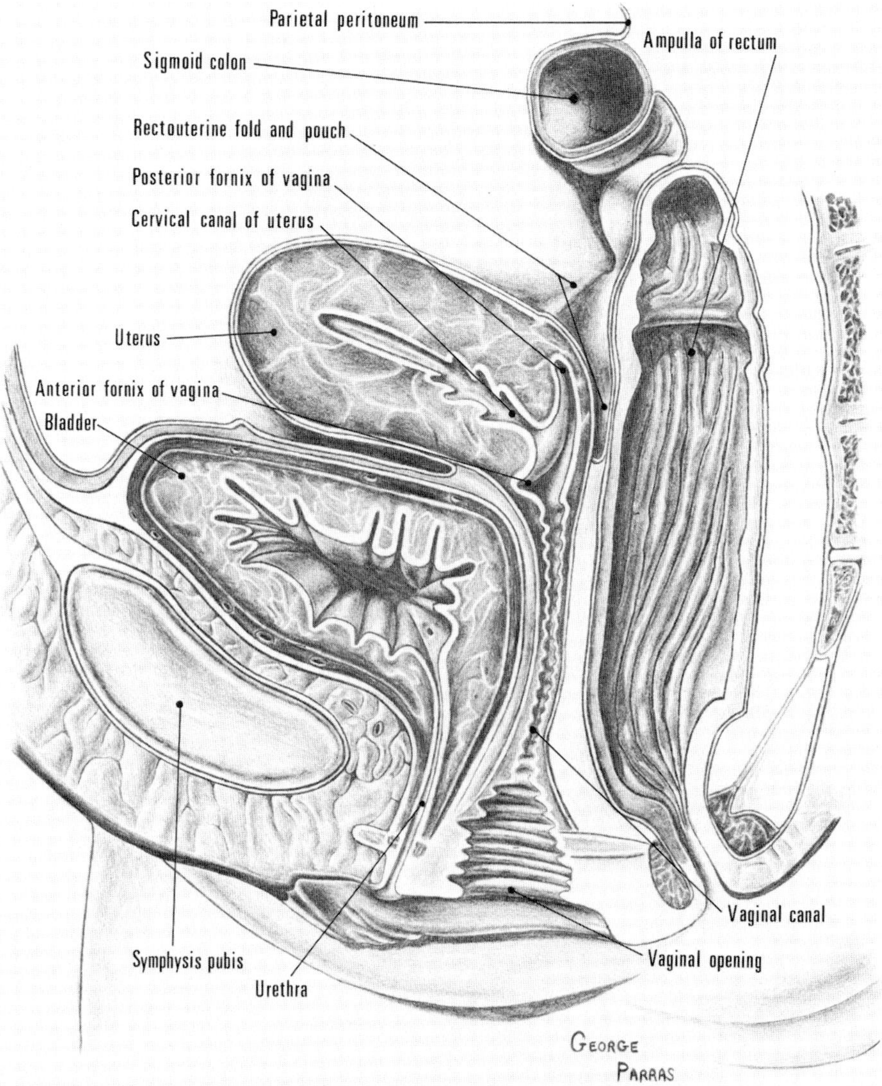

Fig. 5 Median sagittal view of the female pelvis. (Illustration by George Parras, M.D.)

In the normal anatomic stance, the anterior fornix is the lowest in position, the posterior is both the highest and the largest (Fig. 5), while the two lateral ones are located on either side of the cervix uteri (Fig. 7).

Interestingly, the mucosal lining of the vagina, while thick and reinforced by transverse elevations (vaginal rugae), is devoid of glands and virtually free of sen-

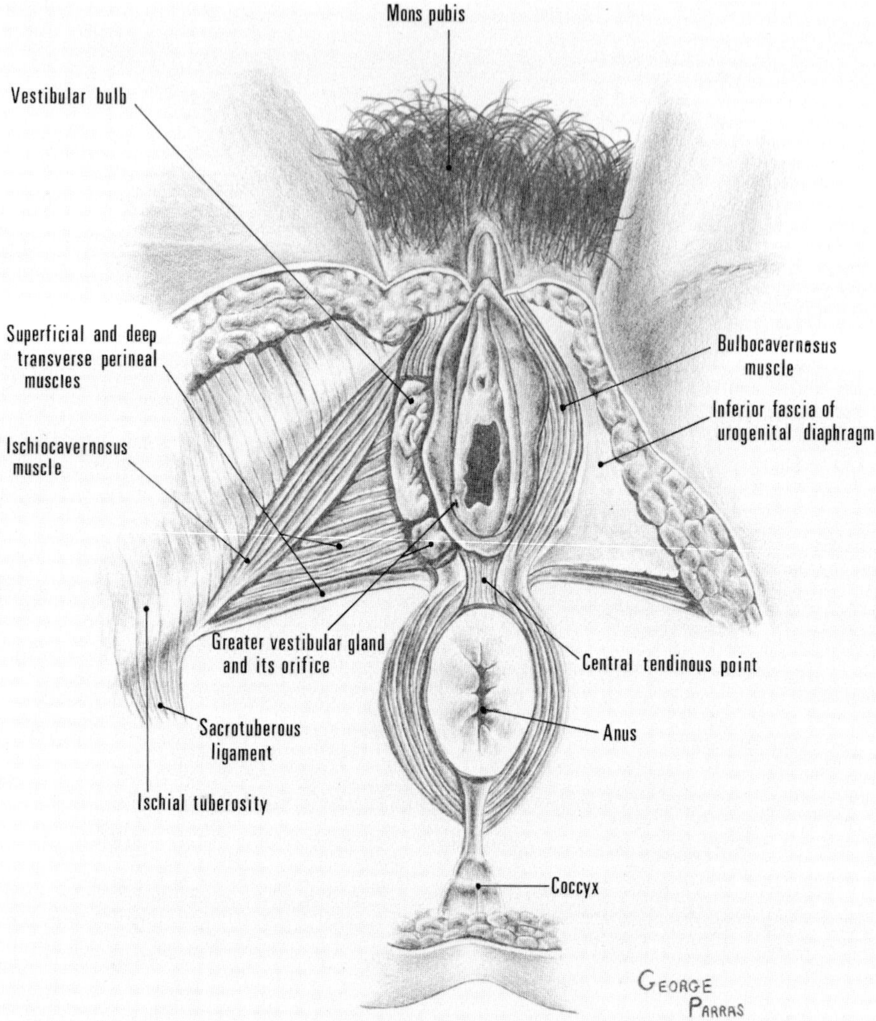

Fig. 6 Superficial muscles of the female perineum. (Illustration by George Parras, M.D.)

sory fibers. The few free nerve endings described by histologists within this area are believed to be primarily pain fibers. In a sagittal view of the region (Fig. 5), the vagina is related anteriorly to the cervix of the uterus, the base of the urinary bladder, and the urethra. Posteriorly the rectouterine peritoneal pouch of Douglas, the ampulla of the rectum, and the perineal membrane abut the vagina along a similar superior-inferior line (Fig. 5).

Because of its muscular nature, the vagina is expandable and can be clinically evaluated by either digital examination or use of a bivalved speculum (with the patient in the lithotomy position).

Besides the singular openings of urethra and vagina, the vaginal vestibule also receives the openings of the greater vestibular glands of Bartholin. Under normal conditions, the opening of the 2-cm-long duct (of each greater vestibular gland) is positioned between the hymen and the labia minora (Figs. 4 and 6). The pea-sized mucus-secreting greater vestibular glands are located on either side of the vagina slightly posterior to and partly covered by the bulbs of the vestibule (Fig. 6). The greater vestibular glands are homologous to the bulbourethral glands of the male. Shaped roughly like a small banana, the bulbs of the vestibule consist of elongated (3 cm) honeycomb-like erectile tissue (Fig. 6). They can be palpated on each side of the vaginal vestibule within the lateral wall of the lower vagina. Externally the two bulbs are covered by the bulbocavernosus muscle, which is located just under the attachment of the labia minora (Fig. 6). Superiorly the two bulbs fuse via connective tissue strands to attach along the midline to clitoris and just in front of the urethral opening. The bulb of the penis and the corpus spongiosum of the male perineum are homologous to the bulbs of the vestibule in the female.

Internal Organs of Reproduction

The internal organs of reproduction consist of two ovaries, two uterine or fallopian tubes, a muscular chamber, the uterus, and a vaginal canal which serves as the birth canal and copulatory organ (Fig. 7).

The two ovaries are the essential glands of reproduction of the female and are homologous to the testes in the male. The mature ovary is solid and ovoid and appears flattened along its anteroposterior aspect, almost like a small rubber ball squeezed between the large and index fingers. The ovary weighs about 3 to 7 g and measures 3 to 5 cm long, 1 to 3 cm in breadth, and 1 to 2 cm thick. The upper part of the ovary is known as the tubal portion, since it is closely associated with the open end of an uterine tube. The lower half of the ovary points toward the muscular uterus and is commonly called the uterine portion. This lower part connects to the uterus via a fibrous band called the ovarian ligament (Fig. 7).

Each ovary is enclosed within a protective layer of peritoneum, the mesovarium (Fig. 7). This peritoneal layer supports and leads blood vessels, nerves, and lymphatic channels to the organ. The suspensory ligament of the ovary, which passes across the iliac vessels and the psoas major muscle, attaches the organ to the lateral pelvic wall (Fig. 7).

Monthly, an ovary of the nonpregnant sexually mature woman produces a follicle which ruptures through the surface of the organ to liberate an egg or ovum. The release of each egg produces a scar on the surface of the organ which, on close examination, appears scarred and pitted, resembling the lunar surface viewed through a telescope. Once the ovary releases the ovum, this latter structure passes through the mesovarium (peritoneal layer) to gain access to the peritoneal cavity.

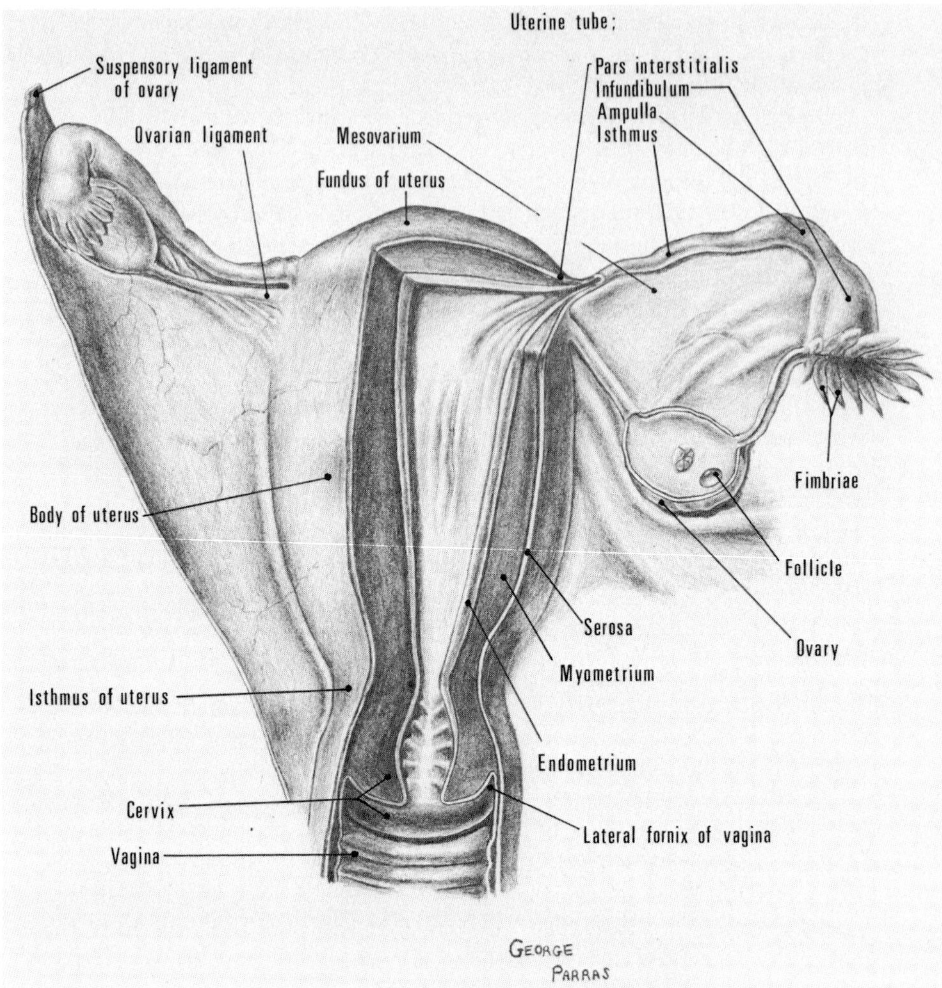

Fig. 7 Female internal organs of reproduction. (Illustration by George Parras, M.D.)

Within this region the ovum can die, if unfertilized by a sperm cell, or, if fertilized, it can lodge anywhere in the peritoneal cavity close to a vascular supply to produce an ectopic (out of place) pregnancy. Normally, the ovum leaves the peritoneal cavity by migrating toward the open or fimbriated end (fimbria, minute finger-like projections) of an uterine tube, being attracted toward this structure by the rhythmic beating of its cilia (hairlike processes) or owing to the release of various chemicals (chemotaxis). Besides its monthly egg production, the ovary secretes progesterone and estrogen, which stimulate the lining of the uterus to undergo its growth and sloughing during each menstrual cycle. The fine balance which exists between these two hormones has been utilized by medical researchers in the production of oral contraceptives. The uterine tubes (oviducts or fallopian tubes) are highly muscular structures capable of motility within the cavity of the lesser or true pelvis. Each tube is about 12 cm long and 1.5 cm in diameter (Fig. 7). The lateral extremity of each tube opens into the peritoneal cavity close to the ovary (to receive the egg or ovum during each ovulation), while its central part connects and opens into the upper side of the cavity of the uterus. For anatomical description, the uterine tube is arbitrarily divided into four parts (Fig. 7). The part which is embedded within the muscular wall of the fundus of the uterus is called the pars interstitialis, since it is related to the interstices of the organ. The second segment of the tube is located just outside the uterine wall and, because of its narrowness, is called the isthmus (Greek, *isthmus* = constriction connecting two larger cavities). The remainder of the tube enlarges gradually as the tube projects laterally toward the ovary, and is called the ampulla (saccular dilatation or canal). The fourth and last segment of the tube is an expansion of the ampulla, and is called the infundibulum (Latin, "funnel"). Normally situated on or near the ovary, the open or free end of the infundibulum possesses fine fingerlike projections called fimbriae (Fig. 7). The entire tube is lined with cells containing very small and fine hairlike structures called cilia. The beating of these cellular processes toward the uterus and the wave of muscular contraction along the tube helps to carry the egg (or the embryo if the latter structure was fertilized by a sperm cell) toward the uterus. The egg is believed to be fertilized, under normal conditions, in either the ampulla or infundibular subdivision of either the right or left tube.

The uterine tubes may become infected with various sexually transmitted organisms, in which case the lining of the tubes becomes inflammed, and scar tissue develops within this region during the healing process. The scarring process may lead to sterility, since it mechanically impairs the advancement of the sperm cells to the ampullary region of the tube and similarly prevents the advancement of the egg along the tube to the uterus.

Infectious processes may also spread via the tubes to the peritoneal cavity leading to severe consequences with inflammation of the peritoneum of both the true (lesser) and false (larger) pelvis called peritonitis.

Because of both obvious and dubious reasons, anatomists and pathologists have frequently compared the organs of the body and their lesions to various fruits. The uterus (womb) has been classically described as a hollow, pear-shaped muscular organ, while most modern medical students have conceptualized it as a flattened or collapsed baseball-shaped organ covered for the most part by peritoneum (Fig. 7).

The organ (8 cm in length, 5 cm in width, 2 to 3 cm in thickness) can be subdivided into four distinct components or parts: the fundus, the body, the isthmus, and the cervix (Fig. 7).

The fundus is the rounded free upper part of the organ which projects from the body of the organ above the openings of the two oviducts. The body consists of the upper two-thirds of the uterus, and it extends between the fundus to the isthmus of the organ.

With an empty urinary bladder, the body of the uterus rests almost in a horizontal position as it lies subperitoneally in the true pelvis (Figs. 5 and 7). Thus one can visualize that its upper part abuts coils of the small intestine and actually pushes the small bowel superiorly toward the diaphragm when greatly enlarged during the last trimester of pregnancy or, to a lesser degree, daily owing to filling of the bladder.

The isthmus is the narrow portion of the organ (1 cm long) connecting the body to the cervix. The neck of the organ or its cervix (2 cm in length) projects through the anterior wall of the vagina into the upper part of this passage. The communication between vagina and the inner cavity of the uterus occurs at the ostium uteri (Latin, "door," "entrance into hollow cavity"), which, when examined through a speculum, appears as a small opening perforating almost centrally the rounded or vaginal extremity of the cervix.

The relatively thick uterine wall can be subdivided into three distinguishable layers (Fig. 7): the outer serosa, or adventitia (Latin, "coming from abroad," "foreign"); the middle or thick smooth muscle layer, called myometrium; and the mucous inner lining, called endometrium.

The endometrium is further subdivided into two distinct regions: (1) the zona functionalis, which forms that portion of the endometrium that is eliminated or sloughed off with the menses (menstruation), and (2) the zona basalis, or the deeper endometrial layer which is retained after the menses to provide new cells (epithelium and lamina propria) for the buildup of the endometrium.

The endometrial lining and its glands are directly influenced by estrogen. In response to this follicle-produced humor(s) (estrogen and 17β-estradiol), the endometrium increases in thickness while its glands undergo a noticeable lengthening process. Following the elimination of the ovum from the follicle, this latter structure changes into a yellowish body known as the corpus luteum. This minute plastic structure represents another hormonal factory which produces estriol and progesterone in response to chorionic gonadotropins. During the progesterone phase the uterine glands become coiled and begin eliminating glycogen and a mucus secreted from their lumina. If the egg is fertilized during this period, it is embedded into the endometrium of the uterus and menstruation ceases. An unfertilized egg, however, dies within either the tube or the uterine cavity, and the built-up endometrium reenters a new menstrual period in which it is sloughed off and eliminated through the vaginal canal.

BIBLIOGRAPHY

Basmajian JV. Grant's method of anatomy. 10th ed. Baltimore: Williams and Wilkins, 1981.

Crafts RC. A textbook of human anatomy. 2nd ed. New York: Wiley, 1979.
Gardner E., Gray, DJ., O'Rahilly, R. Anatomy. 4th ed. Philadelphia: W.B. Saunders, 1975.
Goss CM, ed. Gray's anatomy. 29th American ed. Philadelphia: Lea and Febiger, 1975.
Hamilton WJ. Textbook of human anatomy. 2nd ed. St. Louis: C.V. Mosby, 1976.
Hollinshead HW. Textbook of anatomy. 2nd ed. New York: Hoeber Medical Books, Harper and Row, 1967.
Jones WF. Buchanan's manual of anatomy. 8th ed. London: Bailliere, Tindall and Cox, 1953.
Moore KL. Clinically oriented anatomy. Baltimore: Williams and Wilkins, 1980.
Romanes GJ. Cunningham's textbook of anatomy. 10th ed. London: Oxford University Press, 1964.
Warwick R., Williams PL, eds. Gray's anatomy. 35th British ed. Philadelphia: W. B. Saunders, 1973.
Woodburne RT. Essentials of human anatomy. 7th ed. New York: Oxford University Press, 1983.
Zuckerman S. A new system of anatomy. London: Oxford University Press, 1961.

TWO

Epidemiology of Sexually Transmitted Diseases

Joseph G. Lossick
Division of Sexually Transmitted Diseases
Centers for Disease Control
Atlanta, Georgia
and Venereal Disease Clinic
Columbus Health Department
Columbus, Ohio

INTRODUCTION

During the past two decades, the incidence of gonorrhea has increased sharply in many parts of the world, including the United States. During this period, increased attention to the sexually transmitted diseases (STDs) and technological advances have greatly expanded the scope and sophistication of clinical venereology. The spectrum of STDs has grown from a handful of diseases, such as gonorrhea, syphilis, chancroid, lymphogranuloma venereum, and granuloma inguinale, to include diseases such as nongonococcal urethritis, cervicitis, vaginitis, pelvic inflammatory disease, epidiymitis, infertility, prenatal and perinatal diseases, hepatitis, enteric diseases, herpesvirus disorders, arthritic diseases, pediculoses, immunological disorders, and genital oncogenesis. The number of infectious agents of concern has grown from 5 to approximately 20. Owing to a lack of uniformity in the reporting of these diseases worldwide, it is not possible to readily compare the trends of many of them.Nonetheless, the available data indicate that the gonorrhea epidemic is only the "tip of the iceberg," and that there has been an epidemic of not one, but a variety of sexually transmitted infections. Because of better estimates of gonorrhea incidence and a broader understanding of its epidemiology, it has become acceptable to relate the prevalence of many of the other STDs to that of gonorrhea. As such, gonorrhea disease rates have become the standard by which the prevalence of many of the STDs are compared or estimated.

The field of epidemiology concerns itself with the distribution and determinates of disease in human populations. As a discipline, epidemiological investigations are critical to the control of disease within populations. In contrast to clinical medicine, which concentrates its efforts on symptomatic disease in persons, epidemiologists concern themselves with the control of both symptomatic and asymptomatic disease in populations, which provide the foundation for public health programs designed to control disease. Clinical epidemiology focuses its attention on the biological and molecular etiology and determinants of disease such as host, agent, and environmental interrelationships, whereas descriptive epidemiology addresses the issues of the person, place, and time trend characteristics of various diseases.

This chapter addresses the descriptive epidemiology of some of the sexually transmitted diseases of major public health significance; an intensive discussion of the epidemiology of the STDs, or even a single disease, is beyond its scope. Its major emphasis will be on the reportable diseases such as gonorrhea and syphilis and the descriptive epidemiological features of these diseases in the United States.

DESCRIPTIVE EPIDEMIOLOGY OF GONORRHEA IN THE UNITED STATES

Gonorrhea Morbidity Data Base

The basic foundation of disease control rests on a knowledge of the trends, geographic distribution, and the characteristics of the population involved in the disease process. In the United States, these data are compiled by the Centers for Disease Control (CDC) in Atlanta, Georgia. Using standardized report formats, local health jurisdictions report gonorrhea morbidity to state health departments, who in turn report these data to the CDC. There are a number of features of this process that may confound or bias the perceptions of the descriptive epidemiological features of gonorrhea.

Gonorrhea morbidity in the United States is heavily weighted by a preponderance of morbidity derived from public health clinical facilities such as health department venereal disease clinics (approximately 75%). Data derived from these sources may be significantly influenced by the health-seeking patterns of the populations served. There are no national data describing the average demographic features of patients who seek care in public venereal disease clinics. It is generally accepted that these programs serve a population segment that is less affluent or educated, younger, who do not have a regular source of medical care, and who live within a reasonable traveling distance from the public health facility. As such, these clinics may derive data from only a limited proportion of the population, and its extrapolation to the total population is questionable. Because youth itself can be correlated with income, education, health-seeking care patterns, marital status, multiple sexual partner activity, impetuousness, and the risk of acquiring STDs, the populations served by the public health clinics may provide a reasonable, although clearly limited view, of the distribution of disease in a given community subpopulation.

Gonorrhea morbidity data derived from screening women in various sectors of the medical community provide a broader patient population, and thus a better measure of disease distribution. The data may also be weighted toward specific populations such as those seen in hospital emergency rooms and from geographic areas with higher disease prevalence.

Gonorrhea morbidity from the patient populations seen in the private medical sector are underrepresented in the total morbidity data owing to the tendency of private physicians not to report these cases to the public health sector. It is estimated that only about 10 to 42% of the private medical sector gonorrhea cases appear in the official morbidity statistics [1,2]. Because these unidentified cases may have significantly different demographic and geographic characteristics, it is not possible to say how their lack of representation in the total gonorrhea morbidity data distorts our epidemiological perspective of gonorrhea. If the underreporting of gonorrhea by private physicians is considered, estimates of gonorrhea morbidity would be increased by approximately 30 to 200%. It is probable that the proportion of private physicians' gonorrhea cases that are reported to the public health sector is closer to the higher estimates of physician reporting [3], especially in states that have laws that require laboratories to report all positive gonorrhea cultures.

Trend data are influenced by differences in the various levels of program-funding and case-finding efforts. Because of the increased incidence of disease, there has been an increase in funding, availability of public health clinics, screening, and case-finding efforts over time. These factors confound the relative comparability of morbidity data collected over various time intervals.

The comparability of data relating to the geographic distribution of gonorrhea in the United States is also confounded by different levels of funding directed toward the sexually transmitted diseases, variability in the quality and quantity of clinical services, case-finding efforts, and the presence or absence of laboratory reporting laws, which may differ markedly by state or regions within the states.

Gonorrhea case rates in the United States tend to overestimate population disease prevalence owing to the use of gonorrhea episodes rather than gonorrhea in persons to calculate morbidity rates. Individuals with multiple episodes of gonorrhea are counted as multiple individuals in the calculation of gonorrhea. If gonorrhea repeater rates are between 10 and 15%, gonorrhea prevalence case rates would be overestimated by approximately 11 to 18%. Since this method has been uniformly used over time, it does not affect trend data, but may confound comparisons of subgroups who may have significantly different recidivism rates.

Case identification is potentially confounded by variations in the sensitivity of the culture systems used to identify disease. Some programs have on-site laboratories, while others require the transportation of specimens. There are also potential regional differences in gonorrhea antibiotic susceptibility patterns which may affect the ability of gonorrhea to grow on selective culture media.

The data provided in this section are derived from the data base supplied by the Venereal Disease Control Division at the CDC, Atlanta, Georgia.

Although the gonorrhea morbidity data in the United States are potentially confounded by a number of factors that may influence the time, place, and person variables used in epidemiological analysis, most experts in the field feel that it at least provides a rough description of gonorrhea morbidity, both past and current.

Trend in Gonorrhea Morbidity

Figure 1 shows the epidemic curve of total gonorrhea cases in the United States between 1941 and 1981. An epidemic of gonorrhea of small magnitude and duration occurred following the onset of World War II in 1941. In 1967 gonorrhea cases began to increase and reached peak levels in 1975. In 1975 gonorrhea cases

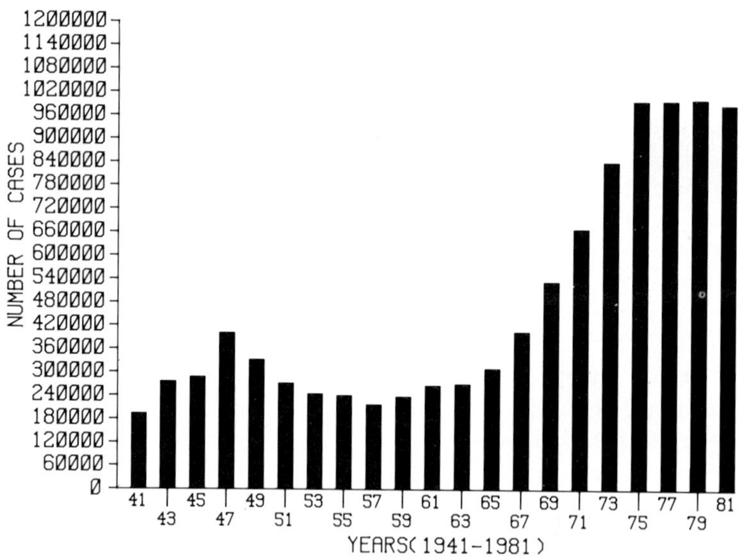

Fig. 1 Gonorrhea morbidity in the United States from 1941 to 1981.

were 3-fold those seen in 1966, and case rates had increased by 2.7-fold. Beginning in 1976, gonorrhea rates leveled off and began to perceptively fall, dropping an average of 1.3% per year. This downward trend has continued into 1982 (not depicted in Fig. 1), with a further decrease in case rates of approximately 4% during that year, with some metropolitan areas documenting gonorrhea case decreases of as much as 20% (Lossick JG, unpublished data). During the first three-quarters of 1983, U.S. gonorrhea cases were down approximately 7%.

Although decreasing, the level of gonorrhea in 1983 continued at major epidemic levels, and the epidemic of gonorrhea which began in 1967 is unprecedented in recorded history in the United States. In 1981 (Fig. 2) gonorrhea was not only the most frequently reported treatable infectious disease in the United States, but was at a level almost eightfold the combined total of the reported prevalence of

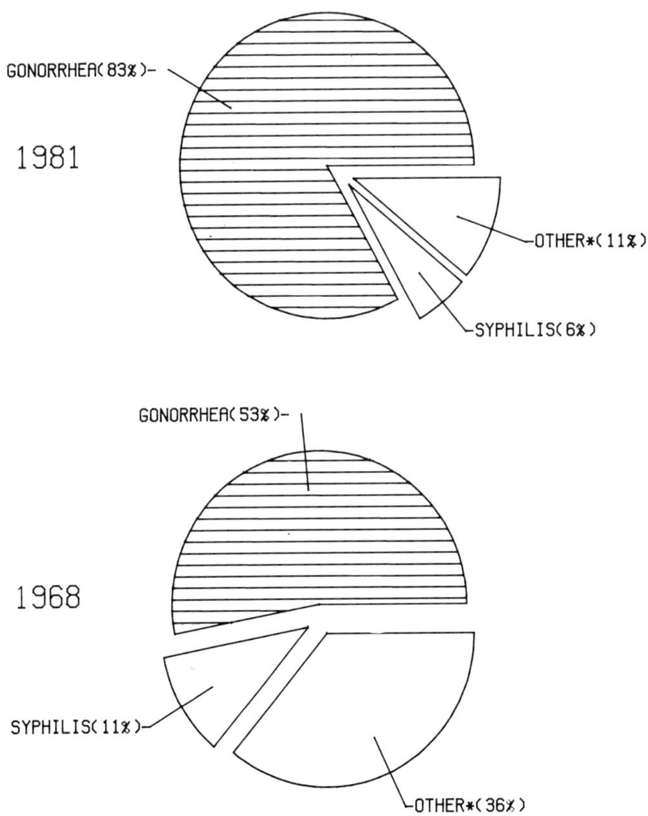

Fig. 2 Reported infectious diseases in the United States, 1968 and 1981 (*, 36 other preventable or treatable infectious diseases).

36 other nonsexually transmissible reportable infections. It is recognized that the data relating to reported infectious diseases may not be all evenly comparable because of differences in the reporting mechanisms, but the data clearly indicate that gonorrhea in the United States has been, and is, the most frequently reported treatable and preventable infectious disorder in the nation. Also, for the first time in history, gonorrhea in 5- to 14-year-old children has exceeded the combined reported prevalence of measles, mumps, and rubella.

The incidence of gonorrhea has a seasonal periodicity, with an increased number of cases reported in the third and fourth quarters of the year, with the highest incidence in the July-September quarter (Fig. 3). Other investigators have reported similar regional seasonal variations in gonorrhea morbidity [4, 5].

Person Variables in Gonorrhea Morbidity

Over 80% of the documented gonorrhea cases in the United States occur in individuals between the ages of 15 and 29 years, with a significant clustering in the 20- to 24-year-old groups. Figure 4 depicts the gonorrhea age group breakdown in the United States in 1981.

Between 1960 and 1980, the 15- to 29-year-old population in the United States increased by 78%, and the 20- to 24-year-old group essentially doubled [6] (Fig. 5). Approximately 88% of the cases are single, divorced, or separated. Between 1965 and 1980, the number of singles 18 years and older in the United

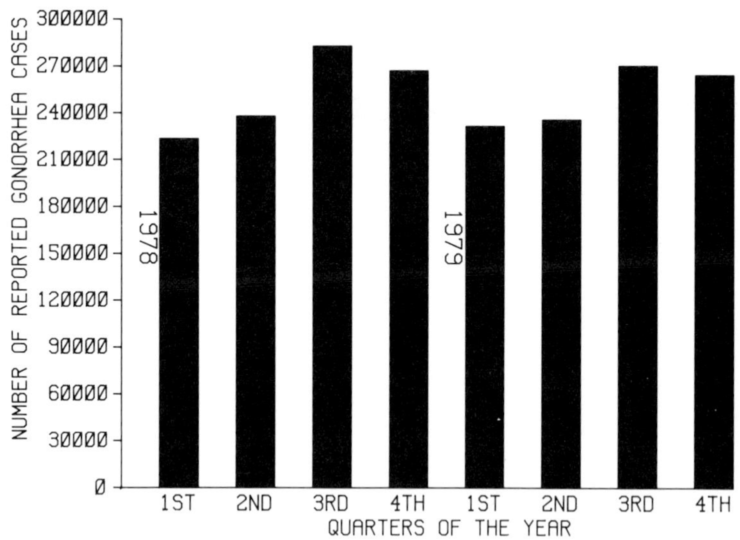

Fig. 3 Seasonal variation in U.S. gonorrhea morbidity from 1978 to 1979.

States grew from 18.2 million to 31.4 million, an increase of 73%. During this same time period, the number of divorced individuals increased by almost threefold, from 3.5 million to 9.7 million. Also, the average age of marriage rose by 2 years. National age-adjusted gonorrhea rates by race and gender for 1967 to 1979 are shown in Figure 6 [7]. The average age-adjusted gonorrhea rates in nonwhite men are approximately 15-fold those of white men, and those of nonwhite women approximately 10-fold those of white women. Gonorrhea rates peaked in 1975 for all groups. Between 1967 and 1975, the gonorrhea rates in white men almost doubled, while the rates only increased 23% in nonwhite men. The average annual rate increase in white men (12%) was more than fourfold that of black men (2.8%). Age-adjusted gonorrhea rates in white women increased by 347%, while those of nonwhite women increased by 157%. The average annual gonorrhea rate increase in white women was more than twofold that of nonwhite women: 43% compared

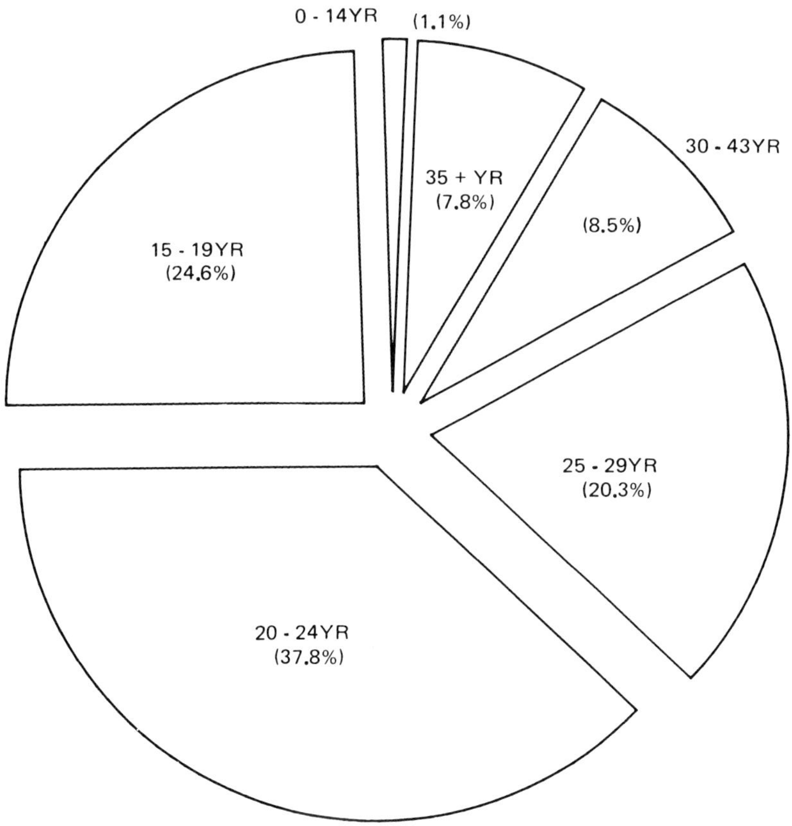

Fig. 4 Gonorrhea in the United States by age groups in 1981.

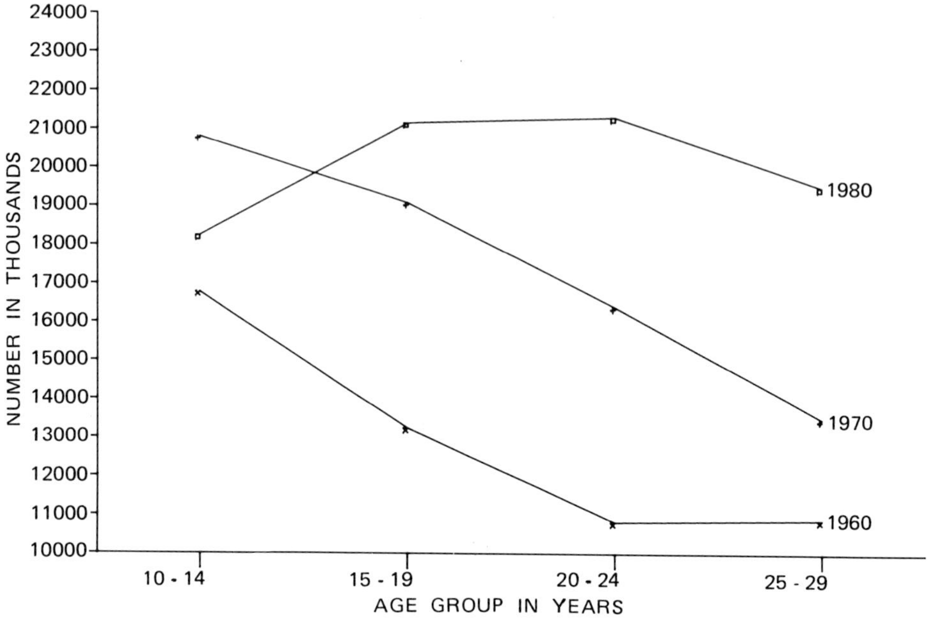

Fig. 5 Population age group changes in the United States from 1960 to 1980.

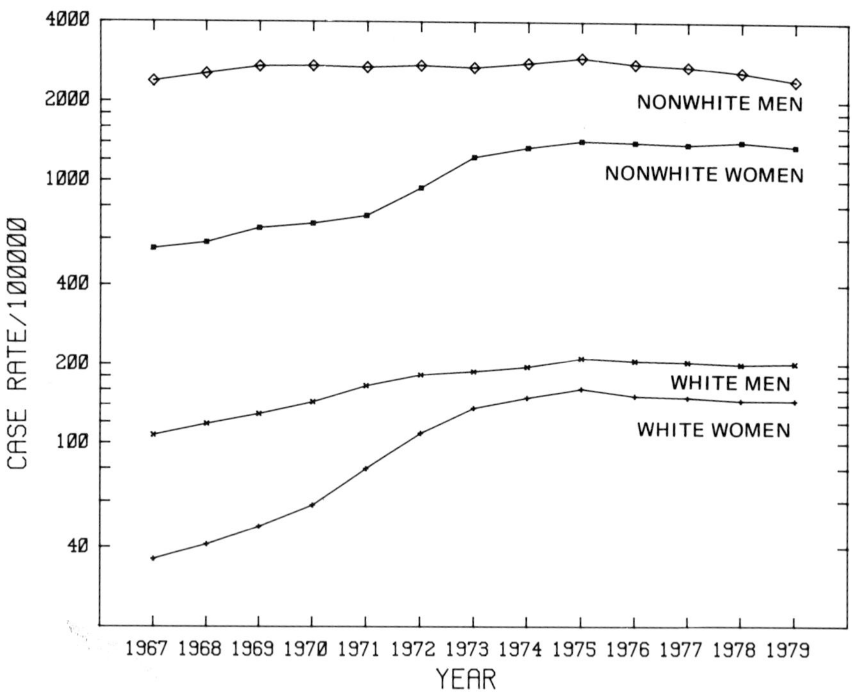

Fig. 6 Gonorrhea rates in the United States by race and sex from 1967 to 1979.

to 20%. After 1975 gonorrhea declined at annual rates of 4.5, 1.1, 2.5, and 1.2% for nonwhite men, white men, nonwhite women, and white women, respectively. If one compares the increases in age-adjusted and unadjusted gonorrhea rates, the proportional increases in total disease morbidity accounted for by changes in the population age groups were 38, 60, 19, and 30% in white men, nonwhite men, white women, and nonwhite women, respectively. By 1979 the age-adjusted rate for nonwhite men approximated that seen in 1967. Figures 7 and 8 show the proportionate rate increases in gonorrhea groups between 1967 and 1975 stratified by age group and race. The largest increases in all races occurred in the population 19 years old or younger.

A sharp increase in gonorrhea morbidity in women occurred in 1972 coincident with the introduction of large-scale national screening of high-risk female populations. Between 1973 and 1981 an average of 7.5 million U.S. women were screened yearly in nonvenereal disease clinic settings, with an average gonorrhea detection rate of 2.7%. Prior to 1973 the average male-to-female gonorrhea ratio was 2.5:1, but between 1973 and 1981 it was 1.5:1, consistent with the sharp increase in newly detected cases in women found by widespread screening programs. Between 1973 and 1984, an average of 52% of the total gonorrhea morbidity in women has come from these screening activities. The highest yields have been found in correctional facilities and manpower agencies, where gonorrhea rates of 4% or higher were encountered. Case detection rates were the highest in the third quarter of the year, similar to the seasonal pattern noted in the

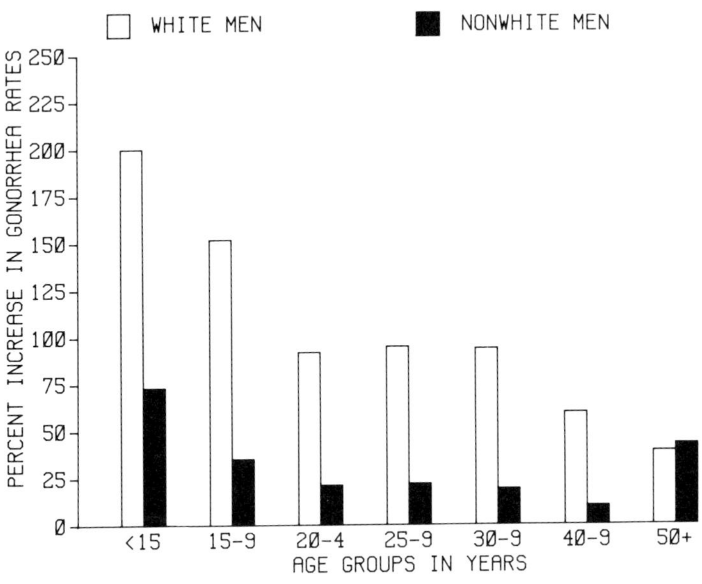

Fig. 7 Gonorrhea rate increases in the United States in men by age group and race from 1967 to 1975.

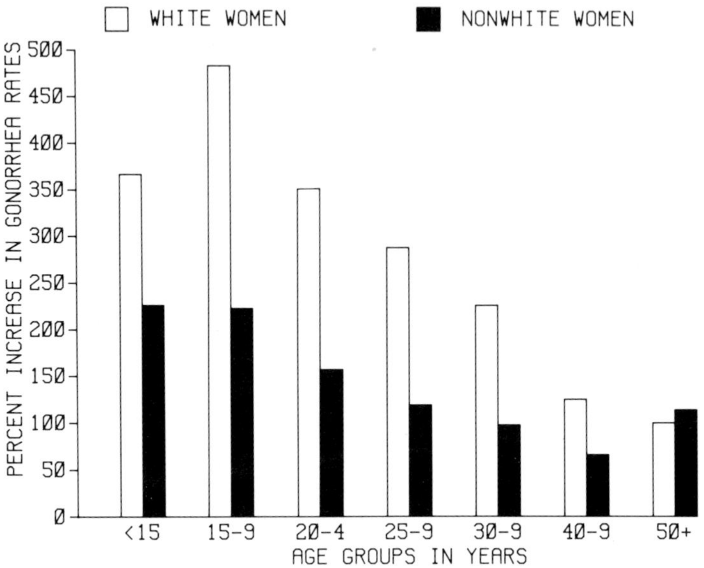

Fig. 8 Gonorrhea rate increases in the United States in women by age group and race from 1967 to 1975.

national gonorrhea morbidity. Approximately 40% of the screening cultures for gonorrhea in women are done in family planning clinics throughout the nation, which have average positivity rates of approximately 2%.

In the past decade, the proportion of urban U.S. white teenaged women who engaged in premarital intercourse rose significantly [8]. Between 1971 and 1979 the proportion of white women between the ages of 15 and 19 years who engaged in premarital sexual activities rose from 26 to 47%, an increase of 77%. Premarital sexual activity in black teenagers increased from 54 to 66% during the same period, an increase of only 23%.

The national gonorrhea rates in homosexual males have not been defined. It is generally felt to be high. Many investigators have identified high rates of gonorrhea in homosexual male populations [9-14]. Darrow et al. [13] found a prior history of gonorrhea in 38.4% of a sample of 4329 homosexual males evaluated by questionnaire. Trend data on gonorrhea in this population are not available, and their contribution to the gonorrhea epidemic has not been defined. In the Columbus, Ohio, Venereal Disease Clinic, the gonorrhea rates in white homosexual males have been historically 1.7 times those of white heterosexual males, whereas the rate in black heterosexual males is 2 times that of white heterosexual males. Although no long-term data are available from this program, the gonorrhea rate in this homosexual population has dropped 38% between January 1, 1981, and September 1, 1983. During this same time period, the gonorrhea rate in heterosexual males dropped only 20%. During the first 8 months of 1983, a statistical decrease in the number of mean sexual partners per month has been noted in white homosexual males frequenting the Columbus program. Sexual partner activity has remained stable in all other male populations. It is tempting to speculate that recent concerns about the acquired immune deficiency syndrome in the homosexual population may have affected the sexual activity patterns in this population and, as a consequence, the rate of acquisition of sexually transmitted infections.

The national trend in the rates of gonorrhea in U.S. prostitutes is not known. It is estimated that the gonorrhea rate in this population is high, and that prostitutes should be considered one of the major reservoirs of gonorrhea in the United States. Potterat et al. [15] estimated that as much as one-third of the gonorrhea in Colorado Springs, Colorado, may be directly or indirectly linked to prostitution. Conrad et al. [16] found gonorrhea infections in 19.8% of the women prostitutes in Atlanta, Georgia. In a prospective unpublished study of 111 massage parlor prostitutes in Columbus, Ohio, followed over a 23-month period between 1978 and 1980, the incidence of gonorrhea was 34%; 51% of these women had gonorrhea at least once during their lifetime.

Geographic Distribution of Gonorrhea

Figure 9 depicts the geographic distribution of gonorrhea in the United States. The highest case rates are seen in the southern and Pacific regions. The mean gonorrhea case rates for U.S. cities are more than twofold the statewide rates, consistent with an urban clustering of gonorrhea morbidity. In 1981 the states with the highest and lowest gonorrhea rates were Georgia and Vermont, respectively, with more than a 10-fold difference in case rates. The cities with the highest and lowest case rates were San Francisco, California, and Omaha, Nebraska, respectively, with a 44-fold difference in case rates. Gonorrhea, like most other infectious diseases, is not diffusely distributed within the population, but tends to be clustered. In Upstate New York, approximately 50% of the gonorrhea cases were derived from 13% of the census tracts (contiguous in location), and from only 9% of the population [17]. The relative risk for gonorrhea was highest in the core census tracts, with a progressive decrease in relative risk as one went from adjacent tracts to those distant from the high gonorrhea density areas. This pattern is consistent with the diffusion theory of the spread of contagious disease [18]. Potterat et al. [19] identified four census tracts (three contiguous and one military base) as responsible for 50% of the gonorrhea morbidity in Colorado Springs, Colorado. In Columbus, Ohio (Lossick JG, unpublished data), 21 contiguous census tracts (10% of the total) account for 43% of the city's gonorrhea morbidity.

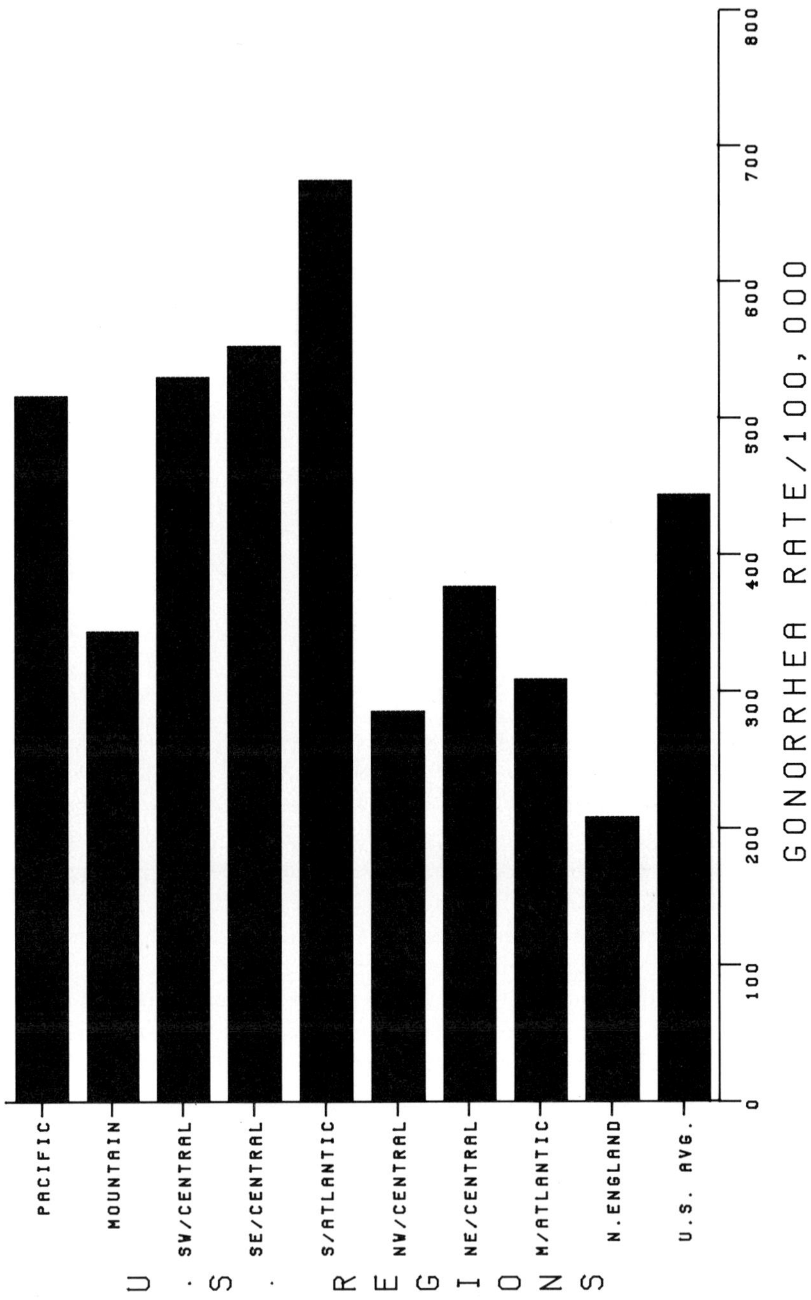

Fig. 9 Gonorrhea rates in the United States by geographic region in 1980.

Pelvic Inflammatory Disease

The major sequela of gonorrhea in women is pelvic inflammatory disease (PID). Curran estimated the cost of PID in the United States in 1979 to be more than $1.25 billion [20]. In 1975 New York State Medicaid spent between $0.55 million and $3.7 million on the treatment of gonorrhea-associated PID, with an average cost of approximately $1280.00 per case [21]. Data regarding hospitalization rates for PID are derived from two sources. Approximately 7500 randomly selected hospitals from throughout the United States are surveyed by the National Center for Health Statistics to provide the Hospital Discharge Survey. The commission on Professional and Hospital Activities maintains hospital discharge summary data from approximately 2200 nonrandomly selected hospitals throughout the nation and provides summary data in the form of the Professional Activity Study. The CDC utilize these data bases to analyze the trends in PID [22]. Figure 10 shows the trend in PID hospitalizations between 1970 and 1977. During this period an average of more than 211,000 women were hospitalized annually for PID. The PID rates in black women were more than threefold those in white women. The trend in black women became relatively stable after 1974, while that of white women showed a slow but steady increase. Black women had an 18.5% decline in PID hospitalization rates between 1973 and 1976; there was a 7.4% increase

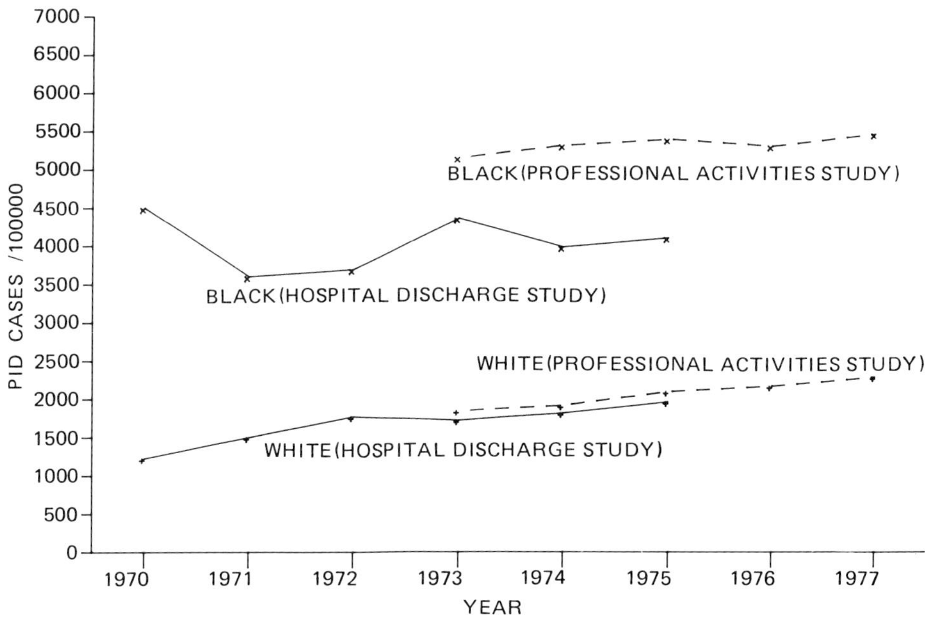

Fig. 10 Number of hospitalizations for pelvic inflammatory disease in the United States from 1970 to 1977.

between 1976 and 1978 (not shown on graph). For white women there was a 26% increase in PID rates between 1970 and 1973 and another 14.5% increase between 1973 and 1977. There is a correlation between hospitalized PID rates and gonorrhea (r = 0.7). Approximately 8% of all gonorrhea cases identified in women are associated with PID. The total of gonorrhea-associated PID in the United States is not known, as the formal data bases do not identify associated etiological agents. The proportion of PID cases associated with gonorrhea infection vary markedly, dependent on the prevalence of gonorrhea in the geographic area, but it is estimated that approximately one-half of the U.S. PID cases are associated with gonorrhea infections [23].

Figure 11 shows the age and race group breakdowns of U.S. PID cases between 1970 and 1975. The disease is predominantly seen in young women in the 15- to 24-year-old group, heavily clustered in black women, with its frequency decreasing with age. About 40% of the PID cases are between the ages of 15 and 24 years, and 74% between the ages of 15 and 34 years.

It has been estimated that only about 20% of women with PID are hospitalized, while the remainder are treated on an outpatient basis [24]. Data regarding outpatient PID are derived from the National Ambulatory Medical Care Survey (NAMCS), a probability sampling of approximately 1900 physicians by the National Center for Health Statistics. Also, a random sample survey is conducted which includes data from 1 in 5000 physician days derived from physicians in the United States in office-based practices: the National Disease and Therapeutic

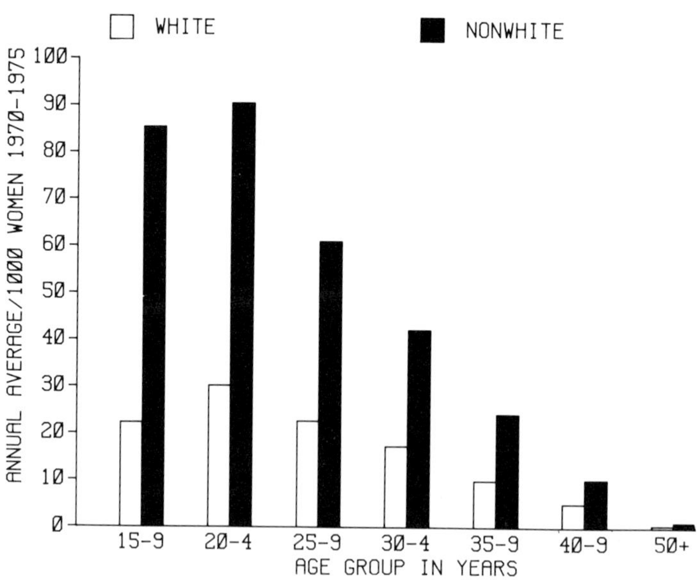

Fig. 11 Age and race breakdown of U.S. pelvic inflammatory disease cases from 1970 to 1975.

Index (NDTI). These data are evaluated by the CDC to provide the trend data on PID physician visits in the United States [25]. Between 1973 and 1977 women made an average of 1.89 million visits per year to physicians during which a diagnosis of PID was made. Nonwhite women, although comprising only 13% of the female population, made 31.4% of these visits, and had race-specific PID rates threefold that of the white women. Figure 12 depicts the trend of physician visits per PID per 100,000 population using combined NAMCS and NDTI survey data. The number of PID visits declined by 42.3% between 1973 and 1977, with the decline beginning after the initiation of widespread gonorrhea screening of women in the United States in 1972. It has been estimated that each episode of PID requires approximately three physician visits, and, based on the average of 1.89 million annual physician visits, approximately 630,000 cases of outpatient PID occurred annually during the study period.

Combining the inpatient and outpatient data, it is estimated that approximately 1 million cases of PID occur annually, of which one-half are associated with gonorrhea infections. Associated with the PID hospitalizations are over 150,000 major surgical procedures, including 53,000 hysterectomies and 83,000 surgical procedures on the fallopian tubes or ovaries.

Penicillinase-Producing *Neisseria gonorrhoeae* Infections

Since their identification in 1976, penicillinase-producing *Neisseria gonorrhoeae* (PPNG) strains have steadily increased in frequency in the United States. The

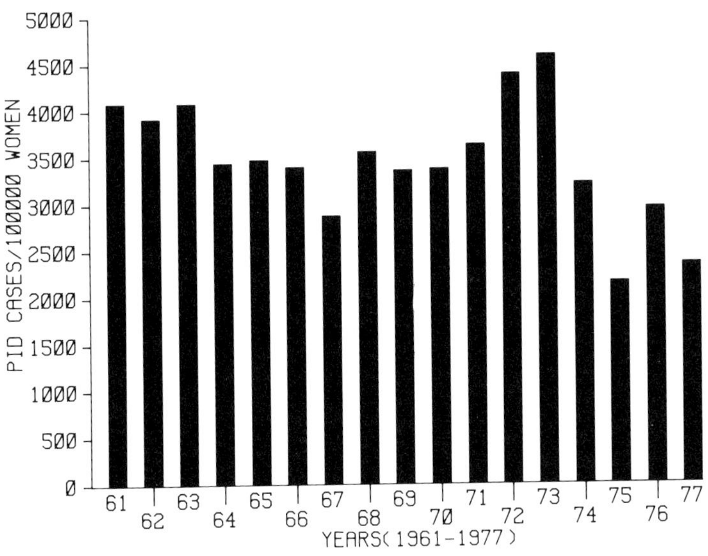

Fig. 12 Physician visits for pelvic inflammatory disease in the United States from 1961 to 1977.

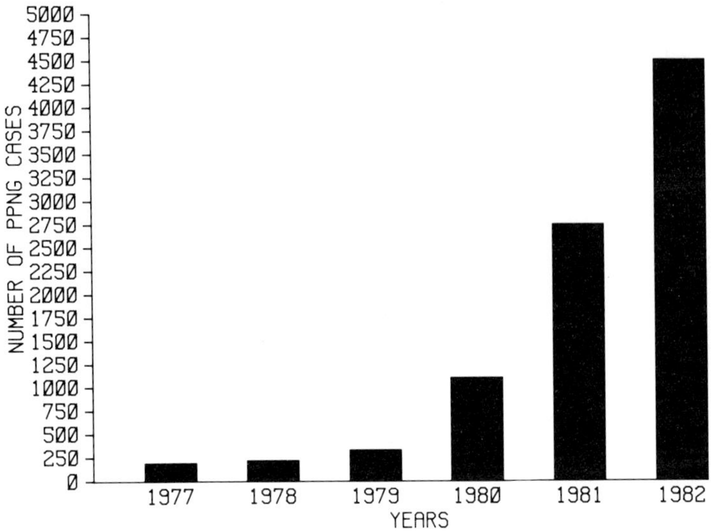

Fig. 13 The trend of penicillinase-producing gonorrhea in the United States from 1977 to 1982.

The number of reported PPNG cases has risen from 190 cases in 1977 to 4507 cases in 1982 (Fig. 13). Between 1979 and 1982 alone there was a 13-fold increase in these strains. The PPNG strains currently constitute approximately 0.5% of all of the gonorrhea infections in the nation. There is a significant clustering of these strains in the United States. The state of California has been the major source of PPNG cases, accounting for more than 40% of the nation's total. Other high-prevalence states, which each contribute approximately 10% of the cases, are Hawaii, Florida, and New York. Sustained long-term endemic transmission of PPNG has been identified in the cities of Los Angeles, New York, and Miami. In the Los Angeles and New York areas, PPNG clustering occurred in the urban poor and the prostitute populations. The epidemic in Miami has been resistant to control measures, with approximately 5% of the gonorrhea isolates in this area found to be PPNG. Although investigation of the Miami epidemic continues, no core transmitter population has been identified. The PPNG strains have been reported from at least 43 states in the United States, with most outbreaks being of acute nature and rapidly brought under control by intense case-finding efforts. The major control strategies that have been employed in PPNG control activities have been intensive contact tracing, selective screening, and the testing of all *N. gonorrhoeae* isolates for the presence of beta-lactamase production. About 11% of the patients with PPNG infection have recently traveled to other states, and 15% of the cases occurred in patients who had recently returned from high PPNG prevalence areas such as the Phillipines, Thailand, and the Republic of Korea. Case importation has been the typical pattern in short, acute outbreaks, while continuing local domestic transmission of the agent characterized the endemic areas. Approximately 14% of women infected with PPNG developed PID. Importation of PPNG from other endemic countries by both civilian and military personnel appears to be increasing.

RISK FACTORS ASSOCIATED WITH GONORRHEA INFECTIONS

The acquisition of gonorrhea by adults requires close intimate contact of susceptible epithelial surfaces such as occurs during sexual activities. It is reasonable to presume that celibacy essentially precludes gonococcal infection. The risk of acquiring infection basically relates to the frequency of unprotected exposure to infected individuals. The ease with which one acquires disease when exposed to infection is mediated by the individual's immune status, the organism's antigenic composition, and the infectious dose of the organism. Individuals in a homologous sexual relationship where the organism is not present at the outset and is not introduced are not at risk for gonorrhea infection. Thus the risk of infection is restricted to individuals who have coital activities with new sex partners. Under these circumstances the risk of acquiring disease is proportional to the statistical likelihood of the sex partner being infected, which, for the most part, is related to the sexual activity history of the partner, and the prevalence of gonorrhea in the population from which he or she is derived. Because of the tendency for gonorrhea infection to be clustered within the population, there appears to be higher, lower, and essentially nonexistent risks associated with sexual activities. It is clear that the risk of acquisition of disease relates to both the quantitative and qualitative sexual activities of either or both of the partners in a sexual liaison. It is also evident that the risk of infection may be very high with a single sexual encounter, and it may also be very low to nonexistent, even with multiple different sexual encounters, depending on the sexual activities of the partners and the prevalence of gonorrhea in their social milieu. The highest risk of acquiring disease occurs in situations where at least one of the individuals is frequently sexually exposed to a community of partners with a high prevalence of gonorrhea. In addition, factors such as the use of protective measures, the type of sexual activities, and the prevalence of symptomatic versus asymptomatic disease modulate, up or down, the risks of acquiring disease. The choice and frequency of new sex partners tend to be the major generic determinants of the risk of acquisition of disease. These factors are conditioned by the psychosocial experiences, cause-and-effect intellectual orientations, basic values, and risk-taking attitudes of the individuals.

PREVALENCE OF DISEASE

The single most important determinant of the risk of gonorrhea acquisition relates to the likelihood with which disease is found in the sex partners. The available data indicates that sexual contact with individuals derived from the high gonorrhea prevalence populations, such as the nonwhite, prostitutes, homosexual-bisexual males, and any individuals from geographically delineated high gonorrhea prevalence core group areas, carries with it a higher probability of acquiring and transmitting gonorrhea than contact with individuals sexually exposed to members of low disease prevalence populations. It is also in this fashion that gonorrhea disease is introduced into sexually active populations relatively free of disease.

Age

The population between the ages of 15 and 24 years have the highest prevalence of gonorrhea. Young age tends to be dependently related to such variables as nonhomologous sexual relationships, increased numbers of different sex partners, increased risk taking, lower economic and educational levels, and sociopathic and impetuous behavior patterns, all of which have been associated as potential risk factors for the acquisition of gonorrhea [26-32].

Number of Sex Partners

The choice of sexual partners may be selective or indiscriminate. Some studies have indicated a correlation between the number of different sex partners and an increased risk of acquiring gonorrhea [13, 26]; other investigators have failed to show such a relationship [31-33]. Ross [34] delineated a relationship between the risk of gonorrhea and the number of sexual partners only if the number of sexual partners exceeded 2 per month. Our own unpublished data, which includes an evaluation of 13,580 individuals with gonorrhea and 50,955 individuals without gonorrhea, all seen in an STD clinic in Columbus, Ohio, indicate that the relationship between the number of recent sex partners and the risk of gonorrhea are correlated, but that the strengths of these correlations vary significantly by population subgroup. Figure 14 compares the relative risk of gonorrhea with the number of different sexual partners within the prior 30 days, by sexual preference and sex. Minimal sexual activity was defined as no sexual partners within the prior 30 days. Between zero and one sex partner, there is clearly an increased risk of acquiring gonorrhea in all subgroups; the relative risk increases by approximately twofold for women and homosexual males, and by fourfold for heterosexual males. Beyond one sex partner per month the relative risk plateaus out for the homosexual male. In women the relative risk of acquiring gonorrhea increases by an additional 22% at the two and three partners per month levels. Although there is a slight increase in the relative risk of gonorrhea in women with more than one sex partner within a 30-day period, it is not dose related, and the statistical relative risk difference beyond two partners is not significant. This is not the situation with heterosexual males. The major increase is seen at the level of one sex partner, and after this the rate of increased risk decreases somewhat but is incrementally increased by each additional sex partner to a level of approxiamtely sevenfold that of the base line at the more than three partner level. Race was not found to be a significant confounder of these findings. The exact meaning of these data is not

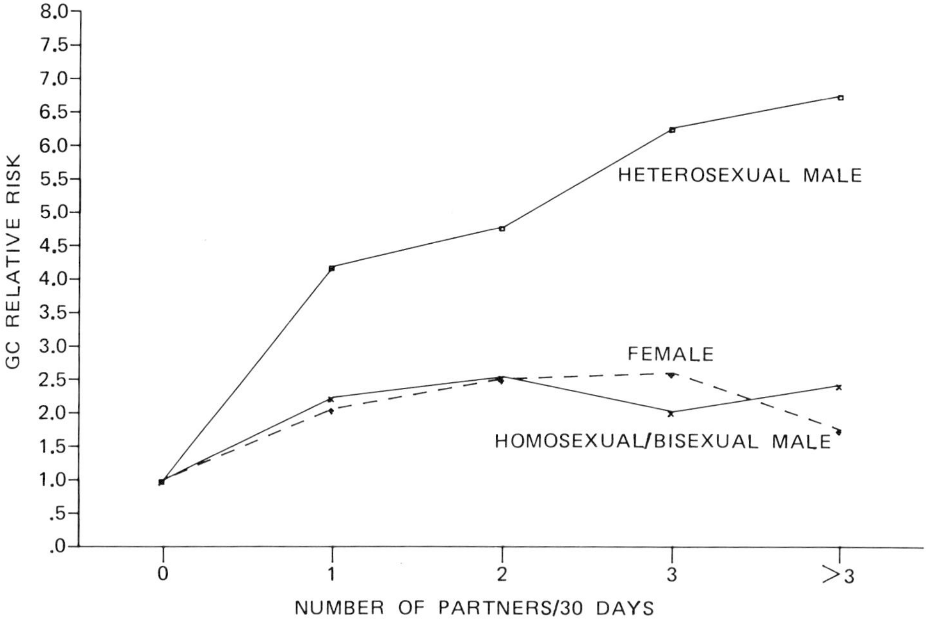

Fig. 14 Number of sex partners within the prior 30 days and the relative risk of gonorrhea.

clear. It is possible that many homosexual males tend to choose their partners selectively. The type of sexual activities may be more significant determinants of disease than the recent number of sex partners. It may also indicate that gonococcal disease in homosexual males is a tightly clustered phenomenon. Darrow et al. [13] found a correlation between the risk of gonorrhea in homosexual males and the type of sexual activities and sexual encounters in bathhouses. Judson et al. [35] have emphasized the high prevalence of gonorrhea in homosexuals who frequent bathhouses. The lack of significant incremental increases in the risk of gonorrhea in women associated with increasing numbers of sex partners may be associated with the low incidence of asymptomatic disease in men. It is possible that this pattern may be different in populations where asymptomatic male carriers of disease are more frequent. Because gonococcal infection in women is predominantly asymptomatic, it is possible that quantitative rather than discriminative factors play a larger role in the acquisition of gonorrhea in heterosexual men.

Our data indicate that there are differences by race, sex preference, and gender in the mean number of sex partners per month. Bisexual and homosexual white males were found to have the most monthly sexual partners. Whites had more partners than nonwhites, and men had more partners than women.

Gonorrhea recidivists tend to be characterized by the presence of multiple risk factors [28,29,31,33]. Our experience with repeaters indicates that they are frequently geographically associated with high gonorrhea prevalence areas. Many investigators have documented the significant effect of gonorrhea recidivists on local morbidity rates [29, 33, 36]. Although the definition of what constitutes a repeater is confounded by the duration of observation in these various studies, repeater rates of 7 to 23% have been shown to account for 23 to 48% of gonorrhea morbidity [29-33]. Between 38 and 50% of the repeat gonorrhea infections occur within 10 weeks of the initial infection [36,37]. In an evaluation of age-specific gonorrhea trends in Scotland, Schofield [38] found that high-risk gonorrhea cohorts with greater risks of infection and reinfection exist and are identifiable in the 10 to 14-year-old group. This cohort influences future gonorrhea morbidity trends at 4-year intervals.

Other Possible Risk Factors for Gonorrhea

Some investigators have identified an increased frequency of personality disorders in patients with gonorrhea or other sexually transmitted diseases [28, 39, 40]. Alcohol and drug abuse has been found more frequently by some [28, 41] and conflicts with the police have been noted [28].

In a currently unreplicated study of prostitutes, Chan et al. [42] hypothesized a possible link between HLA histocompatability types and susceptibility to syphilis and gonorrhea.

Some investigators have found an association between the B blood type or the absence of anti-B isohemagglutinins and the prevalence of gonorrhea [43-45].

NATIONAL PROGRAMS FOR THE CONTROL OF GONORRHEA

The national epidemic of gonorrhea was evident in 1968, and federal money became available for gonorrhea control activities. In 1972 the CDC distributed $3 million throughout the United States for gonorrhea control activities. In 1973 this was increased to $15 million. In 1974 the funding dropped to approximately $12.5 million. The funding remained at this level until 1977, when it was increased, and has steadily increased to approximately $20 million (adjusted for 1972 dollars) in 1980. These monies were provided to the state and local health departments to support STD control activities, including gonorrhea screening of women and contact-interviewing and tracing activities. In 1981 the number of women screened in the U.S. public health clinics and the private sector totaled approximately 9 million, and 361,530 contact interviews were conducted. Centers for Disease Control expenditures support approximately 85% of these activities in the United States. It is estimated that in 1981 gonorrhea screening and contact referral activities throughout the nation prevented over 200,000 gonorrhea cases and averted economic costs for both complicated and uncomplicated disease of over $140 million.

Public Health Clinics

Sexually transmitted disease public health clinics in local communities account for about 75% of reported gonorrhea cases in the United States. The major functions of these programs are to provide low-cost or no-cost clinical STD services and to expedite the contact-tracing process. These programs provide screening, diagnostic, and treatment services for gonorrhea and other STDs. The clinics provide the opportunity for rapid access into the health care system without the deterrent of cost. Because of the short incubation period of gonorrhea and the asymptomatic nature of many infections, rapid access into the primary care system is essential to disease control efforts. Public health clinics provide a milieu for on-site educational counseling and sex partner contact tracing, expediting sex partner treatment in a cost-effective manner. Although traditionally looked upon as a place to go if one could not afford private medical care, more recently some of these programs offer high-quality, comprehensive STD medical services at a level of clinical expertise not available in the private medical community. While in many countries venereology has been an accepted specialty for many years, in the United States this role is filled by public health and academic physicians associated with public sexually transmitted disease programs.

Gonorrhea Interviewing and Contact Tracing

Gonorrhea is frequently spread by individuals with asymptomatic or minimally symptomatic infection. These transmitters may unwittingly infect multiple individuals. Of the 753,953 gonorrhea infections seen in U.S. public clinics in 1981, 44% had contact-tracing interviews. These interviews resulted in the examination of 193,161 additional patients and the discovery and treatment of 73,921 (38%) new infections and the epidemiological treatment of 82,851 others. These disease carriers are only identified if they are fortunate enough to be tested in a screening program or are named as sexual contacts to patients with symptomatic disease or someone with inapparent infection discovered during routine screening. In 1981 a total of 12% of the gonorrhea cases identified by private physician sources were interviewed, yielding 5471 newly discovered infections and the epidemiological treatment of 9421 other patients. The majority of women and as many as 50% of infected male sexual contacts identified by the contact-tracing process have asymptomatic disease. This program has played a major role in diminishing the large reservoir of asymptomatic disease transmitters in the United States.

Gonorrhea Screening of Women

Pelvic inflammatory disease is frequently an early complication of genital gonorrhea in women. Prevention of this sequela requires the identification of gonorrhea prior to the advent of ascending infection. Since 1972, public health officials have formed a liaison with the private medical sector in a national screening "dragnet" that has provided routine, low-cost testing for gonorrhea in approximately 7.5 million women annually. These efforts have identified approximately 206,000 infected women annually and account for more than one-half of all of the gonorrhea morbidity reported in women. Examination of their sex partners has resulted in a large number of infected men brought to treatment, many of which are asymptomatic.

In this program the health department selects various private physicians and clinics as screening sites and provides them with culture media for diagnosis. In most cases the health department laboratory performs the cultures and reports the results to the physicians and makes arrangements for contact tracing by the physician or health department. In many programs the health department provides courier pickup and delivery of culture media and test results.

This program has been a highly efficient and cost-effective method for the discovery of a large number of gonorrhea cases and has contributed measurably to the prevention of PID.

Hospital Emergency Department PID Follow-up

Women with pelvic inflammatory disease often present to the hospital emergency room departments for initial care. Many of these patients do not have family physician, and, if not hospitalized, are treated on an outpatient basis, and do not have ready access back into the health care system. As a natural extension of the screening program, in 1978 the CDC launched a national program to provide gonorrhea culture screening services to all hospital emergency departments and to provide clinical follow-up for gonorrhea-associated PID cases who had no family physicians within 3 to 4 days in local health department STD clinics. The patients are evaluated by the health department clinical staff, counseled, and contact tracing is initiated. Follow-up care is provided and patients are referred back into the health care system for hospitalization or further diagnostic evaluation, as clinically indicated.

About 700 hospitals throughout the nation are participating in this program. Almost 1800 gonorrhea-associated PID cases have been identified monthly in these participating hospitals. Of these patients, 86% have had the benefits of counseling and contact interviews by the health department, and about 7 sexual partners are examined for every 10 PID cases identified. Of the infected male contacts to gonorrhea-associated PID, 42% have been found to be asymptomatic disease transmitters.

The screening programs in hospital emergency departments have yielded a gonorrhea positivity rate of 6 to 9%. In addition to providing screening and clinical follow-up, this program has allowed surveillance of the trends in pelvic inflammatory disease.

In our Columbus, Ohio, program, 70% of the gonorrhea-associated PID patients seen in the hospital emergency departments are seen and followed up in the health department clinic.

GONORRHEA EPIDEMIOLOGY AND THE EPIDEMIC IN PERSPECTIVE

Gonorrhea is caused by not one but a variety of strains of *N. gonorrhoeae*. These strains are antigenically distinct, have variable nutrient requirements, and differ in their virulence and distribution within the population. The virulence of the organism not only varies by strain type, but appears to be mediated to some extent by the host environment. Susceptibility to infection at any given clinical site is dependent on the infectious dose, the strain of gonococci, and the environmental milieu of the clinical site. The organism is highly capable of changing its genetic composition, and in the past four decades there have been significant antigenic shifts and a redistribution of strain types within the population. The major change in the organism has been a progressive increase in antibiotic resistance due to both genetic and plasmid-mediated mechanisms as a response to antibiotic pressures. Natural gonorrhea infection prompts a number of host immune responses at various levels that are polyantigenic and which, for the most part, fail to provide long-term protection against genital reinfection. This is due to the antigenic heterogeneity of the organisms and short-lived local antibody mechanisms. Immunity to systemic gonococcal disease appears to be firmer than that associated with local infection. Host immunity appears to be both inherent and dose related. Both local and systemic immunity appear to be firmer after parenteral injection of gonococcal antigens than that seen in natural genital infections. Although antigenically diverse, gonococcal strains may share common antigens with other strains and some strains demonstrate more cross-reactivity to larger numbers of strains than others. In general, infection and disease occur when the infectious dose of the agent exceeds the immune mechanisms capability.

The current gonorrhea epidemic began in 1967 and, after a threefold increase in disease, peaked in 1975 and began a slow decline. The duration of this epidemic and its intensity have been unprecedented in U.S. history and has involved predominantly white individuals. The sociodemography of this epidemic in the white population has not been well defined.

Epidemics of infectious disease occur primarily because of changes in traditional agent, host, or environmental characteristics. In the gonorrhea epidemic all of these appear to be more or less operative. Changes in the dosages of antibiotics used to treat gonorrhea have kept up with this trend, and current treatment regimens continue to be highly effective. Increasing antibiotic resistance has made it less likely that undiscovered gonorrhea infections would be cured with antibiotic treatment of other unrelated conditions such as respiratory, skin, or urinary tract infections. It is not known, if or by how much, decreasing antibiotic susceptibility has affected gonorrhea morbidity. Because of the magnitude of the incidence increase of gonorrhea, it is unlikely that the changes in antibiotic susceptibility played a major role in the epidemic of disease. There is no firm evidence that the antigenic shifts in *N. gonorrhoeae* during this period have resulted in increases in organism virulence. Thus it appears that although organism changes over time may be contributory to the epidemic, they probably have not been a major factor.

Considerable changes have occurred in the host population in the past two decades. The major component of these changes has served to markedly increase the proportion and total number of individuals at risk for acquiring gonorrhea infections. The population at risk for disease acquisition is those who must make periodic choices as to sexual partners. There has been a large expansion in this susceptible population. The marked increase in the 15- to 29-year-old population, increased divorce rates, and the delaying of marriage have all contributed to the expansion of the population at risk in the United States. During this same period, the proportion of women 15 to 19 years old engaging in premarital sexual activities has significantly increased, especially in white women. These factors influence the total numbers of both cases and, to a lesser degree, case rates. Another factor contributing to the increased rate of disease has been the increasing urbanization of the U.S. society. Between 1960 and 1980 the proportion of individuals living in urban areas has increased by approximately 6% [6].

Beginning in 1972, case detection efforts increased significantly, largely because of widespread screening of women, but also aided by increased efforts in contact tracing and a progressive trend toward shifting resources away from syphilis to gonorrhea case finding. These activities, although effective disease control measures, have tended to artificially elevate the magnitude of the gonorrhea epidemic.

It is evident that host factors have been the major factors in the gonorrhea epidemic. Fortunately, the rate of increase in the high-risk age group population is decreasing, and the rate of urbanization is lessening.

The rapid and sustained increase in gonorrhea incidence in the United States since 1967 regrettably has failed to arouse the enthusiasm or interest of the academic medical communities. During this long-sustained epidemic, there has been little to no commitment by medical educators to prepare American physicians to deal in a knowledgeable and practical fashion with gonorrhea or the rapidly expanding scope of an increasing number of STDs. Between 1966 and 1980 the average total number of teaching hours devoted to venereology in the curricula of U.S. medical schools has dropped from 19.4 to 11.2 hr, a decrease of 42% [46,47]. A total of 70% of U.S. medical schools offer no clinical training in venereology to their students, and in the schools that do only an average of 30% of the students are involved. Residency training programs have fared no better, with only 23% of the programs offering clinical training to approximately 50% of the resident population. There is little evidence that public health schools and preventive medicine departments have provided medical students or graduate students with appropriate orientation as to the extent of the gonorrhea epidemic and the scope and complexity of the expanding spectrum of sexually transmitted diseases. It is not surprising that even academically trained health commissioners, most often responsible for setting public health priorities and managing budgetary disbursements, have little orientation to the problem of STDs. In our local training program for medical students we find graduating students unaware of how to appropriately collect urethral and cervical samples for gonorrhea cultures, and only the rare student passes the precourse rudimentary test in venereology essentially designed for STD clinic nursing personnel. Daily contact with physicians indicates that some still do not believe that asymptomatic gonorrhea exists in males, and inappropriate treatment of gonorrhea is commonly encountered. To what degree this academic void has contributed to the ongoing epidemic is conjectural, but it undoubtedly has been at least contributory.

Cognizant of the paucity of venereology training at the medical school level, and faced with a severe shortage of qualified medical personnel to staff approximately 3000 public health STD clinics throughout the United States, the CDC in 1979 set up nine regional training centers [48]. By 1981 these programs have provided minicourse training of 2 to 14 days duration in clinical venereology for over 970 physicians and 641 nurse practitioners and physician assistants.

The majority of public health STD clinics in the United States still do not have medical directors trained and skilled in the rudiments of venereology. Also, there is strong anecdotal evidence that nonphysician public health personnel in STD clinics have a much broader base of clinical knowledge of the STDs than practicing physicians.

Increased federal appropriations for STD control activities nationwide appear to be decreasing the incidence of gonorrhea in the United States. As of 1981, 39 states had lower gonorrhea rates than they did in 1975. Not all state and local governments have made major commitments to the control of gonorrhea or other sexually transmitted diseases. As a consequence, there is marked variation in both the quality and quantity of STD programs by state and local metropolitan areas within states. This is probably due, at least in part, to the limited orientation to the scope and extent of the STD problem often provided health officials. This is further evidenced by the fact that only a minority (44%) of the gonorrhea patients seen in public clinics received contract illicitation interviews in 1981.

Limited allocation of budgetary resources to local public health clinics and the expanded scope of diseases have forced many STD programs to levy charges in their clinics. Although these charges are usually considerably less expensive than comparable private sector care, it is not known if they deter routine screening or the routine evaluation of patients from high disease prevalence core areas.

Contemporary STD control programs in the United States often fail to utilize geographic disease distributions as guidelines to program priority setting. Screening programs in women are often allocated on the basis of intuition and positivity rates, rather than on data that provide information regarding local morbidity distribution. There remain uncertainties about the cost effectiveness of the contact-tracing process in various patient populations. Many of the STD program managers at both the state and local levels have no formal graduate academic training in epidemiology. There is a need for these managers to obtain additional academic training in data analysis and basic epidemiological concepts.

Even though the current efforts in gonorrhea control appear to be influencing disease rates, it is evident that much more needs to be done. A better understanding of the distribution of gonorrhea strains within communities and their spread patterns is needed. The immunological determinants of infection, disease, and sequelae need to be clarified. Targeting of available resources to clustered populations with the highest prevalence of disease needs to be done. Efforts need to be continually directed at the detection of highly sexually active asymptomatic gonorrhea transmitters. Gonorrhea morbidity data need to be collected in an appropriate fashion using appropriate numerators and denominators and continually evaluated to assist in the formulation of more cost-effective control strategies and the realistic setting of both short- and long-term goals for disease control. A commitment must be made by the academic community to provide increased training to physicians and medical students. A similar commitment must be made by health officials at local and state levels to seriously decrease disease morbidity in their areas. Disease control strategies must be based on time-proven epidemiological principles of disease control. The outlook for vaccine intervention strategies is still conjectural. The available data suggest that a polyantigenic *N. gonorrhoeae* outer membrane protein vaccine composed of "senior" cross-reacting gonorrhea strains may be effective in preventing PID sequelae. It is not known what target populations should be immunized, the cost, and the duration of immunity. Similar caveats apply to pili vaccine preparations under study.

It is apparent that there is no easy or single answer to the gonorrhea problem. Resolution will require considerable effort and dedication to the task by multiple levels of the medical and epidemiological communities. It must be emphasized that the gonorrhea epidemic is only the tip of the iceberg, since a wide variety of other STDs are also at similar epidemic levels in the United States.

WORLDWIDE GONORRHEA TRENDS

Although significant differences exist in the reported sexually transmitted disease surveillance methods between countries, trend data and marked intercountry differences appear to be meaningful. Arya has reviewed the gonorrhea rate trends in England, Poland, Canada, Finland, Denmark, Sweden, and the United States between 1955 and 1975 [49]. Internationally, gonorrhea incidence increased noticeably in all countries between 1959 and 1966. The sharpest increases in the epidemic curves were noted in the United States and Sweden, and the smallest in England and Poland, which demonstrated slow but steady increases during this period. To date, the sharpest decrease in gonorrhea morbidity has been seen in Sweden, where gonorrhea rates are approaching pre-epidemic levels. In contrast, although case rates have been on a slow and steady decline since 1976, the United

States maintains the highest gonorrhea rates internationally. Most countries have noted a similar decline in gonorrhea during the past 5 years. The successful control of gonorrhea in Sweden has been attributed to an increased use of condoms, improved public and medical attitudes toward the disease, and increased detection of asymptomatic gonorrhea in women through screening activities. Most countries, with the notable exception of the United States, have formalized the training and specialization in venereology.

DESCRIPTIVE EPIDEMIOLOGY OF SYPHILIS IN THE UNITED STATES

Syphilis Morbidity Data Base

The national syphilis morbidity data base is collected by the CDC by formal case reporting from the states and is confounded by similar variables that plague the gonorrhea morbidity data. The data provided in this section are derived from this data base. Regional data may vary in accuracy, dependent upon the quality and quantity of the STD control programs. Trend data, particularly those relating to latent disease, may be more influenced than those relating to early infectious syphilis because of a progressive trend over time to concentrate investigational efforts on early disease detection (under 1 year's duration). A significant proportion of the low titer reactive serologies, especially in older patients, which may represent latent (possibly untreated) cases are not investigated. There are no accurate national or local data on the frequency of latent syphilis cases in the United States. The latent syphilis cases currently documented in the morbidity base represent only a portion of the real prevalence of disease, a proportion which varies markedly by regional and STD control program priorities and staffing. Data relating to the incidence of congenital syphilis are particularly confounded by diagnostic errors. One study of 173 reported cases of early congenital syphilis (less than 1 year of age) revealed a definite or probable diagnosis of syphilis in only 14%, 50% were possible but undocumented syphilis cases, and 36% were unlikely to be congenital syphilis [50]. Cases of syphilis in older children, especially the 10- to 14-year-old group, are prone to be labeled congenital disease, rather than be considered the results of sexual activity or abuse. Because public health investigational activites are directed at interrupting infectious syphilis, early syphilis morbidity data tend to be more accurate, especially those relating to the primary and secondary phases, which are associated with signs of disease.

Trend in Syphilis Morbidity

Primary and secondary (P&S) syphilis data provide the best incidence indicators for disease trend comparisons because of their increased reliability and stable criteria for diagnosis. Figure 15 depicts the trend of P&S syphilis in the United States

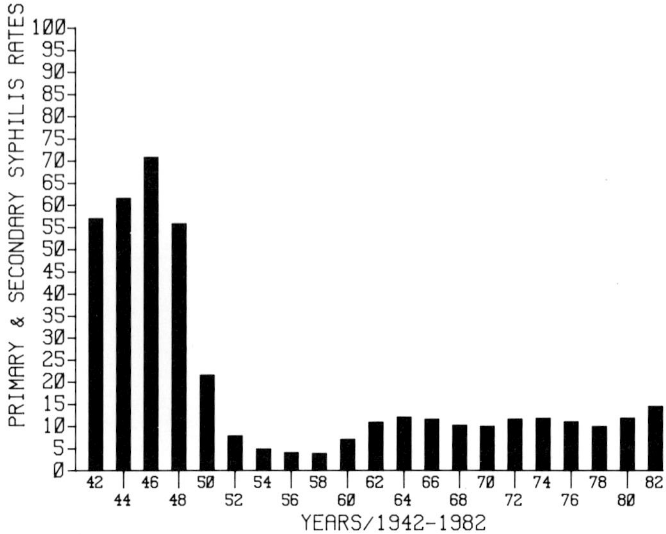

Fig. 15 Rates of primary and secondary syphilis cases in the United States from 1942 to 1982.

over the last 40 years. Following the introduction of the widespread use of penicillin for syphilis treatment, the incidence of the disease dropped markedly. Between 1947 and 1957, P&S case rates declined from 75.6 to 3.9 per 100,000, a decrease of 95%. Total syphilis case rates (including latent cases) between 1941 and 1978 dropped from 368.2 to 30 per 100,000; total cases dropped from 372,963 to 64,875. The incidence of the disease slowly increased in the 1960s and remained relatively stable until 1978. Between 1977 and 1982 case rates of P&S syphilis increased by 54% (from 9.5 to 14.6 per 100,000). This trend is not continuing through 1984. The number of P&S cases identified in the first three-quarters of 1984 was 14% lower than that seen in the comparable 1983 period. The upturn in syphilis beginning in 1978 was anticipated by STD control planners owing to an increasing diversion of program resources toward gonorrhea and pelvic inflammatory disease activities.

Between 1941 and 1981 the number of reported cases of congenital syphilis dropped markedly, demonstrating a more progressive decrease than that of P&S syphilis (Fig. 16). This was probably attributable to the mandatory prenatal screening laws passed by most states and the widespread use of serological screening by the medical community. A notable trend in the annual reported cases of congenital syphilis is the decrease in the proportion of cases over the age of 9 years (Fig. 17). In 1968, 85% of the congenital syphilis cases were identified in youngsters more than 9 years of age. In 1980 only 47% of the reported cases

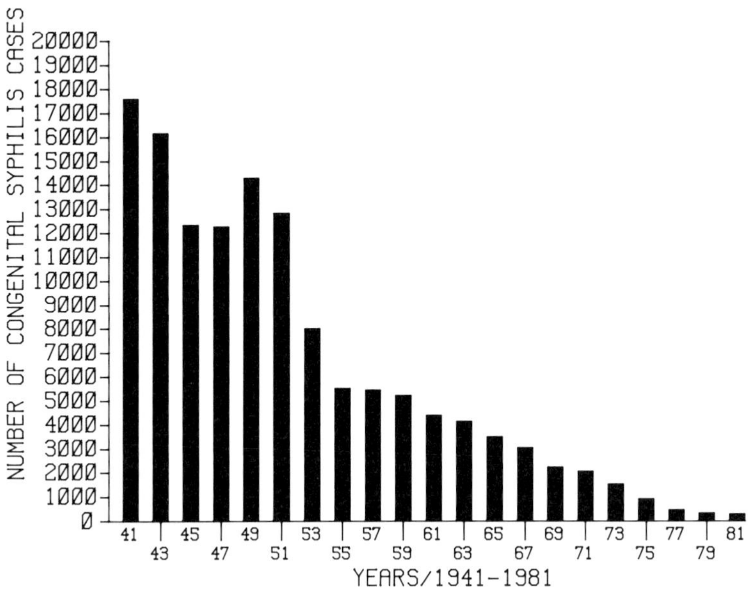

Fig. 16 Number of congenital syphilis cases in the United States from 1941 to 1981.

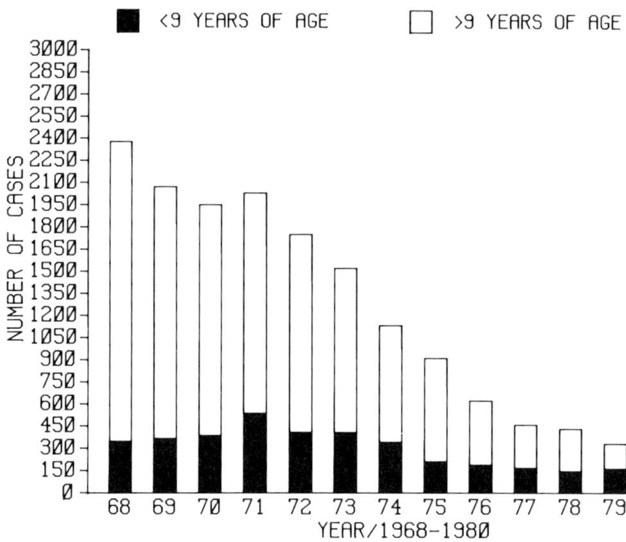

Fig. 17 Number of congenital syphilis cases in the United States from 1968 to 1980.

were in this age group. In addition, in 1968 only 12% of the cases were in infants under 1 year of age, and in 1980 41% of the cases were in this age group. If not a reporting artifact, this suggests a trend in earlier diagnosis of disease.

On the presumption that the reported morbidity data reflect approximately one-half of the true number of congenital syphilis cases born annually in the United States, the incidence of congenital syphilis in 1980 (288 cases) was approximately that of the estimated incidence of phenylketonuria (1 per 15,000 live births), and approximately threefold that of the estimated incidence of congenital rubella syndrome cases (approximately 100).

In spite of the marked decrease in the incidence of syphilis, it remains the third most frequently reported infectious disease in the United States.

Person Variables in Syphilis Morbidity

The highest P&S syphilis case rates occur in the 20- to 29-year-old group. Fichtner et al. [51] evaluated syphilis patient demographical data between 1967 and 1979. During this period, the ratio of male to female cases increased from 1.5:1 in 1967 to 3:1 in 1979. Although the public clinic case detection proportion of total morbidity rose from 65.8% in 1967 to 76.5% in 1979 (a 16% increase), the reported cases in white men utilizing public clinic facilities rose from 4.2 to 18%, an increase of 329%. White males seen in public clinics demostrated a 351% increase in P&S syphilis between 1967 and 1979. The increase reported by the private medical sector was only about 35%, consistent with a significant shift of morbidity to public sector clinical sites. During this same period P&S syphilis continued to decline in nonwhite women by approximately 15 and 36% in public and private sites, respectively. Case rates in nonwhite men seen in public clinics remained stable, while declining approximately 13% in private medical sites. White women showed an increase of approximately 40% from public sources, whereas there was a decrease of a similar magnitude from private sector reporting sites. Between 1977 and 1979, P&S syphilis cases rose by 23%, 85% of which were due to cases in males. The ratio of nonwhite to white P&S cases in 1979 was about 3.5:1 for males and 15:1 for women. The proportion of white males with early syphilis seen in public health clinics who admitted to homosexual activity rose from 37.6 to 69.5% between 1967 and 1979, an increase of 85%.

The overall pattern of P&S syphilis during the period between 1967 and 1979 suggests a changing pattern in the spread of syphilis in the United States. Although the disease continues to be endemic in the nonwhite population, the trend indicates an increasing spread of disease in the white population, particularly in white homosexual males. Even if one conceded the possibility of a homosexuality prevalence of as high as 20% in white males, the fact that 37.6 and 69.5% of the P&S cases in 1967 and 1979, respectively, seen in public clinics were in homosexual males clearly suggests endemic and epidemic syphilis levels in this population. A disproportionate utilization of public clinic facilities is an unlikely explanation of these high levels of disease. Similar conclusions have been reached by other U.S. investigators [13, 52].

The role of prostitution in the spread of syphilis in the United States is poorly documented. Except for local outbreaks associated with prostitution, the disease does not appear to be widespread in this population.

Geographic Distribution of Syphilis

Similar to gonorrhea, syphilis varies significantly in its regional prevalence in the United States (Fig. 18). The highest case rates are seen in the southwest central, southeastern Atlantic, and Pacific states. The highest and lowest P&S syphilis case rates in 1982 were reported from the states of Louisiana and New Hampshire, respectively. As with most communicable infections, the disease tends to be clustered. As with gonorrhea and a variety of other STDs, the disease rates are higher in metropolitan areas.

Syphilis Control Programs

The major public health programs for syphilis control rely heavily on sexual partner tracing of infected individuals and the follow-up of reactive serological tests. In 1981, of the 51,679 syphilis cases identified, 94% were interviewed for sexual contacts. These interviews yielded an average of 1.6 new contacts per patient, and in 32% of the cases the source of the infection could be identified. There were 51,137 contacts examined, 44% within 30 days and 80% within 14 days of the case identification; 17% of these contacts were found to be infected with syphilis, 40% of whom had either primary or secondary syphilis. In addition, 35,655 contacts were prophylactically treated because of potential exposure to infection.

In 1981 there were 1,024,352 positive serological reactions reported. Of these, physician reports or health department investigations yielded 33,272 cases of early syphilis and 22,741 cases of latent disease, a total of 56,013 cases. It is not known what proportion of these cases would have escaped diagnosis or treatment were it not for public health follow-up. Thus, of the over 1 million positive serological tests, approximately 5.5% were associated with newly diagnosed cases of syphilis. What proportion of these reactors were latent syphilis cases brought to treatment is not known. Sixty percent of the cases identified through the reactor follow-up were early cases of syphilis, indicating selective follow-up of the reactors and bias toward the documentation of early infectious syphilis. This selection is usually done by prioritizing case follow-up on the basis of highly positive tests and younger age groups. This contrasts to the usual outcomes of serological screening of apparently healthy populations, where the cases usually discovered are latent, not early, infectious syphilis. Serological screening yielded 11,331 cases, or 22% of the 51,679 early syphilis cases identified in 1982. Premarital (528) and prenatal testing (958) alone accounted for over 13% of the

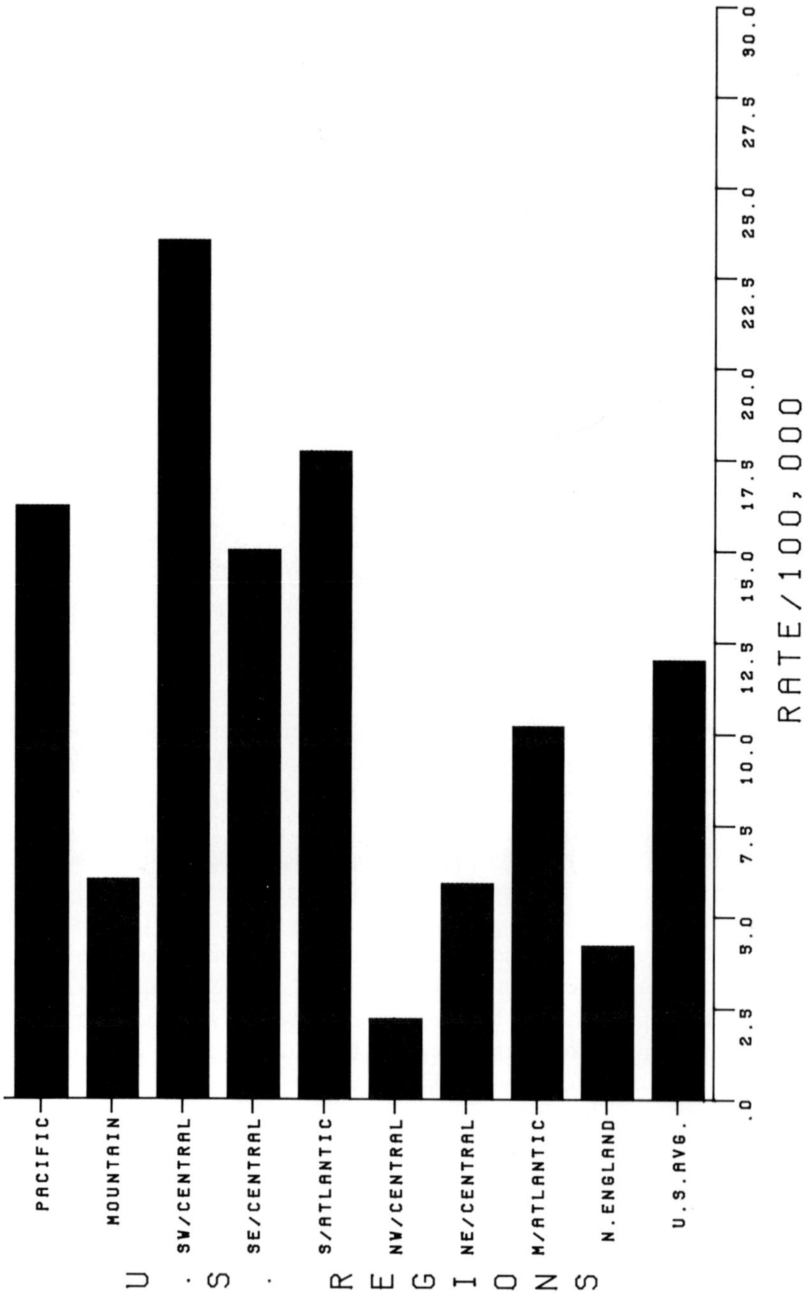

Fig. 18 Rates of primary and secondary syphilis cases in the United States in 1980 by geographic region.

early cases detected by screening. The number of latent syphilis cases identified by serological testing has not been documented, but is undoubtedly significantly higher than the number of early cases detected.

Syphilis in Perspective

The incidence of syphilis in 1982 was only approximately 20% of the level seen in 1947, but fourfold that seen in 1957. The total number of syphilis cases today, including all stages, is less than 50% of the cases seen in 1957. This is due to a marked decrease in the number of latent syphilis cases. In 1957 the total versus the P&S syphilis ratio was 21:1; today that ratio is only 2.2:1. It is not yet clear what proportion of this large decrease in latent cases is due to a true decrease in disease prevalence versus a progressive decrease in case-finding efforts by the public health sector and a significant decrease in routine serological testing in the private medical sector. Undoubtedly, some of the apparent decrease in latent syphilis cases is real, but in light of a progressive increase in the incidence of syphilis over the last 15 years, and known reasons to project decreasing effectiveness in the documentation of latent, asymptomatic disease, the data are questionable. The major problems of syphilis reside in its tendency to produce asymptomatic latent infection with significant neurological or cardiovascular sequelae, or perinatal mortality and morbidity. In spite of highly effective and inexpensive single-dose treatment and low-cost and effective testing for this disease, it persists and has even increased in incidence. Perinatal morbidity, although markedly decreased, has not been eradicated and is as frequent as phenylketonuria and significantly more frequent than that of congenital rubella syndrome. The prevention of perinatal disease and latent syphilis sequelae is relatively inexpensive when compared to most disease prevention measures espoused today.

Although latent disease and its sequelae and perinatal morbidity are the true measures of the importance of syphilis, there is little evidence that the national syphilis control program directly addresses these issues. Accurate data on the frequency of latent disease are not kept, nor has any attempt been made to encourage targeted and more cost-effective screening activities. There are no formal programs to monitor the ultimate diagnostic outcomes of infants with reactive serologies.

The trend of a higher proportion of syphilis in homosexual males may be a fortuitous one, since it does not impact on the congenital syphilis rates. Although a well-defined population, there is little evidence of formal approaches to disease detection in male homosexuals, except on a sporadic basis. There are few who believe contact-tracing activities detect and treat almost all of the individuals exposed to infection. The missing infections will potentially go on to asymptomatic latent disease and possible disease sequelae. Cognizant of the expanding problem of a variety of significant sexually transmitted diseases and the need to spread limited resources farther, often at the expense of syphilis control activities, STD program managers throughout the United States remain uneasy about the future trends of both early and latent syphilis.

GENITAL HERPES SIMPLEX INFECTIONS

Genital herpes is a vesiculoulcerative disease caused by either herpes simplex virus 1 (HSV-1) or herpes simplex virus 2 (HSV-2). In the United States genital herpes is associated with the HSV-2 virus in more than 90% of the cases [53]. Some investigators have found HSV-1 genital infections in 35 to 50% of the cases [54, 55]. Herpes simplex virus 1 is more frequently found in first rather than recurrent episodes of the disease [53, 56].

Because herpes is not a reportable disease and it tends to be recurrent, accurate estimates of its incidence are not possible. Data from the National Disease and Therapeutic Index (NDTI) and from STD clinics suggest that the frequency of genital herpes is approximately 1/10 as frequent as gonorrhea [57]. This would suggest that between 150,000 and 200,000 cases of genital herpes infections occur annually in the United States. Survey data of the NDTI identified 260,890 physician visits for genital herpes in 1979 [58]. In the same study, the National Ambulatory Medical Care Survey (NAMCS) yielded approximately 937,000 cases of genital herpes-related physician visits for the same year. A study conducted in Olmstead County, Minnesota, found an incidence of herpes of 82 per 100,000 between 1975 and 1979 [59]. If this rate were extrapolated nationally, it would yield an annual U.S. incidence of approximately 186,000 cases of genital herpes, similar to that derived from using gonorrhea ratio estimates. Extrapolating the 1979 herpes rates (128 per 100,000) to national figures would yield 270,000 cases, similar to the NDTI herpes-related physician visits for that year. Because type-specific antibody studies have not been available, it is not possible to estimate what proportion of the herpes cases represented new cases versus recurrences. Because the virus often produces latent infection and frequently recurs, the prevalence of herpes infections far exceeds its incidence.

The trend in the incidence of genital herpes has paralleled that of gonorrhea. Physician visits associated with a diagnosis of genital herpes increased ninefold between 1966 and 1979 (NDTI), although NAMCS data indicated only a 12% increase between 1973 and 1979 [58]. The Olmstead, Minnesota, study [59] revealed a sevenfold increase in herpes incidence between 1965 and 1979. It is not known what effect widespread news media attention to herpes simplex had on health-seeking habits and the frequency of the diagnosis of the disease.

There are no representative national data to define the demography of the herpes cases. Corey et al. [53] provided patient profiles on 630 herpes cases seen in Seattle, Washington. The average age was 27.1 years, 96% were white, 32% were men, and 64% were single, with a mean educational status of 15.1 years. These data were remarkably similar to those seen in a nationwide survey of self-selected herpes patients [60]. A prior history of gonorrhea was obtained in 31% of the men and 12% of the women. The mean number of lifetime sexual partners for men was 32.8 and 8.8 for women. Approximately one-half of the patients engaged in orogenital sexual activities. The data from our STD clinic program in Columbus, Ohio, from a predominantly lower- to middle-income population reveal a similar but slightly different population afflicted with herpes. The average patient age was 24.5 years and the mean educational level achieved was 13.1 years. The initial visit case rate for whites is 3.1 per 100, and that for nonwhites 1.8 per 100, with a white-to-nonwhite ratio of 1.7:1. This ratio is identical but reversed for gonorrhea. Chuang et al. [59] found the median age of their patients to be 24 years, with a male-to-female ratio of 1.5:1. The pattern emerges that genital herpes is more frequent in a slightly older and more educated white population, whereas gonorrhea is more frequent in younger, less-educated nonwhites. Herpes patients are more likely to be married than individuals with gonorrhea.

Genital herpes tends to be recurrent. About 55% of patients with HSV-1 infections suffer from recurrences, while 88% of HSV-2 infections recur. The frequency of recurrence is approximately three- to fourfold higher in HSV-2 infections; 25% of recurrences are asymptomatic [53].

The major problem associated with genital herpes is neonatal infection. The prevalence of neonatal infection in the United States has not been established, nor are there national data on neonatal herpes trends. One retrospective hospital record study of the trend of neonatal herpes in Seattle, Washington, suggested a progressive increase in the number of neonatal infections between 1966 and 1981 [61]. Although the case rate numbers were not statistically different, case rates increased from 2.6 per 100,000 live births during the period 1966 through 1969, to 4.8, 7.4, and 11.9 per 100,000 live births for the years 1970 through 1973, 1974 through 1977, and 1978 through 1981, respectively. If the 1980 case rates were extrapolated nationally, an estimated 430 cases of neonatal herpes would have occurred [62]. Neonatal herpes can be prevented by cesarean delivery of the infant. Because most women with symptomatic herpes are delivered surgically, the majority of neonatal herpes cases occur in women with asymptomatic infection. The current dilemma surrounding the prevention of neonatal herpes involves the high cost and low detection rate of routine, repeated last-trimester herpes culture screening. If only patients with a prior history of disease or with a sex partner with herpes were screened, as many as 44% of the infected patients would be missed [62]. In spite of this, these patients should continue to be routinely screened, and all women should be carefully examined to detect clinically evident infection. The future control of neonatal herpes will depend on the development of rapid, sensitive, and inexpensive direct smear testing procedures which could be used prior to the onset of labor.

The geographical distribution of genital herpes infections has not been delineated.

CHLAMYDIA TRACHOMATIS INFECTIONS

There are 15 serotypes of *Chlamydia trachomatis*. Anogenital infections are caused by types D through K [63]. These serotypes have also been associated with neonatal conjunctivitis and pneumonitis [64], epididymitis [65], prostatitis [66], Reiter's syndrome [67], salpingitis [68], and the urethral syndrome [69]. Types L1 through L3 are associated with lymphogranuloma venereum. *Chlamydia trachomatis* is the most frequent pathogen isolated in nongonococcal urethritis cases, occurring in an average of 37% of the cases (range 31 to 47%) studied by U.S. investigators [63]. The organism is also found concomitantly with gonorrhea urethritis in 17.5% of U.S. studies (range 4 to 33%) and accounts for about 50% of the postgonococcal urethritis infections [63].

Because *C. trachomatis* is not a reportable infection and definitive cultures for diagnosis are expensive or unavailable, reliable incidence, prevalence, and trend data are not available. Nongonococcal urethritis (NGU) is frequently used as a proxy to estimate chlamydial infection rates. Although this disorder is also not reportable, at least some data on the disease are available. Data from our Columbus program indicate that NGU case rates in heterosexual males are twofold those seen in homosexual men. This is consistent with the low prevalence of chlamydial infections in homosexual men [70]. Urethritis in white heterosexual males is more likely to be nongonococcal than gonococcal infection [71]. In our program we find that 67% of the urethritis cases in white heterosexuals are nongonococcal in type, while in nonwhite heterosexual men the NGU proportion is 46%, and only 34% in homosexual males. In some populations the proportion of urethritis cases due to NGU has been as high as 87% [63]. These data have led many to believe that case rates of NGU are significantly higher in white males than in nonwhite males. We have not found that to be true in our program, where the NGU case rates per 100 men are 22.9, 22.0, and 11.0 for nonwhite heterosexuals, white heterosexuals, and homosexual males, respectively. The lower proportion of NGU in the nonwhite population in our program is solely due to an increased prevalence of gonococcal disease. The CDC estimates that the prevalence of NGU in the United States is approximately 2.5 million cases annually, or about 2.5 times the frequency of gonococcal urethritis [63]. Males with NGU tend to be of higher socioeconomic status, more educated, and somewhat less sexually active than men with gonorrhea [72]. There is evidence that the incidence of NGU has been increasing. Between 1975 and 1980 Judson [71] reported a 70% increase in the number of NGU cases seen in an STD program. We have seen a similar trend in Columbus, Ohio.

The geographic distribution of NGU is poorly defined. Studies of the prevalence of NGU in STD clinics throughout the United States suggest that higher case rates are seen in the Pacific and northeast regions of the country.

Women with genital chlamydial infections tend to be clinically asymptomatic or present with a vaginal discharge or clinical mucopurulent cervicitis. *Chlamydia trachomatis* has been isolated in 12 to 29% of sexually active women studied in the United States, and in 20 to 40% of women with gonorrhea [63]. The proportional role of chlamydia in PID in the United States is currently unknown, but it is estimated that approximately 250,000 cases of chlamydial PID occur annually [73]. It has been estimated that 60 to 70% of the infants exposed to chlamydia during birth will become infected. A total of 25 to 50% of the infants will develop conjunctivitis, and 10 to 20% will develop pneumonitis [73]. Chlamydial pneumonitis accounts for 30 to 50% of the pneumonia cases reported in the first 6 months of life in the United States.

OTHER SEXUALLY TRANSMITTED AGENTS OF IMPORTANCE

Condyloma acuminatum, the human papillomavirus that causes venereal warts, has demonstrated a dramatic increase in incidence during the last 15 years. Data of the NDTI reveal that physician visits for venereal warts increased from 169,000 in 1966 to 946,000 in 1981, a fivefold increase [74]. Chuang et al. [59] found a similar trend in condyloma acuminatum cases in their study. There is evidence that a significant proportion of venereal warts, particularly those of the flat variety, tend to be asymptomatic, and that case rates for this disease may be even higher than documented. This virus has been strongly linked to cervical malignancy [75]. A similar link has been shown to be associated with HSV-2 [76].

Lymphogranuloma venereum and granuloma inguinale cases in the United States are uncommon, with only 55 and 66 cases reported, respectively, in 1981. It is not known how many of these diagnoses were accurate, and it may be that these diseases are even more uncommon than reported. Chancroid may be increasing in incidence in the United States since 1978, with 850 cases reported in 1981. Between 1978 and 1981 the incidence of this disease has increased by approximately 86%. Like the other two diseases, the accuracy of the diagnoses has been questioned. In 1982 an epidemic of 126 cases of chancroid in Orange County, California, was confirmed by the CDC [77]. It is probable that this disease is increasing in incidence.

CONCLUSIONS

The incidence and prevalence of many sexually transmitted diseases have increased markedly during the last 15 years. These diseases have been and are currently at unprecedented epidemic levels. In addition to the quantity of disease, the clinical spectrum of these diseases has significantly expanded. Many of the STDs are associated with serious sequelae. The case rates of the STDs in the United States currently may be the highest in the developed world.

Control of STDs requires the combined efforts of the academic, private, and public sectors of medicine. It is clearly time to consider the formalization of the specialty of venereology. The increasing complexity of these diseases and the costs of diagnosis and treatment are currently exceeding the capabilities of the public health sector to maintain high-quality clinical services and control programs. It is essential that appropriate liaisons be developed between the public health sector and the academic medical community to address a major effort to curtail the rate of these diseases in the United States and in the world.

REFERENCES

1. Fleming WL, Brown WJ, Donohue JF. National survey of venereal disease treated by physicians in 1968. JAMA 1968; 211:1827-1830.
2. Eisenberg MS, Wiesner PJ. Reporting and treating gonorrhea: results of a statewide survey in Alaska. J Am Vener Dis Assoc 1976; 3:79-83.
3. Rothenberg R, Bross DC, Vernon TM. Reporting of gonorrhea by private physicians: a behavioral study. Am J Public Health 1980; 70:983-986.
4. Dandoy S, Dandoy JR. Seasonality of gonorrhea in Arizona. Ariz Med 1973; 30:486-487.
5. Wright RA, Judson FN. Relative and seasonal incidences of the sexually transmitted diseases. A two year statistical review. Br J Vener Dis 1978; 54:433-440.
6. US Bureau of the Census. Statistical abstract of the United States. Washington, DC, 1981.
7. Zaidi AA, Aval SO, Reynolds GH, Blount JH, Jones OG, Fichter RR. Gonorrhea in the United States: 1967-1979. Sex Transm Dis 1983; 2:72-76.
8. Zelnik M, Kantner JF. Sexual activity, contraceptive use and pregnancy among metropolitan area teenagers: 1971-1979. Fam Plan Perspect 1980; 12:230-237.
9. Ritchey MG, Leff AM. Venereal disease control among homosexuals: an outreach program. JAMA 1975; 232:509-510.
10. Marino HI, Richards JB. An innovative program of venereal disease case finding, treatment and education for a population of gay men. Sex Transm Dis 1977; 4:50-52.
11. Ostrow DG, Shaskey DM. The experience of the Howard Brown Memorial Clinic of Chicago with sexually transmitted diseases. Sex Transm Dis 1977; 4:53-55.
12. Marino HI, Judson FN, Bennett D, Schaffnit TR. Screening for gonorrhea and syphilis in gay bath houses in Denver and Los Angeles. Public Health Rep 1979; 94:376-379.
13. Darrow WW, Barrett D, Jay K, Young A. The gay report on sexually transmitted diseases. Am J Public Health 1981; 71:1004-1011.
14. Ostrow DG, Shaskey D, Steffan G, Altman N. Epidemiology of gonorrhea infections in gay men. J Homosex 1980; 5:285-288.
15. Potterat JJ, Rothenberg R, Bross DC. Gonorrhea in street prostitutes: epidemiologic and legal implications. Sex Transm Dis 1979; 6:58-63.

16. Conrad GL, Kleris GS, Rush B, Darrow WW. Sexually transmitted diseases among prostitutes and other sexual offenders. Sex Transm Dis 1981; 8:241-244.
17. Rothenberg RB. The geography of gonorrhea: empirical demonstration of core group transmission. Am J Epidemiol 1983; 117:688-694.
18. Angulo JJ, Pederneiras CAA, Ebner W, Kimura EM, Megale P. Concepts of diffusion theory and a graphic approach to the description of the epidemic flow of contagious disease. Public Health Rep 1980; 95:478-485.
19. Potterat JJ, Rothenberg RB, Woodhouse D, Muth JS, Pratts CI. Gonorrhea as a social disease: empirical demonstration of the core group hypothesis. In: Programs and abstracts, 5th international meeting of the International Society for STD Research. Seattle, 1983 (Abstract 22).
20. Curran JW. Economic consequences of pelvic inflammatory disease in the United States. Am J Obstet Gynecol 1980; 138:848-851.
21. Pulice RT, Lyman DO. Gonococcal pelvic inflammatory disease. Economic impact in New York. Medicaid 1975 1979; 79:1728-1729.
22. St. John RK, Jones OB, Blount JH, Zaidi AA. Pelvic inflammatory disease in the United States. Epidemiology and trends among hospitalized women. Sex Transm Dis 1981; 8:62-66.
23. Hager DW, Wiesner PJ. Selected epidemiological aspects of acute salpingitis. A review. J Reprod Med 1977; 19:47-50.
24. O'Hare PA, Fiumara NJ, McCormack WM. Pelvic inflammatory disease among women presenting to emergency rooms of hospitals in Massachusetts. Am J Obstet Gynecol 1980; 138:909-912.
25. St. John RK, Blount J, Jones O. Pelvic inflammatory disease in the United States. Incidence and trends in private practice. Sex Transm Dis 1981; 8:56-61.
26. Cooper DL, Bernstein GS, Ivler D, Pinal Y, Nakamura R. Gonorrhea screening program in a women's hospital outpatient department: Results and analysis of risk factors. J Am Vener Dis Assoc 1976; 3:71-75.
27. Levine JB, Erikson JM, Dean LM. Social aspects of venereal disease aboard a U.S. Navy destroyer. J Am Vener Dis Assoc 1976; 3:35-39.
28. Londin RS, Wright MW, Scatliff JN. Behavioral and social characteristics of the patient with repeated venereal disease and his effect on statistics on venereal disease. Br J Vener Dis 1977; 53:140-144.
29. Brooks GF, Darrow WW, Day JA. Repeated gonorrhea: an analysis of important risk factors. J Infect Dis 1978; 137:161-169.
30. Morton WE, Horton HB, Baker HW. Effects of socioeconomic status on incidences of three sexually transmitted diseases. Sex Transm Dis 1979; 6:206-210.
31. Darrow WW. Venereal disease in three ethnic groups in Sacramento. Am J Public Health 1976; 66:446-450.
32. Darrow WW. Social stratification, sexual behavior and the sexually transmitted disease. Sex Transm Dis 1979; 6:228-230.
33. Noble RC, Kirk NM, Slagel WA, Vance BJ, Somes GW. Recidivism among patients with gonococcal infection presenting to a venereal disease clinic. Sex Transm Dis 1977; 4:39-43.

34. Ross MW. Social factors in homosexually acquired venereal disease: comparison between Sweden and Australia. Br J Vener Dis 1982; 58:263-268.
35. Judson FN, Miller KG, Schaffnit TR. Screening for gonorrhea and syphilis in the gay baths – Denver, Colorado. Am J Public Health 1977; 67:740-742.
36. Rothenberg RB. Analysis of routine data describing morbidity from gonorrhea. Sex Transm Dis 1979; 6:5-9.
37. Blackwood LG. Repeated infection with *Neisseria gonorrhoeae* in a population of Alaska natives. Sex Transm Dis 1982; 9:89-92.
38. Schoffield CBS. Gonorrhea in women in Scotland: evidence of cohorts having a higher or lower incidence than expected. Br J Vener Dis 1979; 55:274-277.
39. Hayes J, Prokop CK. Sociopsychiatric characteristics of clinic patrons with repeat gonorrhea infections. J Am Vener Dis Assoc 1976; 3:43-48.
40. Szarmach H, Midro H, Wronski A, Zajac W. Psychological analysis of patients with venereal diseases. Przegl Dermatol 1978; 65:667-672.
41. Medhus A, Hansson H. Alcohol problems among female gonorrhea patients. Scand J Soc Med 1976; 4:141-143.
42. Chan SH, Tan T, Kamarudin A, Wee GB, Rajen VS. HLA and sexually transmitted disease in prostitutes. Br J Vener Dis 1979; 55:207-210.
43. Foster MT, Labrum AH. Relation of infection with *Neisseria gonorrhoeae* to ABO blood groups. J Infect Dis 1976; 133:329.
44. Miller JJ, Novotny P, Walker PHD, Harris JRW, MacLennan IPD. *Neisseria gonorrhoeae* and ABO isohaemagglutinins. Infect Immun 1977; 51:713.
45. Kinane DF, Blackwell CC, Winstanley FP, Weir DM. Blood group, secretor status, and susceptibility to infection by *Neisseria gonorrhoeae.* Br J Vener Dis 1983; 57:44-46.
46. Webster B. Teaching of venereal diseases in medical schools throughout the world: preliminary report. Br J Vener Dis 1966; 42:132-133.
47. Stamm WE, Kaetz S, Holmes KK. Clinical training in venereology in the United States and Canada. JAMA 1982; 248:2020-2024.
48. Margolis M. Initiation of the sexually transmitted diseases prevention/training clinic program. Sex Transm Dis 1981; 8:87-88.
49. Arya OP. Epidemiology of gonorrhoea. In: Harris JRW, ed. Recent advances in sexually transmitted diseases (number II). Edinburgh: Churchill Livingstone 1981: 35-48.
50. Kaufman RE, Jones OG, Blount JH, Wiesner PJ. Questionaire survey of reported early congenital syphilis: Problems in diagnosis, prevention, and treatment. Sex Transm Dis 1977; 4:135-139.
51. Fichtner RR, Aral SO, Blount JH, Zaidi AA, Reynolds GH, Darrow WW. Syphilis in the United States: 1967 – 1979. Sex Transm Dis 1983; 10:77-80.
52. Handsfield HH. Sexually transmitted diseases in homosexual men. Am J Public Health 1981; 71:989-990.
53. Corey L, Adams HG, Brown ZA, Holmes KK. Genital herpes simplex virus infections: clinical manifestations, course, and complications. Ann Intern Med 1983; 98:958-972.
54. Kawana TKT, Sakomoto S. Clinical and virological studies on genital herpes. Lancet 1976; 2:964.

55. Berton IG, Kinghorn GR, Najem S, Al-Omar LS, Potter CW. Incidence of herpes simplex virus types 1 and 2 isolated in patients with herpes genitalis in Scheffield. Br J Vener Dis 1982; 58:44-47.
56. Reeves WC, Corey L, Adams HG, Vontver LA, Holmes KK. Risk of recurrence after first episodes of genital herpes. Relation to HSV type and antibody response. N Engl J Med 1981; 305:315-319.
57. Centers for Disease Control. STD fact sheet. 1977; 34:12.
58. Centers for Disease Control. Genital herpes, United States 1966-1979. Morbid Mortal Week Rep 1982; 31:137-139.
59. Chuang TY, Su WPD, Perry HO, Illstrup DM, Kurland LT. Incidence and trend of herpes progenitalis. Mayo Clin Proc 1983; 58:436-441.
60. Knox SR, Corey L, Blough HA, Lerner AM. Historical findings in subjects from a high socioeconomic group who have genital infections with herpes simplex virus. Sex Transm Dis 1982; 9:15-20.
61. Sullivan-Bolyai J, Hull HF, Wison C, Corey L. Neonatal herpex simplex infection in King County, Washington. Increasing incidence and epidemiological correlates. JAMA 1983; 250:3059-3062.
62. Binkin NJ, Alexander ER. Neonatal herpes: how can it be prevented?. JAMA 1983; 250:3094-3095.
63. Thompson SE, Washington AE. Epidemiology of sexually transmitted *Chlamydia trachomatis* infections. Epidemiol Rev 1983; 5:96-123.
64. Frommell GT, Rothenberg R, San-Pin W, McIntosh K. Chlamydial infection of mothers and infants. J Pediatr 1979; 95:28-32.
65. Berger RE, Alexander ER, Harnisch JP, Paulson CA, Monda G, Ansell S, Holmes KK. Etiology, manifestations, and therapy of acute epididymitis: prospective study of 50 cases. J Urol 750-754:1979.
66. Bruce AW, Chadwick P, Willet WS, O'Shaughnessy M. The role of chlamydiae in genitourinary disease. J Urol 1981; 126:625-629.
67. Ford DK. Reiters syndrome: current concepts of etiology and pathogenesis. In: Hobson D, Holmes KK, eds. Nongonococcal urethritis and related infections. Washington, DC: American Society for Microbiology 1977:64-66.
68. Paavonen J. *Chalmydia trachomatis* in acute salpingitis. Am J Obstet Gynecol 1980; 138:957-964.
69. Stamm WE. Etiology and management of the acute urethral syndrome. Sex Transm Dis 1981; 8:235-238.
70. Bowie WR, Alexander ER, Holmes KK. Etiologies of postgonococcal urethritis in homosexual men and heterosexual men. Sex Transm Dis 1978; 5:151-154.
71. Judson FN. Epidemiology and control of nongonococcal urethritis and genital chlamydial infections: a review. Sex Transm Dis 1981; 8:117-126.
72. Holmes KK, Handsfield HH, Wang HH, Wentworth BB, Turck M, Anderson JB, Alexander ER. Etiology of nongonococcal urethritis. N Engl J Med 1975; 292:1199-1205.
73. Schacter J, Dawson CR. Chlamydial infections, a worldwide problem: epidemiology and implications for trachoma therapy. Sex Transm Dis 1981; 8:167-174.

74. Centers for Disease Control. Condyloma acuminata – United States, 1966: 1981. Morbid Mortal Week Rep 1983; 32:306-308.
75. Reid R, Stanhope CR, Herschman BR, Booth E, Phibbs GD, Smith JP. Genital warts and cervical cancer. Cancer 1982; 50:377-387.
76. Nahmias AJ, Naib ZM, Josey WE. Epidemiological studies relating genital herpetic infection to cervical carcinoma. Cancer Res 1974; 34:1111-1117.
77. Centers for disease Control. Chancroid – California. Morbid Mortal Week Rep 1982; 31:173-175.

THREE

Urethritis Syndromes

Vincent A. Spagna
The Ohio State University
College of Medicine
Columbus, Ohio

DEFINITION

Urethritis can be defined as an inflammatory process affecting the urethra caused by a variety of established, suspected or unknown infectious agents and, rarely, noninfectious agents. Objective evidence for a diagnosis of urethritis requires the presence of an exudative process and/or the demonstration of an arbitrary number of inflammatory cells [1,2]. Urethritis falls into one of two subdivisions on the basis of acquisition: sexually transmitted or nonsexually transmitted. The nonsexually transmitted urethritides can be consequences of urological procedures, foreign bodies, anatomical abnormalities, trauma, or chronic irritation secondary to self-abuse [3]. Traditionally, the sexually transmitted urethritis syndromes have been conveniently categorized as gonococcal or nongonococcal and compared and contrasted as distinct entities. It is now known that "mixed" infections can exist in a substantial minority of cases [4], however, the distinction between gonococcal and nongonococcal urethritis is important for purposes of antibiotic treatment, follow-up evaluation, the disposition of sexual contacts, and the collection of valid epidemiological information in assessing their distribution and control in different populations.

While urethritis can affect both sexes, the following discussion will focus on the disease in males. Urethral disorders of females are covered in Chapter 9.

GONOCOCCAL URETHRITIS

Background

Gonococcal urethritis has been alluded to in the earliest writings of recorded history. Hippocrates is credited with the first scientific observations on urethritis, which included dissections of infected urethrae and examinations of the contents. Galen coined the word *gonorrhoea,* which literally means a "flow of semen" [5]. It was not until the eighteenth century that gonorrhea was shown to be a separate clinical entity and not an early manifestation of syphilis. In 1879 Neisser demonstrated the causative agent in smears of clinical material. The organism was cultivated and shown to fulfill Koch's postulates shortly thereafter by other researchers [6].

Etiology

Neisseria gonorrhoeae, the causative bacterium, is an aerobic, nonmotile, non-spore-forming, oxidase-positive, gram-negative coccal (round) organism which often appears as a kidney bean-shaped pair (diplococcus) with adjacent sides flattened [3,6]. They are fastidious organisms with complex nutritional and environmental growth requirements [6]. Electron micrographs of *N. gonorrhoeae* reveal hairlike filaments, known as pili, extending from the cell surface. These pili play an important role in the attachment of the organism to host cells [7]. Man is the only natural host for *N. gonorrhoeae* [6].

Epidemiology

Gonococcal urethritis continues to defy existing control measures, with annual estimates of world incidence approaching 100 million [8]. In the United States a conservative estimate of 1 million cases of gonococcal urethritis represents the annual incidence [9]. A total of 60 to 70% of gonococcal urethritis cases in the United States are seen in the private sector and are not reported [10]. More reliable figures are available from the United Kingdom, where 95% of the general practitioners refer men to a sexually transmitted disease clinic and the cases are therefore reported.

In 1979 there were more than 30,000 cases of gonococcal urethritis reported in England [11]. The emergence of penicillinase-producing *N. gonorrhoeae* (PPNG) has been an added threat to the containment of gonorrhea throughout the world. Cases of PPNG have been reported from 27 countries [8]. The United States has experienced a 900% increase in the number of PPNG cases from 1979 (300) to 1981 (2700) [12]. Spectinomycin-resistant gonococci have been noted worldwide and may become a significant problem in those areas where spectinomycin is used as the drug of first choice in gonorrhea treatment [13].

Gonococcal urethritis is primarily a disease of 15- to 30-year-old sexually promiscuous men [9]. The complex variables which contribute to the epidemic incidence and prevalence of gonorrhea have been analyzed by numerous researchers [8,14-16]. A categorization of these determinants is illustrated in Table 1 under the headings of sociosexual behavior, sexual climate, and characteristics of the gonococcus. Additionally, there exists a heterogeneous population of infected individuals collectively known as the "core group" [17]. This is a dynamic, constantly changing array of prostitutes, military recruits, "inner city" lower-socioeconomic minorities, vagrants, sociopaths, and promiscuous sexual amateurs [15-17]. The members of this group are sexually promiscuous, difficult to trace by

Table 1 Factors Relevant to the Epidemic Nature of Gonorrhea

Sociosexual behavior[a]
Decrease in early-age marriages
Uninhibited homosexual life-styles
Increase in divorce rates and extramarital sex
Casual sexual relationships are routine
Sexual aggressiveness of women as well as men
Sexual relationships begin during early teen years
Multiple sex partners common for men and women
Sexual climate
Sexual themes prominent in books, movies, and sales promotions
Birth control available to anyone
Homosexuals congregated in organized communities
Prosperity encourages permissiveness and prostitution
Singles bars popular for casual meetings
Virginity is an embarassment, not a virtue
Characteristics of the gonococcus
Causes asymptomatic disease in the majority (60%) of women and a substantial minority (10%) of men
Resistance to standard antibiotic regimens by chromosomal change and plasmid acquisition
Fastidious growth requirements makes cultural isolation difficult at times
Does not stimulate protective immunity by host, allowing repeat infections
High contagion rate
Can infect multiple sites
Short incubation period allows rapid turnover of infected individuals

[a]From *Playboy*, October 1982.

epidemiological interviews, and probably include a large percentage of asymptomatically infected individuals [8,18]. Since untreated gonorrhea does not spontaneously resolve for a considerable time period, asymptomatically infected people have the potential to reinfect treated individuals and are themselves reinfected [19,20]. The average infectious period for men has been roughly estimated to be 10 days and, for women 30 days [21]. These high-risk groups have contributed significantly to gonorrhea morbidity and continue to be the primary targets of control efforts by public health authorities [15,16].

The risk of transmission of the gonococcus is very high as demonstrated by the prevalence of gonorrhea among female contacts (36 to 92%) and male contacts (40 to 90%) of infected individuals [9]. Gonorrhea is a sexually acquired disease in the overwhelming majority of cases [3]. Confusion within the medical profession as to the transmission of gonorrhea is a function of society's constant evolution and expansion of modes of sexual expression. The wide range of calculated risk for gonorrhea acquisition denotes multifactorial variables, including frequency of intercourse, frequency of changing partners, infected sites, percentage of partners who are infected, and the practice of precautions (barrier contraception). Discussions of the various nongenital sites of gonococcal infections in newborn, children, and adults are presented in Chapter 8.

Clinical Manifestations

The clinical spectrum of gonococcal urethritis ranges from an acute anterior urethritis to an asymptomatic carrier state [20]. The incubation period is variable, with a generally accepted average of 2 to 5 days with a range of 2 to 3 weeks [3,20]. In those men who develop signs and symptoms after the incubation period, the classic description is the abrupt onset of severe dysuria soon accompanied by the spontaneous appearance of thick, purulent exudate at the urethral meatus [22]. Unfortunately, this presentation accounts for approximately 40% of the cases, and asymptomatic gonococcal urethral carriage has been recognized as an important mode of disease transmission [19,23]. The signs, symptoms, and demographic features of gonococcal urethritis overlap to a considerable extent with those of nongonococcal urethritis. Therefore both history and physical findings may provide clinical clues in the diagnosis of gonococcal urethritis, but should not be a substitute for laboratory testing [3,24]. Untreated gonococcal anterior urethritis will peak out in 2 to 3 weeks, with subsequent gradual resolution of signs and symptoms [20]. After a period of 6 months, 95% of untreated patients with gonococcal urethritis will be symptom free [25]. The local complications of untreated gonococcal urethritis were common in the preantibiotic era and included posterior urethritis, prostatitis, epididymitis, orchitis, seminal vesiculitis, lymphadenitis, and involvement of the periurethral and Tyson's glands [26]. The advent of antibiotics has allowed the prompt treatment of the majority of symptomatic urethritis cases, with a subsequent decrease of complications.

While the actual incidence of asymptomatic cases (neither symptoms nor signs of urethritis) among all men with gonorrhea is only a few percent, they constitute a substantial reservior of gonococcal infection in the community and figure greatly in disease transmission [9,18,19]. An average of 50% of the named infected sexual contacts of women with symptomatic gonorrhea are found to have asymptomatic urethral gonorrhea [18,27]. Efforts to define those variables associated with asymptomatic urethral carriage have uncovered some interesting facts. Those strains of *N. gonorrhoeae* whose nutritional requirements included arginine, hypoxanthine, and uracil ($Arg^-Hyx^-Ura^-$ auxotype) were isolated from more than 90% of asymptomatic men with urethral gonorrhea, but from only 40% of symptomatic controls [28]. Moreover, homosexuals are rarely found to have either asymptomatic urethral infection or Arg^-Hyx^-Ura strains [29]. Inappropriate or partial antibiotic treatment has also been correlated with asymptomatic urethral infection. Gonococci were isolated from 6% of men rendered asymptomatic by incomplete courses of antibiotic therapy [30].

A commonly recognized sequela of treated gonococcal urethritis is postgonococcal urethritis, which actually represents a "mixed" infection (simultaneous gonorrhea and nongonococcal urethritis). Holmes et al. reported postgonococcal urethritis to occur in 65% of penicillin-treated gonorrhea and 27% of tetracycline-treated gonorrhea within 20 days of antibiotic therapy [31].

Diagnosis

The laboratory diagnosis of gonococcal urethritis is made for the most part on presumptive evidence. The Gram stain of a urethral specimen is considered diagnostic for gonorrhea when gram-negative diplococci with typical "kidney bean" morphology are seen within polymorphonuclear leukocytes (PMNs) [3]. Until recently, the ability of the Gram stain to indicate gonococcal urethritis was assumed to be excellent and divorced from pitfalls that would appreciably affect sensitivity or specificity [32]. However, researchers who critically evaluated the performance of the Gram stain in a clinic for sexually transmitted diseases concluded that stained smears of urethral specimens were equivocal in as many as 15% of cases [22]. The frequency of smears containing typical gram-negative diplococci that are only outside of PMNs was recognized in 10.4% of male patients with urethritis; gonococci were isolated in only 29% of these cases [33]. In other studies the demonstration of extracellular-only gram-negative diplococci varied from 2 to 16% and was correlated with culture-proven gonococcal urethritis in 14 to 50% of cases [22,34,35]. The predictive accuracy of the Gram stain in the diagnosis of gonococcal urethritis has also been shown to be markedly influenced by the expertise of the microscopist interpreting urethral smears and the prevalence of gonorrhea in the population being evaluated for urethritis [33, 36]. Maximal sensitivity (96%) and specificity (95%) of urethral smear interpretation was accomplished only by those technicians who had interpreted more than 200 slides per week for several years [33]. Recent micturition has been shown to make the accurate interpretation of a meatal Gram-stained smear more difficult, with a 10% decrease in sensitivity [37]. The Gram stain also has limited usefulness in the diagnosis of asymptomatic (no signs or symptoms) gonorrhea, with a sensitivity that is less than 70% [19].

With the limitations of the Gram stain apparent, a variety of tests which provide rapid and accurate results have been investigated as potential diagnostic aids in the evaluation of urethritis. Most techniques involve the processing of urethral exudate; however, the potential of serodiagnosis for gonococcal urethritis (detecting antibodies specific for gonococcal antigens) has been applied principally to asymptomatic male patients seen at clinics for sexually transmitted diseases. The results have been disappointing, with the low discriminatory power of serodiagnosis related to persistence of antibody due to previous gonococcal disease and colonization by *Neisseria meningitidis* in the study population [38].

The indirect immunofluorescence technique and the modified hemagglutination test have been utilized in an attempt to detect locally produced antibody in urethral secretions from men with gonorrhea. Secretory IgA was found in 29 of 35 infected men; however, the procedures involved were time-consuming and required highly trained personnel [39]. The same limitations applied to the use of direct immunofluorescence techniques in the identification of gonococci directly in urethral specimens [40]. Gonococcal antigens have been detected in urine by radioimmunoassay with radioactively labeled antibody; however, the procedure required sophisticated technology and identified only 31 (74%) of 42 samples from men with gonorrhea [41].

Recently a solid-phase enzyme immunoassay, the Gonozyme test, has been developed for detecting gonococcal antigens in urethral and endocervical specimens. There was excellent correlation between microscopy and assay results in the 50 urethritis cases that were evaluated [42]. However, the numerous procedural steps, the time period (1 hr), the multiple reagents and the apparent need of a spectrophotometer limit its practical utilization by either private physicians or laboratory personnel.

A method to detect gonococcal DNA (genetic transformation test) has been investigated and appears to be comparable to culture in accuracy [43]. The major disadvantages of this approach include the necessary shipment of specimens to special laboratories and delayed results which may not be available for as long as a week.

Rapid diagnostic methodologies which are not dependent upon the presence of specific gonococcal antigens have also been investigated. The Gonodecten test kit involves the direct testing of urethral exudate with a swab impregnated with N,N,N',N'-tetramethyl-p-phenylenediamine dihydrochloride. This chemical will turn purple within 3 min in the presence of oxidase-positive organisms, which includes *N. gonorrhoeae* [44]. The test would be expected to perform well if oxidase-positive organisms other than *N. gonorrhoeae* were uncommonly associated with urethritis. Unfortunately, the manufacturer quotes a specificity of only 74%, and our experience with the test has revealed a high percentage (40%) of "false positive" reactions. The recent isolation of an oxidase-positive organism in significant quantity from 50% of patients with nongonococcal urethritis may offer a partial explanation for the lack of specificity with the Gonodecten test [45].

The *Limulus* amebocyte lysate assay has been employed in detecting endotoxin in urethral exudate to distinguish gonococcal from nongonococcal urethritis [46]. The gonococci are abundant producers of endotoxin, a cell wall component unique to gram-negative bacteria, while the etiological agents of nongonococcal urethritis produce limited quantities of endotoxin [6,47]. The active component of the *Limulus* amebocyte lysate assay forms a gel in the presence of endotoxin, and the assay has been shown to be rapid (30 min), simple (gel versus no gel), sensitive (98%), and specific (96%) when applied to properly diluted urethral specimens [48]. A self-contained diagnostic kit, Gonoscreen, is commercially available and adapted for use by the private physician as an office test [49]. The only drawback to this test is its inability to detect gonorrhea unless an adequate (0.015 to 0.025 ml) urethral sample is obtained.

The absolute diagnostic modality is the cultural recovery of *N. gonorrhoeae*. Cultural isolation generally requires a selective medium (Thayer-Martin, New York City) which consists of a buffered peptone-starch agar base to which is added blood or hemoglobin and a defined supplement. Selectivity for the gonococcus is accomplished by the addition of antibiotics. For maximal sensitivity, cultures are incubated for 24 to 48 hr in an atmosphere of defined temperature (35°C), humidity, and CO_2 content [50]. Specimen transport systems include a nonnutrient holding medium (Amies) [51] and a selective growth transport medium (Transgow, JEMBEC) [51,52]. Delay in setting up or incubating cultures is associated with failure to recover *N. gonorrhoeae*, especially if more than 24 hr have elapsed in specimen transport [53]. Following incubation, suspicious colonies are Gram-stained and examined microscopically and by the oxidase test [50]. Definitive identification traditionally involved time-consuming fermentation reactions; however, a coagglutination test utilizing antigonococcal antibodies makes it possible to identify suspicious organisms as *N. gonorrhoeae* with a high degree of certainty within minutes [54]. The increasing number of PPNG cases has justified the routine screening of gonococcal isolates for penicillinase production by various methods, including the rapid and economical chromogenic cephalosporin technique [55]. While specimens for culture are usually obtained directly from the urethra, urine samples have been shown to be comparable to urethral samples for the cultural diagnosis of gonorrhea in men [56,57]. While reducing the time that personnel spend in specimen collection and alleviating patient discomfort produced by inserting swabs into the urethra, urine specimens require patient cooperation, separate facilities to obtain specimens, and laboratory processing within a few hours to obtain favorable culture results.

Gonorrhea Treatment

The guidelines for treatment of gonococcal urethritis have been recently updated by the Centers for Disease Control [58]. Those gonococcal strains which are susceptible to penicillin are successfully eradicated by single-dose therapy with either ampicillin, amoxicillin, or aqueous procaine penicillin. Tetracycline hydrochloride or doxycycline hyclate are effective multiple-day regimens. Single-dose therapy has the obvious advantage of ensuring low-cost curative treatment of gonococcal urethritis immediately. The major disadvantage of this approach is its ineffectiveness against *Chlamydia trachomatis* and other possible agents of nongonococcal urethritis [59]. Multiple-day therapy with tetracycline or doxycycline is effective against *C. trachomatis* and most strains of *Ureaplasma urealyticum* [60]. However, success with multiple-day regimens requires patient compliance, without which the emergence of tetracycline-resistant gonococcal strains or asymptomatic gonococcal carriers may be encouraged. A recent study in a public health clinic compared treatment results with 5-day courses of tetracycline and doxycycline. Of those patients who returned for test-of-cure examinations, the compliance rate for tetracycline was 62.2% and that for doxycycline was 78.5% [61]. This suggests that a substantial supply of antibiotics would be available for unprescribed usage by individuals at high risk for sexually transmitted diseases. Moreover, men treated for gonorrhea with tetracycline have been shown to have a significantly lower return rate for test-of-cure cultures than did those treated with penicillin or ampicillin [62].

Since *C. trachomatis* has been recovered from 4 to 32% of men who had gonococcal urethritis and the problem of patient compliance with multiple-day therapy exists, the CDC has proposed a combined regimen which consists of single-dose ampicillin or amoxicillin plus a 7-day treatment course with tetracycline or doxycycline [58,63]. When compared to tetracycline, doxycycline has the advantages of twice-a-day dosage, reliable absorption despite simultaneous food intake, and milder gastrointestinal side effects [61]. However, the wholesale cost of a 7-day course of doxycycline therapy is $12.94, compared to $1.09 for generic tetracycline [59]. This cost factor differential severely limits the practical administration of doxycycline in publicly funded control programs, which operate on frugal budgets despite increased demands for their services.

Patients with documented PPNG urethritis or who have acquired their infection in areas of high PPNG prevalence should be treated with spectinomycin [58, 64,65]. In the event that spectinomycin therapy is ineffective, treatment with cefoxitin is recommended [66-68]. Additionally, PPNG urethritis has been successfully treated with other antibiotics, including cefotaxime [69], and aminoglycosides [70].

Follow-up cultures should be obtained 4 to 7 days after completion of treatment [58].

The development of an effective gonococcal vaccine has been unsuccessful and may ultimately involve the induction of immunity to various virulence factors such as pili, outer membrane proteins, capsular polysaccharide, and lipopolysaccharides [71].

NONGONOCOCCAL URETHRITIS

Background

The inclusion of nongonococcal urethritis (NGU) to sexually transmitted diseases has been a recent event. As recently as 1970, a monograph on venereal disease sponsored by the American Public Health Association failed to discuss NGU, and it is still not a reportable disease under federal law. Nongonococcal urethritis represents a perplexing challenge to research venereologists, who continually attempt to define its etiological agents, diagnostic criteria, epidemiological trends, and treatment approaches. Despite NGU's prominent position as the most common of sexually transmitted diseases, there are few estabilished facts relating to this disease process.

Etiological Agents

The potential etiological agents in NGU have been the focus of intense bacteriological, virological, and serological studies. While various organisms have been associated with NGU, supporting evidence is lacking for the majority of these hypotheses. The microbiological studies of NGU are complicated by our limited understanding of the complex flora of the normal urethra. The myriad of different species of aerobes and anaerobes isolated from urethritis cases and normal controls has made the distinction between commensals and pathogens an incredibly difficult task [72].

Chlamydia trachomatis is an obligate, intracellular, prokaryotic parasite of eukaryotic cells which has been unequivocally established as an etiological agent in NGU [4,73]. The organism has bacterial properties, including replication by binary fission, possession of both deoxyribonucleic and ribonucleic acids, a discrete cell wall biochemically similar to that of gram-negative bacteria, protein synthesis via ribosomes, and susceptibility to certain antibiotics. There exist only primitive enzyme systems, allowing for limited metabolic activities, and cultural recovery requires living cellular media [74]. A complex life cycle includes two distinct forms: an elementary body and a reticulate body. These forms are especially adapted for extracellular survival, and transfer from cell to cell, and for intracellular growth. The smaller, infective elementary body enters a susceptible cell by phagocytosis, where it reorganizes to form a larger, noninfective, metabolically active reticulate body. The reticulate body divides several times over a period of 24 to 48 hr to reform the elementary bodies which are released by cell lysis [75]. The association of *C. trachomatis* with NGU was initially recognized by Dunlop et al. in 1965 [76]. The accumulated serological, clinical, and microbiological evidence from various sources has concluded that the D to K serotypes of *C. trachomatis* are urethral pathogens [77-79]. The summary data of more than 30 separate studies demonstrated that the organism was present in 36.5% (1625 of 4451) cases of NGU, as compared to its presence in only 2.8% (34 of 1210 cases) of "controls" without urethritis [73]. A well-controlled study tested the hypothesis that *C. trachomatis* may exist as a nonpathogenic, sexually transmitted urethral commensal and concluded that the organism was pathogenic and not part of the normal urethral flora of sexually active men [80]. Further proof of the etiological role of *C. trachomatis* in NGU is indirectly provided by its proven association with other sexually transmitted disease syndromes [79,81].

Mycoplasmas are the smallest free-living microorganisms. They share all the physical and metabolic properties of bacteria, with the exception of a cell wall. The lack of a rigid cell wall allows the organisms to assume various morphological configurations (pleomorphism) and makes them susceptible to osmotic conditions in their environment. *Ureaplasma urealyticum* is a mycoplasma which colonizes the genitourinary tract and has the unique ability to metabolize urea [82]. While other mycoplasmas have also been isolated from the genitourinary tract, *U. urealyticum* has been the principal topic of a long-term debate concerning a potential etiological role in NGU. Some of the difficulties encountered in the research of ureaplasmas and NGU include (1) the high prevalence and persistence of the organisms in both sexes as a function of the number of different sexual partners, independent of the presence or absence of disease; (2) the ill-defined variables affecting the type, collection, and handling of specimens; (3) the fastidious cultural requirements; and (4) the lack of sensitive serological tests that indicate infection [83]. Evidence which favors an etiological role for ureaplasmas in NGU involves a number of independent studies where ureaplasmas were isolated significantly more frequently from the genitourinary tract of men with NGU than from control subjects without NGU [83,84]. One study demonstrated both qualitatively and quantitatively the association of ureaplasmas with first-episode chlamydia-negative NGU compared to chlamydia-positive cases or from men without urethritis [77]. Further support for the pathogenicity of ureaplasmas has come from treatment studies with antibiotics which differentiate between chlamydial and ureaplasmal NGU [85,86] and disease production following intraurethral inoculation of the organism into volunteers [87]. Evidence against a pathogenic role for ureaplasmas includes investigations demonstrating similar ureaplasmal isolation rates in both NGU and control groups [88]. One study over a 4-month period involved weekly ureaplasmal cultures of healthy, monogamous, married men with no evidence of urethritis and demonstrated that ureaplasmas were part of the permanent urethral flora in 30% of these volunteers [89]. The accumulated evidence suggests that certain, but not all, strains of *U. urealyticum* can cause NGU [83]. However, it would be impractical and unrewarding to routinely include ureaplasmal cultures in the evaluation of NGU in light of the limited value of this information in decision analysis and patient management.

Trichomonas vaginalis has been a postulated cause of NGU; however, the majority of reports are of limited value because the investigations were performed prior to the availability of chlamydial cultures [90]. More recent studies have attributed no significant role to *T. vaginalis* in NGU [78,91,92]. The majority of men harboring *T. vaginalis* are asymptomatic and shed relatively few trichomonads [93]. One study documented that 59% of men in whom *T. vaginalis* was demonstrated spontaneously eradicated the organism in less than 2 weeks; persistent urethral carriage of *T. vaginalis* was associated with urethroscopy-proven strictures in half of the cases [94]. Another study correlated persistent, recurrent urethritis and prostatitis with *T. vaginalis* isolation [95]. The accumulated data suggest that *T. vaginalis* may be an etiological agent of NGU when anatomical abnormalities or chronic inflammatory conditions compromise the genitourinary tract.

Staphylococcus saprophyticus is a documented etiological agent of the urethral syndrome and cystourethritis in sexually active women. Preliminary evidence suggests a possible role for *S. saprophyticus* in NGU; however, further investigation is necessary before any conclusions about its pathogenic potential can be drawn [96].

Gardnerella vaginalis has been associated with vaginal syndromes, is prevalent (15%) among sexually active men, and has been mentioned as a possible cause of NGU [97,98]. Recent evidence has discounted any role for *G. vaginalis* in NGU and has shown the organism to constitute part of the normal flora of healthy, sexually active males [77,97].

Virological investigations have shown that viruses such as *Herpesvirus hominis* and cytomegalovirus are seldom isolated from NGU patients, which suggests that these organisms are rarely, if ever, etiological agents in that syndrome [1,60,78]. Scattered reports in the scientific literature have implicated various microorganisms as causes of NGU; for the most part, supportive evidence by subsequent research is lacking and their potential roles as agents of NGU must be considered unproven. This applies, as well, to an unclassified gram-negative anaerobic bacillus which was isolated from 50% of men with NGU in contrast to isolation rates of 14 and 13% from men with gonorrhea and no disease, respectively [45].

Epidemiology

Nongonococcal urethritis has been identified as the most common sexually transmitted disease in several European countries and accounts for more than half of the cases of urethritis seen in sexually active men attending venereal disease clinics in the United States [4,99]. The epidemiology of NGU is a matter of speculation and defies precise definition because of (1) the lack of definite diagnostic criteria, (2) ignorance about disease incidence and prevalence secondary to the worldwide absence of systematic recording, and (3) the paucity of information about risk factors and contact tracing [99]. Nongonococcal urethritis has been a reportable disease since 1951 in Great Britain, and there has been a 10-fold increase in the incidence of NGU, with greater than 100,000 cases reported annually. Since 1965 the number of NGU cases has exceeded the number of gonococcal urethritis cases by a ratio of nearly 2 to 1 in Great Britain [100]. Statistics relating to NGU in the United States are only rough estimates. In 1951 the New York City Health Department reported only 149 cases of NGU; by 1978 the number of cases increased to 14,886, and this represented 42% of urethritis diagnoses [4]. In 1974 NGU was responsible for an estimated 450,000 office visits, while the Centers for Disease Control estimate that 2.5 million cases of NGU occurred in 1977 compared to 1 million cases of gonococcal urethritis [99]. Nongonococcal urethritis probably comprises 50 to 70% of all acute urethritis in the United States [24]. One study reviewed the incidence of gonorrhea and NGU in men seen over a 6-year period (1975 to 1980) in a venereal disease clinic and showed that NGU cases exceeded gonorrhea cases by a stable ratio of 5 to 4 [101]. While there is little doubt that NGU is the most common sexually transmitted disease of men in the United States, the accumulated epidemiological evidence has been derived from biasedly selected populations with various diagnostic criteria for NGU. Extrapolation of this information to the general population is impossible without introducing wide margins of error.

Despite the confusion surrounding NGU, certain patterns have emerged which are probably applicable on a universal scale. For example, NGU patients are similar to gonorrhea patients with respect to age, marital status, and the number of different sexual contacts; however, as opposed to gonorrhea patients, individuals with NGU are more likely to be white, educated, and have an established relationship with a private physician [24]. Homosexual men experience NGU significantly less frequently than gonorrhea [101]. Unfortunately, no epidemiological or clinical characteristics can be relied upon as absolute criteria in differentiating NGU from gonococcal urethritis [23,101].

Clinical Manifestations

Clinical characteristics differentiating gonococcal urethritis from NGU have been formulated. Simultaneous discharge and dysuria, a spontaneous purulent discharge, and an abrupt, severe onset suggest gonorrhea. Nongonococcal urethritis patients may note dysuria alone (15%) or discharge alone (47%). The discharge associated with NGU is white, mucoid, and scant. The observation of a discharge only in the morning prior to voiding is reported by 29% of NGU patients [102]. Root et al. [60] noted prostatic enlargement and tenderness in 23% of NGU cases, but questioned the significance of these findings because of the difficulties of diagnosing prostatitis in an objective fashion. While it is apparent that the classic signs and symptoms of gonococcal urethritis differ from those of NGU, there is sufficient clinical overlap so that accurate differential diagnosis can be achieved only by utilizing laboratory tests. Rothenberg and Judson reported that the optimal performance of clinical diagnosis based on the quantity and quality of urethral discharge was 73% (range, 39 to 84%) [23]. Table 2 illustrates the relationship of discharge characteristics to diagnosis from 967 urethritis cases.

An accepted generalization is that the incubation period for NGU is longer than that for gonococcal urethritis, usually 1 to 4 weeks [4]. Schofield reviewed the records of 264 NGU patients and reported a mean incubation period of 7.7 days. This compared to a mean incubation period of 6.2 days for 242 gonococcal urethritis cases [103]. Oriel et al. [104] reported that chlamydial NGU had a longer incubation time than nonchlamydial NGU, and Terho [105] noted a positive correlation between the severity of urethral discharge and chlamydial NGU. However, Ghadirian and Robson found that neither history nor clinical examination was useful in distinguishing chlamydia-positive from chlamydia-negative NGU [106].

The natural history of untreated NGU has not been extensively researched owing to the appearance of complications, especially epididymitis [107]. Untreated NGU has been shown to regress in 1 to 3 months in 50 to 70% of men [108]. Schachter has suggested that untreated chlamydial urethritis will gradually remit with the abatement of symptoms; however, chlamydial infection will persist for months or years in asymptomatic carriers [79]. Swartz and Kraus defined a significant group of asymptomatic NGU patients in a venereal disease clinic population [109]. The isolation of *C. trachomatis* from 24% of these patients substantiated the clinical significance of asymptomatic NGU [1,109].

Laboratory Diagnosis

Nongonococcal urethritis is essentially a diagnosis of exclusion. While there is little disagreement that a diagnosis of NGU be applied to men with a urethral discharge who have negative urethral cultures for *N. gonorrhoeae*, there has been a

Table 2 Clinical Breakdown of Urethral Exudates from 967 Men with Culture-Positive Gonococcal and Nongonococcal Urethritis

		Percent urethral discharge				
Diagnosis	Number evaluated	Profuse[a]	Moderate[b]	Scant[c]	Purulent	Non-purulent
Gonococcal urethritis	603	39	40	21	67	33
Nongonococcal urethritis	364	12	44	44	23	77

[a]Spontaneous discharge visible without penile massage.
[b]Discharge not obvious, but visible upon compression of the glans.
[c]Discharge obtained only after urethral massage.
Source: V.A. Spagna, unpublished data.

chronic debate regarding those criteria that satisfy the diagnosis of NGU for symptomatic individuals without a discernable urethral discharge [2]. Until recently, the observation of 10 polymorphonuclear leukocytes per high-power field (PMN/hpf) on the urethral smear or 20 PMN per high dry field in the urinary sediment was considered indicative of inflammation of the urethra [31,110]. However, clinicians recognized that a significant minority of symptomatic patients did not satisfy these criteria and that their clinical status was in need of definition. One study concluded that the microscopic observation of more than 4 PMN/hpf was objective evidence of NGU, regardless of the presence or absence of a urethral discharge in symptomatic men. Moreover, the number per high-power field was unaffected by the interval since last urination or the time since last intercourse [1]. The same investigators concluded that asymptomatic, sexually active men with urethral smears having at least 4 PMN/hpf at the initial visit and again 1 week later or conversion to at least 4 PMN/hpf were at high risk (approximately 50%) of harboring *C. trachomatis*; however, the semiquantitation of less than 4 PMN/hpf on both evaluations essentially ruled out the possibility of *C. trachomatis* carriage [109]. A comparative study of the sensitivity of the Gram-stained urethral smear and first-voided urine sediment in the diagnosis of NGU concluded that the observation of at least 10 PMN in five fields at 400X magnification in urine sediment was superior to the presence of at least 4 PMN/hpf in urethral exudate [111]. The apparent uselessness of the semiquantitation of PMN per high-power field on the urethral smear was further suggested by a recent investigation where *C. trachomatis* was isolated in 16% of patients with less than 5 PMN/hpf; however, there was no mention of the presence or absence of urethral discharge in this subset of patients [60]. This debate has been further complicated by the effects of intraobserver and interobserver variations on PMN per high-power field reporting and variations in microscopic visual field sizes [112,113]. Experienced microscopists reading the same urethral smears on different occasions reported results which changed the diagnosis of NGU in 14 to 21% of cases [112]. The need for additional research on the criteria for a diagnosis of NGU is mandatory before a unified scientific approach to this disease can be assured.

Treatment

While treatment regimens for gonococcal urethritis are well established and universally accepted, the same does not apply to NGU therapy. Optimal treatment for NGU remains an enigma for several reasons, including (1) the absence of universal criteria for NGU diagnosis and cure, (2) the inability to identify specific etiological agents in 50% of NGU cases, (3) the spontaneous resolution of NGU over time, and (4) the difficulty of assuring patient compliance with multiple-dose regimens and maintaining sexual abstinence during clinical trials [108,114].

The standard antibiotic regimens employed in NGU treatment are 7-day courses of tetracycline hydrochloride (United States) or oxytetracycline (Great Britain) [59]. While the majority of NGU cases are successfully treated with either medication, a significant initial failure rate (⩾10%) and recurrence rate (30% within 6 weeks after therapy) have promoted numerous studies investigating the optimal dosage and duration of therapy with the tetracyclines as well as other antimicrobial agents [31]. NGU recurrence following tetracycline therapy is particularly common in cases not caused by *C. trachomatis* which include the vast majority of homosexual and bisexual men [91,115]. Holmes et al. established the standard dosage of tetracycline hydrochloride (500 mg every 6 hr) and duration of therapy (7 days) in a closely controlled study of 94 NGU patients confined on an aircraft carrier at sea [31]. Bowie et al. noted similar success rates with the above regimen and one employing only half the dosage of tetracycline [116]. A 14-day course of either tetracycline hydrochloride or doxycycline (a long-acting tetracycline) successfully eradicated symptoms and pathogens in 92% of NGU cases; however, no long-term follow-up of these cases was done [60]. Similarly, McNeil et al. utilized a 10-day course of doxycycline (100 mg twice daily) and noted a favorable short-term clinical outcome in 92% of NGU cases whose pretreatment specimens contained *C. trachomatis*, *U. urealyticum*, or both, and in 85% of NGU cases whose pretreatment specimens contained neither organism. Long-term follow-up revealed a microbiological or clinical recurrence in approximately 25% of evaluable cases. Mild dizziness and nausea were the most common adverse reactions during therapy, occurring in 10% of cases [117]. Bowie et al. compared two dosages (100 mg once or twice daily) and two durations (7 or 21 days) of minocycline (a long-acting tetracycline) in a double-blind randomized study of 289 NGU patients. Short-term follow-up (14 to 28 days) demonstrated persistent or recurrent NGU in 31 (27%) of 114 men given 7-day therapy and in only 9 (8%) of 110 men given 21-day therapy. However, long-term follow-up (35 to 63 days) revealed a cumulative percent rate of failure of 30% with all regimens. The most frequent adverse effect (14%) of minocycline therapy was dizziness [91]. Other researchers have reported conflicting results with longer treatment courses and various dosages of the tetracyclines [118,119]. A critical review of the literature regarding tetracycline therapy for NGU noted a general disarray of information weakened by serious flaws in scientific design, including the lack of placebo-treated controls, a high defaulter rate with follow-up evaluations, and the inability to distinguish treatment failure from reinfection [114].

Erythromycin stearate has been utilized in similar dosage regimens as the tetracyclines, with no appreciable differences in clinical results; moreover, the recent recognition of tetracycline-resistant ureaplasmal isolates may have a positive influence on the role of erythromycin in NGU therapy [59,60,120,121]. While erythromycin has the advantage of being effective when taken with dairy products and antacids as opposed to tetracycline hydrochloride, gastrointestinal intolerance complicates therapy in a significant number of cases. Erythromycin treatment is also eightfold more expensive than tetracycline hydrochloride and would result in an unacceptable failure rate if concomitant gonorrhea were present [59,122]. Rosaramicin, related to erythromycin, has been shown to be as effective as tetracycline hydrochloride in the treatment of both chlamydial and nonchlamydial NGU [123]. The advantage over erythromycin has been demonstrated in clinical studies reporting successful results in gonorrhea treatment with rosaramicin [124]. However, Darne et al. reported a considerable incidence (33%) of gastrointestinal side effects associated with its use in NGU therapy [125]. Although other antimicrobial agents have been employed in NGU treatment studies, their relative ineffectiveness against *C. trachomatis*-negative NGU warrants against their routine utilization [59].

While NGU therapy has been a long-debated topic, the proper disposition of sexual partners of men with NGU has also been a controversial issue. Evans found that the treatment of NGU contacts did not relate significantly to the patients who relapsed or to those who did not relapse [126]. In contrast, Arya et al. noted a significant association between the retreatment rate of NGU patients and the resumption of sexual intercourse. Treatment of sexual contacts before resumption of sexual intercourse significantly reduced the retreatment rate, while other variables, including age, race, duration of symptoms, previous infection, and indulgence in alcohol, did not appear to influence results [127]. The strongest argument supporting the epidemiological treatment of female sexual partners is the observation that *C. trachomatis* has been cultured from cervical specimens obtained from 30 to 43% of the female partners of men with NGU [108,127, 128]. Empirical treatment of male sexual partners of homosexual NGU patients seems reasonable, but is of unproven value. Sexual contacts should receive the same antimicrobial regimens used to treat NGU patients [59].

Rational criteria should be met in the decision of NGU treatment. Minimal cost, minimal adverse reactions, maximal compliance, and adequate coverage for chlamydial, ureaplasmal, and gonococcal disease are noteworthy considerations in prescribing antimicrobial therapy for NGU patients and their sexual partners. Refractory or recurrent NGU cases should be evaluated for unusual causes, such as *T. vaginalis*, and anatomical abnormalities of the genitourinary tract if reinfection can be excluded.

Sequelae

A well-recognized complication of NGU is epididymo-orchitis. Circumstantial evidence linking NGU with epididymitis includes serological data and cultural studies of urethral material [129,130]. Berger et al. isolated *C. trachomatis* from the epididymal aspirate of five of six young men with acute epididymitis and firmly established its major causal role in this syndrome in men under 35 years of age [81]. The same investigators failed to isolate *U. urealyticum* from the epididymal aspirate of five epididymitis cases with positive cultures for *U. urealyticum* from the urine or urethra [131]. While the actual frequency of this condition is unknown, estimates from venereal disease clinics in England and the United States suggest that this occurs in less than 1% of untreated NGU cases [132]. The common clinical presentation is one of unilateral pain, tenderness, and swelling of the epididymis with edema and erythema of the overlying scrotal skin. While epididymitis associated with *N. gonorrhoeae* has dysuria and urethral discharge as part of the clinical picture, 35% of chlamydia-associated epididymitis has no evident urethral discharge [131]. Symptomatic acute prostatitis and urethral stricture are rarely consequences of NGU. There has been no evidence to substantiate a relationship between chronic prostatitis and NGU [133].

Recent investigations have demonstrated that *U. urealyticum* colonization of the genital tract is correlated with unexplained infertility or infertility due to a male factor [134,135]. While the possible role of *U. urealyticum* in involuntary infertility remains controversial, semen samples from infertile men containing ureaplasmas have lower spermatozoal counts, greater morphological abnormalities, and lower-level motility as compared to infertile men who do not harbor ureaplasmas [84,136,137]. One study found that the eradication of ureaplasmas by specific antibiotic therapy markedly improved spermatozoal motility, a parameter considered most important in the assessment of semen quality [137]. A subsequent study demonstrated that among 129 couples in which the men were treated successfully for ureaplasmas, the 3-year rate of successful pregnancy was 60%, in contrast to the 5% pregnancy rate among the 32 couples in which the men remained positive for ureaplasmas after treatment [138].

Reiter's syndrome is defined as the triad of arthritis, conjunctivitis, and urethritis occurring simultaneously or sequentially [139]. Reiter's syndrome has been considered a consequence of NGU, and evidence linking *C. trachomatis* infection as a triggering agent of the syndrome has been documented by independent researchers [140,141]. However, the disorder can occur following bacillary dysentery and resembles other seronegative arthropathies which have no association with NGU. The pathophysiology of Reiter's syndrome is still a matter of speculation, but the hypothesis of an idiosyncratic host response to one or more common infectious agents seems to be the prevailing opinion [139]. The strong association (80 to 90%) of Reiter's syndrome and the HLA-B27 gene, a marker common to other rheumatic diseases, supports the concept of a hereditary transmission of the predisposition to develop the manifestations of the disease [142, 143]. Reiter's syndrome has been shown to complicate as many as 2% of NGU cases, and the complication rate is directly related to the frequency of the HLA-B27 gene in the study population [139,140]. The clinical manifestations may be subtle, transient, and overlooked by the patient or the examiner. The complete spectrum of signs and symptoms associated with Reiter's syndrome involves multiple organ systems and shows considerable case-to-case variability [144, 145]. The clinical course is typically one of random relapses and remissions, with the number of manifestations and sites of involvement varying with each relapse, and attack duration varying from weeks to months [146]. Besides the classic triad, additional features of Reiter's syndrome include mucocutaneous lesions (keratodermia blennorrhagia, painless oral ulcers, circinate balanitis, and nail changes), ankylosing spondylitis, "sausage" digits secondary to dactylitis, Achilles tendonitis, and plantar fasciitis [144, 147]. Rare complications include cardiovascular and neurological syndromes [148, 149]. The recent recognition of an "incomplete" Reiter's syndrome characterized by the typical articular pattern and other discriminating clinical features with the absence of urethritis and conjunctivitis attests to the complex continuum of this disease process [150]. There are no specific laboratory findings which are diagnostic for Reiter's disease [139]. Therapy is directed to suppress inflammatory lesions and maintain joint function. Phenylbutazone, indomethacin, and tolmetin have been used successfully, while salicylates and corticosteroids afford little benefit. Tetracycline is often prescribed to treat the urethritis and as prophylaxis against arthritis, but its efficacy remains unproven [145]. Patients followed over a 5-year period revealed that more than 25% were forced to either change jobs or stop working because of significant chronic disability, particularly of an arthritic nature [146].

REFERENCES

1. Swartz SL, Kraus SJ, Herrmann KL, Stargel MD, Brown WJ, Allen SD. Diagnosis and etiology of nongonococcal urethritis. J Infect Dis 1978; 138:445-54.
2. Kraus SJ. Semiquantitation of urethral polymorphonuclear leukocytes as objective evidence of nongonococcal urethritis. Sex Transm Dis 1982; 9:52-5.
3. Handsfield HH. Gonorrhea and nongonococcal urethritis – recent advances. Med Clin North Am 1978; 62:925-43.
4. Felman YM, Nikitas JA. Nongonococcal urethritis – a clinical review. JAMA 1981; 245:381-6.
5. Morton RS. Gonorrhoea. London: WB Saunders, 1977:1-23.
6. Morse SA. Neisseria. In: Braude AI, ed. Medical microbiology and infectious diseases. Vol 2. Philadelphia: WB Saunders, 1981:326-34.
7. Piarce WA, Buchanan TM. Attachment role of gonococcal pili – optimum conditions and quantitation of adherence of isolated pili to human cells in vitro. J Clin Invest 1978; 61:931-43.
8. Arya OP. Epidemiology of gonorrhoea. In: Harris JRW, ed. Recent advances in sexually transmitted diseases. Vol 2. London: Churchill Livingstone, 1981: 35-48.
9. Rein MF. Epidemiology of gonococcal infections. In: Roberts RB, ed. The gonococcus. New York: Wiley, 1977:1-31.

10. Fleming WL, Brown WI, Donahue JF, Branigan PW. National survey of venereal disease treated by physicians in 1968. JAMA 1970; 211:1827-30.
11. Annual report of the chief medical officer of the department of health and social security. Br J Vener Dis 1981; 57:402-5.
12. Mansfield HH, Sandstrom EG, Knapp JS, Perine PL, Whittington WL, Sayers DE, Holmes KK. Epidemiology of penicillinase-producing *Neisseria gonorrhoeae* infections. N Engl J Med 1982; 306:950-4.
13. Spectinomycin-resistant beta-lactamase-producing *Neisseria gonorrhoeae* – England. Morbid Mortal Week Rep 1982; 31:495-501.
14. Brooks GF, Darrow WW, Day JA. Repeated gonorrhea: analysis of importance and risk factors. J Infect Dis 1978; 137:161-9.
15. Conrad GL, Kleris GS, Rush B, Darrow WW. Sexually transmitted diseases among prostitutes and other sexual offenders. Sex Transm Dis 1981; 8:241-4.
16. Kinghorn GR, Pryce D, Morton RS. Repeated gonorrhea in Sheffield: the size of the problem, epidemiologic significance, and personal characteristics of repeaters. Sex Transm Dis 1982; 9:165-9.
17. Yorke JA, Hethcote HW, Nold A. Dynamics and control of the transmission of gonorrhea. Sex Transm Dis 1978; 5:51-6.
18. Thompson SE. The clinical manifestations of gonococcal infections. In: Harris JRW, ed. Recent advances in sexually transmitted diseases. Vol 2. London: Churchill Livingstone, 1981:49-57.
19. Handsfield HH, Lipman TO, Harnisch JP, Tronca E, Holmes KK. Asymptomatic gonorrhea in men – diagnosis, natural course, prevalence and significance. N Engl J Med 1974; 290:117-23.
20. McCutchan JA. Gonorrhea and nongonococcal urethritis. In: Braude AI, ed. Medical microbiology and infectious diseases. Vol 2. Philadelphia: WB Saunders, 1981:1201-10.
21. Barlow D. Gonorrhoea. In: Sexually transmitted diseases – the facts. Oxford University Press, 1979:30-41.
22. Jacobs NF, Kraus SJ. Gonococcal and nongonococcal urethritis in men – clinical and laboratory differentiation. Ann Intern Med 1975; 82:7-12.
23. Rothenberg R, Judson FN. The clinical diagnosis of urethral discharge. Sex Transm Dis 1983; 10:24-8.
24. Volk J, Kraus SJ. Nongonococcal urethritis – a venereal disease as prevalent as epidemic gonorrhea. Arch Intern Med 1974; 134:511-4.
25. Holmes KK. Gonococcal infection – clinical, epidemiologic, and laboratory perspectives. Adv Intern Med 1974; 19:259-84.
26. Handsfield HH. Clinical aspects of gonococcal infections. In: Roberts RB, ed. The gonococcus. New York: Wiley, 1977:58-79.
27. McCormack WM. Clinical spectrum of infection with *Neisseria gonorrhoeae*. Sex Transm Dis 1981; 8:305-7.
28. Crawford G, Knapp JS, Hale J, Holmes KK. Asymptomatic gonorrhea in men: caused by gonococci with unique nutritional requirements. Science 1977; 196:1352-3.
29. Handsfield HH, Knapp JS, Diehr PK, Holmes KK. Correlation of auxotype and penicillin susceptibility of *Neisseria gonorrhoeae* with sexual preference and clinical manifestations of gonorrhea. Sex Transm Dis 1980; 7:1-5.

30. Priser H, Marino AF. Gonorrhea—frequently unrecognized reservoirs. South Med J 1970; 63:198-201.
31. Holmes KK, Johnson DW, Floyd TM, Kvale PA. Studies of venereal disease—II. Observations on the incidence,etiology, and treatment of the postgonococcal urethritis syndrome. JAMA 1967; 202:467-73.
32. Fiumara NJ. The diagnosis and treatment of gonorrhea. Med Clin North Am 1972; 56:1105-13.
33. Goodhart ME, Ogden J, Zaidi AA, Kraus SJ. Factors affecting the performance of smear and culture tests for the detection of *Neisseria gonorrhoeae*. Sex Transm Dis 1982; 9:63-9.
34. Dans PE, Judson F. The establishment of a venereal disease clinic. II. An appraisal of current diagnostic methods in uncomplicated urogenital and rectal gonorrhea. J Am Vener Dis Assoc 1975; 1:107-12.
35. Judson FN. A clinic-based system for monitoring the quality of techniques for the diagnosis of gonorrhea. Sex Transm Dis 1978; 5:141-5.
36. Kleris GS, Arnold AJ. Differential diagnosis of urethritis: predictive value and therapeutic implications of the urethral smear. Sex Transm Dis 1981; 8:110-6.
37. Judson FN, Wright RA, Mann EA. Recent micturition does not affect the detection of urethral gonorrhea. Br J Vener Dis 1977; 53:308-10.
38. Holmes KK, Buchanan TM, Adam JL, Eschenbach DA. Is serology useful in gonorrhea? A critical analysis of factors influencing serodiagnosis. In: Brooks GF, Gotschlich EC, Holmes KK, Sawyer WD, Young FE, eds. Immunobiology of *Neisseria gonorrhoeae*. Washington, DC: American Society for Microbiology, 1978:370-6.
39. Kearns DH, O'Reilly RJ, Lee L, Welch BG. Secretory IgA antibodies in the urethral exudate of men with uncomplicated urethritis due to *Neisseria gonorrhoeae*. J Infect Dis 1973; 127:99-101.
40. Danielsson D, Olcen P, Sandstrom E. Serological methods of diagnosis. In: Skinner FA, Walker PD, Smith H, eds. Gonorrhoea—epidemiology and pathogenesis. London: Academic, 1977:27-48.
41. Thornley MJ, Wilson DV, DeHormaeche RD, Oates JK, Coombs RRA. Detection of gonococcal antigens in urine by radioimmunoassay. J Med Microbiol 1979; 12:161-75.
42. Aardoom HA, DeHoop D, Iserief COA, Michel MF, Stolz E. Detection of *Neisseria gonorrhoeae* antigen by a solid-phase enzyme immunoassay. Br J Vener Dis 1982; 58:359-62.
43. Jaffe HW, Kraus SJ, Edwards TA, Weinberger SS, Zubrzycki L. Diagnosis of gonorrhea using a genetic transformation test on mailed clinical specimens. J Infect Dis 1982; 146:275-9.
44. Package insert: Gonodecten test kit. United States Packaging Corporation: LaPort, Ind., 1979.
45. Fontaine EA, Taylor-Robinson D, Hanna NF, Coufalik ED. Anaerobes in men with urethritis. Br J Vener Dis 1982; 58:321-6.
46. Spagna VA, Prior RB, Perkins RL. Rapid presumptive diagnosis of gonococcal urethritis in men by the limulus lysate test. Br J Vener Dis 1979; 55:179-82.

47. Prior RB, Spagna VA. Comparative evaluation of the tube and microdilution *Limulus* lysate techniques for rapid presumptive diagnosis of gonococcal urethritis in men. J Clin Microbiol 1980; 11:340-2.
48. Prior RB, Spagna VA. Application of a *Limulus* test device in rapid evaluation of gonococcal and nongonococcal urethritis in males. J Clin Microbiol 1981; 14:256-60.
49. Spagna VA, Prior RB. *Limulus* lysate assay for gonorrhea. AFP 1983; 27: 227-31.
50. Wilkinson AE. Cultural methods for the diagnosis of gonorrhoea. In: Skinner FA, Walker PD, Smith H, eds. Gonorrhoea–epidemiology and pathogenesis. London: Academic, 1977:17-25.
51. Chapel T, Smeltzer M, Printz D, Dassel R, Lewis J. An evaluation of commercially supplied Transgrow and Amies medium for the detection of *Neisseria gonorrhoeae*. Health Lab Sci 1974; 11:28-33.
52. Martin JE, Jackson RL. A biological environmental chamber for the culture of *Neisseria gonorrhoeae*. J Am Vener Dis Assoc 1975; 2:28-30.
53. Taylor E, Phillips I. Assessment of transport and isolation methods for gonococci. Br J Vener Dis 1980; 56:390-3.
54. Helstad AG, Bruns MK. Rapid laboratory identification of *Neisseria gonorrhoeae* by coagglutination. J Clin Microbiol 1980; 11:753-4.
55. Sng, EH, Yeo KL, Rajan VS. Comparison of methods for the detection of penicillinase-producing *Neisseria* gonorrhoeae. Br J Vener Dis 1980; 56: 311-3.
56. Feng WC, Medeiros AA, Murray ES. Diagnosis of gonorrhea in male patients by culture of uncentrifuged first-voided urine. JAMA 1977; 327:896-7.
57. Moore G, Pittard WB, Mosca N, O'Brien WM. Gonorrhea detection by urine sediment culture. JAMA 1973; 224:1499-501.
58. Centers for Disease Control. Sexually transmitted diseases: treatment guidelines, 1982. Rev Infect Dis 1982; 4:S729-46.
59. Jaffe HW. Nongonococcal urethritis: treatment of men and their sexual partners. Rev Infect Dis 1982; 4:S772-7.
60. Root TE, Edwards LD, Spengler PJ. Nongonococcal urethritis: a survey of clinical and laboratory features. Sex Trans Dis 1980; 7:59-65.
61. Jordan WC. Doxycycline vs tetracycline in the treatment of men with gonorrhea: the compliance factor. Sex Transm Dis 1981; 8:105-9.
62. Goodhart GL, Kramer M, Zaidi AA. Characteristics of defaulters in treatment for infection with *Neisseria gonorrhoeae*. J Infect Dis 1979; 140:649-51.
63. Judson FN. The importance of coexisting syphlitic, chlamydial, mycoplasmal, and trichomonal infections in the treatment of gonorrhea. Sex Transm Dis 1979; 6:112-9.
64. Berg SW, Harrison WO. Spectinomycin as primary treatment of gonorrhea in areas of high prevalence of penicillinase-producing *Neisseria gonorrhoeae*. Sex Transm Dis 1981; 8:38-9.
65. Arya OP, Rees E, Percival A, Alergant CD, Annels EA, Turner GC. Epidemiology and treatment of gonorrhoea caused by penicillinase-producing strains in Liverpool. Br J Vener Dis 1978; 54:28-35.

66. Washington AE. Update on treatment recommendations for gonococcal infections. Rev Infect Dis 1982; 4:S758-71.
67. Jones RB, Stimson J, Counts GW, Holmes KK. Cefoxitin in the treatment of gonorrhea. Sex Transm Dis 1979; 6:239-42.
68. Berg SW, Kilpatrick ME, Harrison WO, McCutchan. Cefoxitin as a single-dose treatment for urethritis caused by penicillinase-producing *Neisseria gonorrhoeae*. N Engl J Med 1979; 301:509-11.
69. Rajan VS, Sng EH, Pang R, Tan NJ, Thirumoorthy T, Yeo KL. HR756–a new cephalosporin in the treatment of gonorrhoea caused by ordinary and penicillinase-producing strains of *Neisseria gonorrhoeae*. Br J Vener Dis 1980; 56:255-8.
70. Tan NJ, Rajan VS, Pang R, Sng EH. Gentamicin in the treatment of infections due to penicillinase-producing gonococci. Br J Vener Dis 1980; 56:394-6.
71. Robbins JB. Problems posed by potential gonococcal vaccines viewed from the vantage point of a control agency. Br J Vener Dis 1977; 53:170-2.
72. Bowie WR, Pollock HM, Forsyth PS, Floyd JF, Alexander ER, Wang SP, Holmes KK. Bacteriology of the urethra in normal men and men with non-gonococcal urethritis. J Clin Microbiol 1977; 6:482-8.
73. Dunlop EMC. Chlamydial infection: terminology, disease and treatment. In: Harris JRW, ed. Recent advances in sexually transmitted diseases. Vol 2. London: Churchill Livingstone, 1981:101-19.
74. Darougar S, Treharne JD. Chlamydial infections: laboratory aspects. In: Harris JRW, ed. Recent advances in sexually transmitted diseases. Vol 2. London: Churchill Livingstone, 1981: 141-50.
75. Manire GP. The chlamydiae. In: Braude AI, ed. Medical microbiology and infectious diseases. Vol 2. Philadelphia: WB Saunders, 1981:516-22.
76. Dunlop EMC, Al Hussian MK, Garland JA, Treharne JD, Harper IA, Jones BR. Infection of the urethra by TRIC agent in men presenting because of non-specific urethritis. Lancet 1965; 1:1125-8.
77. Bowie WR, Wang SP, Alexander ER, Floyd J, Forsyth PS, Pollock HM, Lin JSL, Buchanan TM, Holmes KK. Etiology of nongonococcal urethritis–evidence for *Chlamydia trachomatis* and *Ureaplasma urealyticum*. J Clin Invest 1977; 59:735-42.
78. Holmes KK, Handsfield HH, Wang SP, Wentworth BB, Turck M, Anderson JB, Alexander ER. Etiology of nongonococcal urethritis. N Engl J Med 1975; 292:1199-205.
79. Schachter J. Chlamydial infections. N Engl J Med 1978; 298:428-35.
80. Vaughan-Jackson JD, Dunlop EMC, Darougar S, Treharne JD, Taylor-Robinson D. Urethritis due to *Chlamydia trachomatis*. Br J Vener Dis 1977; 53: 180-3.
81. Berger RE, Alexander ER, Monda GD, Ansell J, McCormick G, Holmes KK. *Chlamydia trachomatis* as a cause of acute "idiopathic" epididymitis. N Engl J Med 1978; 298:301-4.
82. McGee ZA, Taylor-Robinson D. Mycoplasmas, In: Braude AI, ed. Medical microbiology and infectious diseases. Vol 2. Philadelphia: WB Saunders, 1981:522-9.

83. Taylor-Robinson D, Csonka GW. Laboratory and clinical aspects of mycoplasmal infections of the human genitourinary tract. In: Harris JRW, ed. Recent advances in sexually transmitted diseases. Vol 2. London: Churchill Livingstone, 1981:151-86.
84. Cassell GH, Cole BC. Mycoplasmas as agents of human disease. N Engl J Med 1981; 304:80-9.
85. Coufalik ED, Taylor-Robinson D, Csonka GW. Treatment of nongonococcal urethritis with rifampicin as a means of defining the role of *Ureaplasma urealyticum*. Br J Vener Dis 1979; 55:36-43.
86. Prentice MJ, Taylor-Robinson D, Csonka GW. Non-specific urethritis. A placebo controlled trial of minocycline in conjunction with laboratory investigations. Br J Vener Dis 1976; 52:269-75.
87. Taylor-Robinson D, Csonka GW, Prentice MJ. Human intraurethral inoculation of ureaplasmas. Q J Med 1977; 46:309-26.
88. Taylor-Robinson D, Evans RT, Coufalik ED, Prentice MJ, Munday PE, Csonka GW, Oates JK. *Ureaplasma urealyticum* and *mycoplasma hominis* in chlamydial and non-chlamydial nongonococcal urethritis. Br J Vener Dis 1979; 55:30-5.
89. Viarengo J, Hebrant F, Piot P. *Ureaplasma urealyticum* in the urethra of healthy men. Br J Vener Dis 1980; 56:169-72.
90. Catterall RD. Diagnosis and treatment of trichomonal urethritis in men. Br Med J 1960; 2:113-8.
91. Bowie WR, Alexander ER, Stimson JB, Floyd JF, Holmes KK. Therapy for nongonococcal urethritis. Ann Intern Med 1981; 95:306-11.
92. Wong JL, Hines PA, Brasher MD, Rogers GT, Smith RF, Schachter J. The etiology of nongonococcal urethritis in men attending in a venereal disease clinic. Sex Transm Dis 1977; 4:4-8.
93. Wilson A, Ackers JP. Urine culture for the detection of *Trichomonas vaginalis* in men. Br J Vener Dis 1980; 56:46-8.
94. Weston TET, Nicol CS. Natural history of trichomonal infection in males. Br J Vener Dis 1963; 39:251-7.
95. Kuberski T. *Trichomonas vaginalis* associated with nongonococcal urethritis and prostatitis. Sex Transm Dis 1980; 7:135-6.
96. Hovelius B, Thelin I, Mårdh PA. *Staphylococcus saprophyticus* in the aetiology of nongonococcal urethritis. Br J Vener Dis 1979; 55:369-74.
97. Dawson SG, Ison CA, Csonka G, Easmon CSF. Male carriage of *Gardnerella vaginalis*. Br J Vener Dis 1982; 58:243-5.
98. Dunkelberg WE, Woolvin SC. *Haemophilus vaginalis* relative to gonorrhea and male urethritis. Mil Med 1963; 128:1098-101.
99. Wiesner PJ. Selected aspects of the epidemiology of nongonococcal urethritis. In: Hobson D, Holmes KK, eds. Nongonococcal urethritis and related infections. Washington, DC: American Society for Microbiology, 1977:9-14.
100. Academic department of genitourinary medicine of the Middlesex hospital medical school, the communicable surveillance centre and the communicable diseases unit. Sexually transmitted disease surveillance 1978. Br Med J 1979; 2:1375-6.

101. Judson FN. Epidemiology and control of nongonococcal urethritis and genital chlamydial infections: a review. Sex Transm Dis 1981;8:117-26.
102. Swartz SL. Diagnosis of nongonococcal urethritis. In: Hobson D, Holmes KK, eds. Nongonococcal urethritis and related infections. Washington, DC: American Society for Microbiology, 1977:15-8.
103. Schofield CBS. Some factors affecting the incubation period and duration of symptoms of urethritis in men. Br J Vener Dis 1982;58:184-7.
104. Oriel JD, Reeve P, Powis P, Miller A, Nicol CS. Isolation of chlamydia from patients with non-specific genital infection. Br J Vener Dis 1972;48:429-36.
105. Terho P. *Chlamydia trachomatis* in non-specific urethritis. Br J Vener Dis 1978; 54:251-6.
106. Ghadirian FD, Robson HG. *Chlamydia trachomatis* genital infections. Br J Vener Dis 1979; 55:415-8.
107. Paavonen J, Kousa M, Saikku PA, Vatiaien E, Kanerva L, Lassus, A. Treatment of non-gonococcal urethritis with trimethoprim-sulphadiazine and with placebo. Br J Vener Dis 1980; 56:101-4.
108. Oriel JD. Treatment of nongonococcal urethritis. In: Hobson D, Holmes KK, eds. Nongonococcal urethritis and related infections. Washington, DC: American Society for Microbiology, 1977:38-42.
109. Swartz SL, Draus SJ. Persistent urethral leukocytosis and asymptomatic chlamydial urethritis. J Infect Dis 1979; 140:614-7.
110. Oriel JD, Reeve P, Wright JT, Owen J. Chlamydial infection of the male urethra. Br J Vener Dis 1976;52:46-51.
111. Desai K, Robson HG. Comparison of the Gram-stained urethral smear and first-voided urine sediment in the diagnosis of nongonococcal urethritis. Sex Transm Dis 1982; 9:21-5.
112. Willcox JR, Adler MW, Belsey EM. Observer variation in the interpretation of Gram-stained urethral smears—implications for the diagnosis of non-specific urethritis. Br J Vener Dis 1981; 57:134-6.
113. Aumonier FJ. Some problems in microscopy encountered in clinics for sexually transmitted diseases. Br J Vener Dis 1978;54:346-7.
114. Simopoulos JCH. Tetracycline treatment for non-specific urethritis. Br J Vener Dis 1977; 53:230-2.
115. Handsfield HH, Alexander ER, Wang SP, Pedersen AHB, Holmes KK. Differences in the therapeutic response of chlamydia-positive and chlamydia-negative forms of nongonococcal urethritis. J Am Vener Dis Assoc 1976; 2:5-9.
116. Bowie WR, Yu JS, Fawcett A, Jones HD. Tetracycline in nongonococcal urethritis—comparison of 2 g and 1g daily for seven days. Br J Vener Dis 1980; 56:332-6.
117. McNeil PJ, Fiumara NJ, Caliando JJ, Benes S, McCormack WM. Evaluation of doxycycline hyclate in the treatment of nongonococcal urethritis. Sex Transm Dis 1981; 8:127-31.
118. John J. Efficacy of prolonged regimens of oxytetracycline in the treatment of nongonococcal urethritis. Br J Vener Dis 1971;47:266-7.
119. Thambar IV, Simmons PD, Thin RN, Darougar S, Yearsley P. Double-blind comparison of two regimens in the treatment of nongonococcal urethritis:

seven-day vs 21-day courses of triple tetracycline. Br J Vener Dis 1979; 55:284-8.

120. Stimson JB, Hale J, Bowie WR, Holmes KK. Tetracycline-resistant *Ureaplasma urealyticum*: a cause of persistent nongonococcal urethritis. Ann Intern Med 1981; 94:192-4.
121. Scheibel JH, Kristensen JK, Hentzer B, Secher L, Ullman S, Verdich J, Weismann K. Treatment of chlamydial urethritis in men and *Chlamydia trachomatis*-positive female partners: comparison of erythromycin and tetracycline in treatment courses of one week. Sex Transm Dis 1982; 9: 128-31.
122. Goodhart GL. Treatment of uncomplicated genital gonorrhea. Sex Transm Dis 1979; 6:126-42.
123. Juvakoski T, Allgulander C, Lassus A. Rosaramicin and tetracycline treatment in *Chlamydia trachomatis*-positive and negative nongonococcal urethritis. Sex Transm Dis 1981; 8:12-5.
124. Dacso C, Greenberg S, Martin RR. Rosaramicin treatment of gonococcal urethritis in men. Sex Transm Dis 1980; 7:133-4.
125. Darne JF, Ridgway GL, Oriel JD. Rosaramicin and tetracycline in the treatment of non-gonococcal urethritis–a comparison of clinical and microbiological results. Br J Vener Dis 1982; 58:117-20.
126. Evans BA. The role of tetracyclines in the treatment of non-specific urethritis. Br J Vener Dis 1977; 53:40-3.
127. Arya OP, Alergant CD, Annels EH, Carey PB, Ghosh AK, Goddard AD. Management of non-specific urethritis in men. Br J Vener Dis 1978; 54: 414-21.
128. Tait IA, Rees E, Hobson D, Byng RE, Tweedie MCK. Chlamydial infection of the cervix in contacts of men with nongonococcal urethritis. Br J Vener Dis 1980; 56:37-45.
129. Harnisch JP, Berger RE, Alexander ER, Monda GD, Holmes KK. Aetiology of acute epididymitis. Lancet 1977; 1:819-21.
130. Heap G. Acute epididymitis attributable to chlamydial infection–preliminary report. Med J Aust 1975; 1:718-9.
131. Berger RE, Alexander ER, Harnisch JP, Paulsen CA, Monda GD, Ansell J, Holmes KK. Etiology, manifestations and therapy of acture epididymitis: prospective study of 50 cases. J Urol 1979; 121:750-4.
132. Drotman DP. Epidemiology and treatment of epididymitis. Rev Infect Dis 1982; 4:S788-92.
133. Mårdh PA, Ripa KT, Colleen S, Treharne JD, Darougar S. Role of *Chlamydia trachomatis* in non-acture prostatitis. Br J Vener Dis 1978; 54:330-4.
134. Cassell GH, Younger JB, Brown MB, Blackwell RE, Davis JK, Marriott P, Stagno S. Microbiologic study of infertile women at the time of diagnostic laparoscopy–association of *Ureaplasma urealyticum* with a defined subpopulation. N Engl J Med 1983; 308:502-5.
135. Graber CD, Creticos P, Valicenti J, Williamson HO. T Mycoplasma in human reproductive failure. Obstet Gynecol 1979; 54:558-61.
136. Fowlkes DM, MacLeod J, O'Leary WM. T-Mycoplasmas and human infertility: correlation of infection with alterations in seminal parameters. Fertil Steril 1965; 26:1212-8.

137. Swenson CE, Toth A, O'Leary WM. *Ureaplasma urealyticum* and human infertility: the effect of antibiotic therapy on semen quality. Fertil Steril 1979; 31:660-5.
138. Toth A, Lesser ML, Brooks C, Labriola D. Subsequent pregnancies among 161 couples treated for T-mycoplasma genital-tract infection. N Engl J Med 1983; 308:505-7.
139. Lassus A, Lousa M. Reiter's disease. In: Harris JRW, ed. Recent advances in sexually transmitted diseases. Vol a. London: Churchill Livingstone, 1981:187-99.
140. Kousa M, Saikku P, Richmond S. Lassus A. Frequent association of chlamydial infection with Reiter's syndrome. Sex Transm Dis 1978; 5:57-61.
141. Csonka GW. The course of Reiter's syndrome. Br Med J 1958; 1:1088-90.
142. Khan MA, Askari AD, Braun WE, Aponte CJ. Low association of HLA-B27 with Reiter's syndrome in blacks. Ann Intern Med 1979; 90:202-3.
143. Woodrow JC. Histocompatibility antigens and rheumatic diseases. Semin Arthritis Rheum 1977; 6:257-76.
144. Wilkens RF, Arnett FC, Bitter T, Calin A, Fisher L, Ford DK, Good AE, Masi AT. Reiter's syndrome—evaluation of preliminary criteria for definite disease. Arthritis Rheum 1981; 24:844-9.
145. Strahlman ER. Reiter's syndrome. John Hopkins Med J 1982; 150:39-44.
146. Fox R, Calin A, Gerber RC, Gibson D. The chronicity of symptoms and disability in Reiter's syndrome—an analysis of 131 consecutive patients. Ann Intern Med 1979; 91:190-3.
147. Kulka JP. The lesions of Reiter's syndrome. Arthritis Rheum 1962; 5: 195-201.
148. Good, AE. Reiter's disease: a review with special attention to cardiovascular and neurologic sequellae. Semin Arthritis Rheum 1974; 3:253-86.
149. Ruppert GB, Lindsay J, Barth WF. Cardiac conduction abnormalities in Reiter's syndrome. Am J Med 1982; 73:335-40.
150. Arnett FC, McClusky OE, Schacter BZ, Lordon RE. Incomplete Reiter's syndrome: discriminating features and HL-AW27 in diagnosis. Ann Intern Med 1976; 84:8-12.

FOUR

Cervicitis Syndromes

Richard B. Prior and Vincent A. Spagna
The Ohio State University
College of Medicine
Columbus, Ohio

INTRODUCTION

Cervicitis can be regarded as the "silent" partner of urethritis in males and occurs with similar frequency, although it is more difficult to recognize [1]. Cervicitis is the most common major sexually transmitted disease (STD) syndrome in females and if undetected and untreated can lead to serious complications such as pelvic inflammatory disease (PID). The etiological agents for cervicitis are similar to those which cause urethritis in males. Although cervicitis may accompany vaginitis due to *Candida albicans* or *Trichomonas vaginalis*, cervicitis without vaginitis is caused primarily by *Neisseria gonorrhoeae*, *Chlamydia trachomatis*, or herpes simplex virus [1]. In fact, an abnormal cervical discharge is usually interpreted by the patient as an abnormal vaginal discharge, and up to 25% of women complaining of vaginal discharge have cervicitis caused by one of these three pathogens [2] (see also Chap. 5).

In this chapter the complex normal microbial flora of the cervix is first described followed by a discussion of the three major STD pathogens of cervicitis. The epidemiology, clinical manifestations, diagnosis, and treatment are included for each pathogen. Finally, a brief discussion of the other important microbial cervical pathogens is presented.

THE NORMAL CERVIX AND MICROBIAL FLORA

The cervix, the lower portion (2 to 3 cm) of the uterus, projects into the vagina at an angle of approximately 90° to 100° (see Chap. 1). The central portion of the cervix bears a small depressed aperture, the os of the cervix, which marks the entrance of the endocervical canal. The endocervical canal is lined by two epithelial components, squamous and columnar, and establishes the connection between the vagina and uterine cavity. The squamous epithelium (an extension of the vaginal surface cells) abruptly adjoins the columnar epithelium (an extension of the uterine surface cells) at the squamo-columnar junction which is located immediately within the os of the virgin cervix. Trauma, such as childbirth, can disrupt the normal boundary of squamous and columnar epithelium. The cervix possesses a complex secretory and cellular immunological surveillance system to protect the sterile uterine cavity from contamination by vaginal flora [3]. The normal endocervix is an unfavorable environment for commensal bacteria. While cultures have shown the qualitative bacteriologies of the cervix and of the vagina to be identical, there are significant quantitative differences [4]. Biopsy studies have demonstrated that the mucosal surface of the cervical os is colonized by small numbers of bacteria, approximately 400 per square millimeter, and microorganisms are rarely encountered at a depth of 2 cm within the endocervical canal [5].

"Normal resident flora" refers to those microorganisms inhabiting the internal and external surfaces of healthy individuals and maintaining a commensal or symbiotic relationship. Critical variables in the colonization of epithelial surfaces by bacteria include the strength of adherence (via pili or fimbriae), host factors, and antagonistic components of the indigenous flora [6]. Shortcomings in attempts to define the microflora of the cervix and vagina include difficulties in accurate bacteriological quantitation and the fastidious nature of many reported microorganisms. The majority of investigators have reported that anaerobic and facultative *Lactobacillus* species constitute the predominant bacteria (48 to 80%) isolated from normal cervices [7-9]. Generally, there have been conflicting reports regarding the various aerobic and anaerobic bacteria and their frequency distribution in normal cervices. These discrepancies may be partly explained by culturing during different phases of the menstrual cycle, the influences of various medications (antibiotics, oral contraceptives), and local factors (intrauterine devices). Several investigators have demonstrated a predominance of anaerobic bacteria in cultures from normal cervices. Gorbach et al. [7] noted a predominance of *Bacteroides* species (57%) among anaerobic isolates, while Ohm and Galask [9] isolated anaerobic gram-positive cocci (*Peptococcus* sp., *Peptostreptococcus* sp.) from 74% of prehysterectomy endocervical cultures. *Clostridium, Eubacterium, Veillonella,* and *Fusobacterium* species are other anaerobic bacteria which are usually reported to occur at various frequencies [7-10]. Among the aerobic bacteria, *Escherichia coli* is the predominant gram-negative organism in cultures of the normal cervix [11]. Diphtheroids, staphylococci, and streptococci are the predominant gram-positive organisms colonizing the cervix [4, 7-11]. Other organisms reported to colonize the normal cervix include *Gardnerella vaginalis, Klebsiella pneumoniae, Enterobacter* sp., *Neisseria* sp., *Proteus* sp., *Acinetobacter* (*Herellea vaginicola*), *Candida* sp., *Torulopsis glabrata*, and many other infrequently isolated microorganisms. There appears to be little if any change in the representative flora in conjunction with gonococcal and nongonococcal cervicitis [8, 12]. Lindner et al. [8] noted that lactobacilli occurred at a statistically higher rate (92%) in cervical cultures during pregnancy. Also, aerobic bacteria occurred less frequently, and 61% of cervical specimens yielded only one bacterial species. Most researchers have reported three or more bacterial species colonizing the cervix [4, 7, 9]. Goplerud et al. [13] cultured women during their pregnancy and in the postpartum period and noted that certain bacteria (aerobic gram-positive cocci, aerobic and anaerobic gram-negative rods, anaerobic cocci) decreased during pregnancy. Thadepalli et al. [10] evaluated the cervical flora in 50 healthy women in labor and on the third day postpartum. Gram-positive cocci predominated in all cervical cultures, and an average of four microbial species was present in each specimen. Neither *Bacteroides fragilis* nor *Clostridium* species were isolated from the cervix during labor and the puerperium, suggesting that pregnancy exerts a negative influence, possibly hormonally mediated, on the colonization of the cervix by these bacteria.

The role of the normal endocervical flora in prevention of infection has also been the subject of several studies. Researchers found that aerobic, facultative anaerobic, and strict anaerobic microorganisms inhibit *N. gonorrhoeae* in vitro and therefore may exert a protective effect against gonorrhea [14-16]; however, the role for this antigonococcal effect by microorganisms in the pathogenesis of gonococcal infection in humans is not known.

The cervical flora is a dynamic ecosystem, responsive to various influences. While a detailed analysis of the variables which affect the female genital flora is beyond the scope of this chapter, further information may be found in an article by Larsen and Galask [11].

GONOCOCCAL CERVICITIS

Etiology

Gonococcal cervicitis is caused by *N. gonorrhoeae*, a small gram-negative, oxidase-positive, coccal bacterium that usually occurs in pairs with adjacent sides flattened (kidney bean appearance). The gonococcus is aerobic but requires an increased carbon dioxide (CO_2) tension for growth. Unlike the other *Neisseria* species, the gonococcus will only utilize glucose with a concomitant production of acid. Humans are the only natural hosts for *N. gonorrhoeae*, and transmission is predominantly via sexual contact. Theoretically, gonorrhea may be acquired nonsexually via fomites, since gonococci can survive from several hours to 3 days on certain objects contaminated by urethral secretions [17, 18]; however, fomite transmission of gonorrhea has never been documented.

Certain strains of *N. gonorrhoeae* contain pili, small hairlike appendages protruding from the cell surface, and these structures are associated with the virulence of gonococcus. Pili permit attachment of the organism to epithelial cells, allowing establishment of infection and invasion into the subepithelial tissues [19, 20]. The virulence of the gonococcus is also related to the elaboration of one or more toxic factors [20, 21]. These toxic factors appear at least partially responsible for the damage to human genital mucosa [20-22]. Studies using human fallopian tube organ cultures have shown the toxicity to be due primarily to gonococcal lipopolysaccharides (endotoxin) [21-23].

Epidemiology

Despite existing control measures, gonorrhea remains epidemic, with an estimated world incidence approaching 100 million [24]. In the United States, over 1 million cases are reported annually [25], and it is estimated that four to five times this number are seen in the private sector by practicing physicians and not reported [26-28]. Of the reported cases, over 400,000 occur in women, which translates to approximately 365 cases occurring per 100,000 population [25]. More than half of the reported cases occur in the 15- to 24-year age group. In 1982 there was a slight decrease from the previous year in the number of new cases reported for both sexes (418 versus 435 per 100,000). This leveling off of reported cases is thought to be due to the federally assisted state and local programs to control gonorrhea which were initiated in 1972 [29]. In England there were 86 new cases in women of all ages per 100,000 population seen at hospital clinics in 1979. For women aged 16 to 24 years, the number of new cases per 100,000 population was approximately 450. The total number of cases in women in England during 1979 showed a 4.5% decrease from the previous year [30].

A disturbing feature noted in England was the increase in the number of reports of penicillinase-producing *N. gonorrhoeae* (PPNG). The number of PPNG cases increased 335% (from 31 to 104) from 1978 to 1979 [30]. Similarly, in the United States the number of PPNG cases increased 900% (from 300 to 2700) from 1979 to 1981 [31]. Spectinomycin-resistant gonococci have also been noted worldwide [32], and sporadic cases of spectinomycin-resistant PPNG have occurred among individuals without known contact with patients infected with these organisms [33-35]. In 1982 transmission of spectinomycin-resistant PPNG was documented for the first time [36].

The many factors which contribute to the high prevalence of gonorrhea are varied and complex. A discussion of the "core group," risks of transmission, and other factors such as age, sociosexual behavior, sexual climate, and characteristics of the gonococcus which relate to the epidemic nature of gonorrhea are discussed in Chapters 2 and 3 and categorized in Table 1 of Chapter 3. The most important element in disease transmission is the asymptomatic carrier, and unsuspected gonococcal infection occurs in both males and females. However, women constitute the greatest reservoir of asymptomatic disease. Since many females are routinely screened for gonorrhea, they offer the best means of identifying asymptomatic males [37, 38].

The female is at greater risk of infection than the male. It has been estimated that a male having a single sexual encounter with a gonorrhea-infected female will become infected 20 to 25% of the time, while the female is invariably infected during intercourse with an infected male [39-41]. The risk of transmission from male to female is estimated at 80 to 90% [42]. Hypothetically, 53 to 79% of women seeking treatment because of exposure to gonorrhea will be infected [43].

Women with asymptomatic gonorrhea unsuspectedly transmit the disease and are at risk for complications. Spagna et al. [44] found that 53 of 100 women with unsuspected gonococcal cervicitis admitted having sexual intercourse between the time they were first cultured (for disposition of contraceptives) and the time they recieved therapy. The average delay from the initial culture to therapy was 11 days, and during this interval 7% developed signs and symptoms of PID [44]. Generally, up to 20% of women with untreated gonorrhea will develop PID [27, 45, 46].

Because of the high risk of transmission and serious complications of undetected gonorrhea in women, massive screening programs were begun in the United States in 1973. In 1979 there were approximately 9 million females tested in the United States, and 4.5% were found to be infected with *N. gonorrhoeae*. While such programs are costly, they have resulted in a reduction of gonorrhea [29]. Selective screening cultures should be performed on high-risk individuals such as gonorrhea contacts, prostitutes, rape victims, and those with a history of STDs. In addition, all pregnant women and those seeking contraceptives or requesting abortions should be screened for gonorrhea.

Clinical Manifestations

"Men are treated for gonorrhea; women suffer from it," according to a students' aide-mémoire [27]. Such a statement was prompted by the sharp contrast of gonorrhea in men and in women. Men will usually develop symptoms (dysuria and/or urethral discharge) and seek medical attention; in contrast, early gonorrhea in women produces little or nothing by way of symptoms. Gonorrhea in women is a tale of latency, complications, chronicity, and disability [27].

The major site of primary gonococcal infection in women is the cervix [42]. In the process of sexual transmission, the cervix is bathed in infected male secretions. The surface pH of vaginal epithelium is too low for growth of the gonococci, except for a small area at the external os. Here the gonococci are able to attach to stratified squamous epithelium and thus maintain the carrier state typical of the female [47]. In ultrastructural studies of cervical gonorrhea Evans, using the transmission electron microscope, found that gonococci establish infection of the cervix by focal attachment to squamous epithelium at the squamocolumnar junction [47]. An attempt to semiquantitate the number of gonococci in the cervicovaginal area of women with gonorrhea revealed an average of approximately 10^5 colony-forming units (CFU) per sample, with a range of 10^2 to 10^7 CFU per sample [48]. The number of gonococci was not influenced by the use of oral contraceptives, concurrent infection with *T. vaginalis* and/or *G. vaginalis*, time of douche prior to examination, or phase of the menstrual cycle at which time the women were examined [48].

The incubation period for gonococcal cervicitis has been difficult to determine because of the asymptomatic nature of the disease in many women. Morton, however, suggests that the incubation period in women is the same as for men, that is, 2 to 5 days following exposure [27].

Following establishment of infection, early gonorrhea in women produces few or no symptoms. The percentage of asymptomatic patients varies, dependent on the criteria followed by different authors in their assessment of the asymptomatic state. Wiesner believes that between 40 and 60% of women who have gonorrhea develop some symptoms [49]. Jha et al. [50] found unsuspected gonococcal infection in 10.2% of 410 female patients who attended an obstetric and gynecological outpatient clinic. Of the infected patients, 40.5% had no symptoms. Little and Hartsfield found that in 66 women with gonorrhea, 44% were asymptomatic [51]. Spagna et al. [44] evaluated 100 untreated referral female patients with positive cervical cultures for *N. gonorrhoeae* and found 60% denied symptoms of genitourinary disease. On repeat examination before therapy, visual inspection of the cervix revealed inflammatory changes (erythema and friability) in 57% and purulent (yellow or green) endocervical secretions in 60% of the patients. Morton suggests that between 70 and 80% of women infected with *N. gonorrhoeae* are asymptomatic [27]. Dysuria may be present if the urethra is infected (see Chap. 9), and vaginal discharge may accompany complaints of dysuria, or may be the only symptom. Additionally, the rectum can become infected as a result of perineal contamination with cervicovaginal exudate. About 36% of women with gonococcal cervicitis will have positive rectal cultures for *N. gonorrhoeae* [42] (see also Chap. 8).

Physical examination rarely shows any vulvar, introital, or vaginal inflammation unless some other condition coexists with cervical gonorrhea. The infected cervix can appear perfectly healthy or show a well-marked, intensely inflamed cervical canal with extensive ectocervical erosion [27]. In such cases a cascade of mucopurulent exudate may be found exuding from the cervical canal. In general, however, the signs of gonococcal cervicitis are indistinguishable from other local cervical conditions or even good health [27]. Thus a diagnosis of gonococcal cervicitis can only be made by utilizing laboratory tests.

During the infectious process local antibody production occurs at the cervix. In a study of cervical secretions, gonococcal antibody was detected in 97% of infected women, with 97% being of the IgG class, 95% of the IgA class, and 39% of the IgM class [52]. Neither IgA nor IgM antibodies were detected in noninfected women. In a subsequent study by the same investigators, anti-gonococcal IgA was detected in cervical secretions in only 72% of women with untreated gonorrhea [53], indicating considerable variability in either the antibody response or the test procedure. Humoral antibodies (IgG, IgM, and IgA) are also produced in response to gonococcal infection. Antibodies have been demonstrated to gonococcal pili [54-56] and to gonococcal envelope protein [57]. In addition, a cell-mediated immune response occurs during gonococcal infection [58, 59].

If gonococcal cervicitis goes undetected and untreated, a minority of patients will probably self-cure [42]. In some patients, complications can occur, which include proctitis and the development of the asymptomatic carrier state which may last for months and in some cases years [27]. In a small percentage of patients dissemination of certain nutritionally deficient strains of *N. gonorrhoeae* may occur (see Chap. 8). In other patients overt complications can occur which include infection of Skene's glands (skenitis), infection of the Bartholin gland duct (bartholinitis), and development of PID [27]. The most serious complication is PID, and as many as 20% of patients with untreated gonococcal cervicitis may develop this complication [27, 45, 46] (see also Chap. 7). In addition, gonococcal infection can be transferred to infants born to mothers infected with *N. gonorrhoeae* (see Chap. 15).

Diagnosis

Since many patients with gonococcal cervicitis have no signs or symptoms and others have signs that are clinically indistinguishable from nongonococcal cervicitis, an accurate diagnosis can only be made by utilizing laboratory tests. The Gram stain is the only acceptable immediate diagnostic aid for the evaluation of potential gonococcal infection [60] and culture for *N. gonorrhoeae* is necessary to obtain a definitive diagnosis.

The Gram Stain

For women, Gram staining of cervical smears is less reliable than urethral smears for men, detecting 55 to 65% of patients who subsequently have positive cultures [42, 60]. Experience of the microscopist reading the smears is the greatest factor in obtaining reliable results. In a recent study, Gram stain sensitivities varied from 15 to 59% for cervical smears [61]. Results were dependent upon the microscopist, with the most accurate results obtained by individuals who read more than 200 slides per week for several years. Specificity of the Gram stain also varies with the experience of the reader. In one report the incidence of false positive smears read by physicians was high (18%) [42]. In another study the incidence of false positive smears among five readers who interpreted the same slides varied from 39 to 0%, with the best results obtained by an experienced reader working in an STD clinic [61]. Since the diagnosis of gonorrhea has tremendous psychosocial as well as epidemiological (contact tracing) implications, the use of the Gram stain outside of an STD clinic for the diagnosis of gonorrhea in women, even by experienced gynecologists, is not recommended, in any case the Gram stain should never be used alone [42].

Culture

Culture, which requires an additional 1 to 2 days for incubation, remains the only definitive method of diagnosing gonococcal cervicitis. In all cases the proper collection, handling, and processing of endocervical specimens are extremely important factors in ensuring accurate results. To obtain an endocervical sample, mucoid material from the cervical portio is first removed with a dry cotton-tipped swab. A second dry, sterile cotton-tipped swab is then inserted approximately 2 to 3 cm into the endocervical canal, moved from side to side, and allowed to remain 10 to 30 sec for absorption of the organisms to the swab. Neither method of contraception nor day of menstrual cycle has a significant influence on the recovery of *N. gonorrhoeae* [62]. The collected specimen is then plated onto selective media for *Neisseria* sp. such as Thayer-Martin or New York city media. The plates are then placed in an incubator set at 35 to 36°C under increased CO_2 tension (see Chap. 16). If processing of the culture is to be delayed or if culture facilities are not available, a holding or transport medium should be used. Goodhart et al. [61] summarize the reported losses with these various systems. For transport via "holding" media such as Stuart's, Aime's, or Culturette, a 10 to 79% loss of isolates after 24 hr can occur; for transport via environmental chamber systems (JEMBEC), a 7 to 22% loss of isolates occurs after 1 day and a 4 to 54% loss after 3 days (weekend) of transport. The use of Transgrow medium has not proven to be very practical [42, 60, 63].

For gonococcal cervicitis, a single cervical culture has been reported to be about 80 to 93% sensitive [42, 64, 65]; however, by combining cervical and rectal cultures taken on two separate occasions, sensitivity to detect gonorrhea increases to greater than 95% [42, 60, 66-68]. Use of the rectal culture adds approximately 5 to 6% of patients infected with *N. gonorrhoeae* [42]. The small percentage of false negative results may be due to vancomycin-susceptible strains. In modified New York City medium, vancomycin is replaced with lincomycin, and Young reported 100% sensivity in a limited number of patients using this medium [69].

Following incubation, suspicious colonies should be Gram-stained and tested for oxidase reactivity. A presumptive diagnosis of gonorrhea made on the basis of oxidase-positive, gram-negative diplococci growing on selective medium is approximately 98% accurate for specimens from the endocervix [60, 70]. Further identification is necessary to provide a definitive diagnosis, and additional testing is needed if isolates are to be screened for penicillinase production.

In STD clinics in England and Wales, Belsey recently reported that 96% of gonococcal infections in women were detected by the first set of Gram-stained smears and cultures [71]. In an STD clinic in the United States, Lossick et al. [72] reported a cervical Gram stain sensitivity of 70%. In this setting, use of the cervical Gram stain combined with epidemiological treatment of potentially exposed patients permitted treatment of 91% of infected women at the initial clinic visit. In a high-volume STD clinic where experienced personnel and state-of-the-art materials are available, such high diagnostic accuracy in women during a single evaluation seems feasible. For less optimal situations, diagnostic accuracy decreases owing to many factors. Physicians should appreciate the limitations of endocervical smears and cultures in their practices when interpreting test results.

Other Tests

To improve the detection and/or exclusion of gonococcal infections, many tests have been developed and evaluated. Serological tests have been the most widely studied and have included complement fixation, hemagglutination, immunofluorescence, latex agglutination, flocculation, radioimmunoassay, and the enzyme-linked immunosorbent assay [73, 74]. The antigens most frequently employed were gonococcal pili. Unfortunately, results varied considerably between tests, and the positive and negative predictive values were low [75-80]. In addition, a positive test on a single serum sample may be due to past infection. Thus these serological tests have not been practical for single-case diagnosis.

Recent studies have focused on detecting gonococcal antigen in cervical secretions using gonococcal antibodies. Gonozyme enzyme-linked immunosorbent assay is a solid-phase procedure used for detecting gonococcal antigens in clinical specimens. Such an assay requires sophisticated and costly equipment and involves many procedural steps. Thus it may only have utility in large laboratories and STD clinics. Preliminary reports show that the test's sensitivity varies according to the patient group tested (i.e., gonorrhea contacts and prostitutes), with sensitivities ranging from 81 to 92% [81, 82]. Other antigen detection tests which utilize monoclonal antibodies have been studied and may provide quick and accurate results in the near future [83].

A genetic transformation test was developed and evaluated on mailed clinical samples [84, 85]. (see also Chap. 3). While the published results look promising, such a test on mailed clinical samples suffers from lack of utility, long turnaround time, and excessive cost [86].

Excluding an STD and assuring patients that they are not infected are at least as important as making the proper diagnosis for infected patients [87]. Recently Spagna et al. [44] reported that the *Limulus* amebocyte lysate assay (see Chap. 3) has a negative predictive value of 100% for excluding gonococcal cervicitis. *Limulus* amebocyte lysate assays were performed on endocervical samples taken with depyrogenated cotton-tipped swabs, and results were available within 30 min. Such a procedure was designed for in-office use and as a screening test to exclude the possibility of gonococcal cervicitis. Since there are over 8 million screening cultures performed each year in the United States, with only about 4.5% positive for *N. gonorrhoeae* [25], such a test may prove beneficial; however, further studies are needed to demonstrate the utility of the *Limulus* amebocyte lysate assay as a screening test to exclude cervical gonorrhea.

Treatment

Women with uncomplicated gonococcal infection are treated with the same drug regimens as those recommended for men [88] (see also Chap. 3). Recommended regimens in the United States include (1) tetracycline HCl (500 mg, by mouth, four times daily for 7 days); (2) doxycycline hyclate (100 mg, by mouth, twice daily for 7 days); (3) amoxicillin (3.0 g) or ampicillin (3.5 g), either with 1.0 g probenecid by mouth; or (4) aqueous procaine penicillin G (4.8 million units given intramuscularly with 1.0 g of probenecid by mouth). Combined regimens of amoxicillin or ampicillin plus tetracycline can be used to cover coexisting chlamydial infection [88].

For pregnant women the drug regimen of choice is amoxicillin (3.0 g) or ampicillin (3.5 g), each with probenecid (1.0 g) [88]. Pregnant women who are allergic to penicillin or probenecid should be treated with 2.0 g spectinomycin, intramuscularly. Erythromycin, 500 mg by mouth four times daily on an empty stomach for at least 7 days, can be added to treat coexistent chlamydial infection. For patients who cannot tolerate this erythromycin regimen, a decreased dose of 250 mg by mouth four times daily for at least 14 days should be used; however, the optimal dose and duration of therapy for pregnant women have not been established [88]. Tetracycline should not be used in pregnant women because of potential adverse effects for the fetus. Additionally, all patients treated for gonorrhea should have a serological test for syphilis.

Follow-up cultures, including rectal cultures, should be obtained 4 to 7 days after completion of therapy. For patients in whom gonorrhea persists after treatment with one of the nonspectinomycin regimens, 2.0 g of spectinomycin should be given intramuscularly. Recurrent gonococcal infections after treatment may be due to reinfection or infection with a PPNG strain. Thus all post-treatment isolates should be tested for penicillinase production [88]. Patients with positive cultures after spectinomycin therapy should be treated with cefoxitin (2.0 g intramuscularly plus 1.0 g probenecid) or cefotaxime (1.0 g intramuscularly without probenecid) [88].

All sexual partners of women with gonorrhea should be examined, cultured, and treated at once with one of the regimens for uncomplicated gonococcal infection in adults [88].

In the United States epidemiological treatment of gonorrhea is recommended for all patients exposed to gonorrhea [43, 88]. Epidemiological treatment refers to the use of antibiotic therapy when a diagnosis is considered likely but before confirmatory culture results are obtained [43], and treatment regimens recommended are the same as those for laboratory-confirmed uncomplicated gonorrhea [88]. Such an approach seems warranted because (1) prevalence of gonorrhea in women exposed to gonorrhea is high, (2) rapid methods to evaluate women at the time of their presentation are lacking, and (3) serious complications can occur in patients with undetected and untreated gonorrhea.

However, with epidemiological treatment, individuals not infected also receive therapy, and it is estimated they constitute 21 to 47% of those seeking treatment because of exposure [43]. Treatment of the uninfected (1) needlessly exposes patients to adverse effects of antibiotics, (2) is an unjustified expense, (3) raises the dilemma as to the management of sexual partners, (4) fosters return visits by many patients for therapy to relieve their anxieties, (5) may promote selection of antibiotic-resistant bacteria, and (6) subjects many patients to the psychosocial discomfort of being treated for a venereal disease [43, 87, 89]. In England, Belsey suggests that in view of modern culture techniques and the low default rates among patients attending STD clinics, there is little justification for the use of epidemiological treatment of gonorrhea in this setting [89].

For prevention of gonococcal infection, prophylactic treatment is not recommended [43]. As for vaccines, the development of an effective gonococcal vaccine has not yet been successful. Gonococcal pili, principal outer membrane proteins, a capsule, and lipopolysaccharide are structures currently under study [90, 91].

CHLAMYDIAL CERVICITIS

Etiology

Chlamydial cervicitis is caused by *C. trachomatis*, a member of the genus *Chlamydia*. This genus consists of two species, *C. trachomatis* and *Chlamydia psittaci*, which share certain characteristics such as morphology and a strict requirement for intracellular growth in susceptible cells. The major characteristics differentiating the two species are sulfonamide susceptibility and the formation of distinct inclusion granula in the host cells [92, 93]. *Chlamydia trachomatis* includes (1) the trachoma/inclusion conjunctivitis agents, subdivided into serogroups A to K; (2) the lymphogranuloma venereum agents, subdivided into serogroups (L1 to 3); and (3) the mouse pneumonitis agent.

Chlamydiae are characterized by a special growth cycle involving a characteristic two-stage infection and replication process. The infective form of *Chlamydia* is the elementary body, which can survive extracellularly. The elementary body stimulates phagocytosis by the host cell and then transforms into the reticulate body within the cell. The reticulate body forms small buds which subdivide by simple fission to produce several reticulate bodies within the host cell. The reticulate body then transforms back into the infective elementary body before liberation from the host cell, thereby completing the growth cycle [93]. The chlamydiae are deficient in independent energy metabolism and obtain their supply of ATP and essential building blocks from the host cell cytoplasm. Because *C. trachomatis* is an obligate intracellular parasite, it must be grown in tissue cell cultures using specially treated McCoy cells [94].

Chlamydia trachomatis is primarily a human pathogen. Serogroups A, B, and C usually cause ocular disease, whereas serogroups D to K are primarily involved in genital infections [93]. Intimate contact is required for passage of the infecting particle into the host cell.

Epidemiology

The prevalence of chlamydial cervicitis equals or exceeds the prevalence of gonococcal cervicitis. In Sweden, where cultures for *C. trachomatis* are routine, 3794 consecutive women attending a gynecological outpatient clinic during 1978 with symptoms of lower genital infection were screened for chlamydial and gonococcal infection. *Chlamydia trachomatis* was isolated from 9.2% and *N. gonorrhoeae* from 2.2% [95]. In another study women aged 15 to 24 years were found to comprise the group at greatest risk, and genital chlamydial infection was about four times as common as gonorrhea [96]. Hansson and Danielsson summarized the reported findings of the prevalence of chlamydial infection in the Scandinavian countries [97]. The isolation rate of *C. trachomatis* was (1) 5% in women consulting for general health reasons, (2) 8% in women consulting for contraceptive advice, (3) 9% in women attending a gynecological outpatient clinic, (4) 4 to 9% in puerperal women, (5) 16% in women applying for legal abortion, (6) 16 to 38% in women attending STD clinics, (7) 19% in women with symptoms of lower genital tract infection, and (8) 47 to 66% in women who were sexual partners of men with known chlamydial infection. *Chlamydia trachomatis* was also found to be a concomitant infection with *N. gonorrhoeae* in 19 to 29% of cases [97]. In England 474 women attending a hospital clinic in 1978 and 1979 were cultured for chlamydial infection. *Chlamydia trachomatis* was isolated from (1) 33.3% of all women, (2) 48.3% of women with concomitant gonococcal infection, (3) 43% of women whose sexual partners had nongonococcal urethritis, and (4) 74% of women whose sexual partners were infected with *C. trachomatis* [98]. For pregnant women attending an STD clinic in 1981, 31.8% harbored *C. trachomatis*, in contrast to the isolation rate of 0 to 16% in pregnant women in non-STD clinics [99]. In promiscuous women *C. trachomatis* was isolated from the cervix of 33% of women who admitted to two or more casual sexual contacts, in contrast to 3% who admitted to only one casual contact in the preceding month [100]. In Scotland *C. trachomatis* was isolated from the cervix in 20.4% of women attending a department of genitourinary medicine clinic in 1980 [101]. In Canada *C. trachomatis* was isolated from 23.5% of women attending an STD clinic [102]. In the United States *C. trachomatis* was isolated from 20% of 2000 women who attended an STD clinic during 1983 (M. Smeltzer, personal communication, 1983).

The many factors which contribute to the high prevalence of chlamydial cervicitis are similar to those listed for gonococcal cervicitis. The most important element in disease transmission is the asymptomatic carrier. Chlamydial cervicitis is often subtle, and infected women may not have signs or symptoms of infection [96, 103]. In addition to young age and level of sexual activity, the use of oral contraceptives and the presence of cervical ectopy are other important risk factors for *C. trachomatis* infection [103].

The risk of transmitting genital *C. trachomatis* may be less than that of genital gonorrhea. Lycke et al. [104] found that for women who were sexual partners of men infected only with *C. trachomatis,* 47% had chlamydial infections. In contrast, 80% of women with sexual partners infected only with *N. gonorrhoeae* had gonococcal infection. In other studies [98, 103], however, the isolation rate of *C. trachomatis* was 19 to 27% higher than the 47% reported by Lycke et al. [104]. Because of the many variables associated with chlamydial cultures and the complicated dynamics of disease transmission, further studies are needed to determine the comparative risks of transmitting chlamydial and gonococcal infections.

Clinical Manifestations

The clinical signs and symptoms of chlamydial cervicitis are similar to those noted in patients with gonococcal cervicitis. Since chlamydial cervicitis can also produce little or nothing by way of symptoms, its natural history in women is also a tale of latency, complications, chronicity, and disability.

The major site of chlamydial infection in women is the cervix, although many also harbor chlamydiae in the urethra [103, 105]. During sexual intercourse with an infected male, chlamydiae infect the cervix and grow within columnar epithelial cells. Quantitative studies have shown that cervical samples yield high inclusion counts on inoculated McCoy cell cover slips (⩾120 inclusions per 12-mm cover slip) in 45% of women with chlamydial cervicitis [106]. Female consorts of men with high counts also had high counts, but, overall, high inclusion counts were obtained significantly more often from men than from women. High counts were significantly associated with the presence of ectopy, with very high counts (⩾4500) being found more frequently in patients whose ectopy was hypertrophic. The distribution of inclusion counts in women was not affected by age, marital status, or stage of menstrual cycle [106].

Following establishment of infection, many patients may have neither symptoms nor signs of cervicitis [103]. In one study 49% of *Chlamydia*-positive patients denied any symptoms [105]. Vaginal discharge was noted as the presenting symptom in 32% of the *Chlamydia*-positive patients, with abdominal pain and urinary symptoms each comprising 4% of the cases. In another study 33% of *Chlamydia*-positive patients were totally asymptomatic [103]. Complaints such as urethral symptoms (dysuria/frequency), abnormal vaginal discharge, and abdominal pain were significantly more common among infected patients than among those who were culture negative for *C. trachomatis*. The urethra can also become infected and *C. trachomatis* can be a causative agent in acute urethral (dysuria-pyuria) syndrome [103] (see also Chap. 9).

On physical examination, the infected cervix can appear perfectly healthy or show various degrees of cervicitis. In many cases chalmydial cervicitis is characterized by a hypertrophic follicular appearance, with severe edema, erythema, friability, and endocervical mucopurulent discharge [103]. Of patients with clinically observed cervicitis, 70% were found to have positive cultures for *C. trachomatis* [103]. On the other hand, 22% of the *Chlamydia*-positive women presented with clinically normal cervices [103]. Rees et al. [105] also isolated *C. trachomatis* from cervices exhibiting no clinical signs of infection; however, a higher isolation rate was associated with hypertrophic erosion and endocervical mucopurulent discharge.

Colposcopic examination can be useful in evaluating women with clinically observed cervicitis. Paavonen et al. [107] found exophytic follicular cervicitis in 73% of women with *C. trachomatis*-associated cervicitis. In age-matched controls with nonspecific cervicitis, these findings were absent. An atypical transformation zone was found to occur significantly more often in patients with chlamydial cervicitis [103, 107]. Specific changes observed with the colposcope included white epithelium, punctation, mosaic pattern, leukoplakia, and atypical blood vessels [103]. Because of the frequent association between chlamydial cervicitis and an atypical transformation zone, Paavonen et al. [107] suggest that colposcopic practices be incorporated in STD clinics.

Cytological atypias are also significantly more common in patients with chlamydial infections. Several studies have shown a possible role of *C. trachomatis* in the development of cervical intraepithelial neoplasia [103, 108-110]. While both local (IgA) and humoral (IgG, IgA) antibodies to *C. trachomatis* are produced during chlamydial cervicitis [111]; patients with cervical dysplasia have higher concentrations of chlamydial IgA antibodies in cervical secretions than patients with cervicitis or uninfected controls [112]. In addition, a majority of patients with cervical dysplasia have been shown to have humoral antibodies against *C. trachomatis* [108]. Similarly, increased serum levels of chlamydial antibodies were noted in patients with cervical dysplasia [109]. Thus there appears to be a strong association with chlamydial infections and premalignant or malignant changes of the cervix. Whether this association is etiological or perhaps connected with some other coincidental factors such as differences in sexual behavior is unclear [112]. Researchers have speculated that in the pathogenesis of cervical carcinoma, intracellular (perhaps non infectious) chlamydial antigens might persist in cervical parabasal cells, giving rise later to malignant changes, possibly interfering with host cell DNA [112]. While this seems feasible, further research is needed to resolve this issue. It is suggested that future studies of patients with cytological atypias should include tests for *C. trachomatis* [103].

Undetected and untreated chlamydial cervicitis can persist for up to a year or longer, and various clinical manifestations and complications can occur. Among these are (1) urethritis, (2) acute urethral syndrome, (3) endometritis, (4) acute PID, (5) perihepatitis, (6) sexually acquired reactive arthritis (Reiter's syndrome), and (7) eye infections in adults (usually acquired by autoinoculation from a concomitant genital infection) [113]. Infections can also be transferred to nearly 50% of all infants born to mothers infected with *C. trachomatis* [113] (see also Chap. 15).

Diagnosis

Symptoms of chlamydial cervicitis and clinical examination do not often provide a presumptive diagnosis of chlamydial infection. In many cases there may be no symptoms or signs of infection. While some studies suggest that follicular cervicitis is characteristic of chlamydial cervicitis and mucopurulent discharge, edema, erythema, and friability are features of *C. trachomatis* infections, a definitive diagnosis can only be made by utilizing laboratory tests. Such tests include various microscopical, cultural, and serological procedures. In all suspected cases of cervicitis, the presence or absence of *N. gonorrhoeae* must also be determined.

Microscopic Tests

Direct microscopic examination of stained cervical specimens has not been practical owing to poor sensitivity of the test. While high sensitivity (95%) was noted on samples from conjunctivitis of the newborn, sensitivities of only 41 and 66% have been reported for Giemsa and fluorescent-antibody-stained cervical specimens, respectively [114]. However, recent use of monoclonal antibodies has greatly improved the sensitivity of direct specimen tests. With fluorescent-labeled monoclonal antibodies, a sensitivity of 90% has been reported with a concomitant specificity of 98% when compared to cell culture [115]. A commercial test (MicroTrak, *C. trachomatis* Direct Specimen Test) detects elementary bodies in clinical samples, allowing a diagnosis based on the direct evaluation of infected cervical specimens, and results are available within 30 min after receipt of the specimen in the laboratory. In a female population with a 5% prevalence of chlamydial cervicitis, the positive and negative predictive values of the fluorescein-labeled monoclonal antibody stain would be 70.3 and 99.5%, respectively.

The use of Papanicolaou-stained cervical smears to diagnose chlamydial cervicitis has not been a reliable procedure [116]. Significant overlap exists between the cytological abnormalities seen in connection with cervical inflammation due to *C. trachomatis* and inflammation due to other causes.

Cell Culture

The only definitive way to diagnose chlamydial cervicitis is by cell culture. Since chlamydiae are obligate intracellular bacteria, tissue cultures are required. The successful use of chlamydial cultures depends upon the proper collection, handling, and processing of cervical specimens. To obtain an endocervical sample, the mucoid material from the ectocervix should be removed to reduce contamination. Cotton-tipped swabs on aluminum or plastic shafts should be used to collect the sample, as alginate-tipped swabs and wooden shafts have a toxic effect on chlamydiae [117, 118]. The swab should be inserted into the endocervical canal approximately 2 to 3 cm and rubbed vigorously against the mucosa. When culturing for *C. trachomatis*, adequate specimen collection requires retrieval of cellular material rather than merely body fluids. The collected specimens should be placed in a sucrose-phosphate buffer which contains fetal calf serum or albumin and various antimicrobial agents [117] and then transported to the laboratory for culture. Kallings and Mårdh have shown that specimens can be stored in the sucrose-phosphate buffer transport medium for as long as 2 days at room temperature and for 4 days at 4°C with no appreciable loss of viability of the organisms [118]. In the laboratory the specimens are inoculated onto irradiated or cycloheximide-treated McCoy cells [119]. Following incubation for 2 to 3 days, the monolayers are stained with iodine, Giemsa, or fluorescent antibody reagents and examined for chlamydial inclusions. The sensitivity of cell culture for detecting chlamydial cervicitis is 75 to 80%, with a specificity of 100% [119]. Use of fluorescein-labeled monoclonal antibodies increases sensitivity significantly on the first passage, and results can be obtained in 48 hr [120]. A commercial monoclonal antibody test (MicroTrak, *C. trachomatis* Culture Confirmation Test) is now available. When culturing the cervix for *C. trachomatis*, it is recommended that the urethra also be cultured.

Since cost for chlamydial cultures is high, clinicians should exercise informed judgment when deciding the need for these cultures. Recommendations for chlamydial cultures may be found in Chapter 16. An excellent review on sampling, specimen handling, and isolation techniques in the diagnosis of chlamydial infections may be found in an article by Mårdh et al. [121].

Other Tests

The detection of antibodies to *C. trachomatis* by the microimmunofluorescence test has been of value in certain chlamydial infections such as epididymitis, PID, and neonatal pneumonia. Additionally, serological methods are important in the study of the epidemiology and pathogenesis of *C. trachomatis.*; however, their application in clinical diagnosis has not been too successful [122]. The complement fixation test, using the chlamydial group antigen, is the least sensitive and specific method. Further research is needed to evaluate the diagnostic value of the detection of antibodies in cervical secretions of *Chlamydia*-infected individuals [122].

Treatment

Women with chlamydial cervicitis are treated with the same drug regimens as those recommended for men with nongonococcal urethritis [88] (see also Chap. 3). Drug regimens of choice in the United States include (1) tetracycline HCl (500 mg, by mouth, four times daily for at least 7 days) and (2) doxycycline hyclate (100 mg, by mouth, twice daily for at least 7 days). An alternate regimen for patients in whom tetracyclines are contraindicated or not tolerated is erythromycin, 500 mg, by mouth, four times daily for at least 7 days [88]. Pregnant women should be treated with erythromycin and not tetracyclines.

Follow-up cultures for *C. trachomatis* are advisable. However, positive cultures may not be detectable until 3 to 6 weeks after treatment [88]. When follow-up cultures are positive for *C. trachomatis*, patients should be treated again with one of the recommended regimens for uncomplicated endocervical infection in adults. Poor response to recommended therapy may indicate noncompliance, organism resistance, reinfection, or complicated disease.

All sexual partners of women with chlamydial infection and all women exposed to men with chlamydial infection should be examined for STDs and promptly treated for exposure to *C. trachomatis* with one of the recommended regimens for uncomplicated urethral, endocervical, or rectal infections in adults [88].

For prevention of chlamydial cervicitis, condoms have been shown to be an effective barrier when used properly [123]. There are currently no effective vaccines for the prevention of chlamydial infection.

HERPETIC CERVICITIS

Etiology

Herpetic cervicitis is caused by herpes simplex virus (HSV), a member of the herpesvirus group. These viruses contain double-stranded DNA and are icosahedral viruses surrounded by a glycoprotein envelope. The diameter of the enveloped virion is approximately 180 nm. There are two distinct types of HSV – type 1 (HSV-1) and type 2 (HSV-2) – which are distinguishable by biochemical, immunological, and serological methods. Both types of HSV can cause genital disease, including herpetic cervicitis; however, HSV-2 is responsible for the vast majority of primary and recurrent genital infections.

Epidemiology

In the United States the incidence and prevalence of HSV genital infections are only rough estimates, since there is no systemized reporting to the Public Health Service. A recent survey of private physicians in the United States indicated that patient consultations for HSV genital infections increased from 3.4 per 100,000 in 1960 to 29.7 per 100,000 population in 1979 [124]. A conservative estimate of the total number of new cases of genital HSV infections annually is 500,000, with the prevalence of genital disease being 10 million. In England the number of reported HSV infections for 1980 was 9281, a 5.6% increase from the previous year. Genital infections with HSV are most commonly encountered in sexually active teenagers and young adults, with a substantial representation from the higher socioeconomic groups [125].

Clinical Manifestations

Cervical HSV involvement has been the subject of intensive research regarding sexual transmission, neonatal infection via vertical transmission, and its oncogenic potential. Herpes simplex virus cervical infection is present in 80 to 88% of women with primary genital infections and in 65% of nonprimary (serological evidence of previous herpesvirus infection existent) first-episode HSV-2 infections. During episodes of recurrent genital lesions, HSV cervical shedding occurs in approximately 12% of cases [126]. As opposed to the commonly reported symptoms, including painful ulcers, pruritus, and dysuria, accompanying genital HSV infection, there are usually no symptoms associated with isolated HSV infection of the cervix. A few patients will report the presence of an abnormal vaginal discharge or intermenstrual spotting, and HSV has been isolated from the urethra or cervix in 5% of patients with symptoms of the urethral syndrome (dysuria, frequency) [126, 127]. Clinically, the HSV-infected cervix is visually abnormal in the vast majority (89%) of women during first-episode infections. Ulcerative lesions can involve any portion of the cervix, in conjunction with diffuse friability and a severe purulent cervicitis. Cervical HSV titers range from 10^4 to 10^6 PFU, and viral shedding occurs over a 10 to 12-day period [126]. In contrast, Guinan et al. [128] did not observe any visible abnormalities of the cervix during a longitudinal study of 27 women with recurrent HSV genital infection. A total of 138 pelvic examinations were performed, 74 of which coincided with the presence of external genital lesions. Despite the normal visual appearance of the cervix, HSV shedding from the cervix was documented in 33% of patients during recurrent episodes and in 4% between recurrences. Titers of all positive cervical cultures were less than 10 PFU, and viral shedding lasted only a few days, suggesting a reduced potential of disease transmission via the cervix in these situations. Asymptomatic cervical shedding has also been documented by other investigators both in recurrent HSV genital disease and in the absence of genital signs or symptoms [129, 130]. Vontver et al. [131] investigated recurrent HSV infection patterns in 80 pregnant women. Of 199 total recurrences (112 HSV culture positive), there were 13 asymptomatic episodes. Five episodes were associated with only asymptomatic cervical HSV shedding, two having simultaneous cervical and vulvar HSV shedding, and six with asymptomatic shedding only from the external genitalia. The overall rate of asymptomatic cervical shedding during pregnancy was 0.66%, and a similar isolation rate (0.75%) was noted from labial specimens taken at times during which neither the patient nor the examiner noted clinical lesions.

Complications

Cervical HSV infection has been linked to an increased risk of spontaneous abortion and premature delivery [132]. Contrary evidence regarding HSV infection and these complications requires that further studies be performed to clarify these issues.

Congenital HSV infections (fetal malformations due to utrauterine infections during embryogenesis) are rare, and the evidence that transplacental transmission occurs is limited to a small number of case reports. The more likely outcome of transplacental infection during the early stages of pregnancy would be spontaneous abortion [133, 134]. There is no benefit from amniocentesis in predicting the presence or absence of a congenitally infected infant [126, 134].

Neonatal HSV infection is a complication of ascending infection prior to delivery (following rupture of the membranes) or a result of direct contact with infectious maternal genital surfaces during delivery. The incidence of newborn infection is estimated to be 1 per 3500 to 1 per 30,000 live births [135]. While the greatest predictable hazard to the newborn has been felt to occur in women with initial (as opposed to recurrent) disease during the last trimester of pregnancy, recent studies of neonatal HSV infections have shown that a majority (70%) of infants are born to mothers without signs or symptoms of disease [136]. The fact that both vulvar and cervical asymptomatic shedding of HSV occurs frequently during pregnancy indicates the necessity for routine HSV cultures, regardless of clinical parameters, at or near term [131]. The overall risk of neonatal HSV infection is approximately 10% with vaginal delivery during active maternal HSV infection. However, the range of risk varies considerably and is dependent upon primary genital (40 to 50% neonatal transmission) versus recurrent genital (3 to 5% neonatal transmission) maternal infection [126, 135, 137]. Immunological and environmental factors have also been considered in assessing risk of neonatal HSV infection; however, these parameters need further evaluation in defining their contribution to HSV neonatal infection [133]. Routine monitoring of high-risk pregnancies should include weekly cervical and vulvar cultures for HSV starting at the eighth month of pregnancy [126, 131]. About 1 in 200 to 1 in 2000 women will be found with HSV in the cervix or other genital sites at or near the time of delivery [135]. Cesarean section has been documented to reduce the likelihood of neonatal HSV infection by preventing perinatal viral transfer at parturition [126, 131, 134]. Cesarean section is not an innocuous procedure and should be considered only for those women with clinical or laboratory evidence of HSV shedding at or near the time of delivery [134]. In the past, cesarean section was not recommended if membranes were ruptured for more than 4 to 6 h in the presence of active lesions [132, 138]. Since cervical HSV shedding occurs in only a limited number (2 to 30%) of women with recurrent genital disease, cesarean section should be performed in appropriate situations, regardless of the duration of ruptured membranes [126, 131]. In the absence of cervical shedding, the infant would not be exposed to infected genital secretions until the late stages of labor. Multiple pelvic examinations should be avoided during labor, and monitoring procedures involving trauma to the fetus should be utilized only when absolutely necessary [126, 131].

While the role of HSV cervical infection in its relationship to neonatal disease is firmly established, there is still considerable debate concerning the role of HSV infection in the genesis of cervical malignancy [139, 130]. The evidence for an association between HSV and cervicocarcinoma is supported by a considerable body of published literature, including the cultural isolation of HSV-2 from cervical carcinoma cells [141] the demonstration of HSV-2 antigens in human premalignant and malignant cervical cells and tissue biopsies [142, 143]; and the detection of two HSV-2 proteins in the sera of cervical cancer patients which appear to be tumor specific [144]. Seroepidemiological studies [145] have established a statistically significant relationship between HSV-2 cervical infection and neoplastic disease; Kalimo et al. [112] detected local IgA antibodies to HSV in the cervical secretions in 10 to 35 (28%) patients with malignant or premalignant changes of the cervix, but these antibodies were absent in cervicitis cases or normal controls. Graham et al. [146] reported that the presence of HSV-2 antibodies detected by radioimmunoassay was accompanied by an increase in the risk of cervical cancer independent from the number of sex partners. Barton et al. [147] pointed out the similar rates of cervical isolation of HSV-1 and HSV-2 and hypothesized a role for HSV-1 in the etiology of cervical carcinogenesis.

There is a need for well-controlled longitudinal studies with long-term follow-up and clarification of the vague cause-effect relationship between HSV cervical infection and carcinoma. The recent appreciation of other cervical pathogens (cytomegalovirus, papillomavirus, *C. trachomatis*) with oncogenic potential may alter current concepts of HSV's contribution to cervical malignant changes [148].

Diagnosis

While the presence of characteristic signs and symptoms allows a fairly accurate clinical diagnosis of genital HSV infection, the normal appearance of the cervix in conjunction with HSV cervicitis demands that laboratory tests be utilized to make a diagnosis [128, 129, 131]. Viral isolation on tissue culture represents the optimal method for establishing the diagnosis of HSV cervical infection and is the standard against which other methods are compared. Tissue cultures should be examined over a period of 10 days to categorically exclude the possibility of HSV, since viral titers from cervical specimens are low during recurrent or asymptomatic shedding [128]. The low numbers of infective virions are associated with prolonged incubation periods to produce characteristic cytopathic changes in vitro [134]. A variety of staining techniques have been applied to tissue cultures in order to reduce the time required for the detection of HSV [149]. Serological tests have been developed which employ monoclonal antibody enzyme-linked immunosorbent assay procedures to distinguish between HSV-1 and HSV-2 antibodies [150, 151]. Serological studies in cases of HSV infection require careful interpretation and have limited usefulness in nonprimary first episodes and recurrent disease [152]. Rapid diagnostic techniques applied directly to clinical samples (cytological examination, immunoperoxidase and immunofluorescent tests) are useful if adequate specimens are obtained from early genital lesions, but they are still less sensitive than viral isolation [152, 153].

Prevention

There is no absolute way of preventing HSV transmission during periods of asymptomatic cervical shedding; however, the results of in vitro studies suggest that undamaged, unlubricated condoms provide an effective physical barrier against HSV transmission, especially during those periods of asymptomatic HSV cervical shedding [123, 152]. The anxiety and despair associated with an incurable illness like HSV infection can be successfully counterbalanced by instructing the patients on how they can actively participate in the prevention of HSV complications and transmission. Women should be informed of the epidemiological association between HSV cervical infection and carcinoma of the cervix, and the importance of having yearly cytological testing of the cervix. They should also be made aware of the potential dangers of neonatal infection and the necessity of informing their physicians early in the course of pregnancy.

Finally, the physician should strive to maintain a current appreciation of advances in HSV research, especially regarding the development of effective vaccines against HSV transmission [154].

OTHER IMPORTANT MICROBIAL CERVICAL PATHOGENS

Cytomegalovirus

Cytomegalovirus (CMV) is a member of the herpesvirus group and shares the group's traits of latency, recurrent disease, and oncogenic potential. It is an enveloped, double-stranded DNA virus which measures 180 to 250 nm in diameter. Cytomegalovirus infection of the uterine cervix is relatively common in sexually active women, and the cervix probably represents an important reservoir for venereal and neonatal transmission of infection. Positive endocervical cultures have been obtained from as many as 14% of women in selected populations [155]. Among women evaluated at STD clinics, Willmott [156] reported a cervical CMV isolation rate of 6.6% (35 of 531 women) and Waner et al. [157] reported an 8.3% (10 of 121 women) CMV isolation rate from the cervix. Risk factors for CMV infection of the cervix include pregnancy, lower socioeconomic status, and young (teenager) age [155]. Viral shedding from the cervix may range from being brief and intermittent to prolonged and continuous. Neutralizing secretory IgA antibodies have been discovered in cervical secretions; however, their appearance and concentration are not correlated with cessation of viral excretion [157].

The majority of primary and recurrent CMV infections produce asymptomatic disease in adults, a few patients exhibiting a mononucleosis-like syndrome [158]. The clinical manifestations vary from absent or minimal findings to extensive cervical erosion. The hallmark of CMV infection (characteristic intranuclear and intracytoplasmic inclusions) is rarely evident in cervical biopsies; therefore recovery of CMV is dependent upon culture [159]. Chiang et al. [160] noted that the overall cultural recovery from cervical biopsy was twice as likely as from cervical swabs; however, for the individual patient, biopsies and swabs were both necessary to obtain the greatest CMV recovery. Cell cultures (human fibroblasts) inoculated with virus-containing material will show specific cytopathic effect in 3 or 4 days, or 1 to 2 weeks, depending on the concentration of virus in the specimen [155].

There are two major concerns relating to cervical CMV infection: (1) malignant transformation and (2) neonatal transmission. The oncogenic potential of CMV, a property of all herpesviruses, has been the basis of theories linking cervical infection with the subsequent development of cancer [161]. There is no absolute evidence to substantiate a cause-effect relationship between CMV infection and cervical neoplasia. There is an association between the later stages of pregnancy and CMV cervical shedding in young (under 25 years of age), primiparous women [155]. Among infants whose mothers were shedding CMV from the cervix during the second or third trimester, the infection rates were 12.5 and 37%, respectively. In neonates whose mothers were active CMV cervical shedders at birth, the infection rate was 57% [162]. The severe consequences of congenital (transplacental) CMV infection have not been attributed to the acquisition of disease during perinatal passage through an infected cervical canal [155]. A subclinical infection with no long-term deleterious effects is the rule for these infants; therefore CMV endocervicitis does not indicate a threat to subsequent offspring as does HSV endocervicitis.

Papillomavirus

Genital warts are caused by human papillomavirus (HPV), a member of the papovavirus group. The virology of HPV has been difficult to analyze because it cannot be propagated in cell culture. Recently, multiple strains of HPV have been found to exist, and their specific relationships to clinical syndromes are current topics of investigation [163]. Genital warts, condyloma acuminatum, have been reported with increasing frequency over the last 15 years. From 1966 to 1981, office-based private physicians in the United States noted a 684% increase in the number of women evaluated for genital warts. In 1981, 463,220 women were seen in consultation for genital warts by private physicians in the United States [164]. In England the reported number of women with diagnosed genital warts approached 10,000 for the year 1980 [165].

Cervical HPV infection is characterized by distinct cytological changes (koilocytosis, dyskeratosis, nuclear atypia) and is clinically recognized as a fleshy, exophytic growth [166]. Recently, cervical disease associated with HPV infection has been described in the absence of visible "wartlike" growths. These inconspicuous cervical lesions have been called "flat" or "endophytic" condylomata and are visualized only by colposcopy [167]. It is now apparent that HPV infection of the cervix can occur in the absence of vulvar disease and affects as many as 1% of women [167, 168]. Walker et al. [169] reported that 20 (40%) of 50 women with vulvar warts had cervical changes indicative of HPV infection; however, only 6 patients had exophytic lesions, while 14 had no evidence of HPV infection by naked eye examination of the cervix. These subclinical cervical lesions have a distinct and characteristic cytology (cellular hypertrophy, bi- or multinucleation, hyperchromasia, perinuclear clearing, amphophilia, and dyskeratotic changes) which closely resembles cervical intraepithelial neoplasia [166]. Upon reexamining the cytology of 152 patients previously considered to have mild dysplasia, Meisels and Fortin [166] revised 70% of these diagnoses to that of occult wart virus infection. Of the 50 women with vulvar warts studied by Walker et al. [169], 18 (36%) had cervical abnormalities consistent with cervical intraepithelial neoplasia 1 or 2. A recent report tested the hypothesis that these endophytic HPV cervical lesions were precancerous by studying their prevalence in women treated surgically for invasive or preinvasive cervical neoplasia and a matched control group. A highly significant statistical relationship existed between subclinical HPV infection and cervical malignancy: 73 of 80 women (91%) with cervical neoplasia versus 10 of 80 matched controls (12.5%) [170]. It is premature at this time to conclude that a causal relationship between HPV and cervical neoplasia exists. Coinciding risk factors must be considered and longitudinal epidemiological surveys should demonstrate a relationship between HPV infection and cervical cancer. Presently it is advisable that all women with genital warts or whose sex partners have genital warts have annual cervical cytological examinations. Persistently abnormal Papanicolaou-stained smears should prompt further evaluation by colposcopy.

Group B Streptococcus

The colonization of the cervix with group B streptococci (GBS), *Streptococcus agalacticae*, has its primary importance in relationship to serious disease (meningitis, septicemia, pneumonitis) in the neonate. The prevalence of GBS at any time between conception and delivery is 5 to 25%, and the offspring of colonized mothers harbor the organisms in various sites [171]. Infections develop in approximately 1% of colonized infants [172]; the clinical manifestations being variable and described in detail in Chapter 15. Group B streptococci will account for approximately 15,000 newborn infections annually in the United States [173]. Prospective data from England and reports from other countries suggest that GBS disease may be less common in other parts of the world.

Group B streptococcus is not confined to the cervix, the organism actually being isolated more frequently from the periurethral [171] and perineal-anorectal areas [174, 175]. The possible role of sexual transmission in the spread of

GBS has been extensively researched. There is a high prevalence of GBS carriage among patients attending STD clinics, the isolation rate in women being approximately 40% [175,176].

The male partners of GBS-colonized women have been found to harbor GBS of the same serotype in a significant number of cases [172,177]; however, Jackson et al. [175] reported that only 15% (3 of 20) of couples, where both partners harbored GBS, had identical serotypes and phage types. It has been suggested that female genital colonization with GBS is via the ingress of perineal bacteria, a process promoted by intercourse [171]. A longitudinal prospective study of GBS carriage during pregnancy concluded that the intestinal tract was the primary reservoir for GBS and the likely source of genital colonization in pregnant women [174]. The value of prenatal screening in the identification of GBS carriers has been considered limited in importance, since approximately one-half of prenatal genital carriers will self-eradicate the organism, while an equal number of culture-negative individuals will harbor GBS at or near term [174,178]. One contradictory study found that 90% of all GBS carriers at labor were positive in the first half of pregnancy, and only 7% of women negative at 16 to 20 weeks of pregnancy became persistent GBS carriers in follow-up [179].

Measures for the prevention of GBS carriage and disease have been proposed [180] and include (1) actively immunizing women with capsular polysaccharide antigens of GBS to stimulate type-specific IgG antibody for transplacental protection of the fetus, (2) passively immunizing high-risk infants with type-specific IgG antibody, and (3) administration of intrapartum antibiotics (intravenous ampicillin) to GBS-colonized mothers. There is considerable debate concerning the routine use of penicillin at birth to prevent GBS disease [180].

Detailed discussions of GBS in adults and children can be found in Chapters 14 and 15, respectively.

Mycoplasmas

Mycoplasmas are gram-negative, cell-wall-deficient bacteria which are the smallest and simplest of self-replicating organisms. Eleven species are known to colonize humans as either constituents of the normal flora or as potential pathogens. Two species, *Mycoplasma hominis* and *Ureaplasma urealyticum* (formally referred to as "T-stain mycoplasma" because they produced "tiny" atypical colonies), colonize the genitourinary tract and have been implicated in various disease processes; however, their pathogenic role remains unclear and their pathophysiology remains poorly defined [181].

About one-third of female infants are colonized by mycoplasmas during birth, but the carrier state is transient and rarely lasts longer than 1 year [182]. The colonization of the pubertal female genital tract is a function of sexual activity. Mycoplasmas are rarely recovered from the genital tract of sexually mature virgin females, whereas over 37% of women who have had intercourse with a single partner and 75% of women with multiple (at least three) partners are colonized with *U. urealyticum* [183]. Colonization with *M. hominis* is less prevalent but has similar trends. Other positive epidemiological factors associated with the prevalence of mycoplasmas include race (black), socioeconomic status (lower), and pregnancy [184,185].

Although many reports have documented an association between mycoplasmas and cervicitis, the high prevalence of mycoplasmas among "normal" sexually active individuals and the failure to consider *C. trachomatis* and other potential cervical pathogens limit their value. Hunter et al. [186] failed to demonstrate an association between the presence of *U. urealyticum* and any symptoms or signs of genital tract disease, despite a cervical isolation rate of 50%, in women attending an STD clinic. *Mycoplasma hominis* has been considered a potential pathogen in vaginitis; however, the differential antibiotic approach has not confirmed a significant role for this organism in vaginal syndromes [187].

While *U. urealyticum* appears to be of no importance as an etiological agent of nongonococcal PID, *M. hominis* has been isolated repeatedly from inflamed fallopian tubes and abscesses (tubo-ovarian, cul-de-sac) [188,189]. Serological studies suggest an etiological role for *M. hominis* in a substantial minority (12%) of PID cases [190]. The potential role of mycoplasmas in PID is further discussed in Chapter 7.

As stated earlier, mycoplasmas are isolated from a substantial percentage of pregnant women. The isolation of mycoplasmas from the blood of women with unexplained fever who delivered vaginally has been strong evidence for their pathogenic role in postpartum fever [191,192]. Eschenbach estimates that 10 to 20% of febrile postpartum women have a mycoplasma infection [193]. *Mycoplasma hominis* was isolated from the amniotic fluid of 35% of patients with intra-amniotic infection, as opposed to 8% of controls; however, *M. hominis* was commonly associated with other virulent bacteria and may represent a commensal rather than a pathogen [194]. There is a continuing debate regarding the ability of *U. urealyticum* to cause growth retardation and premature delivery. Placental colonization occurs in conjunction with cervical colonization in a majority of cases and results by an ascending infection after membrane rupture, the isolation rate being higher after prolonged membrane rupture [195]. A recent study of 316 pregnant women failed to demonstrate a significant correlation between *U. urealyticum* and low birth weight or gestational age despite a significant isolation rate of the organism from the cervix and placenta [196]. *Mycoplasma hominis* has been associated with reproductive failure, low birth weight, and recurrent abortions [197,198]. The evidence is largely circumstantial, and conclusive investigations are needed before an etiological association can be established.

The collection of cervical, vaginal, and urine specimens ensures the greatest cultural yield of mycoplasmas. Cotton-tipped swabs should be expressed immediately into mycoplasmal transport medium which can be safely stored for several days at 4°C [199,200]. Mycoplasma and ureaplasma are grown on enriched medium and form small colonies 10 to 100 μm in diameter. Colonies frequently show a "fried egg" appearance. Biochemically, the ureaplasmas hydrolyzed urea, whereas the mycoplasmas do not [199,200]. These microorganisms require highly specialized techniques for cultural isolation and identification. Therefore clinicians should evaluate the information they hope to gain before ordering these costly tests.

REFERENCES

1. Holmes KK, Handsfield HH. Sexually transmitted diseases. In: Petersdorf RC, et al., eds. Principles of internal medicine. Vol. 1. New York: McGraw-Hill, 1983:889-902.
2. Eschenbach DA. Vaginal infections. Clin Obstet Gynecol 1983; 26:186-202.
3. Murdoch AJM, Buckley CH, Fox H. Hormonal control of the secretory immune system of the human uterine cervix. J Reprod Immun 1982; 4:23-30.
4. Corbishley CM. Microbial flora of the vagina and cervix. J Clin Pathol 1977; 30:745-748.
5. Sparks RA, Purrier BG, Watt PJ, Elstein M. The bacteriology of the cervical canal in relation to the use of an intrauterine contraceptive device. In: Insler V, Brettendorf G, eds. The uterine cervix in reproduction. Vol 1. Stuttgart: Georg Thieme Verlag, 1977:271-277.
6. Machowiak PA. The normal microbial flora. N Engl J Med 1982; 307:83-93.
7. Gorbach SL, Menda KB, Thadepalli H, Keith L. Anaerobic microflora of the cervix in healthy women. Am J Obstet Gynecol 1973; 117:1053-1055.
8. Lindner JGEM, Plantema FHF, Hoogkamp-Korstanje JAA. Quantitative studies of the vaginal flora of healthy women and of obstetric and gynaecological patients. J Med Microbiol 1978; 11:233-241.
9. Ohm MJ, Galask RP. Bacterial flora of the cervix from 100 pre-hysterectomy patients. Am J Obstet Gynecol 1975; 122:683-687.
10. Thadepalli H, Chan WH, Maidman JE, Davidson EC. Microflora of the cervix during normal labor and the puerperium. J Infect Dis 1978; 137:568-572.
11. Larsen B, Galask RP. Vaginal microbial flora: practical and theoretic relevance. Obstet Gynecol 1980; 55:100S-113S.
12. Spagna VA, Prior RB, Perkins RL. Rapid presumptive diagnosis of gonococcal cervicitis by the limulus lysate assay. Am J Obstet Gynecol 1980; 137:595-599.
13. Goplerud CP, Ohm MJ, Galask RP. Aerobic and anaerobic flora of the cervix during pregnancy and the puerperium. Am J Obstet Gynecol 1976; 126:858-868.
14. Ingraham LS, Kraus SJ, Brooks GF. Microbial inhibition of *Neisseria gonorrhoeae*. In: Brooks GF, et al., eds. Immunobiology of *Neisseria gonorrhoeae*. Washington, DC: American Society for Microbiology, 1978:350-355.
15. Saigh JH, Sanders CC, Sanders WE. Inhibition of *Neisseria gonorrhoeae* by aerobic and facultatively anaerobic components of the endocervical flora:

evidence for a protective effect against infection. Infect Immun 1978; 19: 704-710.
16. Morin A, Saheb SA, Bisaillon JG, Beaudet R, Sylvestre M. In vitro inhibition of *Neisseria gonorrhoeae* growth by strict anaerobes. Infect Immun 1980; 28:766-770.
17. Gilbaugh JH, Fuchs PC. The gonococcus and the toilet seat. N Engl J Med 1979; 301:91-93.
18. Srivastava AC. Survival of gonococci in urethral secretions with reference to the nonsexual transmission of gonococcal infection. J Med Microbiol 1980; 13:593-596.
19. Pearce WA, Buchanan TM. Attachment role of gonococcal pili–optimum conditions and quantitation of adherence of isolated pili to human cells in vitro. J Clin Invest 1978; 61:931-943.
20. McGee ZA, Johnson AP, Taylor-Robinson D. Pathogenic mechanisms of *Neisseria gonorrhoeae*: observations on damage to human fallopian tubes in organ culture by gonococci of colony type 1 or type 4. J Infect Dis 1981; 143:413-422.
21. McGee ZA, Melly MA, Gregg CR, Horn RG, Taylor-Robinson D, Johnson AP, McCutchan JA. Virulence factors of gonococci: studies using human fallopian tube organ cultures. In: Brooks GF, et al., eds. Immunobiology of *Neisseria gonorrhoeae*. Washington, DC: American Society for Microbiology, 1978:258-262.
22. Melly MA, Gregg CR, McGee ZA. Studies of toxicity of *Neisseria gonorrhoeae* for human fallopian tube mucosa. J Infect Dis 1981: 143:423-431.
23. Gregg CR, Melly MA, Hellerqvist CG, Coniglio JG, McGee ZA. Toxic activity of purified lipopolysaccharide of *Neisseria gonorrhoeae* for human fallopian tube mucosa. J Infect Dis 1981; 143-432-439.
24. Arya OP. Epidemiology of gonorrhoea. In: Harris JRW, ed. Recent advances in sexually transmitted diseases. Vol. 2. London: Churchill Livingstone, 1981: 35-48.
25. Centers for Disease Control. Sexually transmitted disease (STD) statistical letter, issue No. 129. Atlanta, Ga.: Centers for Disease Control, 1979:9-46.
26. Fleming WL, Brown WJ, Donohue JF, Barnigin PW. National survey of venereal disease treated by physicians in 1968. JAMA 1970; 211:1827-1830.
27. Morton RS. Gonorrhoea. London: WB Saunders, 1977:94-122, 204-234.
28. Barlow D. Sexually transmitted diseases, the facts. New York: Oxford University Press, 1979:19-29.
29. Centers for Disease Control. Gonorrhea, annual summary 1982. Morbid Mortal Week Rep 1983; 31:29-33.
30. Chief Medical Officer. Sexually transmitted diseases. Extract from the annual report of the Chief Medical Officer of the Department of Health and Social Security for the year 1979. Br J Vener Dis 1981; 57:402-405.
31. Handsfield HH, Sandstrom EG, Knapp JS, Perine PL, Whittington WL, Sayers DE, Homes KK. Epidemiology of penicillinase-producing *Neisseria gonorrhoeae* infections. N Engl J Med 1982; 306:950-954.
32. Centers for Disease Control. Spectinomycin-resistant *Neisseria gonorrhoeae*-worldwide. Morbid Mortal Week Rep 1982; 31:632, 637-638.

33. Ashford WA, Potts DW, Adams HJ, English JC, Johnson SR, Biddle JW, Thornsberry C, Jaffe HW. Spectinomycin-resistant penicillinase-producing *Neisseria gonorrhoeae*. Lancet 1981; 2:1035-1037.
34. Easmon CS, Ison CA, Bellinger CM, Harris JW. Emergence of resistance after spectinomycin treatment for gonorrhea due to β-lactamase-producing strain of *Neisseria gonorrhoeae*. Br Med J 1982; 284:1604-1605.
35. Centers for Disease Control. Spectinomycin-resistant β-lactamase-producing *Neisseria gonorrhoeae*—England. Morbid Mortal Week Rep 1982;31:495-501.
36. Centers for Disease Control. Spectinomycin-resistant penicillinase-producing *Neisseria gonorrhoeae*. Morbid Mortal Week Rep 1983; 32:51-52.
37. Handsfield HH, Lipman TO, Harnisch JP, Tronca E, Holmes KK. Asymptomatic gonorrhea in men. N Engl J Med 1974; 290:117-123.
38. Rein MF. Epidemiology of gonococcal infections. In: Roberts RR, ed. The gonococcus. New York: Wiley, 1977:2-17.
39. Holmes KK, Johnson DW, Trostle HJ. Estimate of the risk of men acquiring gonorrhea by sexual contact with infected females. Am J Epidemiol 1970; 91:170-174.
40. Willcox RR. What are the chances of catching VD? Resid Staff Physician 1976; 9:51-56.
41. Hooper RR, Reynolds GH, Jones OG, Zaidi A, Wiesner PJ, Latimer KP, Lester A, Campbell AF, Harrison WO, Karney WW, Holmes KK. Cohort study of venereal disease. I: The risk of gonorrhea transmission from infected women to men. Am J Epidemiol 1978; 108:136-144.
42. Dans PE. Gonococcal anogenital infection. Clin Obstet Gynecol 1975; 18: 103-119.
43. Johnson RE. Epidemiologic and prophylactic treatment of gonorrhea: a decision analysis review. Sex Transm Dis 1979; 6:159-167.
44. Spagna VA, Prior RB, Sawaya GA. Sensitivity, specificity, and predictive values of the *Limulus* lysate assay for detection or exclusion of gonococcal cervicitis. J Clin Microbiol 1982; 16:77-81.
45. Eschenbach DA, Holmes KK. Acute pelvic inflammatory disease: current concepts of pathogenesis, etiology, and management. Clin Obstet Gynecol 1975; 18:35-56.
46. Handsfield HH. Gonorrhea and nongonococcal urethritis—recent advances. Med Clin North Am 1978; 62:925-943.
47. Evans BA. Ultrastructural study of cervical gonorrhea. J Infect Dis 1977; 136:248-255.
48. Lowe TL, Kraus SJ. Quantitation of *Neisseria gonorrhoeae* from women with gonorrhea. J Infect Dis 1976; 133:621-626.
49. Wiesner PJ. Gonorrhea. Cutis 1981; 27:249-254.
50. Jha PK, Singh G, Kaur P, Sharma D. Unsuspected gonococcal infection in female patients. Br J Vener Dis 1978; 54:324-325.
51. Little RG, Hartsfield M. Incidence of asymptomatic gonorrhea in women. J Fam Pract 1978; 7:597-599.
52. McMillan A, McNeillage G, Young H, Bain SSR. Secretory antibody response of the cervix to infection with *Neisseria gonorrhoeae*. Br J Vener Dis 1979; 55:265-270.

53. McMillan A, McNeillage G, Young H, and Bain SSR. Detection of antigonococcal IgA in cervical secretions by indirect immunofluorescence: an evaluation as a diagnostic test. Br J Vener Dis 1980; 56:223-226.
54. Buchanan TM, Swanson J, Holmes KK, Kraus SJ, Gotschlich EC. Quantitative determination of antibody to gonococcal pili. Changes in antibody levels with gonococcal infection. J Clin Invest 1973; 52:2896-2909.
55. Reimann K, Lind I. An indirect haemagglutination test for demonstration of gonococcal antibodies using gonococcal pili as antigen. I. Methodology and preliminary results. Acta Pathol Microbiol Scand Sec C. 1977; 85:115-122.
56. Lind I, Reimann K. Indirect hemagglutination test for demonstration of gonococcal antibodies using gonococcal pili as antigen. In: Brooks GF, et al., eds. Immunobiology of *Neisseria gonorrhoeae*. Washington, DC: American Society for Microbiology, 1978:385-386.
57. Glynn AA, Catherine I. Antibodies to a gonococcal envelope protein in acute gonorrhea. In: Brooks GF, et al., eds. Immunobiology of *Neisseria gonorrhoeae*. Washington, DC: American Society for Microbiology, 1978:387-388.
58. Watson RR. Cell-mediated immune responses to *Neisseria gonorrhoeae*. In: Brooks GF, et al., eds. Immunobiology of *Neisseria gonorrhoeae*. Washington, DC: American Society for Microbiology, 1978:290-292.
59. Landolfo PJ, Marrie TJ, Nelson NA, Ronald AR. Cell-mediated immune response in gonococcal infection. Can J Microbiol 1981; 27:76-80.
60. Young H. Advances in routine laboratory procedures for the diagnosis of gonorrhoea. In: Harris JRW, ed. Recent advances in sexually transmitted diseases. Edinburgh: Churchill Livingstone, 1981:59-71.
61. Goodhart ME, Ogden A, Zaidi A, Kraus SJ. Factors affecting the performance of smear and culture tests for the detection of *Neisseria gonorrhoeae*. Sex Transm Dis 1982; 9:63-69.
62. McCormack WM, Reynolds GH, Cooperative Study Group. Effect of menstrual cycle and method of contraception on recovery of *Neisseria gonorrhoeae*. JAMA 1982; 247:1292-1294.
63. Spence MR, Guzick DS, Katta RA. The isolation of *Neisseria gonorrhoeae*: A comparison of three culture transport systems. Sex Transm Dis 1983; 10:138-140.
64. Caldwell JG, Price EV, Pazin GJ, Cornelius CE. Sensitivity and reproducibility of Thayer-Martin culture medium in diagnosing gonorrhea in women. Am Obstet Gynecol 1971; 109:463-468.
65. Holmes KK. The *Chlamydia* epidemic. JAMA 1981; 245:1718-1723.
66. Barlow D, Nayyar K, Phillips I, Barrow J. Diagnosis of gonorrhoea in women. Br J Vener Dis 1976; 52:326-328.
67. Chipperfield EJ, Catterall RD. Reappraisal of Gram-staining and culture techniques for the diagnosis of gonorrhoea in women. Br J Vener Dis 1976; 52:36-39.
68. Jephcott AE, Rashid S. Improved management in the diagnosis of gonorrhoea in women. Br J Vener Dis 1978; 54:155-159.
69. Young H. Cultural diagnosis of gonorrhoea with modified New York City (MNYC) medium. Br J Vener Dis 1978; 54:36-40.

70. Smeltzer MP, Curran JW, Brown ST, Pass J. Accuracy of presumptive criteria for culture diagnosis of *Neisseria gonorrhoeae* in low-prevalence populations of women. J Clin Microbiol 1980; 11:485-487.
71. Belsey EM. Diagnosis of gonorrhoea in women—a national survey. Br J Vener Dis 1983; 59:59-62.
72. Lossick JG, Smeltzer MP, Curran JW. The value of the cervical Gram stain in the diagnosis and treatment of gonorrhea in women in a venereal disease clinic. Sex Transm Dis 1982; 9:124-127.
73. Koransky JR, Jacobs NF. Serologic testing for gonorrhea. Sex Transm Dis 1977; 4:27-31.
74. Low AC, Young H. Modern trends in the laboratory diagnosis of gonorrhea. Med Lab Sci 1979; 36:375-281.
75. Holmes KK, Buchanan TM, Adams JL, Eschenbach DA. Is serology useful for gonorrhea? A critical analysis of factors influencing serodiagnosis. In: Brooks GF, et al., eds. Immunobiology of *Neisseria gonorrhoea*. Washington, DC: American Society for Microbiology, 1978:370-376.
76. Mårdh PA, Buchanan T, Christensen P, Danielsson D, Lind I, Reimann K. Comparison of four serological tests for detection of gonococcal antibodies in patients with complicated gonococcal infection. In: Brooks GF, et al., eds. Immunobiology of *Neisseria gonorrhoeae*. Washington, DC: American Society for Microbiology, 1978:377-381.
77. Williams RP, Childress JR. Variation in responses to four serological tests for gonorrhea. In: Brooks GF, et al., eds. Immunobiology of *Neisseria gonorrhoeae*. Washington, DC: American Society for Microbiology, 1978:382-384.
78. Oranje AP, Reimann K, VanEijk RVW, Schouten HJA, deRoo A, Tideman GJ, Stolz E, Michel M. Gonococcal serology—a comparison of three different tests. Br J Vener Dis 1983; 59:47-52.
79. Oranje AP, Iserief COA, deRoo A, Stolz E, Michel MF. Antibodies to gonococcal pili in women with asymptomatic gonorrhoea—diagnostic value of the ELISA for testing women attending an STD clinic. Br J Vener Dis 1983; 59:85-88.
80. Oranje AP, Reimann K, deRoo A, Schouten HJA, Stolz E, Michel MF. Enzyme-linked immunosorbent assay for detecting gonococcal antibodies using two antigenically different gonococcal pili as antigen. Br J Vener Dis 1983; 59:89-91.
81. Aardoom HA, Hoop D, Iserief COA, Michel MF, Stolz E. Detection of *Neisseria gonorrhoeae* antigen by a solid-phase enzyme immunoassay. Br J Vener Dis 1982; 58:359-362.
82. Hofmann H, Berger V, Petzoldt D. Decreased reliability of an enzyme immunoassay for the detection of gonococcal antigen in routine screening of prostitutes. In: Program and abstracts of the International Society for STD Research, 5th international meeting, Seattle, Washington; 1983 (Abstract 40).
83. Nowinski RC, Tam MR, Goldstein LC, Strong L, Kuo CC, Corey L, Stamm WE, Handsfield HH, Knapp JS, Holmes KK. Diagnosis of sexually transmitted

diseases with monoclonal antibodies. In: Program and abstracts of the International Society for STD Research, 5th international meeting, Seattle, Washington; 1983 (Abstract 88).

84. Zubrzycki L, Weinberger SS. Laboratory diagnosis of gonorrhea by a simple transformation test with a temperature-sensitive mutant of *Neisseria gonorrhoeae*. Sex Transm Dis 1980; 7:183-187.
85. Jaffe HW, Kraus SJ, Edwards TA, Weinberger SS, Zubrzycki L. Diagnosis of gonorrhea using a genetic transformation test on mailed clinical specimens. J Infect Dis 1982; 146:275-279.
86. Spagna VA, Prior RB. Genetic transformation test for diagnosis of gonorrhea. J Infect Dis 1983; 147:1124-1125.
87. Kraus SJ. Semiquantitation of urethral polymorphonuclear leukocytes as objective evidence of nongonococcal urethritis. Sex Transm Dis 1982;9:52-55.
88. Centers for Disease Control. Sexually transmitted diseases treatment guidelines 1982. Morbid Mortal Week Rep Suppl 1982; 31:33S-60S.
89. Belsey EM. Epidemiological treatment of gonorrhoea and non-specific genital infection in female sexual contacts—current practices in STD clinics in England and Wales. Br J Vener Dis 1982; 58:113-116.
90. Robbins JB. Problems posed by potential gonococcal vaccines viewed from the vantage point of a control agency. Br J Vener Dis 1977;53:170-172.
91. Robbins JB. Disease control for gonorrhea by vaccine immunoprophylaxis: the next step? In: Brooks GF, et al., eds. Immunobiology of *Neisseria gonorrhoeae*. Washington, DC: American Society for Microbiology, 1978:391-394.
92. Manire GP. Biological characteristics of chlamydiae. In: Hobson D, Holmes KK, eds. Nongonococcal urethritis and related infections. Washington, DC: American Society for Microbiology, 1977:167-175.
93. Bergan T. Biology of *Chlamydia*. Scand J Infect Dis Suppl 1982;32:11-15.
94. Ripa KT. Biological principles of the culture of *Chlamydia trachomatis* in cell monolayers. Scand J Infect Dis Suppl 1982; 32:25-29.
95. Svensson L, Weström L, Mårdh PA. *Chlamydia trachomatis* in women attending a gynaecological outpatient clinic with lower genital tract infection. Br J Vener Dis 1981; 57:259-262.
96. Weström L, Svensson L, Wølner-Hanssen P, Mårdh PA. Chlamydial and gonococcal infections in a defined population of women. Scand J Infect Dis Suppl 1982; 32:157-162.
97. Hansson H, Danielsson D. Epidemiology of sexually transmitted diseases in the Scandinavian countries. Scand J Infect Dis Suppl 1982; 32:149-156.
98. Arya OP, Mallinson H, Goddard AD. Epidemiological and clinical correlates of chlamydial infection of the cervix. Br J Vener Dis 1981; 57:118-124.
99. Goh BT, Morgan-Capner P, Lim KS. Chlamydial screening of pregnant women in a sexually transmitted disease clinic. Br J Vener Dis 1982; 58: 327-239.
100. Munday PE, Pritchard G, Harris JRW, Taylor-Robinson D. Prevalence of chlamydial infection in promiscuous women. Br J Vener Dis 1983; 59: 103-104.

101. Hunter JM, Smith IW, Peutherer JF, MacAulay AJ. *Chlamydia trachomatis* infection of the cervix: the need for a diagnostic service. Scot Med J 1982; 27:147-151.
102. Embil JA, Thiebaux HJ, Manuel FR, Pereira LH, MacDonald SW. Sequential cervical specimens and the isolation of *Chlamydia trachomatis*: factors affecting detection. Sex Transm Dis 1983; 10:62-66.
103. Paavonen J, Vesterinen E. *Chlamydia trachomatis* in cervicitis and urethritis in women. Scand J Infect Dis Suppl 1982; 32:45-54.
104. Lycke E, Lowhagen GB, Hallhagen G, Johannisson G. The risk of transmission of genital *Chlamydia trachomatis* infection is less than that of genital *Neisseria gonorrhoeae* infection. Sex Transm Dis 1980; 7:6-10.
105. Rees E, Tait IA, Hobson D, Johnson FWA. Chlamydia in relation to cervical infection and pelvic inflammatory disease. In: Hobson D, Holmes KK, eds. Nongonococcal urethritis and related infections. Washington, DC: American Society for Microbiology, 1977:67-76.
106. Mallinson H, Arya OP, Goddard AD. Quantitative study of *Chlamydia trachomatis* in genital infection. Br J Vener Dis 1982; 58:36-39.
107. Paavonen J, Vesterinen E, Meyer B, Saksela E. Colposcopic and histologic findings in cervical chlamydial infection. Obstet Gynecol 1982; 59:712-714.
108. Schachter J, Hill EC, King EB, Coleman VR, Jones R, Meyer KF. Chlamydial infection in women with cervical dysplasia. Am J Obstet Gynecol 1975; 123:753-757.
109. Paavonen J, Vesterinen E, Meyer B, Saikku P, Suni J, Purola E, Saksela E. Genital *Chlamydia trachomatis* infections in patients with cervical atypia. Obstet Gynecol 1979; 54:289-291.
110. Hare MJ, Taylor-Robinson D, Cooper P. Evidence for an association between *Chlamydia trachomatis* and cervical intraepithelial neoplasia. Br J Obstet Gynaecol 1982; 89:489-492.
111. Terho P, Meurman O. Chlamydial serum IgG, IgA and local IgA antibodies in patients with genital-tract infections measured by solid-phase radioimmunoassay. J Med Microbiol 1981; 14:77-87.
112. Kalimo K. Terho P, Gronroos M, Halonen P. *Chlamydia trachomatis* and herpes simplex virus IgA antibodies in cervical secretions of patients with cervical atypia. Br J Obstet Gynaecol 1981; 88:1130-1134.
113. Recommendations for diagnosis and treatment on infections caused by *Chlamydia trachomatis*. In: Mårdh PA, Møller BR, Paavonen J, eds. *Chlamydia trachomatis* in genital and related infections. Scand J Infect Dis Suppl 1982; 32:195-199.
114. Schachter J, Dawson CR. Comparative efficiency of various diagnostic methods for chlamydial infection. In: Hobson D, Holmes KK, eds. Nongonococcal urethritis and related infections. Washington, DC: American Society for Microbiology, 1977:337-341.
115. Stamm WE, Koester CM, Cles L, Cole B, Holmes KK. Diagnosis of *C. trachomatis* cervical and urethral infections by direct immunofluorescence (IF) staining of genital secretions. In: Program and abstracts of the International

Society for STD Research, 5th international meeting, Seattle, Washington; 1983 (Abstract 50).
116. Purola E, Paavonen J. Routine cytology as a diagnostic aid in chlamydial cervicitis. Scand J Infect Dis Suppl 1982; 32:55-58.
117. Mårdh PA, Zeeberg B. Toxic effect of sampling swabs and transportation test tubes on the formation of intracytoplasmic inclusions of *Chlamydia trachomatis* in McCoy cell cultures. Br J Vener Dis 1981; 57:268-272.
118. Kallings I, Mårdh PA. Sampling and specimen handling in the diagnosis of genital *Chlamydia trachomatis* infections. Scand J Infect Dis Suppl 1982; 32:21-24.
119. Ripa KT. Biological principles of the culture of *Chlamydia trachomatis* in cell monolayers. Scand J Infect Dis Suppl 1982; 32:25-29.
120. Stephens RS, Kuo CC, Tam MR. Sensitivity of immunofluorescence with monoclonal antibodies for detection of *Chlamydia trachomatis* inclusions in cell culture. J Clin Microbiol 1982; 16:4-7.
121. Mårdh PA, Weström L, Colleen S, Wølner-Hanssen P. Sampling, specimen handling, and isolation techniques in the diagnosis of chlamydial and other genital infections. Sex Transm Dis 1981; 8:280-285.
122. Saikker P. Chalmydial serology. Scand J Infect Dis Suppl 1982; 32:34-37.
123. Judson FN, Bodin GF, Levin MJ, Ehret JM, Masters HB. In vitro tests demonstrate condoms provide an effective barrier against *Chlamydia trachomatis* and herpes simplex virus. In: Program and abstracts of the International Society for STD Research, 5th international meeting, Seattle, Washington; 1983 (Abstract 176).
124. Centers for Disease Control. Genital herpes infection—United States, 1966-1979. Morbid Mortal Week Rep 1982; 31:137-139.
125. Knox SR, Corey L, Blough HA, Lerner AM. Historical findings in subjects from a high socioeconomic group who have genital infections with herpes simplex virus. Sex Transm Dis 1982; 9:15-20.
126. Corey L, Adams HG, Brown ZA, Holmes KK. Genital herpes simplex virus infections: clinical manifestations, course, and complications. Ann Intern Med 1983; 98:958-972.
127. Stamm WE, Wagner KF, Amsel R, Alexander ER, Turck M, Counts GW, Holmes KK. Causes of the acute urethral syndrome in women. N Engl J Med 1980; 303:409-415.
128. Guinan ME, MacCalman J, Kern ER, Overall JC, Spruance SL. The course of untreated recurrent genital herpes simplex infection in 27 women. N Engl J Med 1981; 304:759-763.
129. Adam E, Kaufman RH, Mirkovic RR, Melnick JL. Persistence of virus shedding in asymptomatic women after recovery from herpes genitalis. Obstet Gynecol 1979; 133:548-554.
130. Rattray MC, Corey L, Reeves WC, Vontver LA, Holmes KK. Recurrent genital herpes among women: symptomatic v. asymptomatic viral shedding. Br J Vener Dis 1978; 54:262-265.
131. Vontver LA, Hickok DE, Brown Z, Reid L, Corey L. Recurrent genital herpes simplex virus infection in pregnancy: infant outcome and frequency of asymptomatic recurrences. Am J Obstet Gynecol 1982; 143:75-81.

132. Nahmias AJ, Josey WE, Naib ZM, Freeman MG, Fernandez RJ, Wheeler JH. Perinatal risk associated with maternal genital herpes simplex virus infection. Am J Obstet Gynecol 1971; 110:825-837.
133. Hanshaw JB. *Herpesvirus hominis* infections in the fetus and the newborn. Am J Dis Child 1973; 126:546-555.
134. Grossman JH. Herpes simplex virus (HSV) infections. Clin Obstet Gynecol 1982; 25:555-561.
135. Nahmias AJ, Visintine AM, Starr SE. Viral infections of the fetus and newborn. In: Drew WL, ed. Viral infections—a clinical approach. Philadelphia. Davis, 1976:47-68.
136. Whitley RJ, Nahmias AJ, Visintine AM, Fleming CL, Alford CA. The natural history of herpes simplex virus infection of mother and newborn. Pediatrics 1980; 66:489-494.
137. Nahmias AJ, Visintine M. Herpes simplex virus. In: Remington JS, Kelin JD, eds. Infectious diseases of the fetus and newborn. Philadelphia: WB Saunders; 1976:156-190.
138. Committee on Fetus and Newborn; Committee on Infectious Diseases: Perinatal herpes simplex virus infections. Pediatrics 1980; 66:147.
139. Cassai E, Rotola A, Meneguzzi G, Milanesi G, Garsia S, Remotti G, Rizzi G. Herpes simplex virus and human cancer. I. Relationship between human cervical tumours and herpes simplex type 2. Eu J Cancer 1981; 17:685-693.
140. Fish EN, Tobin SM, Cooter NBE, Papsin FR. Update on the relationship of *Herpesvirus hominis* type II to carcinoma of the cervix. Obstet Gynecol 1982; 59:220-224.
141. Aurelian L, Stranberg JD, Melendez LV, Marcus RL. Herpesvirus type 2 isolated from cervical tumor cells grown in tissue culture. Science 1971; 174:704-707.
142. Cabral GA, Fry D, Marciano-Cabral F, Lumpkin C, Mercer L, Goplerud D. A herpesvirus antigen in human premalignant and malignant cervical biopsies and explants. Am J Obstet Gynecol 1983; 145:79-86.
143. Rayston I, Aurelian L. Immunofluorescent detection of herpesvirus antigens in exfoliated cells from human cervical carcinoma. Proc Nat Acad Sci USA 1970; 67:204-212.
144. Gilman SC, Docherty JJ, Clarke A. Reaction patterns of herpes simplex virus type 1 and type 2 proteins with sera of patients with uterine cervical carcinoma and matched controls. Cancer Res 1980; 40:4640-4647.
145. Melnick JL, Adam E, Rawls WE. The causative role of herpesvirus type 2 in cervical cancer. Cancer 1974; 34:1375-1385.
146. Graham S, Rawls W, Swanson M, McCurtis J. Sex partners and herpes simplex virus type 2 in the epidemiology of cancer of the cervix. Am J Epidemiol 1982; 115:729-735.
147. Barton IG, Kinghorn GR, Walker MJ, Al-Omer LS, Potter CW, Turner EB. Association of HSV-1 with cervical infection. Lancet 1981; 2:1108.
148. Hulka BS. Risk factors for cervical cancer. J Chron Dis 1982; 35:3-11.
149. Miller MJ, Howell CL. Rapid detection and identification of herpes simplex virus in cell culture by a direct immunoperoxidase staining procedure. J Clin Microbiol 1983; 18:550-553.

150. Pereira LD, Dondero DV, Gallo D, Devlin V, Woodie JD. Serological analysis of herpes simplex viruses 1 and 2 with monoclonal antibodies. Infect Immun 1982; 35:363-367.
151. Coleman RM, Pereira L, Bailey PD, Dondero D, Wickliffe C, Nahmias AJ. Determination of herpes simplex type-specific antibodies by enzyme-linked immunosorbent assay. J Clin Microbiol 1983; 18:287-291.
152. Corey L, Holmes KK. Genital herpes simplex virus infections: current concepts in diagnosis, therapy, and prevention. Ann Intern Med 1983; 98: 973-983.
153. Moseley RC, Corey L, Benjamin D, Winter C, Remington ML. Comparison of viral isolation, direct immunofluorescence, and indirect immunoperoxidase techniques for detection of genital herpes simplex virus infection. J Clin Microbiol 1981; 13:913-918.
154. Skinner GRB, Woodman CBJ, Hartley CE, Buchan A, Fuller A, Durham J, Synnott M, Clay JC, Melling J, Wiblin C, Wilkins J. Preparation and immunogenicity of vaccine Ac NFU, (S^-) MRC towards the prevention of herpes genitalis. Br J Vener Dis 1982; 58:381-386.
155. Ho M. Cytomegalovirus infections and diseases. DM 1978; 24:12-28.
156. Willmott FE. Cytomegalovirus in female patients attending a VD clinic. Br J Vener Dis 1975; 51:278-280.
157. Waner JL, Hopkins DR, Weller TH, Allred EN. Cervical excretion of cytomegalovirus: correlation with secretory and humoral antibody. J Infect Dis 1977; 136:805-809.
158. Griffiths PD, Campbell-Benzie A, Heath RB. A prospective study of primary cytomegalovirus infection in pregnant women. Br J Obstet Gynaecol 1980; 87:308-314.
159. Deppisch LM. Cytomegalovirus inclusion body endocervicitis: significance of CMV inclusions in endocervical biopsies. Mount Sinai J Med 1981; 48: 418-421.
160. Chiang WT, Chen HM, Hsieh CY, Tsai WS, Wei PY, Alexander ER. Cytomegalovirus infection of the uterine cervix: local cervical infection and antibody response. Int J Gynaecol Obstet 1981; 19:177-180.
161. Alexander ER. Possible etiologies of cancer of the cervix other than herpesvirus. Cancer Res 1973; 33:1485-1496.
162. Reynolds DW, Stagno S, Hosty TS, Tiller M, Alford CA. Maternal cytomegalovirus excretion and perinatal infection. N Engl J Med 1973; 289:1-5.
163. Oriel JD. Genital warts. Sex Transm Dis 1981; 8:326-329.
164. Centers for Disease Control. Condyloma acuminatum – United States, 1966-1981. Morbid Mortal Week Rep 1983; 32:306-308.
165. Chief Medical Officier. Sexually transmitted diseases. Extract from the annual report of the Chief Officier of the Department of Health and Social Security for the year 1980. Br J Vener Dis 1983; 59:134-137.
166. Meisels A, Fortin R. Condylomatous lesions of the cervix and vagina. I. Cytologic patterns. Acta Cytol 1976; 20:505-509.
167. Reid R, Laverty CR, Coppleson M, Isarangkul W, Hills E. Noncondylomatous cervical wart virus infection. Obstet Gynecol 1980; 55:476-483.

168. Meisels A, Fortin R, Roy M. Condylomatous lesions of the cervix and vagina. II. Cytologic, colposcopic and histopathologic criteria. Acata Cytol 1977; 21:379-389.
169. Walker PG, Colley NV, Grubb C, Tejerina A, Oriel JD. Abnormalities of the uterine cervix in women with vulvar warts—a preliminary communication. Br J Vener Dis 1983; 59:120-123.
170. Reid R, Stanhope CR, Herschman BR, Booth E, Phibbs GD, Smith JP. Genital warts and cervical cancer. I. Evidence of an association between subclinical papillomavirus infection and cervical malignancy. Cancer 1982; 50:377-387.
171. Anthony BA. Carriage of group B streptococci during pregnancy: a puzzler. J Infect Dis 1982; 145:789-793.
172. Eichenwald JF. Group B streptococcal disease of infancy. Infect Dis 1978; 8:4.
173. Horn KA, Zimmerman RA, Knostman JD, Meyer WT. Neurological sequelae of group B streptococcal neonatal infections. Pediatrics 1974; 53:501.
174. Dillon HC, Gray E, Pass MA, Gray BM. Anorectal and vaginal carriage of group B streptococci during pregnancy. J Infect Dis 1982; 145:794-799.
175. Jackson DH, Hinder SM, Stringer J, Easmon CSF. Carriage and transmission of group B streptococci among STD clinic patients. Br J Vener Dis 1982; 58:334-337.
176. Embil JA, Martin TR, Hanset NH, MacDonald SW, Manvel FR. Group B beta-hemolytic streptococci in the female genital tract: a study of four clinic populations. Br J Obstet Gynaecol 1978; 85:783-786.
177. Weindling AM, Hawkins JM, Coombes MA, Stringer J. Colonization of babies and their families by group B streptococci. Br Med J 1981; 2:1503-1505.
178. Ferrieri P, Cleary PP, Seeds AE. Epidemiology of group-B streptococcal carriage in pregnant women and newborn infants. J Med Microbiol 1977; 10:103-114.
179. Hoogkamp-Korstanje JAA, Gerards LJ, Cats BP. Maternal carriage and neonatal acquisition of group B streptococci. J Infect Dis 1982; 145:800-803.
180. Fischer G, Horton RE, Edelman R. From the National Institute of Allergy and Infectious Diseases: summary of the National Institutes of Health workshop on group B streptococcal infection. J Infect Dis 1983; 148:163-166.
181. McCormack WM, Braun P, Lee YH, Klein JO, Kass EH. The genital mycoplasmas. N Engl J Med 1973; 288:78-89.
182. Foy HM, Kenny GE, Levinsohn EM, Grayston JT. Acquisition of mycoplasmata and T-strains during infancy. J Infect Dis 1970; 121:579-587.
183. McCormack WM, Almeida PC, Bailey PE, Grady EM, Lee YH. Sexual activity and vaginal colonization with genital mycoplasmas. JAMA 1972; 221: 1375-1377.
184. McCormack WM, Rosner B, Lee YH. Colonization with genital mycoplasmas in women. Am J Epidemiol 1973; 97:240-245.
185. Braun P, Klein JO, Lee YH, Kass EM. Methodologic investigations and prevalence of genital mycoplasmas in pregnancy. J Infect Dis 1970; 121:391-400.

186. Hunter JM, Young H, Harris AB. Genitourinary infection with *Ureaplasma urealyticum* in women attending a sexually transmitted diseases clinic. Br J Vener Dis 1981; 57:338-342.
187. Pheifer TA, Forsyth PS, Durfee MA, Pollock HM, Holmes KK. Nonspecific vaginitis: role of *Haemophilus vaginalis* and treatment with metronidazole. N Engl J Med 1978; 298:1429-1434.
188. Eschenbach DA, Buchanan TM, Pollock HM, Forsyth PS, Alexander ER, Lin JS, Wang SP, Wentworth BB, McCormack WM, Holmes KK. Polymicrobial etiology of acute pelvic inflammatory disease. N Engl J Med 1975; 293:166-171.
189. Mårdh PA, Weström L. Tubal and cervical cultures in acute salpingitis with special reference to *Mycoplasma hominis* and T-strain mycoplasmas. Br J Vener Dis 1970; 46:179-185.
190. Mårdh PA, Lind I, Svensson L, Weström L, Møller BR. Antibodies to *Chlamydia trachomatis*, *Mycoplasma hominis*, and *Neisseria gonorrhoeae* in sera from patients with acute salpingitis. Br J Vener Dis 1981; 57:125-129.
191. McCormack WM, Lee Y, Lin J, Rankin JS. Genital mycoplasmas in postpartum fever. J Infect Dis 1973; 127:193-196.
192. Platt R, Lin JSL, Warren JW, Rosner B, Edelin KC, McCormack WM. Infection with *Mycoplasma hominis* in postpartum fever. Lancet 1980; 2:1217-1221.
193. Eschenbach DA. The diagnosis of fever occuring in a postpartum patient. In: Remington JS, Swartz MN, eds. Current clinical topics in infectious diseases. Vol. 4. New York: McGraw-Hill, 1983:186-223.
194. Blanco JD, Gibbs RS, Malherbe H, Strickland-Cholmley M, St. Clair PJ, Castaneda YS. A controlled study of genital mycoplasmas in amniotic fluid from patients with intra-amniotic infection. J Infect Dis 1983; 147: 650-653.
195. Embree JE, Krause VW, Embil JA, MacDonald S. Placental infection with *Mycoplasma hominis* and *Ureaplasma urealyticum*: clinical correlation. Obstet Gynecol 1980; 56:475-481.
196. Naessens A, Foulon W, Volckaert M, Amy JJ, Lauwers S. Cervical and placental colonization by *Ureaplasma urealyticum* in pregnant women and fetal outcome. J Infect Dis 1983; 148:333.
197. Kundsin RB, Driscoll SG. Mycoplasmas and human reproductive failure. Surg Gynecol Obstet 1970; 131:89-92.
198. Braun P, Lee YH, Klein JO, Marcy SM, Klein TA, Charles D, Levy P, Kass EH. Birth weight and genital mycoplasmas in pregnancy. N Engl J Med 1971; 284:167-171.
199. Kundsin RB, Parreno A, Poulin S. Significance of appropriate techniques and media for isolation and identification of *Ureaplasma urealyticum* from clinical specimens. J Clin Microbiol 1978; 8:445-453.
200. Kenny GE. Mycoplasmata. In: Lennette EH, et al., eds. Manual of clinical microbiology. 3rd ed. Washington DC: American Society for Microbiology, 1980:365-370.

FIVE

Vaginal Syndromes

David A. Eschenbach
University of Washington
Seattle, Washington

INTRODUCTION

Complaint of a vaginal discharge is one of the most frequent reasons that symptomatic women visit sexually transmitted disease (STD) clinics. In 1971 an estimated 10.8 million women sought therapy for vaginitis and cervicitis [1]. Although the prevalence varies, depending on the population, the most common causes of infectious vaginitis are bacterial vaginosis (BV), formerly called nonspecific vaginitis (40 to 50%), candidiasis (20 to 30%), and trichomoniasis (20 to 30%) [2].

Despite a seemingly limited number of causes for vaginal discharge, the woman often finds that she is plagued by a lack of symptomatic relief following therapy. There are multiple reasons for the failure to cure a vaginal discharge, which include most commonly diagnostic errors, therapeutic errors, and sexual reacquisition, but also nonsexual recurrence, drug resistance, and depressed cellular immunity. Most

This work was supported by National Institutes of Health Program Project Grant AI-12191.

patients incorrectly assume that the complaint is easily remediable. Failure to effectively treat the vaginal discharge often causes both patient and physician frustration.

BASIC CONCEPTS

Components of Normal Vaginal Discharge

A vaginal discharge consists of several components, including water, electrolytes, microorganisms, epithelial cells, and organic compounds, such as fatty acids, proteins, and carbohydrates [3]. The components combine to produce a vaginal discharge with pH of less than 4.5 [2]. The largest volume of vaginal fluid arises from the egress of a serum transudate through local capillary walls and through the vaginal wall to the vaginal lumen. Smaller amounts of fluid are derived from Bartholin's glands, the cervix, endometrium, and fallopian tubes [3]. Cellular elements are sloughed from both cervical columnar and vaginal squamous epithelium. The normal vaginal flora consists of microorganisms that colonize the vaginal fluid and the epithelial cell. White blood cells (WBCs), though normally present in the secretory phase of the menstrual cycle, are usually found in only small numbers.

Influence of Sex Hormones on Normal Vaginal Discharge

The vaginal fluid and the microbial flora are influenced by sex hormones. An increase in the volume and a decrease in the viscosity of vaginal fluid occur following ovulation [4]. Estrogens also act to increase the level of glucose in vaginal fluid [5]. It is unclear whether estrogen increases glycogen turnover or the glycogen content of epithelial cells, which in turn could influence the types of organisms that colonize the epithelium. Menstruating women have proprotionately more facultative bacteria, including lactobacilli, than women with low estrogen levels. Premenarchal [6] and postmenopausal women with low estrogen levels have more anaerobic bacteria than menstruating women.

Influence of pH and Glucose on the Vaginal Flora

Two other important factors that influence the types of organisms present in the vaginal flora are the pH and the availability of glucose. The glycogen content of the vaginal epithelium is undoubtedly increased in menstruating women. It is the current hypothesis that the vaginal lactic acid content produces a very acidic pH (less than 4.5). Lactic acid is produced not only by the metabolism of lactobacilli, but also by the metabolism of other bacteria and by the metabolism of vaginal epithelial cells. The resultant low pH in turn favors the growth of acidophilic organisms such as lactobacilli. Thus the presence of lactobacilli is probably central in limiting the growth of other bacteria. Heavy vaginal lactobacilli colonization inhibits the growth of other organisms through its own metabolism by maintaining a low pH, through the use of glucose to produce lactic acid, and by producing hydrogen peroxide, which inhibits the growth of anaerobic bacteria.

Among postmenopausal women the lowered cellular glycogen content caused by reduced estrogen levels is believed to be responsible for the rise in the vaginal pH. In a high-pH environment, the inhibitory and competitive effects of lactobacilli are removed and other organisms, most notably anaerobes, proliferate.

Microecosystems of the Vaginal Epithelium

It is becoming increasingly recognized that epithelial cells contain sites to which bacteria attach and that the ability of certain bacteria to occupy these sites varies among patients [7]. Some women are particularly susceptible to infection probably because their cells contain sites to which bacteria readily attach. The normal flora that attaches to vaginal epithelial cells and exists within microecosystems of the vaginal epithelium inhibits the overgrowth of pathological organisms by at least two mechanisms. The normal flora undoubtedly both uses substrate nutrients and produces metabolic products that inhibit the attachment and the proliferation of potentially pathogenic organisms. Analogous to oral microflora, the vagina probably contains many distinctive microbial ecosystems that vary within the few millimeters' distance in the vaginal epithelium [8]. Although these dynamic ecosystems have not been well studied, it is likely that there is a very complex interrelationship between the large variety of organisms that exist within these ecosystems.

Microorganisms Present in Normal Vaginal Discharge

The organisms are recovered from vaginal discharge in concentrations as high as 10^{10} (10 billion) colony-forming units (CFU) per milliliter of fluid [9]. The practitioner does not usually appreciate the tremendous differences in concentration that can exist between organisms in the vagina. Among normal women lactobacillus species account for well over 90% of the total organisms which are present. In disease states increased concentration of other organisms can eliminate the dominant lactobacillus flora. An average of 5 to 10 organisms are recovered from the vagina [9-11]; although repeated sampling could undoubtedly recover even more individual species. The most prominent facultative organisms are species of lactobacilli, corynebacteria, and streptococci, *Staphylococcus epidermitis,* and *Gardnerella vaginalis* [9-11]. Virtually all women have at least one facultative organism, and each one of the individual facultative organisms can be found in 40 to 80% of women. *Escherichia coli,* which is the most common virulent coliform organism, can be recovered from only about 20% of women. The most prominent anaerobic organisms are peptostreptococci, peptococci, anaerobic lactobacilli, eubacteria, and *Bacteroides* species, which together are recovered from virtually all women and individually are recovered from 20 to 60% of women.

Candida albicans, the most common yeast organism, is present in 5 to 10% of women. *Mycoplasma hominis* is present in 20 to 50%, and *Ureaplasma urealyticum* is present in 50 to 70% of sexually active asymptomatic women [12].

Mechanisms of Vaginal Infection

When the complex balance of microorganisms is changed, potentially pathogenic organisms that are part of the normal flora—for example, *C. albicans* in cases of candida infections and *G. vaginalis* and anaerobic bacteria in the case of BV—proliferate to a concentration that is associated with symptoms. In an alternative mechanism of infection , organisms that are sexually transmitted and not part of the normal flora, such as *Trichomonas vaginalis, Neisseria gonorrhoeae,* and *Chlamydia trachomatis,* can produce symptoms when the host mounts an inflammatory response to the infecting organisms by attracting white blood cells and releasing prostaglandins and other components of the inflammatory response.

Symptoms of vaginal discomfort or pruritis result from a local vaginal inflammatory response of *T. vaginalis* or *C. albicans* infection. The organisms that attract white blood cells produce a purulent discharge. Among women with BV, an odor is caused by the presence of amines, which are possibly formed as a result of anaerobic bacterial metabolism [13]. Certain amines, most notably putrescine and cadaverine, are particularly odorous. Others, such as histamine, may produce discomfort by local vasodilatory effects. Still other metabolic products produced in women with BV, such as propionate and butyrate, may damage epithelial cells in a manner analogous to gingival infections [14].

A purulent cervical exudate is most commonly caused by *N. gonorrhoeae, C. trachomatis,* or *Herpesvirus hominis* (herpes simplex virus) [15], because these infecting organisms attract WBCs. The presence of an intrauterine device can result in low-grade endometritis and/or cervicitis in which WBCs are discharged into the vagina through the cervix [16].

DIAGNOSIS

Sensitivity of Microscopic Diagnostic Criteria

Before an attempt is made to make a diagnosis of vaginitis, one should be aware of the sensitivity of the various diagnostic methods. Although the physician considers many physical findings during his examination, a diagnosis based entirely on the physical appearance of the vaginal discharge is too insensitive and too nonspecific to be used as the only basis for diagnosis. The diagnosis of vaginitis is based in large part on microscopic criteria; however, it has been estimated that mycelia and trichomonads are identified microscopically in only 80% of symptomatic women who have candidiasis and trichomoniasis [17]; and the sensitivity of identifying the "clue cell" among women with BV may be at a similar level [18]. Thus 20% of symptomatic women with vaginitis may not be detected by an initial microscopic examination. If a diagnosis cannot be established with certainty, a repeat examination should be made several days later for both symptomatic women with suspected vaginitis (to make a specific diagnosis) and symptomatic women with a presumed normal discharge (to further exclude vaginitis). Two normal examinations would theoretically raise the diagnostic accuracy in both categories to 96%. The use of this plan should reduce the physician's tendency to exclude vaginitis after one "normal" examination among women with infection, but, conversely, two examinations should allow the physician who failed to detect microscopic abnormalities during both examinations to reassure the woman with vaginal discharge that she has no infection.

Physical Examination

Vulvar Appearance

The vulva should be inspected for the geographic erythema that can occur with candidiasis and for the edema that is occasionally present with trichomoniasis. Vulvar and perirectal erythema, placque formation, or fissures may also be present in patients with candidiasis. A thin, introital vaginal discharge is often present with trichomoniasis or BV.

Appearance of Vaginal Discharge

The color, consistency, and location of the discharge should be noted. Women with a normal vaginal discharge usually have a white, floccular, viscous discharge that pools in the dependent recesses of the vagina. In contrast, women with BV have a gray, homogeneous, nonviscous (watery) discharge that is present on the anterior and lateral vaginal walls. Characteristics of other vaginal discharges are also sufficiently different to be helpful in an initial classification attempt (Fig. 1). However, as previously mentioned, a specific diagnosis cannot be made solely from the appearance of the discharge, because of the large variability and the overlap in the appearance of the discharge from one disease to another.

Cervical Appearance

During the early estrogen-dominant phase of the menstrual cycle, a clear mucous discharge is normally present in the endocervix. In the latter progesterone phase of the cycle, this discharge may be very scant or not visible. However, the presence of a purulent-appearing cervical discharge at any point is abnormal, and it should prompt the suspicion of a cervicitis. The cervical portion of women with an anteverted uterus is bathed in the pool of vaginal discharge. Therefore, before a diagnosis of cervicitis can be made with certainty, all the vaginal discharge on the ectocervix must be wiped from the cervical portio by a cotton swab. The presence of a purulent discharge from the endocervix following this procedure establishes the diagnosis of cervicitis. *Neisseria gonorrhoeae* and *C. trachomatis* are two of the most common causes of cervicitis. *Herpesvirus hominis* also causes a cervicitis, but virtually always during a primary infection in association with vulvar herpetic

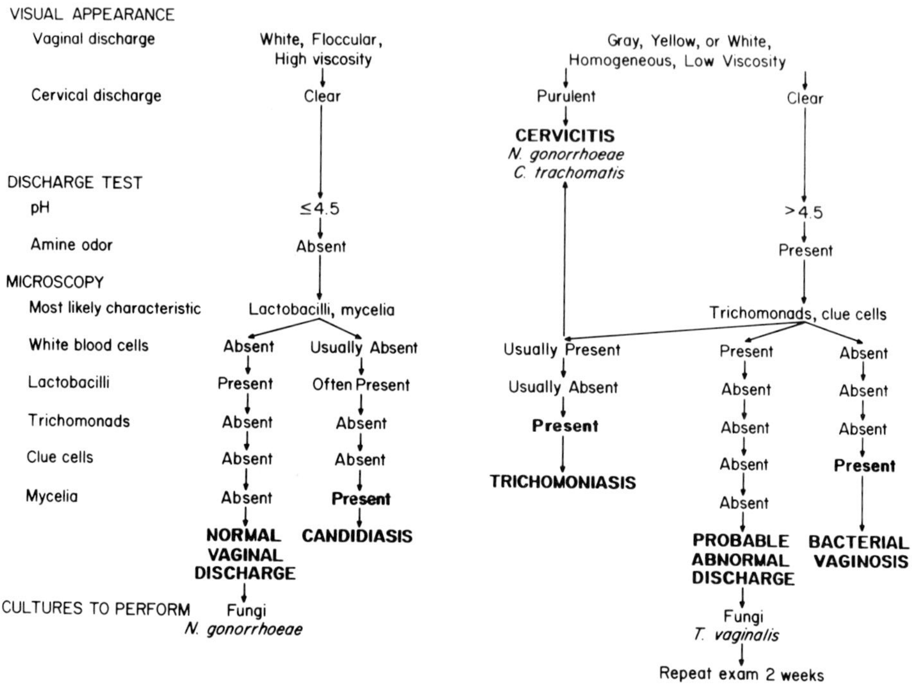

Fig. 1 Algorithm for the diagnosis of vaginitis.

lesions. Patients with cervicitis frequently also have excessive friability and erythema of the columnar epithelium, manifested by endocervical bleeding that occurs when this area is touched with the swab. Among women with chlamydial cervicitis, hypertrophy of the columnar epithelium occurs above the plane of the squamous epithelium.

Chemical Analysis of Vaginal Discharge

pH

The vaginal pH should be tested by placing a drop of the discharge on pH paper. The pH is less than 4.5 among women with candidiasis or normal vaginal discharge. An abnormally elevated pH of more than 4.5 occurs among women with trichomoniasis or BV.

Amine Odor

A large amount of vaginal fluid is mixed with a drop of 10% potassium hydroxide (KOH) and an odor is immediately assessed [19]. A fishy amine odor is present in women with BV and some women with trichomoniasis. Patients with candidiasis or a normal discharge have no odor. The fishy odor is caused by the volatization of amines, most notably putrescine and cadaverine, which are the products of anaerobic metabolism.

Microscopic Analysis of Vaginal Discharge

The slides are observed microscopically. A small amount of vaginal discharge is mixed with normal saline on a glass slide and a cover slip is placed over the preparation. Following the amine odor test, a cover slip is also placed over the KOH preparation. Based on the previous appearance and chemical determinations, the most likely characteristics to be identified by microscopy can be determined (see Fig. 1). The saline portion is first observed for various features.

White Blood Cells

Though a few white blood cells are present in the vagina as a result of physiological cervical discharge, particularly premenstrually, there are usually only one or two cells per field. In an alternative method of quantitating WBCs, the number of WBCs does not exceed the number of vaginal epithelial cells. The presence of a large number of white blood cells should suggest either trichomoniasis or cervicitis and occasionally they are present in candidiasis. Patients with an abnormal vaginal discharge usually caused by an overgrowth of anaerobes also have a large number of WBCs. White blood cells are notably absent in the discharge of patients with BV.

Lactobacilli

The discharge from women with either candidiasis or a normal discharge usually has a predominance of large rods, which, if Gram-stained, are gram positive. These rods generally represent lactobacilli. Women with trichomoniasis may also have lactobacilli, although they are frequently not observed. Lactobacilli have long been thought to be inhibited by the presence of BV, although there is an alternative explanation for their absence. Lactobacilli produce hydrogen peroxide, which inhibits the overgrowth of organisms. However, the diminution of lactobacilli, for whatever reason, may foster the presence of the predominantly anaerobic flora which is observed among patients with BV. Large numbers of small coccobacillary organisms are identified instead of lactobacillus among patients with BV.

Trichomonads

The trichomonad is a motile, flagellated organism that is slightly larger than a white blood cell (Fig. 2). Trichomonads are easily identified when they are fully motile by their characteristic undulating swimming motions. However, white blood cells occasionally surround these organisms, and in 15 to 20% of women with trichomoniasis the motility of the trichomonad is not seen because white blood cells have surrounded the organism. In this case the 400-power objective

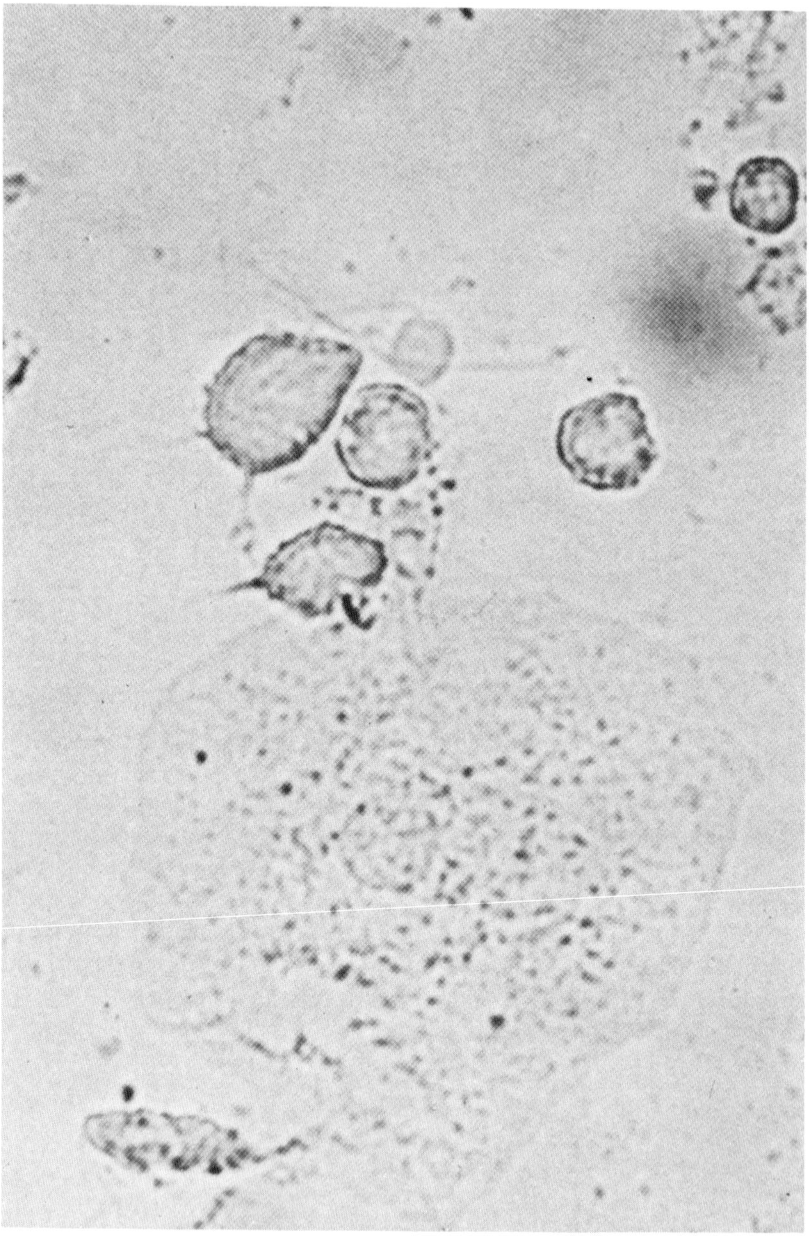

Fig. 2 *Trichomonas vaginalis* on a saline wet mount. (From J. H. Duenhoelter (ed.), *Greenhill's Office Gynecology,* Year Book Medical, Chicago, 1983.)

should be used, and the beating motion of the flagella distinguishes the trichomonad from the white blood cell. Dual infections of trichomoniasis and BV or trichomoniasis and candidiasis occasionally occur, so the potassium hydroxide portion of the slide should also be observed.

Clue Cells

The clue cell is a vaginal epithelial cell to which such a large number of organisms attach that the entire cell border is obscured (Fig. 3). Clue cells are most objectively identified by observing the absence of a clear cell border rather than the so-called granular appearance of the cytoplasmic or nuclear portion. The cell border must be observed through the 400-power objective. Among women with BV, from 5 to 50% of the vaginal epithelial cells are clue cells. Although some investigators have tried to associate the clue cell with the presence of *G. vaginalis,* this correlation is very poor because the clue cell is not present in the 40% of normal women who have *G. vaginalis* but who do not have BV. As mentioned, trichomonads may be seen together with clue cells, although mycelia are almost never seen in the presence of clue cells because of vast pH differences between the fluid in the two infections.

Mycelia

Mycelia cannot usually be seen on the saline portion of the microscopic preparation. They can be identified, however, if a portion of vaginal discharge is mixed with a drop of 10% KOH solution. The mycelia have a very characteristic branching appearance (Fig. 4) which is usually identified through the 100-power objective. The entire surface of the cover slip should be scanned, because even in symptomatic women the mycelia may be clumped in only one area of the slide. Care should be used so that straight strands of cervical mucus are not mistaken for the branching mycelia.

Gram Stain

Vaginal Gram stains can be used in place of the wet mount to detect WBCs, the prominent flora, yeast forms, and "clue cells." The Gram stain is not useful to detect trichomonas; however, it is one of the best methods to detect the presence of the abnormalities present among patients with BV [20] and to detect *Candida* [21].

Vaginal Cultures

Vaginal cultures are of limited use in the diagnosis of vaginitis and they should be used in only specific circumstances. Any woman with a purulent cervical exudate should be cultured for *N. gonorrhoeae* and *C. trachomatis.* A *Candida* vaginal culture should only be obtained from women with suspected candidiasis who have normal KOH preparations. Thus a culture should be obtained from women who have pruritus, an erythematous vulvar rash, or a characteristic vaginal appearance of candidiasis but a normal KOH smear. Trichomonal cultures should also

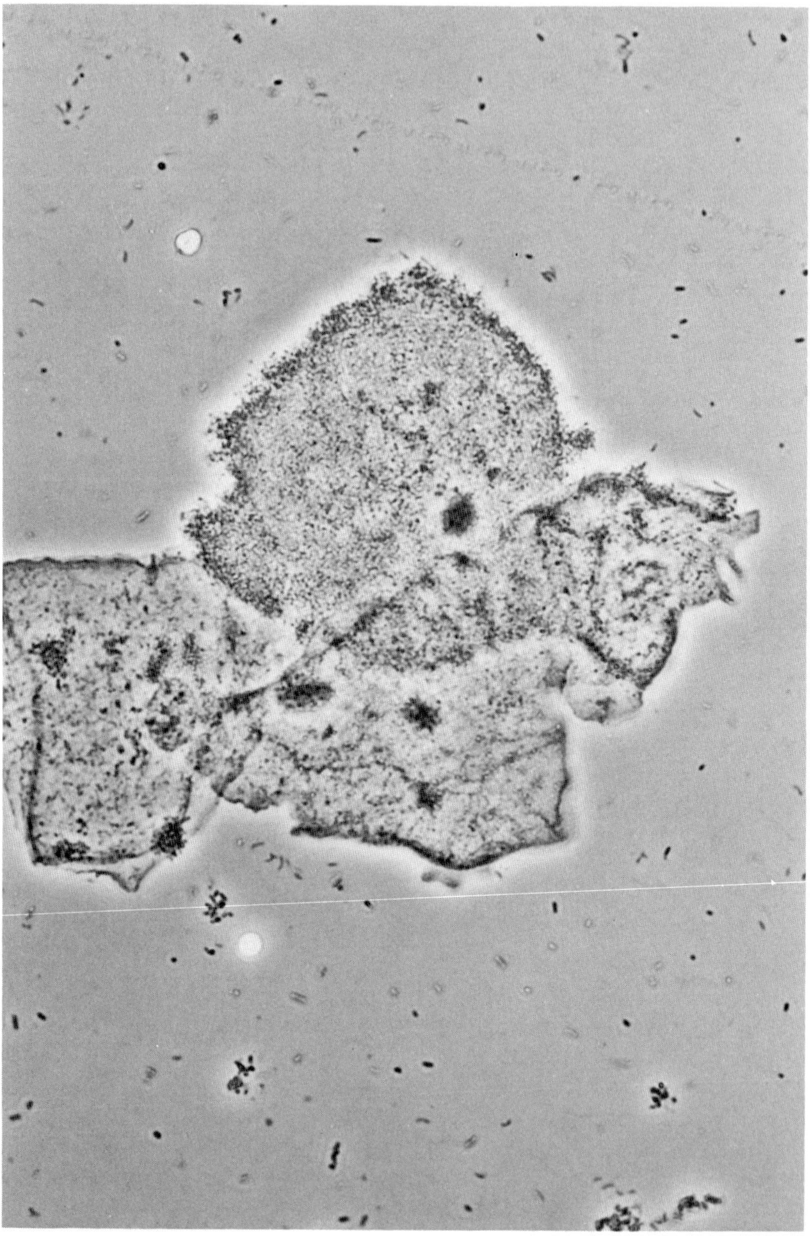

Fig. 3 The clue cell with an indistinct cell border overlapping normal epithelial cells. (From J. H. Duenhoelter (ed.), *Greenhill's Office Gynecology,* Year Book Medical, Chicago, 1983.)

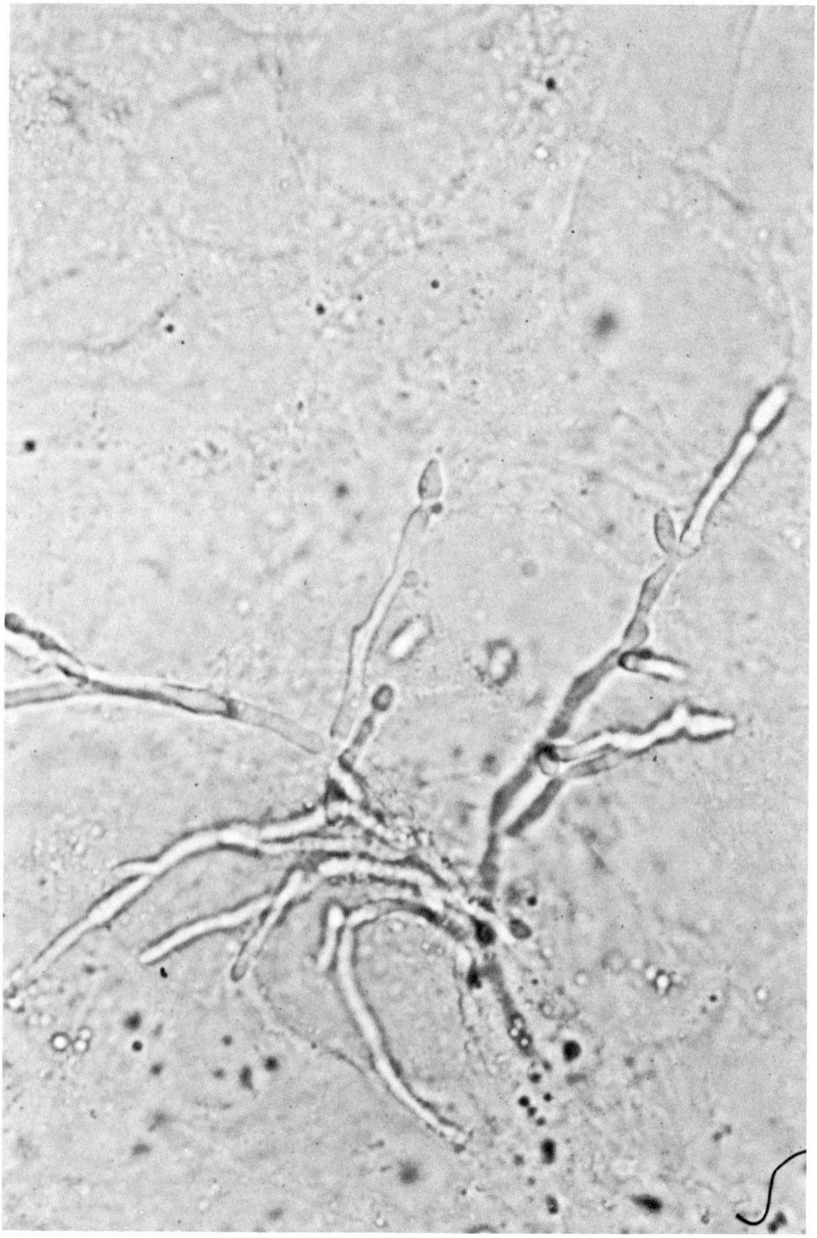

Fig. 4 Pseudohyphae of *Candida* species in a 10% KOH wet mount. (From J. H. Duenhoelter (ed.), *Greenhill's Office Gynecology,* Year Book Medical, Chicago, 1983.)

be performed on a purulent vaginal discharge when repeated microscopic examinations fail to identify the organism. Trichomonads are microscopically identified in 80% of symptomatic women who have *T. vaginalis* recovered by culture. Although trichomonas is microscopically identified in only 50 to 70% of asymptomatic women with trichomoniasis [22]; routine cultures are not generally advocated to identify asymptomatically infected women except in some high-risk groups who attend STD clinics where routine cultures could be cost effective.

Vaginal cultures for *G. vaginalis* (formerly called *Haemophilus vaginalis*), other normal vaginal flora bacteria, or genital mycoplasma are of almost no benefit in making a diagnosis of vaginitis. These organisms are isolated with such a high frequency among asymptomatic women without vaginitis that their presence is correlated either poorly or not at all with vaginitis [23]. Because *Chlamydia* causes a vaginal discharge only from a cervial discharge, *C. trachomatis* cultures are not useful for symptomatic women who have no cervical discharge.

CAUSES OF VULVOVAGINAL DISCHARGE

Physiological Vaginal Discharge

The clinician's first objective is to distinguish a physiological from a pathological vaginal discharge by clinical, laboratory, and microbiological criteria. About 10% of women who complain of vaginal discharge have a physiological increase in the amount of either normal cervical mucus or normal vaginal epithelial discharge [24]. Women with a physiological discharge usually have no vulvar abnormalities. The discharge is not usually present at the introitus (see Fig. 1). A normal vaginal discharge is white and has a nonhomogeneous, floccular appearance because of epithelial cellular clumping. The discharge is very viscous and it pools in the dependent portion of the vagina. The vagina and cervix appear normal. The pH of the discharge is usually less than 4.5, and there is no amine odor when KOH is applied. Microscopically, there are no clue cells, trichomonads, and mycelia, and WBCs are found infrequently. The most striking microscopic finding is an abundance of vaginal epithelial cells and large rods representing gram-positive lactobacilli (see Fig. 1).

Cervical mucus is a second cause of a physiological discharge. A large quantity of cervical mucus is produced by some women, particularly those with a large area of cervical columnar epithelium. These women typically complain of an excessive mid-cycle discharge. Examination of the cervix mid-cycle reveals a large amount of clear cervical mucus and usually a large zone of columnar epithelium. A Gram strain of the cervical discharge reveals only an occasional WBC and organism. The microscopic appearance of vaginal discharge is that of the physiological vaginal discharge. A cervical gonococcal culture should be obtained from all women who complain of a vaginal discharge.

For most women who have a physiological discharge, reassurance is the only necessary therapy. Symptomatic patients who still suspect they have infectious vaginitis should be reexamined within 1 or 2 weeks. Chronic tampon use should be avoided when a persistent physiological discharge is present to prevent vaginal ulceration, which causes a discharge from the tampon per se [25]. Although the practice should generally be discouraged, some women insist on douching; mild vinegar solutions or water should be used. The repeated drying effect of multiple douches may actually increase the amount of discharge, and douching with commercial or harsh preparations frequently produces even more discharge by damaging vaginal cells.

Local vaginal antimicrobial regimen administration to women with a physiological vaginal discharge should be discouraged. It is costly and nonbeneficial. A physiological discharge is only infrequently diminished with local vaginal regimens. Women are easily led to believe that the normal but excessive amount of vaginal discharge is abnormal, particularly when the discharge persists after attempted therapy. Other patients with a physiological discharge are erroneously diagnosed to have *"Monilia"* or "nonspecific vaginitis." When relief is not achieved, sometimes after repeated attempts by several physicians, it becomes extremely difficult to convince the patients that what they observe is normal. Often, as the result of overzealous "hygiene" or the use of soaps, nonprescription or prescription products, and douches, the vulvar and perianal skin and mucous membranes become red, dry, and cracked. It is necessary to stop the application of these products to alleviate this iatrogenic vulvitis. A reduction of these symptoms will often convince the patient that her physiological discharge is normal.

I favor educating the patient to accept an excessive, clear mucoid cervical discharge rather than surgical measures to ablate columnar epithelium. Cryocautery, laser cautery, electrical cautery, silver nitrate application, and acidification are usually unnecessary. The occasional salpingitis caused when a cervical infection is disseminated to the fallopian tubes by these measures creates an unfavorable cost-benefit ratio for the procedures.

Candida Vaginitis

Candida albicans causes 80 to 90% of vaginal fungal infections; other *Candida* and *Torulopsis* species cause the remaining infections [26]. These saprophytic fungi can be isolated in small numbers from 10 to 25% of asymptomatic women; however, symptomatic infection usually results only when these organisms are present in large numbers.

Several factors have been associated with candidal overgrowth and resultant infection. Candidal overgrowth is favored by high blood glucose levels, and diabetics are susceptible to infection. *Candida* organisms also overgrow the normal vaginal bacteria when the latter are suppressed by the administration of broad-spectrum antibiotics. Oral contraceptive use probably does not cause candidiasis [27]. Cellular and not humoral immunity is required for the eradication of candidal infections [28]. Patients with depressed cell-mediated immunity due to pregnancy or immunosuppresive drug administration are predisposed to candidiasis.

Women with candidal infection usually experience intense vulvar and vaginal pruritus. External dysuria caused by the vulvar inflammation is also common. External dysuria is the pain caused when urine passes over the inflamed vulva. Internal dysuria is urethral pain with urination caused by urethritis. Internal dysuria is uncommon. A nonodorous or even a "sour milk"-smelling vaginal discharge may occur, but vaginal or foul-smelling discharge is not usually present.

On examination, an erythematous geographic vulvar rash is often present. The vulva may also be edematous or even fissured. There may also be an erythematous perianal rash. The appearance of the vagina is quite varied. The characteristic vaginal discharge consists of gray to white, dry, viscous, "cottage cheese"-appearing placques that adhere to all sides of the vaginal wall; however, most women have a minimal amount of noncharacteristic discharge. The appearance of the vaginal walls also varies widely from erythematous to normal.

The vaginal pH is usually less than 4.5, and there is no odor from the discharge when KOH is added. Mycelial forms of the organism are identified under the 100-power microscopic objective from material mixed with KOH. Vaginal samples from plaques or vulvar scraping from the edge of the erythema are the best areas to obtain material for examination, although the organism can also be identified from pooled vaginal discharge. The sensitivity of candidal identification by a KOH preparation (80%) [17] is increased by Gram-staining the material (up to 100%) [21] .Papanicolaou smears identify organisms in less than half of patients.

Candida organisms are easily recovered on a variety of media, but because they are part of the normal vagina flora, the recovery of fungi does not necessarily prove that an infection exists. Therefore cultures should be limited to women in whom *Candida* is suspected on the basis of pruritus or abnormal signs, but in whom the diagnosis cannot be confirmed by the KOH preparation. In fact, in some studies cultures performed on symptomatic women identified 50% more patients than microscopic methods.

The local application of antifungal agents is used in the therapy for vaginal fungal infection because, to date, none of the approved agents are absorbed when taken orally. In Table 1 the response of vaginal candidiasis to various locally applied antifungal agents is listed. The studies were selected because the inclusion and cure criteria were clearly stated, the mycology determination were satisfactory, and either a large number of patients were treated or the study was unique. All of the women entered met the inclusion criteria of positive symptoms and either a positive KOH wet mount or a positive fungal culture or both prior to therapy. In all of the studies but one [38] ; a negative culture was required for the patient to be cured, usually 21 to 42 days after the beginning of therapy. In most of the studies the women also had to be without symptoms to be considered cured, although there were no appreciable changes in the cure rates if the latter criterium was not used.

From 33 to 65% of women treated with nystatin were cured using doses which ranged from twice daily for 6 days to twice daily for 15 days. There was no trend

Table 1 Response of Vaginal Candidiasis to Various Locally Applied Antifungal Agents

Authors	Reference	Positive inclusion criteria[a]	Cure criteria	Days followed	Number cured/number treated: Placebo	Nystatin	Miconazole	Clotri-mazole	Boric acid	p	Dose[b]
Proost et al.	29	Sx + cult	Cult	Unknown	1/8					.5	hs × 14 days
						7/21				.001	hs × 14 days
							127/140[c]				Various
Davis et al.	30	Sx + KOH + cult	Sx + sign + KOH + cult	30		46/60				<05	hs × 15 days
							51/56				hs × 14 days
Culbertson	31	Sx + KOH + cult	Sx + KOH/cult	30		23/24				NS[d]	bid × 15 days
							37/45				hs × 14 days
McNellis et al.	32	Sx + KOH + cult	Sx, KOH, cult	8-35		130/244				<01	hs × 15 days
							243/291				hs × 14 days
Robertson	33	Sx + KOH + cult	Sx + cult	21-42			15/24				Daily × 14 days
										NS	Placebo × 7 days
								15/20			Daily × 7 days
Marks	34	Sx + cult	Sx + cult	28		47/60				NS	bid × 5 days,
								54/60			then, hs × 2 days
Tan et al.	35	Sx + cult	Cult	35		7/22				<005	hs × 6 days
								21/22			hs × 6 days
Masterson et al.	36	Sx + sign + KOH + cult	Cult	28				93/103		–	(2) hs × 3 days
Brown et al.	37	Sx + KOH	KOH + cult	28				73/92		–	hs × 7 days
Swate and Weed	38	Sx + KOH + cult	Sx + KOH	30					38/41	–	bid × 14 days
Van Slyke et al.	39	Sx + KOH + cult	Sx + KOH + cult	30		26/52				.02	hs × 14 days
									36/50		hs × 14 days
Range of response (%)						32-65	63-91	75-95	72-95		

[a]Sx, symptoms; KOH, potassium hydroxide; cult, culture.
[b]hs, at bedtime; bid, twice daily.
[c]Includes only the more effective 2% miconazole dose.
[d]NS, not significant.

to indicate that 15 days of therapy was more effective than short-term therapy. However, for the entire group, the range of cure rates for women treated with nystatin was less than the range of cure rates for women treated with either miconazole, clotrimazole, or boric acid. In a number of studies, a statistically significant increase in the cure rates was achieved by miconazole [29,30,32], clotrimazole [35], or boric acid [39] therapy compared to nystatin therapy. Although nystatin therapy was the preferred method, the new, more active antifungal agents that are now available should be used instead of nystatin.

Miconazole, clotrimazole, and boric acid capsules all have excellent activity against *C. albicans*, and they are clinically effective in treating candidiasis. The response rates ranged from 60 to 90%, and it does not appear that any one of these agents is more effective than the other (Table 1). Miconazole and clotrimazole can be administered in a suppository or cream form twice daily for 3½ days or once at night for 7 days. Although the data are not entirely clear on this point, the 7-day therapy may achieve fewer recurrences than the 3½-day regimen. Prolonged therapy is rarely beneficial. Gentian violet therapy has been advocated, but it is rarely necessary because of the effectiveness of these active agents.

Although it is well established that patients with frequent recurrences are the most difficult to cure, physicians often choose nystatin, the least active agent, to treat the most difficult cases of candidiasis. There is a parallel (but not a direct) relationship between the presence of *C. albicans* following therapy and the development of recurrent symptomatic infection. The cure rates are the same after a second course of miconazole therapy as they are after a first course. In contrast, if a second antifungal course was required and nystatin was chosen for treatment, only a minority of women (10 to 30%) responded [29,31,32]. In addition, women who previously had vaginal candidiasis respond better to the more active drugs than to nystatin. The proportion of women cured with miconazole was similar whether or not they had had prior candidiasis; however, fewer women were cured with nystatin if they had prior candidiasis (44%) than if they had no prior candidiasis (57%), and miconazole was clearly better than nystatin for women with prior candidiasis [32]. Clotrimazole also achieves high success rates in women with prior candidiasis.

Boric acid, 600-mg capsules placed high in the vagina once daily for 14 days, has also been found to be highly effective therapy [38,39]. Boric acid capsules can be used repeatedly in the patients with frequent recurrence or persistent symptoms. While pregnant women can be safely treated with nystatin, miconazole, or clotrimazole, boric acid therapy should not be used during pregnancy. Although borate may be poorly absorbed, its absorption [40], particularly during pregnancy, is uncertain.

Vulvitis can be treated with the cream form of miconazole or clotrimazole. Temporary and adjunctive benefit can be gained from sitz baths and superdrying of the skin with a hair dryer. Fungi grow poorly in dry areas. Women should be questioned about symptoms among their sexual partners. At least 10% of male partners have symptomatic urethritis or balanitis caused by *Candida* organisms [41]. Symptomatic men should be treated both to provide symptomatic relief of the man and to prevent recurrent infection in the woman.

Women with recurrent candidiasis should be treated with either miconazole, clotrimazole, or boric acid, and not with nystatin (see Table 4). Their sexual partners should be examined and at least, if symptoms or signs of candidiasis are present, the males should be treated locally. Unfortunately, oral nystatin tablets to eliminate fungi from the stools has not been effective. In fact, even the usually held concept that *Candida* recolonizes from the stool or rectum has been challenged [39] and it is possible that the organism recolonizes from other skin sites.

A minority of women with vaginal candidiasis will develop such frequent recurrences that they virtually always have symptoms. These women are not usually diabetic and they have not evidence of general immunosuppression. It has been difficult to explain the almost continual candidiasis. However, recently it was reported that these women may produce *Candida*-specific suppressor lymphocytes which are able to block the cellular immunity to only this organism [42] while having otherwise normal immunity.

The treatment of individuals with frequent recurrences or women unresponsive to local therapy is most challenging. Many of these women remained with chronic, severe, and often debilitating symptoms. Recently women in these two categories have responded to ketoconazole, 400 mg orally daily for 14 days. This drug is still investigative for the treatment of vaginal candidiasis, in part because of hepatotoxic reactions which have occurred among the women [43]. It has also become apparent that recurrences are still common after the symptoms and candidiasis have been eradicated, and further work is still required.

Trichomonas vaginalis

Trichomonas vaginalis is an ubiquitous sexually transmitted anaerobic parasite. A median of 40% of women who attend STD clinics carry the organism [44]. *Trichomonas vaginalis* has been associated with atypical cytological smears, a rare cause of reversible sterility, and other sexually transmitted infection. In fact, half of women with gonorrhea also have trichomoniasis. Trichomoniasis, and not gonorrhea or *Chlamydia*, is often the cause of a symptomatic discharge when *Trichomonas* and the other two organisms exist together so it is necessary to scrutinize most individuals attending an STD clinic for trichomoniasis [45].

Trichomonas vaginalis can be recovered from the prostatic fluid of up to 70% of male contacts of women with trichomoniasis [46]. Men may be better able to eliminate *Trichomonas* over time from the urinary tract than women, but a significant number of men carry the organism for a prolonged time. Male contacts are particularly likely to harbor *Trichomonas* (>60%) if they are identified within 6 days of their last exposure, but over 33% of male contacts carry *Tricho-*

monas from 6 to over 60 days after the last exposure [47]. From 14 to 60% of male contacts of women with trichomoniasis had the organism in 10 studies reviewed [44]. These data confirm the sexual spread of the infection and further emphasize the necessity of male partner therapy to prevent female reinfection.

Perhaps only 50% of the women infected with *Trichomonas* are symptomatic [48]. In fact, in STD clinics a very high proportion of women with trichomoniasis may be asymptomatic or have symptoms attributed to other agents; however, trichomoniasis is most often identified, even in STD clinics, among symptomatic women who characteristically complain of a profuse, malodorous, and often uncomfortable or pruritic vaginal discharge that causes both internal and external dysuria. The frequently purulent discharge results from the inflammatory response, which most likely is responsible for the symptoms. A sense of vulvar vaginal fullness and even lower abdominal tenderness may also be present. Symptoms typically exacerbate during or following menses.

Trichomonas vaginalis is considered to be an agent which causes lower genital infection only. It can infect the vagina, Bartholin glands, urethra, or periurethral glands, and bladder. In men the organism is present in the urethra and prostate. Trichomoniasis has been associated with an increased rate of postpartum endometritis [49], but this observation has not been confirmed. *Trichomonas vaginalis* has not usually been recovered from infected uterine or intra-abdominal sites, although it has been a rare cause of pyelonephritis. Some women with trichomoniasis have an increase in their anaerobic flora analogous to women with bacterial (nonspecific) vaginosis. The metabolic by-products of anaerobic *T. vaginalis* and of the other anaerobes that increase in concentration during trichomoniasis probably cause the malodorous discharge.

On examination, the vulva may be slightly edematous and the vaginal walls may be covered with the discharge. The classic gray, green, or yellow, purulent, frothy, and odorous discharge is present in only about one-third of women. Small subepithelial hemorrhages of the vagina and cervix usually require colposcopy for identification, but occasionally the hemorrhages are identified on the cervical epithelium by the naked eye (strawberry cervix).

The discharge has a pH greater than 4.5, and after the addition of KOH an amine odor can often be detected. Motile trichomonads vary in size but are larger than WBCs. They are identified by their rapid, jerking motility under a 100 to 400-power microscopic objective. Polymorphonuclear leukocytes may be so abundant that they are able to surround the trichomonad, limiting its motility. The beating flagellar motion can be used to identify the organism in these circumstances, even if the remainder of the organism is stationary. The wet mount identifies trichomonads in 80% of symptomatic women [17], but in probably less than 50% of asymptomatic women because of a smaller number of organisms present and a reduction of the motility among asymptomatic women [48]. Trichomonads are also incidentally detected on Papanicolaou smears, but high false positive rates of identification have been reported and the presence of the organism on Pap smear should usually be confirmed by wet mount and/or culture.

Trichomonas cultures have been advocated to increase the rate of diagnosis, particularly among the asymptomatic women who tend to have a few nonmotile organisms. The culture is easy to perform, but it has limited practicality because fresh media are required for consistent results. Current use is limited to cases in which the diagnosis is suspected but the organism cannot be identified or in populations with large rates of asymptomatic trichomoniasis, such as exist in STD clinis. Diamond's and Feinberg-Whittington media are the most commonly used for culture [48]. Women with *Trichomonas* should also have an *N. gonorrhoeae* culture because of the frequent association of these organisms.

Because *T. vaginalis* resides not only in the vagina but also in the urethra and bladder [44], systemic rather than local therapy is necessary. Both symptomatic and asymptomatic women should be treated. A single 2-g metronidazole dose is preferred because cure rates are not increased with an extended 7-day course. A summary of selected studies in which a 2-g STAT dose was compared to a 7-day metronidazole dose is presented in Table 2. Although differences in detection methods and duration of follow-up occur, there is a remarkable similarity in the cure rates of different investigators using either regimen. Patients should be advised not to drink alcohol for 24 hr after the last dose, and they should be warned of possible nausea and a metallic taste. Simultaneous treatment of the male partner with a 2-g dose of metronidazole is recommended (see Table 2).

At present more than 90% of patients are cured with the single-dose regimen. Male reinfection was totally avoided in only two of the studies in Table 2 [54,55] in which incarcerated women with trichomoniasis had a 97% response rate to both the 2-g one-time dose and the 7-day dose. Thus the achievable cure rate without the factor of male reinfection would be expected to be 97%. Patients with persistent trichomoniasis should be scrutinized for sexual reinfection, and untreated male partners must be simultaneously treated. The recurrence rate was 5% among women whose partners were also treated, compared to 24% among women whose partners were not treated [56]. Both partners can be retreated with a single-dose regimen. In the patient who fails to respond to a second course, a longer 500-mg, twice-a-day regimen for 7 days should be tried (see Table 4).

The treatment is controversial for the patient who does not respond to these measures. Although reports of *T. vaginalis* resistant to metronidazole in vitro have been published [57], we found that absolute metronidazole resistance is an unusual cause of treatment failure. However, a relatively higher resistance to metronidazole [58] has been a factor in some women who do not respond to usual doses. Very high metronidazole levels achieved by 1 g of metronidazole administered orally every 12 hr and the simultaneous intravaginal administration of metronidazole 500 mg every 12 hr may cure patients with susceptible organisms but who fail to respond to the usual oral doses.

Because of the mutagenic and carcinogenic potential of metronidazole [59], its use during pregnancy should be limited to the second half of pregnancy, and then only for symptomatic women who do not become asymptomatic after a

Table 2 Treatment of Vaginal Trichomoniasis with Metronidazole

Authors	Reference	Trichomoniasis determination method[a]	Days followed	Treatment results, cured/total (%) 2 g		7 g		Male Partners treated (2 g)
Csonka	49	M, C	7-30	29/36	(82)	46/49	(94)	Not stated
Woodcock	50	M	7-84	63/73	(86)	51/60	(85)	No
Underhill and Peck	51	M, C	7-21	58/65	(89)	43/55	(78)	Treated
Hager et al.	52	M, C	7-21	80/93	(86)	76/83	(92)	Yes
Aubert and Sesta	53	M	7-21	90/96	(94)	72/74	(97)	As female
Pereyra and Lansing	54	M	~42			932/950	(98)	Not exposed
			~84			933/950	(98)	
Lossick	55	M	28-84	229/237	(97)			Not exposed

[a]M, microscopy; C, culture.

vaginal acidifying cream. One cannot usually achieve the reported 50% cure rate when pregnant women are treated with clotrimazole [60], but this drug could have a temporary effect. Asymptomatic or minimally symptomatic pregnant women can be given a 2-g dose the day of delivery and little of the drug would be present in breast milk. The low carcinogenic potential is, of course, of concern for the nonpregnant woman as well. Although there is no evidence of an increase in cancer among women treated with metronidazole [61], the studies are too small and of too short a duration to be certain.

Bacterial (Nonspecific) Vaginosis

The term "nonspecific vaginitis" is a misnomer that implies that nonspecific organisms cause discharge, or that nonspecific diagnostic criteria are used in its definition and diagnosis. This condition results when there is an overgrowth of both anaerobic bacteria and *Gardnerella vaginalis*, formerly called *Haemophilus vaginalis* [62]. Although both anaerobes and *G. vaginalis* are part of the normal flora, their overgrowth produces this most common form of symptomatic vaginitis. Thus the term "bacterial" should replace "nonspecific." The term "vaginitis" implies that a vaginal inflammatory reaction exists and the distinctive feature in this vaginal condition is the absence of inflammation. Thus the term "vaginosis" should replace "vaginitis," because it best characterizes the most common manifestation of the condition, the malodorous discharge, and bacterial vaginosis (BV) is the precise term to describe this entity. Bacterial vaginosis causes between one-third and one-half of all infectious vaginal conditions [2]. The frequency of this cause of vaginitis is even better illustrated by the finding of symptomatic BV among 12 to 19% of gynecological patients [2]. With the knowledge that an additional number of women have asymptomatic BV, this is indeed a common vaginal infection.

The microbiology of this complex infection remains controversial despite several recent advancements. Previously *G. vaginalis* was believed to be the sole cause of the infection. In the classic study by Gardner and Dukes, *G. vaginalis* was recovered from 92% of symptomatic patients and from none of the asymptomatic patients [2]. However, other investigators isolated *G. vaginalis* from only 30 to 60% of symptomatic women and from 10 to 50% of asymptomatic patients [23] and the role of *G. vaginalis* in BV was questioned. The wide discrepancies between these studies is best explained by the diverse set of diagnostic criteria used by various investigators. Many investigators included into the group with BV either women with other forms of vaginitis or, more commonly, women with a normal physiological discharge. Therefore it was difficult to compare the results of different studies, and the inclusion of women without BV made the bacteriological results innaccurate. In addition, it has been recently appreciated that *G. vaginalis* is an organism present in the vagina of normal women. *Gardnerella vaginalis* can be recovered from 40% of asymptomatic women who have no signs of vaginitis or vaginosis [63]. *Gardnerella vaginalis* is recovered from a higher proportion (more than 95%) of women with BV. The concentration increases from a mean of less than 10^5 CFU/cm^3 of vaginal fluid in women without BV to more than 10^8 CFU/cm^3 of vaginal fluid among women with BV [62].

A similar shift in anaerobic flora occurs among women with BV. The prevalence of anaerobic bacteria increases from 50% in normal women to over 95% in women with BV [62,64]. This increased prevalence is undoubtedly due to increased anaerobe concentrations. The concentration of total anaerobic bacteria increases 1000-fold in women with BV, compared to women without vaginitis, to reach levels of 10^7 CFU/cm^3 of vaginal fluid. The most common anaerobes are members of the *Bacteroides* and *Peptococcus* genera.

It has recently been appreciated that anaerobic curved gram-negative rods are associated with BV. The organisms are only infrequently isolated, but they are observed by Gram stain in one-half of women with BV and in none of the women without vaginitis [65]. The presence of high concentration of these organism together with other anaerobes and *G. vaginalis* attests to the complex microbiology of this form of vaginosis.

It has been known that *Lactobacillus* is infrequently identified by Gram stain or culture among women with BV. The vast majority of lactobacilli isolated from normal women are facultative, while the majority of lactobacilli isolated from women with BV are anaerobic. The factors which control the lactobacillus concentration in the vagina are largely unknown.

The most common characteristic symptom is a foul-smelling, fishy vaginal odor. The fishy odor is caused by the volatization of amines, most notably putrescine and cadaverine, which are produced by bacterial metabolism [13]. The amines are not produced by *G. vaginalis* alone, but by a combination of organisms. This amine odor often increases with menses and after intercourse, when the amines are volatilized by alkalinization. The gray, homogeneous, thin vaginal discharge may be present at the introitus [63], and it usually adheres to the anterior and lateral vaginal walls in addition to pooling beneath the cervix. The vaginal walls and cervix appear normal.

The diagnosis of BV is based on the characteristic homogeneous, nonviscous appearance of the discharge, which has a pH greater than 4.5, produces a fishy amine odor with the addition of KOH, and contains clue cells. Bacterial vaginosis can be diagnosed when three of these four criteria are present [63]. Clue cells can also be identified on Gram stain or Papanicolaou smears. In fact, Gram stains can be used alone to accurately diagnose BV [20]. White blood cells and lactobacilli are usually absent in the smears of women with BV. Because both anaerobes and *G. vaginalis* are recovered from normal women, routine cultures are not useful in the diagnosis. As mentioned, although *G. vaginalis* is recovered from 95% of women with BV, *G. vaginalis* is also recovered from 40% of normal asymptomatic women without vaginitis. Thus the isolation of *G. vaginalis* does not prove that the patient has BV. The culture is also not useful following therapy. *Gardnerella vaginalis* is recovered from 40% of women who have been successfully treated for BV [66,67,69]. Expensive quantitative and anaerobic cultures should be limited to investigative studies.

Recently the diagnosis of BV has been made by gas-liquid chromatography analysis of the vaginal fluid. Gas-liquid chromatography analysis identifies metabolic organic acid by-products of the organisms. Volatile fatty acids other than acetic acid were present in the vaginal discharge of 79% of women with BV and none of the women without BV [62]. The fact that *G. vaginalis* produces some acetic acid but none of the other acids (propionic, butyric, isobutyric, succinic) further emphasizes the presence of other organisms in women with BV.

It is generally believed that this vaginosis produces only local vaginal difficulties. A high concentration of potentially virulent anaerobic bacteria, however, might be expected to cause other morbidity. Recently BV has been associated with postpartum endometritis and prematurity [67]. These observations need to be confirmed, but the data suggest that BV may be important for the development of consequences other than a vaginal discharge.

The therapy of BV has been controversial mainly because there has not been a clear understanding of the cause or the diagnosis, both of which are necessary to provide criteria to determine a cure. Thus a wide variety of cure rates have been reported. The absence of three of four clinical criteria can now be used to establish a cure. In Table 3 the treatment results of BV from several studies are given with various regimens. While most investigators clearly identified and treated BV, in some of the studies the presence of *G. vaginalis* was treated and the presence of BV was not defined. In these later studies an unknown number of women would not have had BV. The studies of *G. vaginalis* therapy are separated from studies of BV therapy in Table 3.

Metronidazole, 500 mg twice a day for 7 days, has been the most effective drug for the treatment of BV, with a cure rate usually ranging from 85 to 95% (Table 3). A 2-g STAT dose of metronidazole is less effective than the 7-day dose [69]. Tinidazole, an imidazole of similar activity, is also effective. Although metronidazole has only modest activity against *G. vaginalis*, it is highly active against anaerobic bacteria, and its effectiveness is undoubtedly due to the anaerobe inhibition. The hydroxymetronidazole metabolite even has good activity against *G. vaginalis* [67,76].

Ampicillin has been used to treat BV, but, as seen from Table 3, ampicillin cures only 33 to 43% of women with BV. Ampicillin is more effective in reducing the concentration of *G. vaginalis*. While *G. vaginalis* was eradicated from 50 to 100% of women treated with ampicillin in the studies listed in Table 3, selective media were not used and the actual cure rates would have been lower had the selective media been used. Small concentrations of the *G. vaginalis* are not as readily detected by nonselective as by selective media [63].

Table 3 Treatment of BV or *Gardnerella vaginalis* with Various Regimens

Drug	Author	Reference	Positive inclusion criteria[a]	Negative cure criteria[a]	Days followed	Number cured/ number treated (%)	
Metronidazole[b]	Pheifer et al.	19	1-4	1-4	14-35	81/81	(100)
	Balsdon et al.	68	1,4	1,4	14-28	16/17	(94)[c]
	Amsel et al.	66	1-5	1-5	>29	(26)	(88)[d]
	Eschenbach et al.	69	1-5	1-5	>29	31/38	(82)[c]
						24/35	(69)[c] (2 g)
	Malouf et al.	70	6	7	>30	20/22	(91)[e]
	Minkowski et al.	71	1,6	1,7	5-7	505/531	(95)[e] (2 g)
Tinidazole[f]	Piot et al.	72	3-5	3-5	8-21	24/26	(92)[c]
Ampicillin[g]	Pheifer et al.	19	1-4	1-4	7	9/27	(33)
	Amsel et al.	66	1-5	1-5	>29	(65)	(43)[d,h]
	Lee and Schmale	73	6	7	30	21/21	(100)[e]
	Rogers et al.	74	1,2,6	7	14-35	19/24	(79)[e]
			1,2	1,2	14-35	18/24	(75)[e]
	Malouf et al.	70	6	7	>30	11/23	(48)[e]
Vaginal triple sulfa[i]	Gardner and Dukes	2	1-4	7	>30	10/13	(77)
	Pheifer et al.	19	1-4	1-4	14-35	1/7	(14)
	Piot et al.	72	3-5	3-5	8-21	4/9	(44)[c]
	Malouf et al.	70	6	7	>30	10/18	(56)[e]

Oral tetracycline[j]	Gardner and Dukes	2	1-4	7	>30	12/17	(71)
	Pheifer et al.	19	1-4	1-4	7	2/15	(13)
Oral doxycycline[k]	Malouf et al.	70	6	7	>30	21/33	(64)
Vaginal tetracycline suppository[l]	Gardner and Dukes	2	1-4	7	>30	26/27	(96)
Erythromycin[m]	Durfee et al.	75	1-4	1-4	7-21	2/11	(18)

[a]1, symptoms of vaginal discharge; 2, signs of abnormal vaginal discharge; 3, pH; 4, clue cells, wet mount or Gram stain; 5, amine odor; 6, culture, presence of *G. vaginalis*; 7, culture, absence of *G. vaginalis*.
[b]500 mg twice daily for 7 days.
[c]Randomized blind treatment trials.
[d]Cumulative percentage, cured.
[e]*Gardnerella vaginitis* was treated, but proportion with BV is unknown.
[f]650 mg twice daily for 5 days.
[g]500 mg every 6 hr for 5 to 7 days.
[h]Treated with ampicillin or amoxicillin.
[i]Twice daily for 7 to 10 days.
[j]250 mg every 6 to 12 hr for 2 to 5 days.
[k]100 mg twice daily for 7 days.
[l]100 mg every 24 hr for 10 days.
[m]500 mg four times daily for 7 days.

Triple sulfa vaginal cream preparations were successfully used by Gardner and Dukes [2], but recently investigators have reported that only 15 to 50% of women with BV are cured, although the concentration of *G. vaginalis* may be reduced. Oral tetracycline and erythromycin are also of limited benefit in treating BV, although both antimicrobials have in vitro activity against some of the organism present among women with BV.

It is of interest that intravaginal tetracycline was very successful in the treatment of BV [2]. The treatment fell out of use because it usually induces vaginal candidiasis, but 100 to 200 mg of tetracycline administered in a cream base one to two time daily is particularly helpful in the treatment of women unresponsive to metronidazole or women who have BV recur immediately after therapy (see below). Patients given vaginal tetracycline should also simultaneously receive a prescription for possible candidiasis.

The male role in BV is not clear. From 80 to 90% of male sexual contacts of women with BV have *G. vaginalis* recovered from the urethra [2,19]. Although one report suggested that male treatment prevents recurrent BV [19], we have not confirmed this in several large subsequent studies. At present the male contact should at least be treated when recurrent disease occurs, but male treatment is not routinely advocated.

Symptomatic women with recurrent BV can usually be successfully treated with metronidazole for 7 days. However, multiple recurrences do occur in perhaps 10 to 15% of women and, although therapy may only be temporarily successful, other regimens which can be used include metronidazole, 1 g twice daily for 7 days; cephalexin, 500 mg four times daily for 7 days; and intravaginal tetracycline for 7 days. Symptomatic pregnant women with BV should not be treated at the present time with metronidazole because of the unknown benefits and the possible risks. Ampicillin could be used during pregnancy.

Asymptomatic women usually need not be treated. The natural course of BV is unknown at present, and thus data are not available on how many women eventually become symptomatic and how many women spontaneously resolve the vaginosis. Similarly, women with *G. vaginalis* identified on culture or Pap should not be treated if they are asymptomatic. If women with *G. vaginalis* identified by these means are symptomatic, they, of course, should be examined for the presence of BV, but in no circumstance should treatment be given for vaginal *G. vaginalis* per se.

Atrophic Vaginitis

Atrophic vaginitis is a symptomatic vaginal inflammatory condition caused by the infection of an estrogen-deficient vaginal epithelium. Women who attend STD clinics are not usually estrogen deficient unless they have undergone bilateral oopherectomies or are in the postmenopausal age range. The thin layer of estrogen-deficient vaginal epithelium is particularly susceptible to infection. Symptoms include vaginal bleeding and soreness, external dysuria, pruritus, and dyspareunia. The diagnosis of atrophic vaginitis can be confirmed by demonstration of a smooth, pale-pink vaginal surface without rugae. A predominance of parabasal and only a few superficial vaginal epithelial cells are observed on a Papanicolaou smear. Moderate vulvar irritation may be present. The discharge is usually slight and has an elevated pH. Microscopy usually reveals no abnormal organisms, although the bacteriology of atrophic vaginitis has not been well defined. Neoplasm, foreign bodies, and other infectious causes of the symptoms should be excluded. Atrophic vaginitis is treated with topical estrogens, which thicken the vaginal epithelium and reduce the susceptibility of the surface to infection. Estrogen cream can be inserted into the vagina once daily for 2 weeks and then every other day for 2 weeks. In the majority of patients, estrogen therapy can be completely stopped without recurrence of symptoms. Because vaginal estrogens are readily absorbed, prolonged vaginal estrogen use has the same disadvantages as systemic estrogens in the postmenopausal woman, and therapy is not usually necessary beyond 4 weeks for the majority of patients.

Cervicitis

Although cervicitis is distinct from vaginitis, cervicitis commonly causes a symptomatic vaginal discharge. As many as 25% of women who complain of vaginal discharge have cervicitis [77]. At the present time, *N. gonorrhoeae, C. trachomatis,* and *H. hominis* are the only established causes of cervicitis [15,77].

The diagnosis is made by demonstrating a mucopurulent cervical exudate after vaginal material is wiped from the cervical portio. The columnar epithelium of women with infectious cervicitis is friable and frequently bleeds on contact. A Gram stain of the endocervical mucus reveals a large number of white blood cells and usually an absence of organisms, except for *N. gonorrhoeae*, among women with gonorrhea. Cultures should always be obtained for *N. gonorrhoeae* and, if possible, *C. trachomatis* (see Fig. 1; see also Chap. 4).

At present 500 mg of tetracycline four times a day for 7 to 10 days is advocated to treat cervicitis. A total of 40% of women with *C. trachomatis* and the women with *N. gonorrhoeae* dramatically respond to tetracycline therapy [77], but the remaining women without either organism may not respond. The cause and the therapy of the remaining cases of vaginitis remain to be determined. Destruction of the columnar epithelium by cryocautery, laser therapy, or conization is not usually necessary to treat this condition, and it frequently causes salpingitis.

Other Causes of Vaginal Discharge

Perhaps 5% of women with vaginitis have a constellation of a foul-smelling discharge with a pH greater than 4.5 and a purulent appearance, confirmed by the presence of a large number of white blood cells on the wet mount with or without clue cells. A large number of anaerobic bacteria but usually no *G. vaginalis* have been isolated from these women. They have often had previous metronidazole treatment and, perhaps because of prior therapy, relative clinical metronidazole resistance seems to exist. Some have responded to local tetracycline, 100 to 200 mg, given intravaginally twice daily for 7 days. An additional group of women have a purulent vaginitis without an increase of anaerobic bacteria. Treatment of the predominant facultative organism should be attempted, but failure rates are high.

Uncommon causes of vaginal discharge should be sought among patients with unusual presentations or findings or patients with persistent symptoms. Chronic tampon use by women who have persistant vaginal discharge or bleeding may cause vaginal ulceration and persistent symptoms. Occasionally women with vaginal adenosis have intermittent vaginal spotting. A history of drug use, which could cause a fixed drug reaction or a localized allergic dermatitis, should be sought among women with unusual findings. Many of the women who complain of a chronic, unresponsive discharge have a normal vaginal flora and no evidence of vaginitis.

A summary of the treatment regimens is provided in Table 4.

Table 4 Treatment Regimens for Women with Vaginitis

	Initial	Recurrent
Normal vaginal (physiological) discharge	Reassurance	Reexamination
Candidiasis	Miconazole: 7 g once daily for 7 days Clotrimazole: 100-mg tablet or 7 g of cream once daily for 7 days Boric acid: 600 mg daily for 7 to 14 days	Miconazole, clotrimazole, or boric acid
Trichomoniasis	Metronidazole: 2 g in a one-time dose; also treat male sexual partner	Metronidazole: 500 mg twice daily for 7 days; retreat male sexual partner
Bacterial (nonspecific) vaginosis	Metronidazole: 500 mg twice daily for 7 days Ampicillin: 500 mg four times daily for 7 days	Metronidazole or intravaginal tetracyclines; treat male sexual partner
Cervicitis	Tetracycline: 500 mg four times daily for 7 days	

REFERENCES

1. National Disease and Therapeutic Index. Ambler, Pa.: Lea, 1971:13-15.
2. Gardner HL, Dukes CD. *Haemophilus vaginalis* vaginitis. Am J Obstet Gynecol 1955; 69:962-976.
3. Huggins GR, Preti G. Vaginal odors and secretions. Clin Obstet Gynecol 1981; 24:355-377.
4. Moghissi KS, Syner FN, Evans TN. A composite picture of the menstrual cycle. Am J Obstet Gynecol 1972; 114:405-416.
5. Huggins GR, Preti G. Volatile constituents of human vaginal secretions. Am J Obstet Gynecol 1976; 126:129-136.
6. Hammerschlag M, Alpert S, Onderdonk AB, Thurston P, Drude E, McCormack WM, Bartlett JG. Anaerobic microflora of the vagina in children. Am J Obstet Gynecol 1978; 131:853-856.
7. Schaeffer AF, Jones JM, Dunn JK. Association of in vitro *Escherichia coli* adherence to vaginal and buccal epithelial cells with susceptibility of women to recurrent urinary-tract infections. N Engl J Med 1981; 304:1062-1066.
8. Bartlett JG, Moon NE, Goldstein PR, Goren B, Onderdonk AB, Polk BF. Cervical and vaginal bacterial flora: ecologic niches in the female lower genital tract. Am J Obstet Gynecol 1978; 130:658-661.
9. Levison ME, Trestman I, Quach R, Sladowski C, Floro CN. Quantitative bacteriology of the vaginal flora in vaginitis. Am J Obstet Gynecol 1979; 133:139-144.
10. Gorbach SL, Menda KB, Thadepalli H, Keith L. Anaerobic microflora of the cervix in healthy women. Am J Obstet Gynecol 1973; 117:1053-1055.
11. Larson B, Galask RP. Vaginal microbial flora: practical and theoretical relevance. Obstet Gynecol 1980; 55:100S-113S.
12. McCormack WM, Rosner B, Lee YH. Colonization with genital mycoplasmas in women. Am J Epidemiol 1973; 97:240-245.
13. Chen KCS, Forsyth PS, Buchanan TM, Holmes KK. Amine content of vaginal fluid from untreated patients with nonspecific vaginitis. J Clin Invest 1979; 63:828-835.
14. Singer RE, Buchner BA. Butyrate and propionate: important components of toxic dental placque extracts. Infect Immun 1981; 32:458-463.
15. Rees E, Tait IA, Hobson D, Johnson FWA. Chlamydia in relation to cervical infection and pelvic inflammatory disease. In: Hobson D, Holmes KK, eds. Washington, DC: American Society for Microbiology, 1977:67-76.
16. Burnhill MS. Syndrome of progressive endometritis associated with intrauterine contraceptive devices. Adv Fam Plan 1972; 8:144-147.
17. McLennon MT, Smith JM, McLennon CE. Diagnosis of vaginal mycosis, trichomoniasis. Reliability of cytologic smear, wet smear and culture. Obstet Gynecol 1972; 40:231-234.
18. Smith RF, Rogers HA, Hines PA, Ray RM. Comparison between direct microscopic and cultural methods of recognition of *Corynebacterium vaginale* in women with vaginitis. J Clin Microbiol 1977; 5:268-272.

19. Pheifer TA, Forsyth PA, Durfee MA, Pollock HM, Holmes KK. Nonspecific vaginitis: Role of *Haemophilus vaginialis* and treatment with metronidazole. N Engl J Med 1978; 298:1429-1434.
20. Spiegel CA, Amsel R, Holmes KK. Diagnosis of bacterial vaginosis by direct gram stain of vaginal fluid. J Clin Microbiol 1983; 18:170-177.
21. Eddie DAS. The laboratory diagnosis of vaginal infection caused by *Trichomonas* and *Candida* (*Monilia*) species. J Med Microbiol 1968; 1:153-156.
22. Nielsen R. *Trichomonas vaginalis* II laboratory investigation in trichomoniasis. Br J Vener Dis 1973; 49:531-535.
23. Vontver LA, Eschenbach DA. The role of *Gardnerella vaginalis* in nonspecific vaginitis. Clin Obstet Gynecol 1981; 24:439-460.
24. Fleury FJ. Adult vaginitis. Clin Obstet Gynecol 1981; 24:407-438.
25. Friedrich EG, Siegesmund KA. Tampon-associated vaginal ulcerations. Obstet Gynecol 1980; 55:149-156.
26. Oriel JD, Partridge BM, Denny MJ, Coleman JC. Genital yeast infections. Br Med J 1972; 4:761-764.
27. Spellacy WN, Zaias N, Buhi WC, Birk SA. Vaginal yeast growth and contraceptive practices. Obstet Gynecol 1971; 38:343-349.
28. Syverson RE, Buckley H, Gibian J, Ryan GM. Cellular and humoral immune status in women with chronic *Candida* infection. Am J Obstet Gynecol 1979; 134:624-627.
29. Proost JM, Maes-Dockx FM, Nelis MO, van Cutsem JM. Miconazole in the treatment of mycotic vulvovaginitis. Am J Obstet Gynecol 1972; 112:688-692.
30. Davis JE, Frudenfeld JH, Goddard JL. Comparative evaluation of monistat and mycostatin in the treatment of vulvovaginal candidiasis. Obstet Gynecol 1974; 44:403-406.
31. Culbertson C. Monistat: a new fungicide for treatment of vulvovaginal candidiasis. Am J Obstet Gynecol 1974; 120:973-976.
32. McNellis D, McLeon M, Lawson J, Pasquale SA. Treatment of vulvovaginitis candidiasis in pregnancy: a comparative study. Obstet Gynecol 1977; 50: 674-678.
33. Robertson WH. Vulvovaginal candidiasis treated with clotrimazole cream in seven days with fourteen-day treatment with miconazole cream. Am J Obstet Gynecol 1978; 132:321-323.
34. Marks HJ. A double-blind comparison of clotrimazole and nystatin vaginal tablets in candida vaginitis. Postgrad Med J Suppl 1974; 1:105-106.
35. Tan CG, Milne LJR, Good CS, Loudon JDO. A comparative trial of six day therapy with clotrimazole and nystatin in pregnant patients with vaginal candidiasis. Postgrad Med J Suppl 1974; 1:102-105.
36. Masterson G, Napier IR, Henderson JN, Roberts JE. Three-day clotrimazole treatment in candidal vulvovaginitis. Br J Vener Dis 1977; 53:126-128.
37. Brown D, Binder GL, Gardner HL, Wells J. Comparison of econazole and clotrimazole in the treatment of vulvovaginal candidiasis. Obstet Gynecol 1980; 56:121-123.
38. Swate TC, Weed JC. Boric acid treatment of vulvovaginal candidiasis. Obstet Gynecol 1974; 43:893-895.

39. Van Slyke KK, Michel VP, Rein MF. Treatment of vulvovaginal candidiasis with boric acid powder. Am J Obstet Gynecol 1981; 141:145-148.
40. Cooke CW. Vulvovaginal candidiasis: to editor. Obstet Gynecol 1976; 48: 631.
41. Oriel JD, Partridge BM, Denny MJ, Coleman JC. Genital yeast infections. Br Med J 1972; 4:761-764.
42. Witkin SS, Yu IR, Ledger WJ. Inhibition of *Candida albicans*-induced lymphocyte proliferation by lymphocytes and sera from women with recurrent vaginitis. Am J Obstet Gynecol 1983; 147:809-811.
43. Peterson EA, Alling DW, Kirkpatrick CH. Treatment of chronic mucocutaneous candidiasis with ketoconazole: a controlled clinical trial. Ann Intern Med 1980; 93:791-795.
44. Krieger JN. Urologic aspects of trichomoniasis. Invest Urol 1981; 18:411-417.
45. Lossick JG. Treatment of *Trichomonas vaginalis* infections. Rev Infect Dis Suppl 1982; 4:S801-S818.
46. Block E. Occurrence of trichomonas in sexual partners of women with trichomoniasis. Acta Obstet Gynecol Scand 1959; 38:398-401.
47. Weston TET, Nicol CS. Natural history of trichomonal infection in males. Br J Vener Dis 1963; 39:251-257.
48. Fouts AC, Kraus SJ. *Trichomonas vaginalis*: reevaluation of its clinical presentation and laboratory diagnosis. J Infect Dis 1980; 141:137-143.
49. Csonka GW. Trichomonas vaginitis treated with one dose of metronidazole. Br J Vener Dis 1971; 47:456-458.
50. Woodcock KR. Treatment of *Trichomonas vaginalis* with a single oral dose of metronidazole. Br J Vener Dis 1972; 48:65-68.
51. Underhill RA, Peck JE. Causes of therapeutic failure after treatment of trichomonal vaginitis with metronidazole: comparison of single-dose treatment with a standard regimen. Br J Clin Pract 1974; 28:134-136.
52. Hager WD, Brown ST, Kraus SJ, Kleris GS, Perkins GJ, Henderson M. Metronidazole for vaginal trichomoniasis. JAMA 1980; 244:1219-1220.
53. Aubert JM, Sesta HJ. Treatment of vaginal trichomoniasis: single 2 gram dose of metronidazole as compared with a seven-day course. J Reprod Med 1982; 27:743-745.
54. Pereyra AJ, Lansing JD. Urogenital trichomoniasis: treatment with metronidazole in 2002 incarcerated women. Obstet Gynecol 1964; 24:499-508.
55. Lossick JG. Single-dose metronidazole treatment for vaginal trichomoniasis. Obstet Gynecol 1980; 56:508-510.
56. Lyng J, Christensen J. A double-blind study of the value of treatment with a single-dose tinidazole of partners to female with trichomoniasis. Acta Obstet Gynecol Scand 1981; 60:199-201.
57. Meingassner JG, Thurner J. Strain of *Trichomonas vaginalis* resistant to metronidazole and other 5-nitromidazoles. Antimicrob Agents Chemother 1979; 15:254-257.
58. Lossick JG. Metronidazole. N Engl J Med 1981; 304:735.
59. Rustia M, Shubik P. Induction of lung tumors and malignant lymphomas in mice by metronidazole. J Nat Cancer Inst 1972; 48:721-729.

60. Schnell JD. The incidence of vaginal candidiasis and trichomonas infections and treatment of trichomoniasis vaginitis with clotrimazole. Postgrad Med J Suppl 1974; 1:79-81.
61. Beard C, Noller K, O'Fallon W, Kurland LT, Dockerty MB. Lack of evidence of cancer due to use of metronidazole. N Engl J Med 1979; 301:519-522.
62. Spiegel CA, Amsel R, Eschenbach DA, Schoenknecht F, Holmes KK. Anaerobic bacteria in nonspecific vaginitis. N Engl J Med 1980; 303:601-606.
63. Amsel R, Totten PA, Spiegel CA, Chen KCS, Eschenbach D, Holmes KK. Nonspecific vaginitis: diagnostic criteria and microbiol and epidemiologic associations. Am J Med 1983; 74:14-22.
64. Blackwell AL, Fox AR, Phillips I, Barlow D. Anaerobic vaginosis (nonspecific vaginitis): clinical microbiological and therapeutic findings. Lancet 1982; 2:1379-1382.
65. Spiegel CA, Eschenbach DA, Amsel R, Holmes KK. Curved anaerobic bacteria in bacterial (nonspecific) vaginosis and their response to antimicrobial therapy. J Infect Dis 1983; 148:817-822.
66. Amsel R, Critchlow CW, Spiegel CA, Chen KCS, Eschenbach D, Smith K, Holmes KK. Comparison of metronidazole, ampicillin and amoxicillin for treatment of bacterial vaginosis (nonspecific vaginitis): possible explanation for the greater efficacy of metronidazole. In: Finegold SM, ed. First United States metronidazole conference. New York: Biomedical Information, 1982; 225-237.
67. Eschenbach DA, Gravett MG, Chen KCS. Complication of nonspecific vaginosis during pregnancy. Scand J Urol Nephrol (in press).
68. Balsdon MJ, Taylor GE, Pead L, Maskell R. *Cornyebacterium vaginalae* and vaginitis: a controlled trial of treatment. Lancet 1980; 1:501-503.
69. Eschenbach DA, Critchlow CW, Watkins H, Smith K, Spiegel CA, Chen KCS, Holmes KK. A dose duration study of metronidazole for the treatment of nonspecific vaginitis. Scand J Infect Dis Suppl 1983; 40:73-80.
70. Malouf M, Fortier M, Morin G, Dube JL. Treatment of *Haemophilis vaginalis* vaginitis. Obstet Gynecol 1981; 57:711-714.
71. Minkowski WL, Baker CJ, Alleyne D, Baghai M, Friedlander L, Schultz B. Single oral dose metronidazole therapy for *Gardnerella vaginalis* vaginitis in adolescent females. J Adol Health Care 1983; 4:113-116.
72. Piot P, Van Dyck E, Godts P, Vanderheyden J. A placebo-controlled, double blinded comparison of tinidazole and triple sulfonamide cream for the treatment of nonspecific vaginitis. Am J Obstet Gynecol 1983; 147:85-89.
73. Lee L, Schmale JD. Ampicillin therapy for *Corynebacterium vaginalae* (*Haemophilus vaginalis*) vaginitis. Am J Obstet Gynecol 1973; 115:786-788.
74. Rogers HA, Hesse FE, Pulley HC, Hines PA, Smith RF. *Haemophilus vaginalis* (*Corynebacterium vaginalae*) vaginitis in women attending public health clinics: response to treatment with ampicillin. Sex Transm Dis 1978; 5:18-21.
75. Durfee MA, Forsyth PS, Hale JA, Holmes KK. Ineffectiveness of erythromycin for treatment of *Haemophilus vaginalis*-associated vaginitis: possible relationship to acidity of vaginal secretion. Antimicrob Agent Chemother 1979; 16:635-637.

76. Ralph ED, Amatnieks YE. Relative susceptibility of *Gardnerella vaginalis* (*Haemophilus vaginalae*), *Neisseria gonorrhoeae* and *Bacteroides fragilis* to metronidazole and its two metabolites. Sex Transm Dis 1980; 7:157-160.
77. Paavonen J, Brunham RC, Kiviat N, Stevens C, Kuo CC, Stamm WE, Holmes KK. Cervicitis: etiologic, clinical and histopathologic findings. In: Mårdh PA, ed. Chlamydial infection. Amsterdam: Elsevier Biomedical, 1982:141-145.

SIX

Genital Ulcer Syndromes

Michael F. Para
The Ohio State University
College of Medicine
Columbus, Ohio

Ian M. Baird
Riverside Methodist Hospital
Columbus, Ohio

INTRODUCTION

Genital ulceration is a morphological feature of a multitude of infectious and noninfectious diseases. The differential diagnosis of this type of genital lesion is listed in Table 1. This chapter will detail an approach to the patient with a genital ulceration and review the more common etiologies. An algorithm outlining an approach to the patient with genital ulceration has recently been published [1] and is shown in Figure 1.

Successful diagnosis and therapy of any sexually transmitted disease (STD) require sensitivity and discretion on the part of the physician and a nonjudgmental approach to the patient. The physician must elicit an accurate and thorough history, perform a careful examination, and utilize the appropriate laboratory studies. In addition, a knowledge of which STDs are prevalent in the community and the antibiotic sensitivities of the genital pathogens is necessary.

Table 1 Causes of Genital Ulceration

Infectious	
	Syphilis
	Herpes simplex genitalis
	Chancroid
	Lymphogranuloma venereum
	Granuloma inguinale
	Excoriations ± superinfection associated with lice, scabies, molluscum contagiosum, genital warts
Noninfectious	
	Trauma
	Behçet's syndrome
	Drug allergy or chemical exposure
	Erythema multiforme
	Malignancy

While this chapter deals mainly with those STDs which cause genital ulceration, the practitioner must remember that multiple pathogens may infect a single patient. Management of a patient with a genital ulcer should not necessarily end with a single diagnosis and treatment. Coexistent infections should be considered likely and ruled out even if other characteristic features are absent.

History

As with many infectious diseases, the patient's history often provides the major clues to the diagnosis of a genital ulcer. When the lesion was first noted relative to any recent sexual contact and its initial manifestation and evolution prior to presentation to the physician will give a needed longitudinal perspective. The patient should be asked about any local symptoms such as burning or itching which may have preceded the lesion and whether the lesion is painful or tender. Previous genital lesions and STDs should also be reviewed.

The details of recent sexual exposures need to be delineated. Inquiries concerning the patient's sexual practices, including active or passive orogenital and anogenital contact, are necessary and should be made with the utmost discretion. Recent use of topical or systemic drugs such as antibiotics or chemicals such as vaginal deodorants should be investigated. Medical treatment for an STD or the presence of genital lesions on a sexual partner may also provide an important clue to the diagnosis of any genital ulcer. The patient should be asked about oral or anal lesions on the sexual partner if there was orogenital or anogenital contact.

Since genital ulceration may be a manifestation of systemic illnesses, the presence of constitutional symptoms (fever, malaise, arthralgias) and ophthalmic or oral lesions must be considered. Dysuria, genital itching, and discharge should

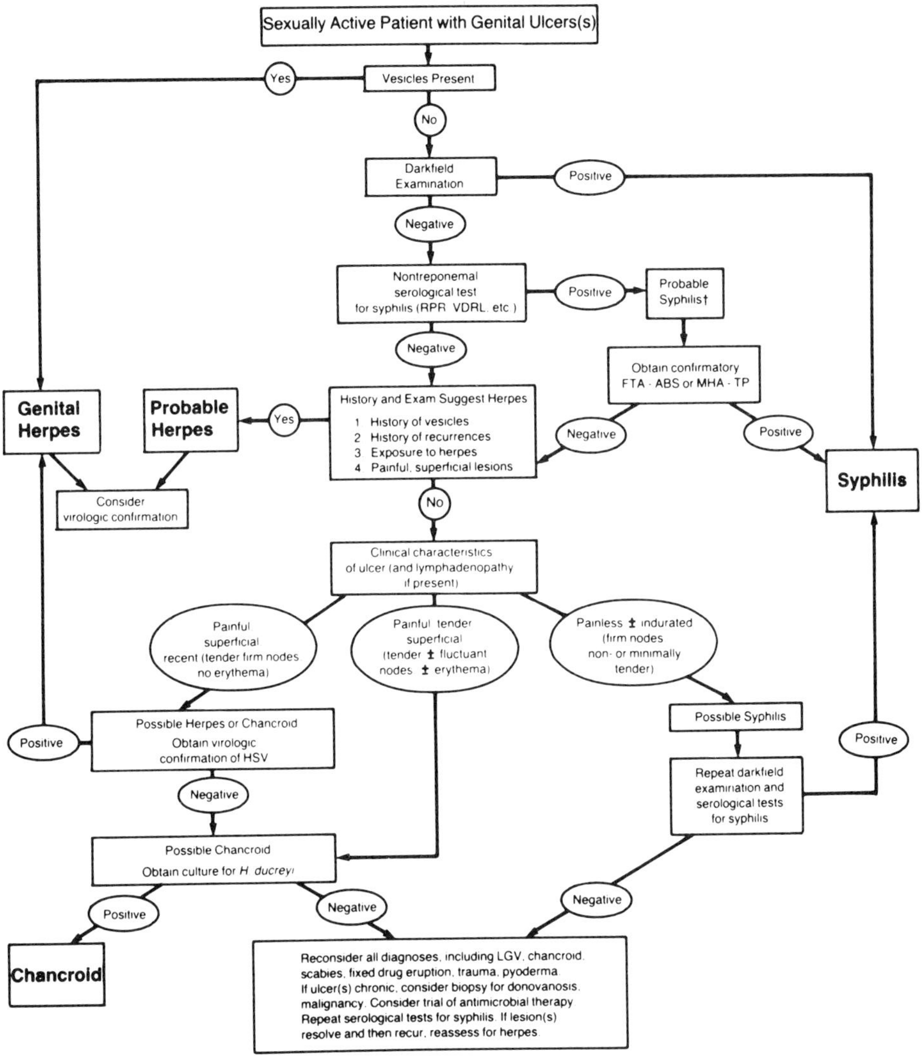

Fig. 1 Algorithm outlining an approach to managing the patient who presents with a genital ulceration (FTA-ABS, fluorescent treponemal antibody absorption; MHA, microhemagglutination assay for *Treponema pallidum*). (From Ann Intern Med 1983; 98:975.)

also be documented. Women should be questioned about birth control practices and the possibility of an early pregnancy.

The etiologies of genital ulceration vary widely throughout the world. The physician must know when and where the patient has traveled and whether there was sexual contact in these locations. State health officials in the STD divison can provide the practitioner with the details of diseases which are prevalent in different areas of the country or world.

The patient must be asked about all sexual contacts since the onset of the lesion to ensure the proper epidemiological management of these individuals.

Physical Examination

Thorough inspection of the lesion, genitals, and perineum is necessary. A complete physical examination may also reveal a critical diagnostic finding if the diagnosis is more doubtful. The history of the patient's sexual practices should also lead to closer inspection of extragenital sites involved in sexual contact. The number and size of genital ulcerations have some diagnostic usefulness. A single ulcer is most commonly seen with primary syphilis, but multiple chancres are not rare. Ulcers should be palpated to determine if there is tenderness or induration. Close inspection of the ulcer base will reveal whether it is clean or necrotic and whether an exudate is present or absent. Hypertrophic tissue which may be ulcerated is seen with granuloma inguinale. Groups of vesicles on an erythematous base are highly suggestive of herpes simplex infections. Herpetic lesions may also form a crust. While careful physical examination is necessary, morphological analysis of genital ulceration alone is inadequate even in the most experienced hands [2]. Clinical findings may be helpful, but the temptation of making a diagnosis solely on these criteria should be avoided.

The presence of inguinal and femoral adenopathy is also helpful in the evaluation of genital ulceration. The duration, presence or absence of tenderness and erythema, and consistency and mobility of nodes should be noted.

Extragenital sites which require particular attention include the oropharynx, rectum, and skin. Herpetic vesicles can be seen on the lips and intraorally, as well as on the skin some distance from the genitalia. Anal intercourse may also cause herpetic proctitis. Similarly, syphilitic lesions can occur at any body site. Recurrent oral and genital ulcerations suggest Behçet's disease and the patient must be carefully questioned and examined for multisystem involvement. Eye, joint, skin, gastrointestinal, and central nervous systems may show manifestations of this illness.

Laboratory Evaluation

Genital ulcers which cannot be accurately diagnosed by history and physical examination may require a more definitive laboratory evaluation. The physician must be guided by his clinical impression in deciding what studies should be performed. The details of performing these tests are discussed with the individual pathogens in the latter sections of the chapter. What follows is a brief description of the laboratory studies which should be considered in the evaluation of a genital ulcer. These can be divided into microbiological and serological studies.

Microbiology

Dark-field microscopic examination of the mobile spirochete *Treponema pallidum* should be performed on any ulcer where diagnostic uncertainty exists. This examination may need to be repeated if negative initially. While clinical diagnosis of a herpes infection is usually adequate, viral cultures provide the most definitive and sensitive diagnostic test. Cytological examination of cells scraped from the base of the lesion (Tzanck preparation) can easily be performed in the office and is diagnostic for herpesvirus when positive (see Chap. 16). Cervical Pap smears may also reveal typical cytological changes associated with herpes involvement of the cervix.

Ulcerations which are compatible with chancroid can be examined by Gram stain of exudate swabbed from the undermined edge of a lesion. Fluctuant nodes can also be aspirated and this material can also be Gram stained and inspected for the typical gram-negative coccobacilli in the "school of fish" configuration. Both the swab and aspirate should be cultured, and although the causative organism, *Haemophilus ducreyi*, is difficult to grow, recent development of a selective culture media makes culture feasible.

The diagnosis of granuloma inguinale can be made by demonstration of the intracytoplasmic bacteria *Calymmatobacterium granulomatis* in the macrophages of tissue smears or biopsies. Culture is not practical at the present time.

Genital ulceration is a transient manifestation of lymphogranuloma venereum. Microbiological diagnosis can be made by culture or immunofluorescence of material aspirated from an affected lymph node. Gram stain of this material should be examined for pyogenic bacteria.

Since patients may harbor multiple infectious agents, gonorrhea cultures should be routinely performed. Uretheral smears should also be considered if there is discharge.

Serology

Serological assays are available for several of the infectious diseases which cause genital ulceration. The wide availability of the treponemal and nontreponemal serological tests for syphilis make assays routine for most patients with genital ulceration. In primary syphilis, the specific fluorescent treponemal antibody-absorbed (FTA-ABS) test is frequently more positive than the nonspecific Venereal Disease Research Laboratory (VDRL) test (85 versus 70%) [3].

Serological assays for herpes simplex virus are also available; however, extensive cross-reactivity between the type 1 virus and the type 2 virus decreases the utility of these tests in diagnoses of genital herpes infections. Antibodies to type 1 virus are not reliably distinguished from antibodies to type 2 virus [4].

If the clinical picture is compatible with lymphogranuloma venereum, a diagnosis can be made by use of a complement fixation test. A titer of 1:64 or a fourfold rise in titer is found in the great majority of patients [5].

HERPES SIMPLEX GENITALIS

Background

The most common infectious etiology of genital ulceration in the United States is infection by herpes simplex virus (HSV) [6]. The Centers for Disease Control have recently reported that an epidemic of genital HSV is occurring in this country [7]. In the United States there are an estimated 300,000 new cases of genital HSV annually and over 20 million patients with recurrent disease. This infection can be caused by either of the two serotypes of HSV: type 1 (HSV-1) or type 2 (HSV-2). In studies performed in this country over 80% of initial and 98% of recurrent genital infections are due to HSV-2.

Like all the human herpesviruses (Epstein-Barr virus, herpes zoster virus, and cytomegalovirus), HSV-1 and HSV-2 have the ability to enter the latent state in the host and to intermittently undergo reactivation with lytic infection and virus replication. This capacity to cause recurrent infections is the major clinical problem of an HSV infection.

The development of the latent state by HSV is not fully understood. With primary HSV infection the virus quickly enters nerve axons and travels directly up to the cell body located in the dorsal root ganglion [8]. During this initial infection the virus may multiply in the ganglia and cause a local neuritis which can be manifest clinically as numbness in the dermatome or bladder or bowel dysfunction. As the immune response develops, the lytic infection in the skin is suppressed and the virus in the nerve enters the quiescent latent state. At some later time the latent virus will reactivate spontaneously or in response to certain stimuli such as fever, menses, local trauma, or emotional upset. With reactivation viral particles move down the axon [9] and cause a cutaneous recurrence with lytic infection and local virus production. This pattern can be repeated indefinitely and is typical of HSV-1 and HSV-2 infections at all mucocutaneous sites.

Herpes simplex virus types 1 and 2 share approximately 50% DNA homology and have multiple common surface antigens [10]. The cross-reactivity among the antigens of these viruses has made serological distinction of the two serotypes difficult. Monoclonal antibodies to the type-specific antigens are now commercially available for typing laboratory-cultivated HSV isolates [11]. There is no reliable and generally applicable test which can distinguish human antibodies to HSV-1 from those to HSV-2.

Epidemiology

Within HSV-1 and HSV-2 serotypes each viral isolate can be further subdivided and characterized by its "DNA fingerprints." The DNA fingerprint is the fragmentation pattern of the viral DNA after cleavage or digestion with restriction endonuclease. Each viral strain has a unique fingerprint unless it has a direct epidemiological link to another strain [12]. Although determination of the virus DNA fingerprint is currently performed only in research laboratories, this technique provides a very powerful epidemiological tool for relating HSV infections [13].

With the use of DNA fingerprinting, more detailed analysis of the epidemiology and communicability of HSV is now possible. There are well-documented cases of intrafamily and nosocomial transmission of a single HSV strain [13, 14]. Genital reinfection with a second HSV-2 strain has also been demonstrated [15]. Not surprisingly, orogenital sex has been implicated in transmission of these viruses [16,17]. Herpes simplex virus may be transmitted by formites, since infectious virus can survive on wet surfaces for several hours [18]; however, this mode of spread has never been proven. Many questions remain unanswered concerning the degree of communicability of symptomatic and asymptomatic genital HSV infections.

Clinical Manifestations

Genital infection with HSV can elicit a wide range of clinical manifestations. Primary genital infection (in the absence of acute phase HSV-1 or HSV-2 antibodies) is generally considered more severe than recurrent infection; nevertheless, primary genital infections may be asymptomatic.

Corey and associates have done extensive investigations of the clinical course of genital HSV infection and have published recent reviews of this topic [19,20]. Patients usually present with multiple, small (1 to 2 mm), vesicular or ulcerated lesions which are painful or pruritic [Fig. 2 (see Plate I, facing p. 168)]. They are most often located on the labia or penis. Other sites include the cervix, fourchette, buttocks, and thighs. The vesicles may coalesce into larger ulcerations. Tender, nonfluctuant inguinal adenopathy, uretheral and vaginal discharge, and dysuria are frequently present. In the symptomatic primary episode, systemic manifestations include fever, headache, photophobia, and malaise in over half of the cases [19]. Viremia, aseptic meningitis, urinary retention, whitlow (involvement of the finger), and pharyngitis are also seen in 5 to 10% of patients.

Clinically, primary episodes due to either HSV-1 or HSV-2 are indistinguishable. On the average, the patient will have pain and shed virus during the initial 10 to 14 days [19]. During the subsequent 1 to 2 weeks there will be gradual healing either by crust formation or re-epithelialization from the lesion margin

[21]. If prior HSV antibodies are present (i.e., from previous "cold sores"), the clinical course of the episode (termed "initial") of genital herpes tends to be milder [22].

Recurrent genital HSV infections develop after approximately 88% of HSV-2 and 55% of HSV-1 primary infections [19]. These episodes are genrally less severe and of shorter duration than the primary or initial infection. Approximately half of the patients who develop recurrences have prodromal symptoms which may include itching, tingling, or aching of the genital area, buttocks, or leg. The lesions of recurrent disease generally occupy less area and are more often pruritic than painful. Dysuria, discharge, cervicitis, and tender adenopathy occur less often than during primary disease. In recurrent infections pain and viral shedding last 4 to 5 days and lesions resolve in approximately 10 days. Nonetheless, there is considerable variation in the severity of primary and recurrent genital HSV infection. Asymptomatic shedding of virus from the cervix, vulva, and the semen has been demonstrated in 0.25 to 8% of patients attending STD clinics [23,24]. In these cases the average number of infectious viral particles is 10- to 1000-fold less than in symptomatic cases and the duration of shedding is shorter [25].

Laboratory Diagnosis

The "gold standard" of laboratory diagnosis of HSV infection is viral culture. Herpes simplex virus is often isolated within 24 hr of culture. Isolation of virus is most frequent in the vesicular phase and decreases with duration of lesion. Only 25% of crusted lesions have culturable virus present [26]. Although tissue culture facilities are limited, HSV is rather stable, and refrigerated specimens will lose little titer over a 3-day storage period in transport media [27]. We use Virocult swabs to collect a small amount of vesicular fluid or to swab the base of an ulcer. These swabs come supplied with transport media.

Other laboratory studies which detect HSV antigens or infected cell membranes include indirect immunoperoxidase and direct immunofluorescence. Both assays can be performed quickly if adequate numbers of infected cells are present. The sensitivity of these studies is approximately two-thirds that of virus isolation [26]. Cytological examination of clinical samples for multinucleate giant cells will be positive in about half the cases. The serological diagnosis of HSV is possible only when there is a seroconversion from a negative titer in the acute serum to an elevated titer in the convalescent serum.

Treatment

The great array of therapeutic modalities which have been recommended for genital HSV infections attests to the lack of an effective treatment. Only with the release of acyclovir is there now an agent which has proven efficacy.

Therapy for genital HSV can be divided into treatment and prophylaxis. Treatment efficacy of the acute primary or recurrent episode is determined by

Plate I

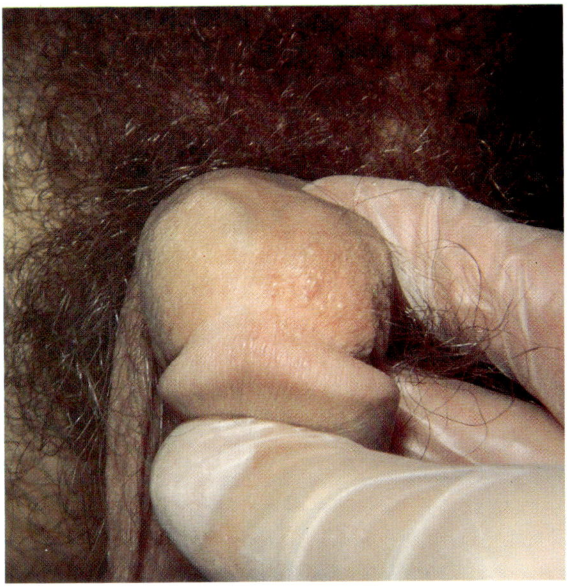

Fig. 2 Vesicular lesions of herpes simplex virus adjacent to glans penis.

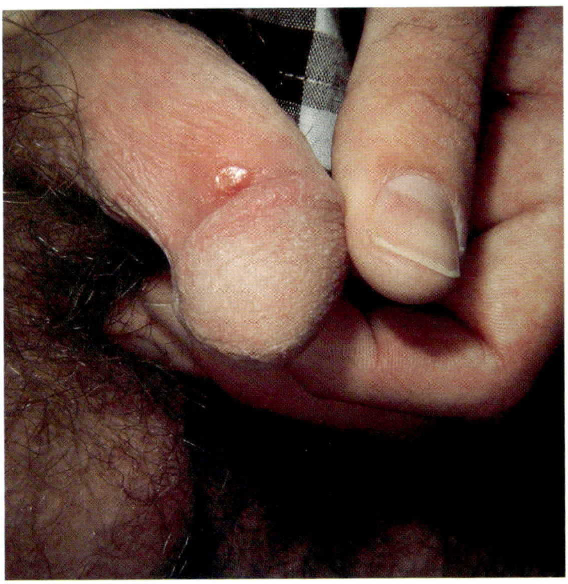

Fig. 3 Solitary chancre of primary syphilis adjacent to glans penis.

decrease in pain, viral shedding, lesion size, and time in healing. A 5% acyclovir topical preparation in polyethylene glycol has been shown to shorten the duration of viral shedding (2.3 versus 5.6 days) and accelerate lesion healing (11.2 versus 15.8 days) in primary genital HSV. In recurrent disease viral shedding was significantly decreased, but lesion duration was slightly decreased only in men [28]. Because of this limited efficacy, the drug is not recommended in recurrent genital HSV. However, acyclovir may be of some benefit in severe protracted recurrences. Topical acyclovir should be applied as early as possible to the involved area and should be used six times per day until the lesions have crusted. It should not be applied intravaginally.

Intravenous acyclovir (5 mg/kg every 8 hr for 5 days) has been shown to be much more effective than topical drug. Virus shedding is decreased from 13 to 2 days and the time till complete healing of genital lesions is reduced from 21 to 9 days [29]. Oral acyclovir (200 mg five times a day for 10 days) appears to be as effective as the intravenous form [30].

Patient-initiated therapy with oral acyclovir during the prodromal phase of recurrent genital HSV showed a decrease in viral shedding (2.1 versus 3.9 days) and accelerated healing (5.7 versus 7.2 days), but no difference in the duration of pain [31]. There is no substantial evidence that acyclovir can decrease the time to or frequency of subsequent recurrences.

Acyclovir has been evaluated in recent studies relative to the prevention of genital HSV recurrences [32-35]. In the reported trials patients with frequent recurrent genital HSV were given 200 mg of oral acyclovir three to five times a day or a placebo. During the studies, lasting 3 to 4 months, there were significantly fewer recurrences in the acyclovir group and little significant toxicity was noted. Oral acyclovir was approved for therapeutic and prophylactic use in the United States by the U.S. Food and Drug Administration in January 1985.

A variety of measures have been used to ease the symptoms of genital HSV. Narcotic derivations may be used to control lesion pain; however, these agents can inhibit sphincter function and should not be generally recommended. Aspirin, when given every 3 to 4 hr, often gives adequate relief. Topical anesthetics have also been used but provide only temporary pain control.

To promote healing the lesions should be kept clean and dry. Sitz baths with Burow's solution or other drying agents can be helpful if limited to 5 to 10 min of soaking. The skin must not become macerated. These baths can be followed by drying the lesions with a blow dryer. Loose-fitting underwear is also recommended. Some patients believe unroofing blisters speeds healing. There are no data to support this practice, and patients should be aware of the infectious nature of the vesicular fluid.

Severe dysuria can be managed by drinking extra fluids to dilute the urine. Women may find that pouring water over the genital area during micturation relieves pain. The deluge of horror stories about genital HSV which have recently appeared in the media has created great anxiety and fear in patients with newly diagnosed HSV infections. Many patients will need counseling and support. This can be provided by the Herpes Resource Center of the American Social Health Association, which has organized local chapters in many cities.

Complications

Herpes simplex virus infection of the neonate has an 80% mortality when untreated [36]. With few exceptions, this infection is acquired by the infant during delivery. Although the exact risk to the infant is unknown, delivery through an actively infected birth canal should be avoided. The exact management of the pregnant female with a history of genital herpes is debatable and a detailed discussion is beyond the scope of this chapter. A balanced review of opinions is presented by Corey and Holmes [1]. A reasonable approach would be weekly viral cultures of the cervix beginning at the 32nd week of pregnancy in all women with either a history of genital herpes or whose sexual contacts have genital herpes. These women should be carefully examined early in labor and a cervical smear for the rapid detection of viral antigens should be done immediately. Any evidence of active infection would require a cesarean section. Management of the infant is also controversial and the directions of the local hospital infection control team should be followed [37].

Several seroepidemiological studies have indicated a relationship between genital HSV infection and the development of cancer of the cervix [38]. The antibody assays, selection of controls, study settings, and results have varied greatly and raised legitimate questions about the validity of these observations. Experimental techniques capable of detecting herpes viral DNA in individual malignant cervical cells have been recently developed [39]. In a series of reports Galloway and McDougall [40] have demonstrated several fragments of HSV DNA within the tissues from 30 to 50% of cervical carcinoma patients. Because no consistent single fragment has been found, these investigators and others have suggested that HSV may induce carcinogenesis by a "hit and run" mechanism whereby the virus induces a malignant alteration in the cell (e.g., critical mutation) and is then shed from the cell [40]. Patients with a history of genital HSV or whose contacts have HSV should have Pap smears at yearly intervals.

Prevention

Herpes simplex virus vaccines have been used in Europe for a number of years. These vaccines consisted of inactivated virus including viral DNA and were never proven to be effective. More recently, subunit vaccines containing viral glycoprotein antigens have been developed and are considered safer than DNA-containing vaccines [41]. These vaccines do elicit antiviral antibodies [42]. The effectiveness of such a vaccine to prevent or modify primary genital HSV infection must be documented in carefully controlled studies and such evaluation is currently underway. Limited studies have shown protection of vaccinated patients at high risk for genital HSV [43]. There has been no convincing evidence to date that any HSV vaccine will modify the course of HSV recurrences.

At the present time prevention is best accomplished by avoiding contact with infectious lesions. Because of the potential for asymptomatic viral shedding, the patient may be infectious and not be aware of it. Unfortunately, the infectious potential of asymptomatic HSV shedders is not known. Because of the low titers of virus shed in the absence of lesions, asymptomatic shedding of HSV is likely to have a reduced infectious potential. Condoms may provide limited protection from acquisition of HSV [44]. Patients who understand the mode of spread of genital HSV and are familiar with the manifestations of their infection are less likely to spread the virus [1].

SYPHILIS

History

While a lengthy discussion of the history of syphilis in Europe and the Americas is not within the scope of this chapter, a brief summary of this disease's significant role in history is in order [45]. There exists a continuing debate whether the disease existed in Europe before the fifteenth century or whether it was introduced by the return of Columbus and his men. During the Middle Ages syphilis was responsible for considerable morbidity, premature mortality, and chronic insanity. Early descriptions of the clinical course indicated that syphilitic infection may have resulted in a more rapidly fatal illness in the sixteenth century than was described in the nineteenth and early twentieth centuries [46].

Since the introduction of penicillin, both early and late forms of syphilis have decreased significantly in developed countries; however, recent studies have shown a gradual increase in the total number of newly diagnosed cases since 1977 [47].

Etiology and Pathology

Initially identified in the early twentieth century, *T. pallidum* is the etiological agent of syphilis. The susceptible host can acquire this organism from an individual with primary, secondary, or early latent (up to 1 year) disease. This spirochete is capable of penetrating intact skin or mucosa. Transfusion-related disease is possible but unlikely, because all donors are tested for serological evidence of syphilis. Sexual intimacy and congenital acquisition are the only practical explanations for transmission of this infection.

While *T. pallidum* is a strictly anaerobic spirochete which has never been grown in vitro, it can be cultured in laboratory animals. A variety of silver impregnation stains have been used to demonstrate the organisms in tissue [48]. At the site of initial inoculation the spirochete multiplies and produces a granulomatous tissue reaction (the chancre) with involvement of the regional lymph nodes. There is a striking endarteritis in all luetic lesions, including the primary chancre. This primary lesion resolves spontaneously within 3 to 6 weeks and is followed in several weeks by the generalized organ involvement of secondary syphilis. This stage of the infection is also self-limiting. Secondary syphilis may eventually be followed by locally destructive or wasting lesions of tertiary disease. Up to 65% of untreated patients with primary and secondary disease fail to develop tertiary infection [46].

Epidemiology

The incidence of primary syphilis in the United States fell dramatically after 1945 but has been slowly increasing since 1977 [47]. Currently syphilis is generally seen in the sexually promiscuous. In a recent report 25% of cases of primary and secondary disease were encountered in the male homosexual population [49]. It is also seen in protitutes and other sexually active persons, but may occasionally be acquired by more sexually naive individuals. Since the only important means of acquiring primary syphilis is by intimate contact, it is important to interview the patient with a primary lesion to determine the sexual contacts in the preceding 3 to 4 months.

Clinical Manifestations

The incubation period of syphilis ranges from 12 days to 12 weeks after exposure, the average time being 2 to 4 weeks. The length of the incubation period is a function of several variables such as inoculum size, organism virulence, and intrinsic host defense. A sore or "hard chancre" develops at the site where *Treponema* invasion has occurred. Although there are some "typical" characteristics of the primary chancre, the appearance of these lesions is often atypical and all genital and anal lesions should be suspected as primary syphilitic lesions until proven otherwise. The "typical" characteristics are listed in Table 2 and a primary chancre is shown in Figure 3 (see Plate I, facing p. 168).

Genital lesions are more commonly observed in males than in females, since female infection often occurs in unexposed areas of the vagina or cervix. Careful speculum examination is necessary to detect such infection. Extragenital lesions are most frequent around the anus and mouth, but may be found on the nipple, the axilla, and the oropharynx. Anal involvement is commonly seen in the male homosexual population.

The differential diagnosis of primary syphilis includes all the diseases which can cause genital ulceration listed in Table 1.

In the absence of treatment the chancre of primary syphilis heals within 3 to 6 weeks, characteristically without scar formation. A latent phase of several weeks usually precedes the widespread clinical manifestations of secondary syphilis; however, approximately 25% of patients may experience this phase of the

Table 2 Characteristics of "Typical" Primary Syphilitic Chancres

A single lesion
An eroded painless papule which is firm and indurated
Variable size, from a few millimeters to 1 to 2 cm
Regional lymph nodes that are frequently enlarged, firm, and nontender

disease while the primary lesion is still present. The secondary stage of syphilis actually represents the invasion of all major organ systems by blood-borne treponemes; however, the clinical manifestations of this process are usually evident only as skin and mucous membrane lesions. The cutaneous lesions may be macular or roseolar, papular, maculopapular, follicular, papulosquamous, pustular, or psoriasiform [50]. A recent study of the signs and symptoms of 105 patients with secondary syphilis noted that maculopapular lesions were predominant (69.5%) and the distribution of lesions was widespread and symmetrical. The palms and soles were the most frequently involved anatomical sites (>50%), mucosal lesions were present in approximately 21%, and lymphadenopathy occurred in approximately 86%. A significant observation was the history of pruritus in 42% of cases, a symptom traditionally unassociated with syphilitic dermatitis [51]. Secondary syphilis may consist of a single episode lasting for several weeks or a series of recurrent episodes. The natural history of this stage of syphilis is the spontaneous cessation of manifestations after a period of 2 to 3 years [50].

Following the secondary stage, the asymptomatic latent stage of syphilis occurs and can remain quiescent for the life of the patient or manifest as cardiovascular or neurosyphilis after 10 years or more. These complications are rarely encountered in developed countries since the advent of penicillin and screening serological testing. Detailed descriptions of these pathological states are found in older medical textbooks [52]. Latent syphilis has been conveniently divided into early latent (confined to the first 2 years of infection and considered contagious) and late latent disease (duration over 2 years and considered noninfectious except for congenital transmission) [50].

Special consideration should be given to the occurrence of syphilis in pregnancy. Historically, *T. pallidum* was thought not to be able to cross the placental barrier until the 15th to 18th week of pregnancy. Therefore detection of disease and appropriate therapy by the end of the fourth month of pregnancy were considered protective to the fetus. However, more recent data suggest that this may not be the case and infections in the first trimester may lead to increased fetal loss. Failure to detect and appropriately treat the disease may cause infection of the fetus, with catastrophic consequences. Treatment of the mother during pregnancy will likely cure the infected fetus; however, all these infants should be examined carefully at birth and at frequent intervals thereafter.

Diagnosis

Since culture of the organism is not possible, diagnosis of early syphilis rests with demonstration of the microorganism by dark-field microscopy. With the infrequency of primary syphilis, this is a technique which few physicians have performed in recent decades. Most larger hospital laboratories will have a dark-field microscope and a technician who is familiar with the technique.

Acquisition and preparation of the specimen to be examined will be the responsibility of the physician. Necessary equipment includes a clean slide, cover slip, petroleum jelly, and a sterile cotton sponge. With gloved hands the examiner should cleanse the suspected lesion with normal saline, allow it to dry, and gently abraid the lesion with the cotton gauze until minimal bleeding occurs. Pressure should be applied until the bleeding stops and clear serum can be expressed from the lesion. This serum is applied to a slide directly or by pipette, and a cover slip sealed at its periphery with petroleum jelly is applied over the exudate. The slide must then be examined immediately. A satisfactory positive control may be obtained by examining a small specimen of saliva (nonsyphilitic spirochetes are part of normal mouth flora).

The agent of syphilis can be identified both by its typical morphology and by its characteristic motion. The organism is 6 to 15 μm in length, very slender, approximately 0.1 to 0.2 μm in diameter, and with 6 to 14 tightly bound spirals. The movement of *T. pallidum* consists of a rocking to-and-fro motion with rotation about its long axis like a corkscrew. In the interpretation of specimens examined by dark-field microscopy, specimens from the mouth will contain nonpathogenic spirochetes and should be interpreted as positive for *T. pallidum* with great caution.

Serological testing is the cornerstone for the diagnosis of secondary, latent, and tertiary syphilis, but has limited value in primary disease. Reaginic tests do not become positive until the fourth to sixth week of the illness, but specific treponemal tests (FTA-ABS) may be positive by the end of the second week. Because diagnostic laboratories do not routinely perform FTA-ABS as a screening test on specimens which are negative for reagin, a special request should be made to the laboratory to perform this test in a patient who has a lesion suggestive of a primary chancre. Following successful therapy, the titers of the nontreponemal tests drop while the treponemal specific titers do not. The nontreponemal tests [VDRL, rapid plasma reagin (RPR)] are positive with high titers (at least 16 dilutions) in secondary syphilis with such consistency that completely negative serological tests exclude the possibility of this entity [53]. Latent syphilis is characterized by low-titer nontreponemal tests. Treponemal-specific tests [FTA-ABS and *Treponema pallidum* hemagglutination (TPHA)] should be performed to establish the diagnosis, since low-titer VDRL or RPR tests may be indicative of other processes. Common causes of transient biological false positive reactions include viral illnesses, malaria, and pregnancy. Chronic biological false positive reactions are associated with certain chronic diseases (tuberculosis, systemic lupus erythematosus, sarcoidosis, rheumatoid arthritis) and narcotic addiction [50].

All individuals with latent syphilis should have a lumbar puncture to evaluate the possibility of neurosyphilis. Cerebrospinal fluid (CSF) demonstrating pleocytosis, elevated protein concentrations, and a reactive VDRL is diagnostic of active neurosyphilis. However, the VDRL is relatively insensitive in the detection of neurosyphilis, and most researchers recommend that a CSF FTA-ABS or CSF TPHA be done, since they are superior indicators of neurosyphilis [54,55].

Treatment

Primary and secondary syphilis are effectively treated with benzathine penicillin G (2.4 million units given intramuscularly at a single session). Patients who are allergic to penicillin and not pregnant should receive tetracycline (500 mg by mouth four times a day for 15 days). If the patient cannot tolerate tetracycline, therapy with erythromycin (500 mg by mouth four times a day for 15 days) is appropriate. Patient compliance with the oral regimens should always be a concern, and considerable effort should be expended to assure that adequate therapy is achieved.

At all stages of pregnancy patients with primary and secondary syphilis should receive penicillin parenterally as recommended for the treatment of nonpregnant patients. Pregnant patients who are documented as having an allergy to penicillin should receive erythromycin (500 mg by mouth four times a day for 15 days) [56]. The efficacy of erythromycin in this situation has never been fully documented, and infants of mothers treated with erythromycin for early syphilis during pregnancy should receive benzathine penicillin, 50,000 units/kg intramuscularly in a single dose shortly after birth. All pregnant women who have been treated for primary syphilis should have monthly quantitative nontreponemal serological tests (VDRL or RPR) for the remainder of the pregnancy. Any woman who shows a fourfold or greater rise in titer should be retreated.

Early latent syphilis with normal CSF findings and adequate opportunity for clinical and serological follow-up is treated with any of the regimens used for primary or secondary syphilis [57]. For late latent syphilis the CDC recommends benzathine penicillin G (7.2 million units total dose intramuscularly, given in three single doses of 2.4 million units each, once every 7 days). The treatment of pregnant women is the same as that for nonpregnant patients. Nonpregnant patients who are allergic to penicillin can receive either tetracycline or erythromycin in dosages of 500 mg by mouth four times a day for 30 days. Pregnant patients allergic to penicillin should be treated with the erythromycin regimen [56].

The treatment of neurosyphilis has been the subject of considerable debate. The lack of detectable penicillin in the CSF after recommended intramuscular doses of benzathine penicillin G and even after aqueous penicillin G (2.4 million units intravenously daily for 10 days) has prompted a reevaluation of the treatment strategy for neurosyphilis. Treponemicidal concentrations of penicillin in the CSF have been demonstrated with aqueous penicillin G (2.0 million units intravenously daily) together with oral probenecid (500 mg by mouth four times a day) for 20 days [58]. While further studies are necessary to resolve this issue, it is obvious that benzathine penicillin is not ideal for the treatment of any patient with established or possible neurosyphilis.

CHANCROID

Epidemiology

This ulcerative disease of the genitalia is caused by *H. ducreyi* and was first recognized as distinct from syphilis in 1852. The etiological agent was first isolated by Ducrey in 1889 [59]. Chancroid is most common in the Far East and was seen regularly in American soldiers during the Korean and Vietnam conflicts. More recently it has been seen in California among men who had recent sexual contact with prostitutes [60]. It is described most commonly in males (>90%). The relative paucity in females is probably the result of asymptomatic vaginal and cervical lesions.

Pathology

The lesions of chancroid are usually confined to those genital sites more often traumatized by sexual intercourse. Hence they are found on the internal surface of the prepuce and frenulum in men, and on the labia, clitoris, and fourchette in women. Trauma facilitates the entry of the causative organism. A small papule develops and is surrounded by a zone of erythema. This lesion enlarges and then erodes to produce a sharply circumscribed soft lesion with a base of granulation tissue. Histologically the lesions show a superficial inflammatory exudate below which there is considerable edema with endothelial proliferation, and at the base of the lesion there is a dense infiltrate of lymphocytes and plasma cells. The histopathology of involved lymph nodes demonstrates acute and severe inflammation with polymorphonuclear infiltration and necrosis.

Clinical Manifestations

Following an incubation period of 1 to 14 days (average, 4 to 5 days) the primary lesion appears. Initially it is an inflamed macule, which rapidly progresses to form a vesicle and then a pustule. The usual clinical presentation is a painful lesion that has eroded to leave a ragged ulcer (3 to 20 mm) with a granulating base. Satellite ulcers, the result of autoinoculation, may occur. As many as 10 have been reported, but usually there are only 1 or 2 [61]. A bubo develops in

25% of patients and has a characteristic appearance. It is usually unilateral, painless, more likely or as likely tender, and unilocular with marked erythema of the overlying skin. The bubo appears 7 to 10 days after the initial lesion, eventually softens and becomes fluctuant, and may rupture spontaneously. Systemic spread does not occur, but local superinfection with aerobic and/or anerobic bacteria has been described [59].

Diagnosis

A Gram stain of the exudate from a clean, dry lesion may demonstrate the typical morphology of a gram-negative coccobacillus 1 to 2 μm long with rounded ends. Typically the organism is seen singly or in small clumps along strands of mucus. Aspirate of the bubo may show the same coccobacillary forms. The sensitivity of either stained specimen is approximately 50%. The organism may be cultured, but it is fastidious and the growth and isolation of the organism are not routinely done in general diagnostic laboratories. Reference laboratories in areas where the disease is seen with regularity usually have the necessary expertise.

Diagnosis should be made on positive grounds and should not be made solely by the exclusion of other recognizable and diagnosable illnesses. A blood-free selective medium consisting of gonococcal medium base, enriched with 1% hemoglobin and Isovitalex, and to which vancomycin (3 μg/ml) is added has been a valuable contribution to the laboratory diagnosis of chancroid [62]. A compatible clinical lesion plus ragged ulceration in the coronal sulcus or severe multiple erosive lesions or a unilateral bubo is also considered diagnostic. Skin tests, serological techniques, and autoinoculation experiments are not useful.

Treatment

Fluctuant lymph nodes should be aspirated through healthy adjacent normal skin. Incision and drainage or excision of nodes will result in delayed healing and are contraindicated. Local cleansing of the ulcers is indicated. The drug of choice for treatment of chancroid is trimethoprim (160 mg) together with sulfamethoxazole (800 mg) twice daily for 10 days. Sexual partners should be treated with a similar regimen. Erythromycin (500 mg by mouth four times a day for 10 days) is a suitable alternative form of treatment.

LYMPHOGRANULOMA VENEREUM

Practitioners are unlikely to see genital ulceration due to lymphogranuloma venereum for two reasons: First, the painless genital ulcers often go unnoticed in this disease and, second, the disease is unusual in the United States. The usual presentation is that of inguinal lymphadenopathy which has a differential diagnosis that is distinct (from Table 1) and includes additional diseases such as cat scratch fever, tularemia, and malignancies.

Etiology and Epidemiology

The etiological agent of lymphogranuloma venereum (LGV) is *Chlamydia trachomatis*. This species is currently divided into 15 serogroups of which only 3 (L-1, L-2, and L-3) are responsible for LGV. These three serogroups appear to have greater tissue invasiveness than the other serogroups, which cause disease generally limited to mucous membranes [63].

Lymphogranuloma venereum has worldwide distribution, but is most frequently seen in tropical areas. Central and South America, Indochina, India, and East Africa have the greatest prevalence of disease [64]. There are approximately 350 cases of LGV reported per year in the United States [65]. The majority of the cases are men. The sex differential may partly be explained by the pelvic lymph drainage, which in women leads to inconspicuous deep iliac rather than inguinal adenopathy [66].

Clinical Manifestations

The clinical manifestations of LGV have been divided into primary, secondary, and tertiary stages. After a 3- to 30-day incubation period a primary lesion may develop on the genitalia. This lesion (5 to 6 mm) is painless and may be vesicular or papular. It may erode to become an ulcer, but heals within a few days without scar formation. This primary sore goes unnoticed by the majority of patients and uncommonly leads to physician consultation. Primary rectal inoculation may be associated with diarrhea, discharge, and ulceration [67].

The secondary stage develops 1 to 4 weeks after the primary stage and manifests as inguinal adenopathy. The lymph nodes are more commonly unilateral and are initially firm, limited in number, discrete, and often tender. Over the next week a more extensive adenitis develops, with matting of nodes and adherence and discoloration of the overlying skin. This is followed by the suppuration and multiple draining sinuses from necrotic foci within the nodes. The process usually resolves spontaneously over weeks or months, with scar formation. The inguinal ligament which divides the femoral and inguinal nodes can create a groove between the nodes if they are both involved. This is called the "groove sign" and is seen in 10 to 20% of cases. During the secondary stage constitutional symptoms such as fever, myalgias, headache, and arthralgias are common [59].

The tertiary phase is remarkable for the continued tissue destruction and scarring. This stage may be seen particularly in women without previous inguinal adenopathy. Sinuses, fistula, and strictures may be found in the vulva, perineum, and rectum. Both women and men may develop elephantiasis. Homosexual men and women with proctitis may develop rectal strictures.

Diagnosis

The diagnosis of LGV can be made by isolation of the organism or serology. When *Chlamydia* culture facilities are available, aspiration and culture of the pus from

2. Chapel TA, Brown WJ, Jeffries C, Stewart JA. How reliable is the morphological diagnosis of penile ulcerations? Sex Transm Dis. 1977; 4:150-653.
3. Sparling PF. Diagnosis and treatment of syphilis. N Engl J Med 1971; 284: 642-653.
4. McClung H, Seth P, Rawls WE. Relative concentrations in human sera of antibodies to cross-reacting and specific antigens of herpes simplex virus types 1 and 2. Am J Epidemiol 1976; 104:192-201.
5. Thorsteinsson SB. Lymphogranuloma venereum: review of clinical manifestations, epidemiology, diagnosis and treatment. Scand J Infect Dis 1982; 14:127-131.
6. Caine VA, Handsfield HH, Corey L, Wang SP, Holmes KK. Prospective study of the etiology of genital ulcers. Program of the First Sexually Transmitted Diseases World Congress. San Juan, Puerto Rico: Latin American Union Against Venereal Diseases, 1981 (Abstract 052).
7. Centers for Disease Control. Genital herpes infections–United States, 1966-1979. Morbid Mortal Week Rep 1982; 31:137-139.
8. Stevens JG. Latent herpes simplex virus and the nervous system. Curr Top Microbiol Immunol 1975; 70:31-50.
9. Cook ML, Stevens JG. Pathogenesis of herpetic neuritis and ganglionitis in mice: evidence of intra-axonal transport of infection. Infect Immunol 1973; 7:272-288.
10. Nahmias AJ, Roizman D. Infection with herpes simplex virus 1 and 2. N Engl J Med 1973; 289:667-674, 719-725, 781-789.
11. Balachandran N, Frame B, Chernesky M, et al. Identification and typing of herpes simplex viruses with monoclonal antibodies. J Clin Microbiol 1982; 16:205-208.
12. Buchman TG, Roizman B, Adams G, Stover BH. Restriction endonuclease fingerprinting of herpes simplex virus DNA: a novel epidemiological tool applied to a nosocomial outbreak. J Infect Dis 1978; 138:488-498.
13. Linnemann CC Jr, Buchman TG, Light IJ, Ballard JL, Roizman B. Transmission of herpes simplex virus type 1 in a nursery for the newborn: identification of viral isolates by DNA fingerprinting. Lancet 1978; 1:964-966.
14. Halperin SA, Hendley JO, Nosal C, Roizman B. DNA fingerprinting in investigation of apparent nosocomial acquisition of neonatal herpes simplex. J Pediatr 1980; 97:91-93.
15. Buchman TG, Roizman B, Nahmias AJ. Demonstration of exogeneous genital reinfection with herpes simplex virus type 2 by restriction endonuclease fingerprinting of viral DNA. J Infect Dis 1979; 140:295-304.
16. Evrard JR. Orogenital transmission of herpes simplex type 1. Obstet Gynecol 1974; 44:593-595.
17. Chang TW. Herpetic angina following orogenital exposure. J Am Vener Dis Assoc 1975; 1:163-164.
18. Turner R, Shebab Z, Osborne K, Hendley JO. Shedding and survival of herpes simplex virus from fever blisters. Pediatrics 1982; 70:547-549.
19. Corey L, Adams HG, Brown ZA, Holmes KK. Genital herpes simplex infections: clinical manifestations, course and complications. Ann Intern Med 1983; 98:958-972.

20. Corey L. The diagnosis and treatment of genital herpes. JAMA 1982; 248: 1041-1049.
21. Pazin G, Harger JH, Breinig MC, Armstrong JA, Ho M. Signs, sexual relationships and source contacts of women with initial genital herpes. Twenty-second ICAAC, Miami Beach, Florida, 1982 (Abstract 549).
22. Reeves WC, Corey L, Adams HG, Vontver LA, Holmes KK. Risk of recurrence after first episodes of genital herpes: relation to HSV type and antibody response. N Engl J Med 1981; 305:315-319.
23. Vontver LA, Hickok DE, Brown ZA, Reid L, Corey L. Recurrent genital herpes simplex virus infection in pregnancy: infant outcome and frequency of asymptomatic recurrences. Am J Obstet Gynecol 1982; 142:75.
24. Adam E, Kaufman RH, Mirkovic RR, Melnick JL. Persistence of virus shedding in asymptomatic women after recovery from herpes genitalis. Obstet Gynecol 1979; 54:171-173.
25. Guinan ME, MacCalman J, Kern ER, Overall JC, Spruance SL. The course of an untreated recurrent genital herpes simplex infection in 27 women. N Engl J Med 1981; 304:759-763.
26. Moseley RC, Corey L, Benjamin D, Winter C, Remington ML. Comparison of viral isolation, direct immunofluorescence, and indirect immunoperoxidase techniques for detection of genital herpes simplex virus infection. J Clin Microbiol 1981; 13:913-918.
27. Yeager AS, Moris JE, Prober CG. Storage and transport of cultures for herpes simplex virus, type 2. Am J Clin Pathol 1979; 72:977-979.
28. Corey L, Nahmias AJ, Guinan ME, Benedetti JK, Critchlow CW, Holmes KK. A trial of topical acyclovir in genital herpes simplex infection. N Engl J Med 1982; 306:1313-1319.
29. Corey L, Fife KH, Benedetti JK, Winter CW, Fahnlander A, Connor JD, Hintz MA, Holmes KK. Intravenous acyclovir for the treatment of primary genital herpes. Ann Intern Med 1983; 98:958-972.
30. Bryson JY, Dillon M, Lovett M, Acuna G, Taylor S, Cherry JD, Johnson BL, Wiesmeier E, Growdon W, Cregh-Kirk T, Keeney R. Treatment of first episodes of genital herpes virus infection with oral acyclovir: a randomized double-blind control trial in normal subjects. N Engl J Med 1983; 308:916-921.
31. Reichman RC, Badger GJ, Mertz GJ, Corey L, Richman D, Oxman M, Connor J, Bryson Y, Tyrrell D, Portnoy J, Dolin R. Patient-initiated therapy of recurrent herpes simplex genitalis with orally administered acyclovir. Abstract. Fortieth Annual National Meeting of American Federation of Clinical Research, Washington, D.C., 1983; 373A.
32. Straus S, Seidlin M, Takiff H, Bachrach S, DiGiovanna J, Western K, Cregh-Kirk T, Lininger L, Alling D. Suppression of recurrent genital herpes with oral acyclovir. Abstract. Ninety-Sixth Annual Meeting of Association of American Physicians, Washington, D.C., 1983; 543A.
33. Douglas J, Critchlow C, Benedetti J, Mertz G, Remington M, Fahnlander A, Winter C, Corey L. Double-blind placebo-controlled trial of prophylactic oral acyclovir for frequent recurrences of genital herpes. In: Program and

abstracts of the International Society for STD Research, 5th International Meeting, Seattle, Washington, 1983 (Abstract 183).
34. Halsos AM, Fiddian AP, Gabrielsen BO. Suppression of recurrent genital herpes infections with oral acyclovir. In: Program and abstracts of the International Society for STD Research, 5th International Meeting, Seattle, Washington, 1983 (Abstract 184).
35. Kinghorn GR, Barton IG, Potter CW, Fiddian AP. Oral acyclovir prophylaxis of recurrent genital herpes. In: Program and abstracts of the International Society for STD Research, 5th International Meeting, Seattle, Washington, 1983 (Abstract 185).
36. Whitley RJ, Nahmias AJ, Visintine AM, Fleming CL, Alford CA. The natural history of herpes simplex virus infection of mother and newborn. Pediatrics 1980; 66:489-494.
37. Committee of Fetus and Newborn and Committee on Infectious Diseases. Perinatal herpes simplex virus infections. Pediatrics 1980; 66:147.
38. Nahmias AJ, Naib ZM, Josey WE, Franklin E, Jenkins R. Prospective studies of the association of genital herpes simplex virus infection and cervical anaplasia. Cancer Res 1973; 33:1491-1497.
39. McDougall JK, Crum CP, Fenoglio CM, Goldstein LC, Galloway DA. Herpesvirus-specific RNA and protein in carcinoma of the uterine cervix. Proc Nat Acad Sci USA 1982; 79:3853-3857.
40. Galloway DA, McDougall JK. The oncogenic potential of herpes simplex viruses: evidence for a "hit and run" mechanism. Nature 1983; 302:21-24.
41. Hilleman MR, Larson VM, Lehman ED, Salerno RA, Conard PG, McLean AA. Subunit herpes simplex 2 vaccine. In: Nahmias AJ, Dowdle WR, Schinazi RF, eds. The human herpesviruses. New York: Elsevier, 1981:503-506.
42. Ashley RL, Clark H, Schick M, Corey L. Antibody response to herpes simplex virus type 2 (HSV-2) vaccine in humans. Abstract. Fortieth Annual Meeting of American Federation of Clinical Research, Washington, D.C., 1982; 358A.
43. Skinner GRB, Woodman CBJ, Hartley CE, Buchan A, Fuller A, Durham J, Synnott M, Clay JC, Melling J, Wiblin C, Wilkins J. Preparation and immunogenicity of vaccine Ac NFU (S^-) MRC towards the prevention of herpes genitalis. Br J Vener Dis 1982; 58:381-386.
44. Judson FN, Bodin GF, Levin MJ, Ehret JM, Masters HB. In vitro tests demonstrate condoms provide an effective barrier against *Chlamydia trachomatis* and herpes simplex virus. In: Program and abstracts of the International Society for STD Research, 5th International Meeting, Seattle, Washington, 1983 (Abstract 176).
45. Dennie CC. A history of syphilis. Springfield, Ill.: Charles C. Thomas, 1962.
46. US Department of Health, Education and Welfare. Syphilis: a synopsis. Public Health Service Publication 1660. Washington, DC: US Government Printing Office, 1967.
47. Centers for Disease Control. Annual summary 1981: reported morbidity and mortality in the United States. Morbid Mortal Week Rep 1982; 30:82-86.
48. Luna LG. Manual of histologic staining methods of the Armed Forces Institute of Pathology. New York: McGraw-Hill, 1968:238-240.

49. Centers for Disease Control. Syphilis trends in the United States. Morbid Mortal Week Rep 1981; 31:441-444.
50. Arya OP, Osoba AO, Bennett FJ. Syphilis. In: Arya OP, Osoba AO, Bennett FJ, eds. Tropical venereology. 1st ed. Edinburgh: Churchill Livingstone, 1980:26-98.
51. Chapel TA. The signs and symptoms of secondary syphilis. Sex Transm Dis 1980; 7:161-164.
52. Youmans JB. Syphilis and other venereal diseases. Med Clin North Am 1964; 48:571-824.
53. Sequeira PJL. Serological diagnosis of untreated early syphilis: importance of the differences in THA, TPHA, and VDRL test titers. Br J Vener Dis 1983; 59:145-150.
54. Luger A, Schmidt BL, Steyrer K, Schonwald E. Diagnosis of neurosyphilis by examination of the cerebrospinal fluid. Br J Vener Dis 1981;57:232-237.
55. McGeeney T, Yount F, Hinthorn DR, Liu C. Utility of the FTA-ABS test of cerebrospinal fluid in the diagnosis of neurosyphilis. Sex Transm Dis 1979; 6:195-198.
56. Centers for Disease Control. Sexually transmitted disease, treatment guidelines 1982. Morbid Mortal Week Rep Suppl 1982; 31:50S-54S.
57. Panconesi E, Zuccati G, Cantini A. Treatment of syphilis: a short critical review. Sex Transm Dis 1981; 8:321-325.
58. Polnikorn N, Witoonpanich R, Vorachit M, Vejjajiva S, Vejjajiva A. Penicillin concentrations in cerebrospinal fluid after different treatment regimens for syphilis. Br J Vener Dis 1980; 56:363-367.
59. Hart G. Chancroid, donovanosis and lymphogranuloma venereum. US Department of Health and Human Services Publication No. (CDC) 82-8302. Washington, DC, 1982.
60. Centers for Disease Control. Chancroid California. Morbit Mortal Week Rep 1982; 31:173-175.
61. Asin J. Chancroid: a report of 1,402 cases. Am J Syph Gonorrhea Vener Dis 1952; 36:483-487.
62. Hammond GW, Chang JL, Wilt JC, Ronald AR. Comparison of specimen collection and laboratory techniques for isolation of *Haemophilus ducreyi*. J Clin Microbiol 1978; 7:39-43.
63. Grayston JT, Wang SP. New knowledge of chlamydiae and the diseases they cause. J Infect Dis 1975; 132:87-105.
64. Willcox RR. International aspects of the venereal diseases and nonvenereal treponematoses. Clin Obstet Gynecol 1975; 18:207-222.
65. Felman YM, Nikitas JA. Lymphogranuloma venereum. Cutis 1980; 35: 264-288.
66. Schachter J. Lymphogranuloma venereum and other nonocular *Chlamydia trachomatis*. In: Hobson D, Holmes KK, eds. Nongonoccal urethritis and related infections. Washington, DC: American Society for Microbiology, 1977: 91-97.
67. Bolan RK, Sands M, Schachter J, Miner RC, Drew WL. Lymphogranuloma venereum and acute ulcerative proctitis. Am J Med 1982; 72:703-706.

68. Schachter J, Smith DE, Dawson CR, Anderson WR, Deller JR, Hoke AW, Smart WH, Meyer KF. Lymphogranuloma venereum. I. Comparison of the Frei test, complement fixation test, and isolation of the agent. J Infect Dis 1969; 120:372-375.
69. Stephens RS, Tam MR, Kuo CC, Nowinski RC. Monoclonal antibodies to *Chlamydia trachomatis*: antibody specificities and antigen characterization. J Immunol 1982; 128:1083-1089.
70. Schachter J. Chlamydial infections. N Engl J Med 1978; 298:428-435, 490-495, 540-549.
71. Felman YM, Mikitas JA. Granuloma inguinale. Cutis 1981; 27:364-377.
72. Kuberski T. Granuloma inguinale (donovanosis). Sex Transm Dis 1980; 7:29-36.
73. Marmell M. Donovanosis of the anus in the male. An epidemiological consideration. Br J Vener Dis 1958; 34:213-218.
74. Lal S, Garg BR. Further evidence of the efficacy of the co-trimoxazole in granuloma venereum. Br J Vener Dis 1980; 56:412-413.

SEVEN

Pelvic Inflammatory Disease

Richard C. Bump and Robert J. Fass
The Ohio State University
College of Medicine
Columbus, Ohio

INTRODUCTION

Pelvic inflammatory disease (PID) is unquestionably the most significant consequence of sexually transmitted disease in the industrialized world. The toll PID extracts from the young female population and society in general is enormous in terms of acute morbidity, hospital and medical facility utilization, economic drain, and long-term health effects. McCormack has pointed out that in comparison to the severe complications suffered by women, sexually transmitted infections in males are mainly trivial [1].

Jones et al. determined that between 1970 and 1975 over 212,000 women were admitted annually to acute care hospitals in the United States with a primary diagnosis of PID, utilizing 897,000 hospital days or the equivalent of six 400-bed hospitals [2]. More recent estimates place the annual number of admissions for PID at 250,000, paralleling the general increase in incidence of sexually transmitted diseases [3]. A total of 1% of nonobstetrical female admissions are for PID, making it a more frequent source of infectious morbidity in the 15- to 25-year-old age group than all other serious infections combined. Over 50% of women with PID who are hospitalized undergo a surgical procedure for the disease, with half of the procedures being hysterectomy. In addition, it is calculated that another 1.89 million outpatient visits are made annually by an estimated 630,000 women for recognized PID [4].

The economic price of PID is equally staggering. Curran calculated the direct and indirect cost of PID and PID-associated ectopic pregnancy in the United States in 1979 at $1.25 billion [5]. Costs for subsequent management of chronic pain and infertility cannot be determined. No price can be attached to more intangible losses such as deprivation of parenthood, absenteeism, or marital discord.

But the most dramatic measure of the magnitude of the PID problem lies in the estimates of its long-term sequelae [5,6]. At current rates, close to 15% of reproductive age women will be in the post-PID state. One out of four of these women will suffer one or more of the sequelae of chronic abdominal pain, infertility, or ectopic pregnancy. In the United States 90,000 women are added to the chronic pain pool, 60,000 are rendered infertile, and 25,000 develop ectopic pregnancies as a result of PID every year. Of every 1000 females born in 1950, by 1980, 138 had PID at least once, 26 were infertile secondary to PID, and 9 suffered an ectopic pregnancy due to PID [6]. While the hospital death rate for PID is quite low (4.2 per 1000 hospitalized women), an average of 897 women hospitalized for PID die each year [5].

These numbers serve vividly to underscore the tragic proportions of PID. Much of the recent explosion of interest and research in PID and sexually transmitted disease is a response to the magnitude of the problem. Many of the controversies that have arisen as a result of this explosion in knowledge are a reflection of the extreme complexity of what was once thought of as a simple, monoetiological, clinically diagnosable, and easily treatable disease. The aim of this chapter is to condense and distill these recent advances into a clinically useful form.

There is considerable justified criticism of the term PID in the literature as having too imprecise an interpretation and too broad an implication to be medically meaningful and useful. Indeed, one prominent authority in gynecological infectious disease refuses to use the term, preferring to utilize the designators ES (endometritis-salpingitis) or ESP (endometritis-salpingitis-peritonitis) instead [7]. While the term PID is often used carelessly and has unquestionable ambiguities, we feel it is so thoroughly ingrained both in daily clinical use and in the medical literature that introducing a variety of personal preference alternatives does little to clarify the issue. In this chapter we will rarely use the term PID without a qualifier (e.g., acute, chronic, subclinical) in an attempt to minimize confusion.

MICROBIOLOGY AND PATHOPHYSIOLOGY

Neisseria gonorrhoeae was discovered by Albert Neisser in 1879 and was first isolated from the fallopian tubes of a patient with acute PID in 1886 by the Swedish gynecologist Westermark. For nearly the next century *N. gonorrhoeae* was accepted as the preeminent cause of virtually all acute PID and was the only unquestionably accepted cause of the entity. Until recent years the only etiological classification of sexually transmitted (nontuberculous) PID was the dichotomous gonococcal and nongonococcal PID system. Cases of nongonococcal PID were felt to represent technical problems in *N. gonorrhoeae* localization or isolation techniques and other etiological agents were not widely accepted. Since the 1970s, however, initiated by the pioneering studies of Scandanavian investigators and confirmed by others worldwide, the role of *Chlamydia trachomatis* in the genesis of some cases of acute PID has been established. American researchers have contributed greatly to our understanding of the role of anerobic bacteria and of the polymicrobial nature of PID during this same period. A role for *Mycoplasma hominis, Ureaplasma urealyticum, Actinomyces israelii*, as well as other microorganisms has also been proposed.

Neisseria gonorrhoeae

The gram-negative aerobic diplococcus *N. gonorrhoeae* is a pathogen for transitional and columnar epithelium [8] and has been established as an important etiological agent for acute salpingitis since Koch's postulates were fulfilled 3 years after its isolation. *Neisseria gonorrhoeae* has been isolated from the endocervix in 7.7 to 80% of cases of PID [9-13]. The isolation rate from intra-abdominal sites via culdocentesis or laparoscopy is consistently lower, however, varying between 0 and 65% in recent series [8,11,13-18].

Most gonococcal infections in women are asymptomatic and involve sites in the lower genitourinary system, such as the urethra, periurethral glands, Bartholin's glands, and most commonly the endocervix. Under certain circumstances *N. gonorrhoeae* ascends canalicularly from the endocervix to involve the endometrium and endosalpinx, ultimately involving the pelvic and abdominal peritoneum and contiguous organs. This acute endometritis, salpingitis, and peritonitis most often presents as a dramatic medical emergency, classic acute PID. Ascent of the gonococcus from the endocervix into the upper reproductive tract typically occurs in close temporal proximity to the menstrual flow, possibly due to diminished resistance of the cervical mucus and enhanced receptivity of the endometrium, as well as to menstrual reflux [10,19]. Some extrinsic factors, such as uterine instrumentation or the presence of an intrauterine device, may increase the frequency of ascent, whereas others, such as oral contraceptives, may decrease the frequency of ascent [20].

The exact reasons why only 2 to 20% of women who have endocervical *N. gonorrhoeae* develop upper tract invasion and PID are unknown [19]. Draper et al. [21] have demonstrated that nutritional requirements (auxotypes) can be used to differentiate *N. gonorrhoeae* that ascends into the upper tract from *N. gonorrhoeae* that remains endocervical. Once reaching the fallopian tubes, the gonococcus attaches to the secretory cells of the endosalpinx, penetrates these epithelial cells, and causes cell destruction [10,19]. Gregg et al. [22] have demonstrated that a gonococcal lipopolysaccharide endotoxin can damage adjacent but uninfected human fallopian tube ciliated cells in organ culture. The loss of the tubal mucociliary wave may impair tissue resistance to further or subsequent invasion. It is the epithelial destruction and the resultant purulent exudate exuding from the initially open distal tube that results in peritoneal and contiguous organ involvement in the inflammatory process. The consequence of epithelial destruction below the level of the basement membrane is healing by fibrosis [23], a distortion of tubal architecture and a compromise of tubal function [24,25].

Polymicrobial and Anaerobic PID

One of the early cracks in the *N. gonorrhoeae* monoetiological theory of most PID was the infrequency with which the organism could be isolated from the tubes or cul de sac even when it was present in the endocervix. Beginning in the mid-1970s a series of reports from California and Washington, utilizing laparoscopy, culdocentesis, and newly developed anaerobic bacteriological techniques, began to appear [11,14,17,26]. These studies established the fact that both aerobic and anaerobic organisms endogenous to the gastrointestinal tract and the vagina could be isolated from the upper reproductive tract in patients with acute and recurrent PID. While these other microorganisms would sometimes be isolated concurrently with *N. gonorrhoeae*, more often the gonococcus was absent. Several reports [18,27,28] established a continuum from pure gonococcal to mixed gonococcal/nongonococcal to only nongonococcal isolation from fallopian tubes and peritoneal fluid in patients with acute PID. Monif et al. [18] theorized a progressive anaerobic superinfection initiated by *N. gonorrhoeae* effecting tubal epithelial damage and altering the upper tract's oxidation-reduction potential allowing recruitment of enteric and vaginal organisms into the disease process. As these bacteria replicate, the microbiological environment of the tube is characterized by a further decrease in redox potential and the relative absence of molecular oxygen, which further enhances polymicrobial proliferation and results in inhibition of gonococcal replication [7,18]. The findings of Sweet et al. supported this hypothesis when they showed that *N. gonorrhoeae* was the most frequent isolate from upper tract sites when culture material was obtained by culdocentesis and laparoscopy within the first 24 hr of the onset of symptoms. Beyond 48 hr the most frequent isolates were anaerobic bacteria, and no cultures were positive for *N. gonorrhoeae* after 7 days from symptom onset [14]. This same study showed that isolation of *N. gonorrhoeae* became less likely with each subsequent attack of PID, being most likely with the first episode and being absent from all women suffering third or subsequent attacks.

In many instances the initial attack of acute PID is caused by *N. gonorrhoeae*. As the time from the onset of symptoms increases, multiple endogenous aerobic and anaerobic organisms become involved in the infectious process, often displacing the gonococcus. The organisms most frequently isolated have been *Escherichia coli*, streptococci, and the anaerobes *Peptococcus, Peptostreptococcus*, and *Bacteroides*, most notably *Bacteroides fragilis*. With subsequent attacks it appears that polymicrobial infection can become established without prior *N. gonorrhoeae* invasion, possibly due to damage effected by preceding infections rendering the upper tract less resistant to invasion. There is evidence that both aerobic and anaerobic microorganisms can migrate with sperm through cervical mucus and thus gain access to the upper tract [29]. Polymicrobial infection can be initiated without prior gonococcal infection in approximately 15% of cases following some type of instrumentation such as dilatation and curettage, induced abortion, hysterosalpingography, or intrauterine device (IUD) insertion [6,30]. It has not been established whether polymicrobial PID can be established de novo in a normal uninstrumented reproductive tract.

Polymicrobial PID may not have the classic temporal relationship to menstruation typical of gonococcal PID, particularly if it follows instrumentation or represents a repeat episode. Women with anaerobic organisms are particularly prone to abscess formation with extensive tissue destruction; however, there is minimal peritoneal irritation and therefore often few overt clinical signs [30].

Chlamydia trachomatis

The evidence that has accumulated in recent years overwhelmingly supports the role of *C. trachomatis* as a major factor in the genesis of acute PID [24,31-40]. This evidence has been the subject of several excellent reviews [9,19,30,41,42] and consists of endocervical and tubal isolations in women with PID, positive antibody titers in active and chronic PID, the demonstration of seroconversion with acute PID, and significantly greater serological evidence of prior chlamydial infection in patients with tubal infertility and pelvic adhesive disease than in normal controls. Animal model studies have confirmed the pathogenicity of *C. trachomatis* for the fallopian tube epithelium. While early reports eminated primarily from Scandanavia, most notably from Weström and Mårdh in Lund, Sweden, later reports from France, Canada, and the western and midwestern United States all support the important role of *C. trachomatis* in the genesis of acute and chronic PID in the industrialized world. While there is an appreciable incidence of concurrent *C. trachomatis* and *N. gonorrhoeae* infection in the same women [43,44], the evidence does not support a commensal or subordinate role for chlamydia analogous to that of genital mycoplasmas or endogenous anaerobes in the etiology of PID; rather, it seems firmly established that *C. trachomatis* is the major cause of nongonococcal PID and in some areas has replaced *N. gonorrhoeae* as the major identifiable cause of nontuberculous PID. At least 40% of acute PID in Scandanavia and 20% in the United States are caused by *C. trachomatis* [30].

Chlamydia (the only genus of the order Chalmydiales) are bacteria-like organisms and obligatory intracellular parasites sensitive to the action of some antibiotics [45]. They display a strict tissue tropism for columnar epithelium and have the ability to cause inapparent or indolent infection [46]. Once phagocytized by the host cell, chlamydiae direct the cell's metabolic capabilities to their own metabolic requirements to allow production of more chlamydiae. Once the 48-hr multiplication cycle of the chlamydia is completed, cell rupture results in the release of more infectious particles [45]. Like *N. gonorrhoeae*, they are capable of infecting the endocervix with mild or absent symptoms before they spread canalicularly into the uterus and tubes. The stimulus for ascent and the frequency of ascent are not known, but ascent seems to be temporally random with respect to menstrual cycles. Like *N. gonorrhoeae, C. trachomatis* has been associated with perihepatitis (Fitz-Hugh-Curtis syndrome) [47,48], as well as endometritis/salpingitis.

One of the most confounding aspects of chlamydial PID is its atypical and often subclinical presentation [19,32,49]. It is often characterized by relatively mild symptoms and an indolent course that belies the considerable tubal damage that it can effect. Patients often have prolonged vague symptomatology and have suffered destruction of tubal architecture before a diagnosis is made. Indeed, evidence is accumulating that a considerable portion of patients with tubal infertility have experienced previous subclinical chlamydial salpingitis [37,39].

Genital Mycoplasmas

The mycoplasmas, the smallest known free-living organisms in nature, differ from bacteria in that they lack cell walls. Since mycoplasmal organisms of human origin were first isolated in 1937 from a Bartholin's abscess, their role as possible pathogens in PID has been postulated and debated [50,51]. Two mycoplasmas have been the primary focus of interest, *M. hominis* and *U. urealyticum*. The mycoplasmas are found quite commonly in the lower genital tract (more often from vaginal than from endocervical sites) in women, the frequency of isolation increasing with sexual activity and with the number of sexual partners [52]. It is this frequency of isolation in normal control populations combined with the mycoplasma's common association with other sexually transmitted organisms in infected individuals that make its true role in PID difficult to establish.

A number of investigators have isolated *M. hominis* from the fallopian tube in a small percentage (2 to 16%) of women with acute PID [11,19,52] and additionally have shown serological evidence of an association of *M. hominis* with PID [11,31,52]. Cervical and vaginal isolation studies have yielded contradictory results, with some studies showing higher isolation rates in patients with PID [11,31] than in controls and others showing no difference [3,15]. Eschenbach et al. [11], however, point out that *M. hominis* recovery rates from the lower reproductive tract were positively correlated with *N. gonorrhoeae* isolation rates in their study and were no different in the *N. gonorrhoeae*-positive population with PID than in the *N. gonorrhoeae*-positive population without PID. *Ureaplasma urealyticum* is so common in women both with and without PID that no difference in the groups has been demonstrated, although it has occasionally been isolated from the tubes of patients with salpingitis [52].

In vitro studies have demonstrated that while *M. hominis* can grow and replicate in fallopian tube explant systems, epithelial damage does not result, in contrast to the effect of *N. gonorrhoeae* on the same systems. The isolation of in vitro systems from the host immune system, which may play an important role in the pathogenesis of PID, must be taken into consideration when interpreting these results [3]. In vivo studies using grivet monkeys demonstrated that *M. hominis* can spread from endocervical sites to cause a parametritis and an "exo-salpingitis" [36]. *Mycoplasma hominis* seems to differ from both *N. gonorrhoeae* and *C. trachomatis*, both of which spread canalicularly along luminal epithelium, in that it spreads via lymphatics and blood vessels to the parametria, producing a parametritis rather than an overt salpingitis and peritonitis [19,30,31,36,41]. To date, animal studies have not demonstrated a similar role for *U. urealyticum* in PID.

While there is far from universal agreement, it seems that *M. hominis* is associated with a small proportion of cases of PID [30] and that *U. urealyticum* does not have as convincing an association. Whether *Mycoplasma*'s association is causal or simply commensal with the true pathogen is uncertain, although the latter role seems more likely in most instances.

Actinomyces

Actinomyces are gram-positive, non-acid-fast anaerobic bacteria that are obligate parasites; *A. israelii* is the most common species. The suppurative, granulomatous PID caused by *A. israelii* is a unique form of nongonococcal PID related to the use of IUDs [51,53-55]. While vaginal colonization with *A. israelii* is unusual, it is probably more common in IUD users or recent users [54]. More significantly, ascent of *A. israelii* from the vagina to the upper reproductive tract is virtually limited to IUD users. The PID that results is often indolent and runs a subacute or mild course, although damage may be severe [51,53]. There is a significantly increased risk of both unilateral and bilateral tubo-ovarian abscesses when PID develops in IUD users with actinomycosis than in those without the organism [55]. It thus seems that *A. israelii* is an unquestionable but unusual primary cause of PID that can be thought of as an example of the IUD potentiating the spread of an endogenous vaginal organism into the upper tract. The IUD may additionally increase the vaginal colonization rate.

Miscellaneous Etiological Agents

Group A β-hemolytic streptocococcus (*Streptococcus pyrogenes*), the classic pathogen of the gravid woman, has been identified in rare instances as the only identifiable infectious agent in acute PID [11,56]. This virulent bacterium typically requires an inciting event and disruption of a mucosal barrier to initiate infection [51]. Monif feels that menstruation can qualify as such an event and that *S. pyrogenes* can be considered an extremely rare cause of acute perimenstrual PID.

Grimes [51] and Mårdh [19] have briefly reviewed other uncommon etiological agents. A variety of primary respiratory tract pathogens such as *Haemophilus influenzae* and *Mycoplasma pneumoniae* have been isolated from fallopian tubes. *Enterobius vermicularis* has been shown capable of invading tubes also. While there has been some suggestion of a role for viruses in acute PID, further study is indicated. Finally, genital tuberculosis still rarely occurs in industrialized nations today, invariably attributed to hematogenous spread from a pulmonary focus.

Microbiological Summary

The importance of *N. gonorrhoeae* and *C. trachomatis* as primary etiological agents of acute PID seems irrefutable. Much of the controversy surrounding their relative importance can be attributed to regional differences in the incidence of *Chlamydia* and in the control of gonorrhea, as well as to differences in specimen collection procedures, culture techniques and reliance on laparoscopy to diagnose PID. While the role of polymicrobial anaerobic infection as a primary cause of acute PID is in some doubt, its role in advanced gonococcal PID and in recurrent PID seems well established. The role of *Mycoplasma* as a significant tubal pathogen is questionable, while the role of *A. israelii* in some IUD-associated PID seems certain. Figure 1 is a diagram of some of the important aspects of the primary agents of PID.

A basic understanding of the microbiological basis of PID is essential to an understanding of its diagnosis and management. A knowledge of differences in the pathophysiology of the various etiological agents also allows one to better appreciate the vast clinical scope of PID. This explosion of research and information does not make clinical management any easier, but hopefully it will make management more thoughtful, appropriate, and successful.

EPIDEMIOLOGY OF PID

While PID must be considered in virtually any patient with gynecological complaints, there are identifiable factors that place certain individuals at a significantly increased risk of developing the disease. Table 1 lists the factors that are

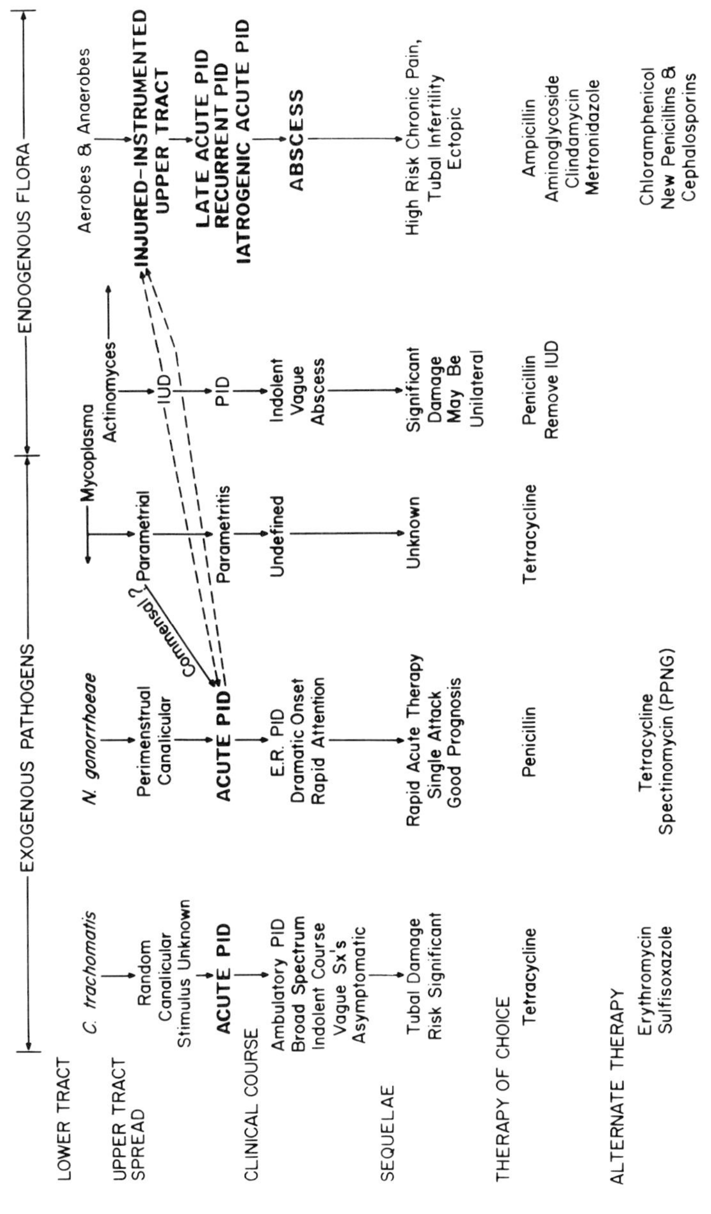

Fig. 1 Overview of pelvic inflammatory disease.

Table 1 Risk Factors for Acute PID

Age (teenage to young adult)
Multiple sexual partners
Colonization with sexually transmitted infections
Previous PID
Uterine instrumentation
IUD usage
Lower socioeconomic status
Menstruation

generally accepted as significantly affecting the likelihood of PID being present in a given patient.

Age is one of the most important identifiable factors related to PID and shows an inverse relationship to the risk of the disease. Put simply, the younger the patient, the greater her risk of developing PID as a consequence of sexual activity. This is particularly tragic, since the young woman is least likely to have fulfilled her childbearing desires and frequently experiences the long-term sequelae of PID. St. John et al. have demonstrated that 75% of patients hospitalized with acute PID in the United States between 1970 and 1975 were below the age of 30 [57]. In Weström's series [6] 74.4% of PID victims were nulliparous. He also determined that the very young sexually active girl's risks were generally underestimated, since only a portion of adolescents are sexually active. Taking these factors into account, Weström calculated the risk of sexually active 15-year-olds acquiring acute PID at 1 in 8, declining to 1 in 80 for 24-year-olds. A total of 33% of women who developed PID had their first episode before age 19, while 70% of cases occurred before age 25. Recent reviews have emphasized the problem of acute PID in the young woman [10,58] and have noted the difficulty in separating the factor of young age from two other interrelated factors, notably, multiple sexual partners and sexually transmitted infections.

Nearly 50% of 15-year-old girls with coital experience in Weström's series had four or more partners per year [6]. Women with multiple sexual partners are 4.6 times more likely to develop PID than women with single partners, independent of age [58]. Likewise, the likelihood of acquiring one of the two sexually transmitted organisms most likely to cause PID, *N. gonorrhoeae* and *C. trachomatis*, is greater in younger sexually active women and in women with multiple partners [30]. Acquisition of either of these organisms in the lower genital tract is directly correlated with the likelihood of spread to the upper tract. An individual who has experienced a prior episode of PID, particularly gonococcal PID, is at an increased risk of developing another episode [1,3,10,58].

A variety of extrinsic factors are also related to the development of PID, most notably uterine instrumentation and contraceptive practices. A variety of diagnostic and therapeutic procedures have been enumerated as contributing to iatrogenic PID, including dilatation and curettage, abortion induction, hysterosalpingography, hysteroscopy, and IUD insertion [6,30]. Approximately 15% of diagnosed instances of PID develop following some such procedure. In some instances the procedures are undoubtedly performed in patients with subclinical disease (e.g., the hysterosalpingogram as part of an infertility evaluation in a patient with unsuspected chronic salpingitis), but in certain instances it is apparent that these procedures can initiate infection in a previously normal upper reproductive tract.

There is little doubt that the IUD plays a role in the development of PID. This risk seems maximum in the immediate postinsertion period (first 30 days) [59], but remains elevated for the duration of use. The estimated relative risk of PID developing in an IUD wearer is two to four times that of a nonwearer utilizing no contraceptive method and may be as high as seven- to ninefold greater in nulliparous women [58,60]. This higher risk in the nulliparous woman has not been confirmed by all investigators [61]. Earlier estimates of the relative risk with the IUD were even higher because many authors failed to realize the protective qualities of some alternative contraceptive methods [20,58]. The IUD risk with respect to PID includes facilitation of ascent of gonococcal, endogenous anaerobic, and actinomycotic organisms from the lower reproductive tract into the tubes [58,60].

Several studies have shown a decreased risk of PID in users of oral contraceptives [20,60,62]. Senanayake and Kramer [20] reviewed 11 studies and found that 10 confirmed the protective effect of oral contraceptives with a relative risk of 0.3 to 0.9. While the risk of lower tract colonization is probably no less in oral contraceptive users, the increased density of cervical mucus due to the pill's progestational effects might be responsible for inhibiting entry of organisms into the uterus. Likewise, the decreased volume and duration of menstrual flow may protect against ascent of infection. Eschenbach et al. [60] have documented the effect of menstruation upon precipitating acute symptoms of gonococcal PID and include this as a risk factor when entertaining the diagnosis. Barrier method contraceptives also display a protective effect (relative risk = 0.6) when compared to no contraceptive use [63,64]. This protection seems to exist for both mechanical and chemical barrier methods and probably is achieved by preventing colonization with pathogenic sexually transmitted organisms.

Socioeconomic factors and their effects on the incidence of PID are extremely complex and difficult to define. St. John et al. demonstrated a threefold greater risk of both hospitalized [57] and ambulatory [4] PID among nonwhite compared to white patients. The great drawback to these studies is that the criteria for a diagnosis of PID was not critically examined. Chatman [65] has shown how unintentional bias (i.e., failure to consider alternative diagnoses such as endometriosis) can prejudice the diagnosis of PID in black women and in the

Table 2 Protective Factors for PID

Celibacy
Pregnancy
Oral contraceptive usage
Barrier contraceptive use
Tubal sterilization
Premenarche
Postmenopause

process potentiate further epidemiological bias. Eschenbach [58] has pointed out that social factors may play a role in the patient's recognition of early PID, her adherence to antibiotic schedules, her seeking therapy for her partner, and her ability to utilize and accept health care.

Several other factors may protect against PID. Celibacy all but eliminates the diagnosis from consideration, as only tuberculous salpingitis and PID secondary to appendicitis have been observed in nuns [6]. Salpingitis in pregnancy is extremely rare, particularly after the 15th week, although there have been some case reports [66,67]. It is felt that the tenacious cervical mucus plug, intact fetal membranes, absence of menstruation, and decidua covering the uterine tubal ostia act as barriers to ascent. On the rare occasions when salpingitis has occurred in pregnancy, it has typically been misdiagnosed. Tubal sterilization is also felt to protect against PID owing to obstruction of the tube and prevention of peritoneal spillage. In 1946 Falk reported treating 1000 recurrent PID patients with fallopian tube interruption and reported no further recurrences of salpingitis. A 1978 study from Chicago reported no admissions for PID among over 3500 postlaparoscopic sterilization patients who represented a predominantly indigent but stable population [68]. On the other hand, tubal sterilization occasionally will initiate an episode of acute PID. Finally, it is quite rare for acute PID to develop at either age extreme outside the reproductive era, although there have been reports of both nongonococcal and gonococcal PID in prepubertal children [69-71]. Table 2 summarizes recognized protective factors.

CLINICAL DIFFERENTIAL DIAGNOSIS

The classic presentation for acute "emergency room" PID is that of a young girl presenting menstrually or just postmenstrually with acute onset of severe lower abdominal pain and fever or chills. Other symptoms might include gastrointestinal or urinary complaints and abnormal vaginal bleeding. On physical exam there is marked pelvic and adnexal tenderness with exquisite pain on cervical movement and signs of pelvic peritonitis with rebound tenderness and guarding. A purulent cervical discharge may be noted. If peritonitis has progressed, right upper quadrant pain signifying perihepatic involvement in the inflammatory process (Fitz-Hugh-Curtis syndrome) may be elicited. Laboratory testing would reveal a polymorphonuclear leukocytosis and an elevated erythrocyte sedimentation rate. In its classic form, PID has never been considered a particularly difficult diagnosis to establish, and most experienced clinicians were confident in their clinical diagnostic abilities. Since 1969, however, a number of findings have shaken this confidence.

In a classic study published in 1969, Jacobson and Weström reported their experience with the clinical diagnosis of PID by objectively confirming the diagnosis with laparoscopic visualization of the fallopian tubes [72]. They demonstrated that a diagnosis established by traditional clinical criteria was confirmed in only 65% of 814 cases. In 23% no pathological condition was encountered, and in the remaining 12% other diagnoses were established such as acute appendicitis or pelvic endometriosis. While some parameters, such as fever and chills, were more common in confirmed PID patients, they were present in only the minority of cases of true PID. Only 20% of visually confirmed cases had the constellation of findings noted above. An additional 91 cases of acute salpingitis were encountered in patients being laparoscoped for other provisional diagnoses such as acute appendicitis, ectopic pregnancy, or ovarian tumor.

Not so overtly sensational, but more unsettling to most thoughtful clinicians, have been the many reports that have documented the prevalence and the damaging sequelae of "ambulatory" PID. This term applies to the many women with extremely vague pelvic complaints who in fact have chlamydial salpingitis. This syndrome is of extreme importance, because, as was mentioned earlier, the vague and mild course belies the extensive tubal damage that may be incurred [13,24, 32,40,49]. There is mounting evidence that some chlamydial salpingitis may be totally subclinical and discovered only during evaluation of one of its sequelae, tubal infertility [33,38,39].

These studies and many others condemn the predictive value of both normal and abnormal signs and symptoms in establishing or ruling out the diagnosis of acute PID. Insistence upon rigid criteria results in a great many cases of salpingitis being overlooked, misdiagnosed, or inappropriately treated [10]. Use of extremely liberal criteria has the opposite effect of giving inappropriate therapy for other potentially life-threatening disorders or giving needless, expensive, and potentially hazardous therapy for absent disease. Table 3 lists the differential diagnosis of acute pelvic pain. The Scandinavians [24,72,73] recommend and utilize routine and universal laparoscopy to establish the diagnosis of PID; however, this policy has been criticized as impractical on organizational and economic grounds in the United States. The following sections will attempt to propose alternative aids to diagnosis and also suggest guidelines for the liberal utilization of laparoscopy.

It must be emphasized that signs and symptoms are not to be totally discounted in the evaluation of suspected PID. Table 4 lists important indicators of acute PID. As the incidence of typical acute gonococcal PID increases in a given population, the greater the predictive value of these symptoms and signs becomes.

Table 3 Differential Diagnosis of Acute Pelvic Pain

Emergency room pelvic pain
Acute PID
Acute appendicitis
Ovarian bleeding, rupture, or torsion
Ectopic pregnancy
Endometriosis
Acute peritonitis
Septic abortion
Pelvic thrombophlebitis
Acute pyelonephritis
Acute cholecystitis
Acute pancreatitis
Colitis
Kidney stone
Leiomyoma degeneration
Chronic PID
Mesenteric lymphadenitis
No pathological diagnosis
Ambulatory pelvic pain
Atypical acute PID
Endometriosis
Chronic PID
Ovarian cyst or tumor
Early ectopic pregnancy
Dysmenorrhea
Premenstrual syndrome
Vague functional complaints
Affective mood disorders
Gastrointestinal dysfunction
Urinary tract disease
IUD symptoms
No pathological diagnosis

As more atypical or indolent cases predominate, as is the case in populations with a higher incidence of chlamydial infection, signs and symptoms become relatively less predictive and the clinician must maintain a high index of suspicion. In this population laparoscopy may be necessary to confirm a suspected atypical presentation. The history and physical may also be less predictive in certain subsets of a population, such as those with previous episodes of acute PID or those with an intrauterine contraceptive device. It is important for physicians and researchers in any single locality to recognize the relative frequencies of different sexually transmitted infections within various segments of the population.

Table 4 Clinical Diagnostic Parameters (PID)

Symptoms
Lower abdominal pain
Abnormal bleeding
Fever/chills
Nonspecific gastrointestinal and urinary symptoms (e.g., frequency, urgency, nausea, vomiting, diarrhea)
Vaginal discharge
Signs
Pelvic tenderness
Cervical motion tenderness
Peritoneal signs (rebound, rigidity, referred pain)
Right upper quadrant tenderness
Purulent vaginal or cervical discharge
Fever $>38^{o}C$
Vaginal bleeding

AIDS TO CLINICAL DIAGNOSIS

Examination of Vaginal/Cervical Secretions

Many clinicians are quite skeptical of the value of a subjective assessment of abnormal discharge from the cervix and pay little heed to their own and no heed to another's interpretation of secretions in a patient with suspected PID. While such examination is rarely diagnostic, it may often increase the predictive value of a clinical impression and sometimes suggest another diagnosis. Vaginal secretions may be examined without staining to look for inflammatory cells and for motile *Trichomonas vaginalis*, a sexually transmitted disease that may alert one to the potential existence of a second such disease. Epithelial clue cells and the liberation of an intense amine odor on addition of 10% KOH is typical of nonspecific vaginitis, a disorder that is associated with anaerobic overgrowth of the vagina [74]. Aspiration of cervical mucus for microscopic examination may be valuable. The complete absence of white blood cells in vaginal and cervical secretions is not consistent with acute PID, although their presence has no diagnostic value [73]. Copious, wattery, ferning (creating a fern pattern microscopically after air drying) cervical mucus indicative of an estrogen-stimulated preovulatory state virtually rules out the diagnosis of a complication of pregnancy. Gram staining of cervical secretions to look for gram-negative intracellular diplococci is not absolutely diagnostic, but is highly presumptive for the presence of gonoccal PID in the symptomatic patient. Also of value is cervical cytology to look for typical intracytoplasmic chlamydial inclusions with standard Papanicolaou staining [75,76] if cultures are not available or while cultures are incubating. The future availability of monoclonal antibody immunofluorescence of cytological specimens promises more sensitive identification of chlamydia. Cytological specimens may also be the most reliable way to confirm a suspicion of pelvic actinomycotic infection. Finally, once the pelvic examination is completed, Monif has stressed the value of obtaining serial temperatures afterward [7]. A febrile response to this "pelvic challenge test" is typical of acute PID.

Blood Tests

The classic confirmatory tests of infection are the white blood count (WBC) and the erythrocyte sedimentation rate. A leukocytosis in excess of 10,000 with an often impressive increase in band forms plus an elevation of the ESR over 20 mm/hr is characteristic of acute bacterial infection. Marked elevation of the erythrocyte sedimentation rate (>30) in contrast to a relatively mild clinical presentation has been described with chamydial PID [31]. C-Reactive protein, an acute phase reactant not found in normal serum, has been found to differentiate inflammatory from noninflammatory pelvic processes. In addition, C-reactive protein seems to more accurately and more acutely predict adequacy of clinical response to antibiotic therapy for acute PID [77,78]. Hyperamylasemia has also been described in association with acute salpingitis, a finding that is more likely to obscure than confirm the diagnosis in atypical cases felt to represent pancreatitis. The amylase clearance/creatinine clearance ratio, elevated in pancreatitis, is normal (2.0 to 4.2%) when hyperamylasemia is secondary to PID [79].

Another blood test that is extremely helpful in assessing acute PID is the rapid and sensitive qualitative β-subunit human chorionic gonadotropin determination in serum. The utilization of this serum pregnancy test and real-time ultrasonography have revolutionized the diagnosis of suspected ectopic pregnancy and represent a significant improvement in differentiating this condition from PID in atypical cases.

A variety of serological evaluations for the detection of various classes of antibodies against *N. gonorrhoeae, C. trachomatis, M. hominis,* and *U. urealyticum* have been utilized as research tools in the investigation of PID. While these tests have been valuable in helping to accumulate evidence as to the role of certain organisms and strains of organisms in the pathogenesis of acute PID, it is generally felt that serum or cervical secretory antibody studies cannot be substituted for agent isolation when diagnosing individual cases [19].

Culdocentesis

In most instances the diagnosis of pelvic peritonitis can be confirmed by the performance of a needle aspiration of the posterior cul-de-sac. Many physicians are reluctant to add a decidedly uncomfortable procedure to the evaluation of an already uncomfortable patient. The clinical situation and the patient's ability to tolerate the procedure will often dictate its desirability and feasibility. Culdocentesis should be performed after analgesic premedication and after the patient has been sitting upright for at least 10 min to allow maximum dependent pooling [7]. A gentle antiseptic cleansing of the vagina should be accomplished prior to culdocentesis and care should be taken to avoid gross vaginal contamination of the needle. The procedure is contraindicated in the presence of a cul-de-sac mass or uterine retroversion.

In addition to bacteriological cultures (see below), culdocentesis specimens can be microscopically examined for organisms and white blood cells indicative of peritonitis. The finding of markedly reduced levels of tubal isoamylases in cul-de-sac aspirates in patients with PID seems to be more predictive of salpingitis than leukocytosis or elevated erythrocyte sedimentation rate or C-reactive protein in the blood [19,73] and offers some promise as a diagnostic method. The degree of isoamylase decrease seems directly correlated to the severity of tubal inflammation and is independent on tubal obstruction. The aspiration of blood from the cul-de-sac does not preclude PID, since retrograde menstruation may be a concurrent finding. A significant hematocrit in a bloody tap, however, should alert one to the possibility of an alternative diagnosis, such as ectopic pregnancy or ruptured corpus luteum.

Microbiological Testing

One of the greatest problems in the clinical management and in the investigation of PID is the inaccessibility of the organs most directly involved, the fallopian tubes, to direct microbiological sampling [80]. Given the multiple organisms that can be involved plus the significant liklihood of a polymicrobial infection in any given case, this inaccessibility often makes the choice of antibiotic either a shot in the dark (single agent) or a shotgun in the dark (triple agent or more). In an effort to make therapy more specific and hopefully more effective, a number of potential culture sites and types of cultures should be entertained.

It is unfortunate that microbiological testing from the lower reproductive tract, the easiest site to sample, is also the least accurate. Most reviews note the poor correlation between endocervical and concurrent tubal cultures even when exogenous pathogens such as *N. gonorrhoeae* are recovered from the cervix [11, 12,26,80]. This is particularly true the further the patient is from the onset of her acute illness. Still there are a number of cultures that should be obtained from the lower genital tract, including endocervical *N. gonorrhoeae* cultures and, if available, *C. trachomatis* tissue cultures of abraded endocervical specimens. In addition, urethral and rectal swabs should be assessed for *N. gonorrhoeae*. *Mycoplasma hominis* cultures are more often positive from the posterior fornix vaginal pool than from endocervix, but their clinical value is not well established. Anaerobes and coliforms may be retrieved from the healthy vagina and endocervix and thus their presence is not an aid to diagnosis [19]. While culture of the endometrial cavity seems entirely logical, given the intraluminal canalicular spread of virtually all etiological agents of PID, transcervical sampling has the obvious probability of contamination with endocervical organisms. Protected sheathed endometrial culture devices have been developed, but their reliability has not been demonstrated. While Ledger et al. has reported suprapubic transabdominal uterine aspiration for suspected postpartum endometritis [81], this technique would not seem feasible in the normally sized nonpuerperal uterus.

Few studies mention utilization of blood cultures in attempting to establish a bacterial etiology for PID. While blood cultures are reasonable in any acutely infected and febrile patient, they seem less useful in the management of PID than in postoperative or postpartum infections.

Needle aspiration of the cul-de-sac has been advocated as an important tool in the evaluation of PID. Indeed, Monif has proposed a clinical staging system to determine optimal therapy based largely on culdocentesis findings [82]. While culdocentesis specimens are more reliable than endocervical specimens, they are still of limited value for two reasons. First, it has been demonstrated that when transvaginal cul-de-sac aspirates are compared with laparoscopically obtained specimens, the former contain a greater number of organisms [15,17]. This indicates that vaginal contamination is not infrequent despite careful attention to technique. Second, it has also been demonstrated that laparoscopically obtained tubal specimens have greater numbers of isolates than laparoscopically obtained cul-de-sac specimens in the same patient, indicating that certain organisms, particularly those that are attached to cells or are obligate intracellular parasites, are less likely to be found in peritoneal fluid [17,19] than in the tube. These findings should not lead one to conclude that culdocentesis is without value. Certainly it can be an extremely valuable aid to the diagnosis of PID and provides useful information as to probable etiology. Culdocentesis should be considered in any patient who is not considered a laparoscopy candidate. Direct procurement of specimens from the tube is the most reliable and elegant way of confirming the etiological diagnosis of PID. Specimens obtained from within the lumen of the tube by use of an infant feeding catheter or by needle puncture are more reliable than tubal exudate samples from the fimbria, particularly if culture for *C. trachomatis* is to be performed [19].

Mårdh emphasizes the importance of staining and immediate direct microscopic examination of all cul-de-sac and fallopian tube specimens [19]. Undue delay in staining may result in certain anaerobes losing their ability to absorb stain. Bacteria visualized on microscopic exam but not grown on aerobic culture are presumptive evidence of an anaerobic infection. This may be useful in clinical management, since the results of anaerobic cultures are frequently available too late to be of clinical use. Microscopically visualized bacteria that are not detected with either aerobic or anaerobic techniques suggest flaws in culture technique. In addition, these same clinical specimens can be analyzed directly by gas-liquid chromatography for volatile and nonvolatile organic acids that characterize anaerobic infections [83].

The review by Mårdh of infectious agents of salpingitis [19] provides an excellent reference to current techniques, pitfalls, and future techniques in the microbiological evaluation of PID. He emphasizes that immediate inoculation and incubation of *N. gonorrhoeae* cultures on specific media results in a higher isolation rate. The sensitivity of a single Thayer-Martin endocervical culture is approximately 80% [51]. Anaerobic specimens require meticulous handling and processing. The best anaerobic specimen is frank pus aspirated from an abscess cavity and transported in a glass syringe bled of all air. *Chlamydia trachomatis* cultures are becoming more widely available and may cost little more than a routine bacterial and less than a complete anaerobic identification workup. Specimens can be transported in recently thawed sucrose phosphate buffer which should be refrozen in the laboratory at −80°C until cycloheximide-treated McCoy cell tissue cultures can be inoculated. Iodine staining is used to identify *C. trachomatis* intracytoplasmic inclusions [84,85]. Because *C. trachomatis* is an obligate intracellular parasite, specimens obtained by gentle abrasion or needle puncture are more likely to contain cells and provide the greatest cultural yield. Svensson et al. have demonstrated that patients with extremely high *C. trachomatis* IgG antibody titers were less likely to have positive cultures, possibly owing to antibody inhibition of organism invasion of tissue culture cells [19,86].

Because the initial microbiological evaluation of acute PID is frequently done on an unscheduled basis, it is important for the gynecologist to establish a good working relationship with the clinical microbiology laboratory. One should consult the laboratory to ensure proper collection techniques and handling of specimens for culture.

Pelvic Ultrasonography

Recently the value of ultrasonography in the evaluation of PID has received considerable attention. Two recent reviews cover well the typical ultrasonographic characteristics of PID and stress the benefits as well as the limitations of the technique [87,88]. Uhrich [87] describes two main patterns: the small, round adnexal or cul-de-sac mass with a slightly irregular border and the complex, large rough-bordered multilocular mass that obscures the uterus. The ultrasonographic diagnosis of a pelvic abscess must be interpreted with a knowledge of the limitations of the specificity of the findings. There is no absolute way to distinguish between a true abscess and a complex inflammatory mass composed of inflamed tube, ovary, omentum, and bowel loops [88]. A number of other clinical entities such as ruptured appendix, chronic ruptured ectopic pregnancy, endometriosis, or ovarian malignancy may present an identical ultrasonographic pattern as PID [87].

However, pelvic ultrasonography may be a valuable adjunct in defining an inflammatory mass in a patient whose discomfort precludes an adequate pelvic examination. Spirtos et al. [89] have shown that the severity of PID as documented by laparoscopy is proportional to the severity of ultrasonographic abnormalities. Serial sonograms may be valuable in objectively following response to therapy and resolution of the process when serial pelvic exams may be undesirable, unsatisfactory, or highly subjective [87,89,90]. Real-time ultrasonography is sometimes superior to static scanning in that observed peristaltic activity by part of an inflammatory mass may help to define a bowel component [88]. The increasing availability of real-time equipment and familiarity with its use make it a valuable and readily accessible tool in many cases. Combining real-time ultrasound with a simultaneous bimanual exam (with the transducer acting as the abdominal hand) is a useful technique that many gynecologists have intuitively adopted [91].

Laparoscopy

Jacobson and Weström [72] have demonstrated the imprecision of the clinical diagnosis of PID when compared to the laparoscopically confirmed diagnosis. Other researchers have confirmed the poor correlation between pelvic exam and laparoscopic findings in a variety of gynecological situations [65,92-94]. While the value of laparoscopy is unquestionable both in establishing the diagnosis and in securing the most reliable culture specimens, there are a number of considerations that need to be addressed before recommending laparoscopy for the evaluation of every suspected case of PID. First, the cited laparoscopic studies did not employ other useful evaluation aids. Notably, there is a lack of utilization of culdocentesis, sensitive human chorionic gonadotropin determinations and ultrasonography. The accuracy of diagnosis may have been enhanced significantly with these techniques. Second, the most convincing laparoscopic studies were performed in Scandanavia, where the incidence of chlamydial infection and atypical PID may be higher than in other geographic areas.

Laparoscopy has been proven safe for patients with PID and concerns of worsening the condition by iatrogenically spreading the infection throughout the abdomen have not been realized. Still, as Ledger points out, the procedure is not devoid of risk: There will be 4.6 major complications per 1000 laparoscopies performed under general anesthesia and 5.2 deaths per 100,000 cases [80]. If all patients diagnosed as having PID in the United States underwent laparoscopy, an additional 880,000 laparoscopies would be performed annually, with 46 predicted deaths. Some women with PID are not laparoscopy candidates owing to a variety of factors ranging from extreme hyperthermia to profound ileus with resultant abdominal distension. However, laparoscopy's benefits are too significant to avoid utilizing the technique in appropriate circumstances. In addition to providing an immediate diagnosis with an accuracy of 95 to 99% [73], Weström and others have shown that laparoscopy has value in establishing a prognosis for future tubal function and fertility [24,72]. By hastening diagnosis in obscure cases, therapeutic delay should be avoided and tubal damage minimized [72]. Performance of well-designed laparoscopic studies of PID in different geographic areas will enhance our understanding of the microbiological aspects of PID. Table 5 lists some clinical indications for laparoscopy in the patient with suspected PID. The greatest values are in identifying the patient with atypical PID early in its course and removing the erroneously labeled "chronic PIDer" from this category and sparing repeated course of useless, expensive, and potentially toxic therapy. A significant percentage of the latter patients will have either no pelvic abnormality or unsuspected endometriosis.

Table 6 enumerates Jacobson and Weström's minimal laparoscopic criteria for acute PID diagnosis. With these criteria an accurate diagnosis is easily obtainable in 95% of cases [72]. In the remaining cases adhesions or borderline changes (perhaps due to perimetritis rather than frank salpingitis) make observation impossible or equivocal. Double-puncture laparoscopy with a separate manipulative site enhances the chance for successful diagnosis and facilitates specimen procurement. While some researchers have suggested that anatomical findings were more important than bacteriological testing [93], this should not be misinterpreted to mean that cultures are unnecessary. To subject a patient to laparoscopy without achieving a complete microbiological workup from the best culture site available is inexcusable.

Table 5 Indications for Laparoscopy

Confusing acute presentation
Unanticipated response to antibiotic therapy
Equivocal or conflicting data from other screening procedures
Multiple equivocal PID episodes
Persistent vague gynecological complaints
Prospective large-scale risk/benefit studies

Table 6 Laparoscopic Criteria for Acute PID Diagnosis

Minimum criteria
Fallopian tube erythema
Fallopian tube edema and swelling
Serosal surface or fimbrial end seropurulent exudate
Scoring
Mild: minimum criteria; freely movable patent tube
Moderate: more marked minimum criteria; decreased movement; patency (?)
Severe: inflammatory mass

Source: Refs. 72, 73.

TREATMENT OF PID

Therapeutic Aims and Challenges

The aim of therapy of acute PID is to prevent the sequelae of tubal damage, infertility, and chronic pain by eradicating the infection in its earliest stage. In the preantibiotic era it was recognized that acute PID was usually not fatal but a self-contained disease which left half of its victims infertile. The success of any therapeutic regimen or approach lies in its ability to prevent sequelae. While there are a plethora of therapeutic recommendations in the literature, there are no valid randomized clinical trials which evaluate long-term sequelae to suggest the most effective antibiotic regimens, route of therapy, or duration of therapy.

The early diagnosis of acute PID coupled with the most effective antibiotic for the specific pathogen would ideally minimize the likelihood of anatomical distortion and functional compromise. Monif has championed the hypothesis that deviation from the expected therapeutic response is a plausible predictor of treatment efficacy with respect to avoiding sequelae [7,23]. Prompt and appropriate treatment should effect normalization of temperature and white blood cell count and markedly ameliorate symptoms within 36 to 48 hr. If response deviates from this schedule, Monif theorizes that prolonged morbidity translates into progressive distortion of normal tubal architecture. The obvious problems facing clinicians are (1) the diagnosis of PID may not be obvious and thus delayed and (2) the precise pathogen(s) are seldom known initially (if ever). Two plausible reasons why initial episode acute gonococcal PID has a lower rate of chronic sequelae compared to nongonococcal PID are (1) most patients become acutely ill early in the course of the upper tract infection, quickly seek medical care, and are diagnosed accurately and (2) acute PID antibiotic regimens are usually directed against *N. gonorrhoeae* [3]. Since the proposed etiological agents of nongonococcal PID are associated with atypical clinical presentations and display resistance to penicillin, they present a challenge to proper management. An additional confounding factor is the not uncommon coexistence of *C. trachomatis* and *N. gonorrhoeae* in the same patient. Severe acute symptoms caused by *N. gonorrhoeae* may be alleviated with penicillin-based regimens for gonococcal PID, but residual indolent infection with penicillin-resistant chlamydia may effect tubal damage [95].

Role of Inpatient and Parenteral Therapy

Two aspects of therapy that have not been adequately evaluated are the relative merits of inpatient versus outpatient therapy and of parenteral versus oral antibiotic administration [3,10,51]. Inpatient therapy offers the dual advantages of guaranteed patient compliance and constant monitoring of therapeutic response versus the obvious disadvantage of drastically increased immediate cost. If sequelae are more effectively avoided, however, ultimate cost may be decreased. Inpatient management also allows parenteral administration of antibiotics. Some antibiotics are only available in parenteral forms, while others are better tolerated parenterally, particularly in high doses. It is generally possible to obtain more rapid and higher blood and tissue levels of an antibiotic when it is administered intravenously, although there are some notable exceptions (e.g., metronidazole [96]). Intense inpatient parenteral therapy and monitoring would appear to be the ideal approach to PID. Thus most authorities encourage liberal criteria for hospitalization [10,51] and some make a valid case for inpatient therapy for all recognized cases of acute PID [24,72].

Table 7 lists some of the most widely accepted criteria for hospitalization of patients with acute PID. Pelvic or tubo-ovarian abscess, fever, generalized peritonitis, and marked leukocytosis have been standard criteria for a number of years and are fairly objective in their determination. Parenteral therapy in the setting of severe pain or nausea and vomiting also seems quite reasonable. Since IUD-associated PID is prone to complication by pelvic abscess and may be an iatrogenic form of PID, most physicians elect inpatient management initially. Pregnancy and PID are unusual concurrent conditions where the prognosis for the pregnancy is so poor [67] that inpatient management seems mandatory. Uncertainty of diagnosis should be considered an indication for hospitalization and pretreatment laparoscopy. Inpatient therapy is also indicated when patient compliance is questionable. The clinician's perception of patient compliance is entirely subjective, often inaccurate, and no better than chance alone [10]. Adolescents are felt to have a higher noncompliance rate than older PID patients and are better managed as inpatients. They represent that subset of the PID population in which ignorance and mental immaturity disallow an appreciation of the consequences of this serious disease. The efficacy of outpatient therapy is traditionally challenged when there is a failure of resolution of signs and symptoms within 48 hr of the onset of therapy. As noted earlier, this prolonged delay of a thera-

Table 7 Indications for Inpatient Therapy

Suspected abscess
Generalized peritoneal signs
Temperature $>38^{\circ}$C
Failure to respond to outpatient therapy
Pregnancy
IUD in place
Conditions precluding oral intake
Severe pain requiring parenteral analgesics
Uncertain diagnosis
Perceived risk of lack of compliance
All adolescents
Marked leukocytosis

Source: Refs. 3, 10, and 51.

peutic response is considered unacceptable for maximizing prognosis by at least one authority [7]. In summary, the most conservative approach to PID treatment would be inpatient therapy, unless the clinical presentation is extremely benign, the patient is judged unquestionably reliable, and close follow-up is guaranteed.

Antibiotic Selection

Inpatient antibiotic therapy of acute PID must be based on a consideration of the various potential pathogens. The antibiotic susceptibilities of the primary causes of PID are noted in Figure 1. A number of different antibiotic options and combinations have been proposed for inpatient therapy of PID. Which regimen represents treatment of choice is open to speculation and has yet to be established.

Penicillin G and semisynthetic penicillin derivatives, particularly ampicillin and amoxicillin, have been mainstays of PID therapy, chiefly because of their effectiveness against *N. gonorrhoeae*. They are still considered excellent selections in cases of PID where the probability of infection with *N. gonorrhoeae* is felt to be high. In addition, they have significant activity against streptococci and many anaerobes and are drugs of choice for *A. israelii*. The main advantages of ampicillin over penicillin G are enhanced activity against certain strains of *E. coli* and enterococci and its effectiveness as an oral medication [97]. The dosage for intravenous ampicillin is 1 to 2 g every 4 to 6 hr. When switching from intravenous to oral therapy (see below), amoxicillin may be preferred, since it is better tolerated orally and maintains therapeutic blood and tissue levels longer at lower dosages than ampicillin [98].

The aminoglycosides are widely used in treating PID as a component of combination therapy with a penicillin and/or an anaerobic antibiotic. They provide optimal coverage for the gram-negative coliforms that contribute to progressive polymicrobial superinfection. They have no useful activity, however, against streptococci or anaerobes. Aminoglycoside coverage is indicated when more than 48 hr have elapsed from the onset of acute gonococcal PID and for patients with recurrent or instrumentation-associated PID. Failure to achieve an anticipated response to single- or double-agent therapy would also be a reason to consider adding an aminoglycoside. The main limitation of aminoglycoside usage is their ineffectiveness as oral agents. Monif states that since the elimination of gram-negative aerobic rods occurs rapidly, aminoglycoside coverage can be discontinued after 36 to 48 hr [7]; however, therapy is usually continued until it is felt advisable to stop all parenteral therapy and institute oral therapy. The dosage and interval of administration are dictated by the specific aminoglycoside and the patient's size and renal status. The metabolic turnover of an aminoglycoside is influenced by the patient's pathological state, necessitating dosage modifications which are best monitored by obtaining serum levels of the drug at specific intervals [99].

The indications for anaerobic coverage parallel those for aminoglycoside utilization. When an abscess is suspected either from physical exam or ultrasonography, anaerobic coverage should be initiated. While many anaerobes are quite sensitive to penicillin or ampicillin, the notable exception is *B. fragilis*. This organism's insensitivity to penicillin dictates inclusion of either clindamycin, chloramphenicol, or metronidazole to provide maximal anaerobic coverage [3]. Bone marrow toxicity (chloramphenicol), bowel toxicity (clindamycin), and mutagenic properties (metronidazole) [96] are potential reactions which should be considered prior to administration. Their judicious use, particularly in advanced disease, will obviate the need for acute surgical intervention in an estimated 70% of PID-associated pelvic abscesses [3,100].

Tetracycline is the drug of choice for *C. trachomatis* and *M. hominis* and also is considered the alternative of choice for *N. gonorrhoeae*. For these reasons and its broad spectrum, including many of the aerobes and anaerobes of polymicrobial PID, a case can be made for treating all PID with tetracycline either alone or in combination with other antibiotics [7,51]. Because of its convenient dosage interval both orally and parenterally, doxycycline, 100 to 200 mg intravenously every 12 hr after a 200-mg loading dose, is considered the tetracycline of choice. Care should be taken to avoid extravescular extravasation. Oral dosage in PID is 100 mg every 12 hr. Tetracycline therapy should also be considered for uncomplicated gonococcal infection owing to the high concurrence rate of *C. trachomatic* with *N. gonorrhoeae* [95]. This is particularly indicated if *C. trachomatis* cultures are not available. Tetracyclines should be avoided in children and pregnant women owing to their detrimental effects on dentition development.

The role of spectinomycin as the agent of choice for treating asymptomatic *N. gonorrhoeae* infection in penicillin-allergic patients is based on its single-dose (and therefore high compliance) schedule. For the same reason it is utilized in combating outbreaks of *N. gonorrhoeae* infection due to penicillinase-producing strains of the organism [101,102]. Spectinomycin has a narrow spectrum of antibacterial activity and should not be used in treating symptomatic PID and particularly nongonococcal PID [103,104].

It is predictable that the flood of recently approved new β-lactam antibiotics (penicillins and cephalosporins) would be followed by reports of their usefullness in treating female pelvic infections, including PID [105-108]. Their attractiveness as therapeutic alternatives lies in their extended activities against gram-negative enteric organisms paralleling that of the aminoglycosides, while being less nephrotoxic than the aminoglycosides [109]. However, the penicillins (mezlocillin, azlocillin, piperacillin) have no activity against *Staphylococcus aureus*, and the cephalosporins (cefotaxime, moxalactam, cefoperazone) have little or no activity against enterococci. None are active against chlamydia or mycoplasmas. They are available only as parenteral drugs and are appreciably more expensive than the older derivatives [109]. The prospect of single-agent therapy for PID with these newer agents remains to be established in randomized prospective clinical trials [108].

The duration of parenteral therapy is determined by the patient's clinical and laboratory response. Therapy is generally continued until the patient has been afebrile and has experienced a significant amelioration of symptoms for 24 to 48 hr. Normalization of white blood cell count and of C-reactive protein is also a frequently employed criterion. Once parenteral antibiotics are discontinued, the patient is usually maintained on oral coverage for 7 to 10 days as an outpatient. Commonly employed oral agents include amoxicillin, doxycycline, and metronidazole alone or in combination.

When outpatient therapy of PID is elected, it should consist of currently recommended Centers for Disease Control schedules for uncomplicated *C. trachomatis* or *N. gonorrhoeae* infection followed by at least 7 days of oral therapy with single or multiple agents. Close follow-up at 24 to 48 hr is mandatory to assess adequacy of response. In all situations, a deviation from the expected response pattern mandates a thorough reappraisal of the patient, the diagnosis, and the choice of antibiotics.

Abscess Therapy and Surgical Intervention

The initial hospital management of the patient with a pelvic abscess should consist of initial triple antibiotic therapy (penicillin, aminoglycoside, anaerobic antibiotic) and serial ultrasonographic follow-up exams to assess resolution. Most authorities advocate removal of an IUD from a patient with a pelvic abscess [7, 51,110]. Surgical intervention is mandated by a failure of response to conservative therapy, worsening symptoms in the face of an adequate antibiotic regimen, and suspected rupture of the abscess. A failure to intervene operatively for ruptured abscess results in mortality in as many as 80 to 100% of cases [111]. A pelvic abscess (cul-de-sac) may be successfully drained via colpotomy and, if the patient remains asymptomatic and desires future fertility, further surgical intervention should not be undertaken routinely. Approximately 10% of such patients will ultimately conceive [112] and others may become in vitro fertilization candidates. Surgical management of tubo-ovarian abscesses necessitates laparotomy. Occasional predominant involvement of only one side (more frequently found with IUD-associated abscesses) may allow unilateral salpingoophorectomy and theoretical fertility preservation [3,113]. Only the rare patient with bilateral involvement will ever conceive and more than half of patients with pelvic abscess ultimately will require sterilizing surgery [100].

Contact Tracing and Patient Education

Two essential concerns in the management of acute PID that are often ignored, especially in the inpatient setting, are patient counseling and contact tracing. Most patients are released after inpatient therapy for PID without having been advised of the basic nature, mode of transmission, or seriousness of the disease. Volkin et al. found a general lack of comprehension on the part of 58 patients with PID with respect to these factors [114] and found that many had no knowledge of the possibility of an asymptomatic male contact. Since the risk of tubal damage and infertility increases with each PID episode [25], patients experiencing their first acute episode should be thoroughly advised of the sexually transmitted nature of the disease and of the likelihood of permanent sequelae with repeated attacks. They should be given information regarding the most effective modes of preventing disease transmission, including the theoretical advantage of combining barrier contraception with oral contraception. Finally, victims of PID should realize the importance of contact identification, examination, and treatment. Contact tracing for women with positive *N. gonorrhoeae* cultures is well established in the United States and other developed countries. Approximately 60% of infected male contacts are asymptomatic, with an estimated one-third of these having been infected for over 1 month [115,116]. A surveillance system of contact tracing, epidemiological treatment, screening cultures for case finding, preventive measures, health education, and health worker training has been credited with some success in the control of *N. gonorrhoeae*. A similar surveillance system has not developed for *C. trachomatis* and thus its efficacy is not proven [117]. The finding that nearly 70% of male contacts of *C. trachomatis* culture-positive women with PID were also chlamydia positive [44] indicates the need to develop an organized schedule for contact tracing.

SEQUELAE

Several sequelae of PID have received relatively little attention. Hagenfeldt and Szanto identified sacroiliitis with sensitive quantitative scanning techniques in 68% of post-PID patients as opposed to 3% of controls. They associated the increased frequency of acute PID in Sweden with an unusually high frequency of sacroiliitis in women [118]. Weiner and Wallach correlated the degree of ovarian inflammatory involvement in cases of PID with menstrual dysfunction [119]. Patients with no history of dysfunctional uterine bleeding most often had no microscopic evidence of ovarian inflammation. When ovarian inflammatory changes and decreased follicular function were noted in patients with chronic PID, dysfunctional bleeding was more prevalent. Finally van Nagell et al. described a significantly increased risk of enteric obstruction and fistula formation in patients with previous PID treated with irradiation for invasive cervical carcinoma [120]. This complication may be particularly important, since many of the epidemiological risk factors for PID and cervical cancer are the same.

The three major sequelae of PID—tubal infertility, ectopic pregnancy, and chronic pelvic pain—have already been extensively discussed. Two points should be reemphasized. First, the risk of tubal occlusion increases as the severity of the acute inflammatory process increases. When the severity of the laparoscopically graded inflammatory reaction worsens (see Table 6), tubal obstruction rates increase [24,72]. The frequencies of tubal occlusion were 2.6, 13.1 and 28.6%, respectively, for mild, moderate, and severe changes in Weström and Mårdh's report [24]. Second, as the number of episodes increases, the likelihood of tubal occlusion increases. Weström reported occlusion rates of 12.8, 35.5, and 75% after one, two, and three or more infections, respectively [25]. These two facts underscore the critical importance of early diagnosis and effective therapy combined with efforts to prevent recurrence in the ideal management of acute PID.

REFERENCES

1. McCormack WM. Sexually transmitted diseases: women as victims. JAMA 1982; 248:177-8.
2. Jones OG, Zaidi AA, St. John RK. Frequency and distribution of salpingitis and pelvic inflammatory disease in short-stay hospitals in the United States. Am J Obstet Gynecol 1980; 138:905-8.
3. Sweet RL. Pelvic inflammatory disease: etiology, diagnosis, and treatment. Sex Transm Dis Suppl 1981; 8:308-15.
4. St. John RK, Blount J, Jones O. Pelvic inflammatory disease in the United States: incidence and trends in private practice. Sex Transm Dis 1981; 8: 56-61.
5. Curran JW. Economic consequences of pelvic inflammatory disease in the United States. Am J Obstet Gynecol 1980; 138:848-51.
6. Weström L. Incidence, prevalence, and trends of acute pelvic inflammatory disease and its consequences in industrialized countries. Am J Obster Gynecol 1980; 138:880-92.
7. Monif GG. Endometritis-salpingitis-peritonitis (acute salpingitis). In: Moniff GG, ed. Infectious diseases in obstetrics and gynecology. Philadelphia: Harper and Row, 1982:542-68.
8. Monif GG. *Neisseria gonorrhoeae*. In: Monif GG, ed. Infectious diseases in obstetrics and gynecology. Philadelphia: Harper and Row, 1982:136-51.
9. Thompson SE, Hager WD, Wong KH, Lopez B, Ramsey C, Allen SD, Stargel MD, Thornsberry C, Benigno BB, Thompson JD, Shullman JA. The microbiology and therapy of acute pelvic inflammatory disease in hospitalized patients. Am J Obstet Gynecol 1980; 136:179-86.
10. Shafer MAB, Irwin CE, Sweet RL. Acute salpingitis in the adolescent female. J Pediatr 1982; 100:339-50.
11. Eschenbach DA, Buchanan TM, Pollock HM, Forsyth PS, Alexander ER, Lin JS, Wang SD, Wentworth BB, McCormack WM, Holmes KK. Polymicrobial etiology of acute pelvic inflammatory disease. N Engl J Med 1975; 293: 166-71.
12. Creatsas GK, Pavlatos MP, Koumantakis E, Zolotas J, Kaskarelis DB. Bacteriologic aspects of pelvic inflammatory disease in gynecologic patients. Gynecol Obstet Invest 1982; 13:1-8.
13. Gjonnaess H, Dalaker K, Anestad G, Mårdh PA, Kvile G, Bergan T. Pelvic inflammatory disease: etiologic studies with emphasis on chlamydial infection. Obstet Gynecol 1982; 59:550-5.

14. Sweet RL, Draper DL, Hadley WK. Etiology of acute salpingitis: influence of episode number and duration of symptoms. Obstet Gynecol 1981; 58: 62-8.
15. Sweet RL, Draper DL, Schachter J, James J, Hadley WK, Brooks GF. Microbiology and pathogenesis of acute salpingitis as determined by laparoscopy: what is the appropriate site to sample? Am J Obstet Gynecol 1980; 138: 985-9.
16. Ripa KT, Svensson L, Treharne JD, Weström L, Mårdh PA. *Chlamydia trachomatis* infection in patients with laparoscopically verified acute salpingitis. Am J Obstet Gynecol 1980; 138:960-4.
17. Sweet RL, Mills J, Hadley KW, Blumenstock E, Schachter J, Robbie MO, Draper DL. Use of laparoscopy to determine the microbiologic etiology of acute salpingitis. Am J Obstet Gynecol 1979; 134:68-74.
18. Monif GRG, Welkos SL, Baer H, Thompson RJ. Cul-de-sac isolates from patients with endometritis-salpingitis-peritonitis and gonococcal endocervicitis. Am J Obster Gynecol 1976; 126:158-61.
19. Mårdh PA. An overview of infectious agents of salpingitis, their biology and recent advances in methods of detection. Am J Obstet Gynecol 1980; 138: 933-51.
20. Senanayake P, Kramer DG. Contraception and the etiology of pelvic inflammatory disease: new perspectives. Am J Obstet Gynecol 1980; 138:852-60.
21. Draper DL, James JF, Hadley WK, Sweet RL. Auxotype and antibiotic susceptibilities of *Neisseria gonorrhoeae* from women with acute salpingitis: compatison with gonococci causing uncomplicated genital tract infections in women. Sex Transm Dis 1981; 8:43-50.
22. Gregg CR, Melly MA, McGee ZA. Gonococcal lipopolysaccharide: a toxin for human fallopian tube mucosa. Am J Obstet Gynecol 1980; 138:981-4.
23. Monif GRG, Welkos SL, Baer H. Clinical response of patients with gonococcal endocervitis and encometritis-salpingitis-peritonitis to doxycycline. Am J Obstet Gynecol 1977; 129:614-22.
24. Weström L, Mårdh PA. Epidemiology, etiology, and prognosis of acute salpingitis: a study of 1,457 laparoscopically verified cases. In: Hobson D, Holmes KK, eds. Nongonococcal urethritis and related infections. Washington: American Society for Microbiology, 1977:84-90.
25. Weström L. Effect of acute pelvic inflammatory disease on fertility. Am J Obstet Gynecol 1975; 121:707-13.
26. Chow AW, Malkasian KL, Marshall JR, Guze LB. The bacteriology of acute pelvic inflammatory disease. Am J Obstet Gynecol 1975; 122:876-9.
27. Monif GRG, Baer H. Impact of diverging anaerobic technology on cul-de-sac isolates from patients with endometritis-salpingitis-peritonitis. Am J Obstet Gynecol 1982; 142:896-900.
28. Cunningham FG, Hauth JC, Gilstrap LC, Herbert WNP, Kappus SS. The bacterial pathogenesis of acute pelvic inflammatory disease. Obstet Gynecol 1978; 52:161-4.
29. Toth A, O'Leary WM, Ledger W. Evidence for microbial transfer by spermatoza. Obstet Gynecol 1982; 59:556-9.
30. Eschenbach DA. New concepts of obstetrics and gynecologic infection. Arch Intern Med 1982; 142:2039-44.

31. Møller BR, Mårdh PA, Ahrons S, Nussler E. Infection with *Chlamydia trachomatis, Mycoplasma hominis,* and *Neisseria gonorrhoeae* in patients with acute pelvic inflammatory disease. Sex Transm Dis 1981; 8:198-202.
32. Mårdh PA, Svensson L. Chlamydial salpingitis. Scand J Infect Dis Suppl 1982; 32:64-72.
33. Henry-Suchet J, Catalan F, Loffredo V, Serfaty D, Siboulet A, Perol Y, Sanson MJ, DeBache C, Pigeau F, Coppin R, DeBrux J, Poynard T. Microbiology of specimens obtained by laparoscopy from controls and from patients with pelvic inflammatory disease or infertility with tubal obstruction: *Chlamydial trachomatis* and *Ureaplasma urealyticum*. Am J Obstet Gynecol 1980; 138:1022-5.
34. Paavonen J. *Chlamydia trachomatis* in acute salpingitis. Am J Obstet Gynecol 1980; 138:957-9.
35. Sweet RL, Banks J, Sung M, Donegan E, Schachter J. Experimental chlamydial salpingitis in the guinea pig. Am J Obstet Gynecol 1980; 138:952-6.
36. Møller BR, Freundt EA, Mårdh PA. Experimental pelvic inflammatory disease provoked by *Chlamydia trachomatis* and *Mycoplasma hominis* in grivet monkeys. Am J Obstet Gynecol 1980; 138:990-5.
37. Moore DE, Foy HM, Daling JR, Grayston JT, Spadoni LR, Wang SD, Kuo CC, Eschenbach DA. Increased frequency of serum antibodies to *Chlamydia trachomatis* in infertility due to distal tubal disease. Lancet 1982; 11:574-7.
38. Henry-Suchet J, Catalan F, Loffredo V, Jose Sanson M, Debache C, Pigeau F, Coppin R. *Chlamydia trachomatis* associated with chronic inflammation in abdominal specimens from women selected for tuboplasty. Fertil Steril 1981; 36:599-605.
39. Jones RB, Ardery BR, Hui SL, Cleary RE. Correlation between serum antichlamydial antibodies and tubal factor as a cause of infertility. Fertil Steril 1982; 38:553-8.
40. Bowie WR, Jones H. Acute pelvic inflammatory disease in outpatients: association with *Chlamydia trachomatis* and *Neisseria gonorrhoeae*. Ann Intern Med 1981; 95:685-8.
41. Holmes KK, Eschenbach DA, Knapp JS. Salpingitis: overview of etiology and epidemiology. Am J Obstet Gynecol 1980; 138:893-900.
42. Sweet RL, Schachter J, Landers DV. Chlamydial infections in obstetrics and gynecology. Clin Obstet Gynecol 1983; 26:143-64.
43. Johannisson G, Lowhagen GN, Lycke E. Genital *Chlamydia trachomatis* infection in women. Obstet Gynecol 1980; 56-671-5.
44. Osser S, Persson K. Epidemiologic and serodiagnostic aspects of chlamydial salpingitis. Obstet Gynecol 1982; 59:206-9.
45. Schachter J. Chlamydial infections (first of three parts). N Engl J Med 1978; 298:428-35.
46. Terho P. *Chlamydia trachomatis* and clinical genital infections: a general review. Infection Suppl 1982; 10:5-9.
47. Wang SP, Eschenbach DA, Holmes KK, Wager G, Grayston JT. *Chlamydia trachomatis* infection in Fitz-Hugh-Curtis syndrome. Am J Obstet Gynecol 1980; 138:1034-8.

48. Wølner-Hanssen P, Weström L, Mårdh PA. Perihepatitis in chlamydial salpingitis. Lancet 1980; 1:901-3.
49. Paavonen J, Vesterinen E, Mårdh PA. Infertility as a sequela of chlamydial pelvic inflammatory disease. Scand J Infect Dis Suppl 1982; 32:73-6.
50. Taylor-Robinson D, McCormack WM. The genital mycoplasmas (first of two parts). N Engl J Med 1980; 302:1003-10.
51. Grimes DA. Nononococcal pelvic inflammatory disease. Clin Obstet Gynecol 1981; 24:1227-43.
52. Mårdh PA, Weström L. Tubal and cervical cultures in acute salpingitis with special reference to *Mycoplasma hominis* and T-stain mycoplasmas. Br J Vener Dis 1970; 46:179-86.
53. Doberneck RC. Pelvic actinomycosis associated with use of intrauterine device: a new challenge for the surgeon. Am Surg 1982; 48:25-7.
54. Burkman R, Schlesselman S, McCaffrey L, Gupta PK, Spence M. The relationship of genital tract actinomycetes and the development of pelvic inflammatory disease. Am J Obstet Gynecol 1982; 143:585-9.
55. Keebler C, Chatwani A, Schwartz R. Actinomycosis infection associated with intrauterine contraceptive devices. Am J Obstet Gynecol 1983; 145: 596-9.
56. Monif GRG, Williams BT, Dase DF. Group A streptococcus as a cause of endometritis/salpingitis/peritonitis in a nongravid female. Obstet Gynecol 1977; 50:509-10.
57. St. John RK, Jones OG, Blount JH, Zaidi AA. Pelvic inflammatory disease in the United States: epidemiology and trends among hospitalized women. Sex Transm Dis 1981; 8:62-6.
58. Eschenbach DA. Epidemiology and diagnosis of acute pelvic inflammatory disease. Obstet Gynecol Suppl 1980; 55:142-52.
59. Nilsson CG, Vartiainen E, Widholm O. Bacterial cultures from intrauterine devices removed from patients with pelvic inflammatory disease. Acta Obstet Gynecol Scand 1981; 60:563-6.
60. Eschenbach DA, Harnisch JP, Holmes KK. Pathogenesis of acute pelvic inflammatory disease: role of contraception and other risk factors. Am J Obstet Gynecol 1977; 128:838-50.
61. Osser S, Liedholm P, Sjoberg NO. Risk of pelvic inflammatory disease among users of intrauterine devices, irrespective of previous pregnancy. Am J Obstet Gynecol 1980; 138:864-7.
62. Burkman RT, Women's Health Study. Association between intrauterine device and pelvic inflammatory disease. Obstet Gynecol 1981; 57:269-76.
63. Kelaghan J, Rubin GL, Ory HW, Layde PM. Barrier-method contraceptives and pelvic inflammatory disease. JAMA 1982; 248:184-7.
64. Senanayake P, Kramer DG. Contraception and pelvic inflammatory disease. Sex Transm Dis 1981; 8:89-91.
65. Chatman DL. Endometriosis in the black woman. Am J Obstet Gynecol 1976; 125:987-9.
66. Genadry RR, Thompson BH, Niebyl JR. Gonococcal salpingitis in pregnancy. Am J Obstet Gynecol 1976; 126:512-3.

67. Odendaal H, DeKock M. Acute salpingitis in pregnancy. S Afr Med J 1973; 47:21-2.
68. Hajj SN. Does sterilization prevent pelvic infection? J Reprod Med 1978; 20:289-90.
69. Auman GL, Waldenberg LM. Gonococcal periappendicitis and salpingitis in a prepubertal girl. Pediatrics 1976; 58:287-8.
70. Touloukian RJ. Acute coliform salpingitis in a premenstrual child with severe vulvovaginitis. J Pediatr 1974; 85:281.
71. Caruso PA. Pelvic inflammatory disease: rare sequela of battered-child syndrome. NY State J Med 1975; 75:2405-6,2415.
72. Jacobson L, Weström L. Objectivized diagnosis of acute pelvic inflammatory disease: diagnostic and prognostic value of routine laparoscopy. Am J Obstet Gynecol 1969; 105:1088-98.
73. Jacobson L. Differential diagnosis of acute pelvic inflammatory disease. Am J Obstet Gynecol 1980; 138:1006-11.
74. Spiegel CA, Amsel R, Eschenbach D, Schoenknecht F, Holmes KK. Anaerobic bacteria in nonspecific vaginitis. N Engl J Med 1980; 303:601-7.
75. Gupta PK, Lee EF, Erozan YS, Frost JK, Geddes ST, Donovan PA. Cytologic investigations in chlamydia infection. Acta Cytol 1979; 23:315-20.
76. Tilton RC. Getting a fix on chlamydia. Diag Med 1980; Sept-Oct:46-52.
77. Angerman NS, Evans MI, Moravec WD, Schumacher GFB, Hajj SN. C-Reactive protein in the evaluation of antibiotic therapy for pelvic infection. J Reprod Med 1980; 25:63-6.
78. Angerman NS, Moravec WD, Hajj SN. C-Reactive protein in treatment and diagnosis of pelvic disease. Surg Forum 1979; 30:478-9.
79. Chow AW, Soll BA, Targan SR, Guze LB. Hyperamylasemia associated with gonococcal salpingitis and perihepatitis. Obstet Gynecol Suppl 1976; 48: 29-30.
80. Ledger WJ. Laparoscopy in the diagnosis and management of patients with suspected salpingo-oophoritis. Am J Obstet Gynecol 1980; 138:1012-6.
81. Ledger WL, Gee CL, Pollin PA, Lewis WP, Sutter VL, Finegold SM. A new approach to patients with suspected anaerobic postpartum pelvic infections. Transabdominal uterine aspiration for culture and metronidazole for treatment. Am J Obstet Gynecol 1976; 126:1-6.
82. Monif GRG. Clinical staging of acute bacterial salpingitis and its therapeutic ramifications. Am J Obstet Gynecol 1982; 143:489-95.
83. Gorbach SL, Mayhew JW, Bartlett JG, Thadepalli H, Onderdonk AB. Rapid diagnosis of anaerobic infections by direct gas-liquid chromatography of clinical specimens. J Clin Invest 1976; 57:478-84.
84. Smith TF, Weed LA, Peltersen GR, Segura JW. Recovery of chlamydia and genital mycoplasma transported in sucrose phosphate buffer and urease color test medium. Health Lab Sci 1977; 14:30-4.
85. Thomas BJ, Evans RT, Taylor-Robinson D. Early detection of chlamydia inclusions combining the use of cycloheximide-treated McCoy cells and immunofluorescence staining. J Clin Microbiol 1977; 6:285-92.
86. Svensson L, Weström L, Ripa KT, Mårdh PA. Differences in some clinical and laboratory parameters in acute salpingitis related to culture and serologic findings. Am J Obstet Gynecol 1980; 138:1017-21.

87. Uhrich PC, Sanders RC. Ultrasonic characteristics of pelvic inflammatory masses. J Clin Ultrasound 1976; 4:199-204.
88. Berland LL, Lawson TL, Foley WD, Albarelli JN. Ultrasound evaluation of pelvic infections. Radiol Clin North Am 1982; 20:367-82.
89. Spirtos NJ, Bernstine RL, Crawford WL, Fayle J. Sonography in acute pelvic inflammatory disease. J Reprod Med 1982; 27:312-20.
90. Spaulding LB, Gelman SR, Wood SD, Monif GRG. The role of ultrasonography in the management of endometritis/salpingitis/peritonitis. Obstet Gynecol 1979; 53:442-6.
91. Platt LD, Manning FA, Hill LM. Simultaneous real-time ultrasound scanning and pelvic examination in assessment of pelvic disease. Am J Obstet Gynecol 1980; 5:693-4.
92. Chaparro MV, Ghosh S, Nashed A, Poliak A. Laparoscopy for the confirmation and prognostic evaluation of pelvic inflammatory disease. Int J Gynaecol Obstet 1978; 15:307-9.
93. Hein K, Kleinhaus S, Mayers M, Cohen MI, Litt IF, Boley SJ. Laparoscopy for presumed nonacute salpingitis: a new look at an old problem. J Adolesc Health Care 1980; 1:96-100.
94. Lundberg WI, Wall JE, Mathers JE. Laparoscopy in evaluation of pelvic pain. Obstet Gynecol 1973; 42:872-6.
95. Rees E. The treatment of pelvic inflammatory disease. Am J Obstet Gynecol 1980; 138:1042-7.
96. Robbie MO, Sweet RL. Metronidazole use in obstetrics and gynecology: a review. Am J Obstet Gynecol 1983; 145:865-81.
97. Monif GG. Group D streptococci (enterococci). In: Monif GG, ed. Infectious diseases in obstetrics and gynecology. Philadelphia: Harper and Row, 1982:219-20.
98. Onsrud M, Bergan T, Gjonnaess M. Antibiotic levels in plasma and peritoneal fluid after amoxycillin, ampicillin, and bacampicillin treatment for pelvic inflammatory disease. Acta Obstet Gynecol Scand 1982; 61:247-51.
99. Zaske DE, Cipolle RJ, Strate RG, Malo JW, Koszalka Jr. MF. Rapid gentamicin elimination in obstetric patients. Obstet Gynecol 1980; 56:559-64.
100. Ginsburg DS, Stern JL, Hamod KA, Genadry R, Spence MR. Tubo-ovarian abscess: a retrospective review. Am J Obstet Gynecol 1980; 138:1055-8.
101. Handsfield HH, Sandström EG, Knapp JS, Perine PL, Whittington WL, Sayers DF, Holmes KK. Epidemiology of penicillinase-producing *Neisseria gonorrhoeae* infections: analysis by auxotyping and serogrouping. N Engl J Med 1982; 306:950-4.
102. Sidhu S, Barnes R. Penicillinase-producing *Neisseria gonorrhoeae*—Los Angeles. JAMA 1983; 249:2300.
103. McCormack WM, Nowroozi K, Alpert S, Sackel SG, Lee YH, Lowe EW, Rankin JS. Acute pelvic inflammatory disease; characteristics of patients with gonococcal and nongonococcal infection and evaluation of their response to treatment with aqueous procaine penicillin G and spectinomycin hydrochloride. Sex Transm Dis 1977; 4:125-31.
104. Gibbs RS. A trial of spectinomycin hydrochloride compared with aqueous penicillin G plus kanamycin for treatment of severe pelvic inflammatory disease. Sex Transm Dis 1980; 7:21-3.

105. Poindexter AN. Comparative studies of mezlocillin, carbenicillin and ampicillin in the treatment of acute pelvic infection. J Antimicrob Chemother Suppl 1982; 9:159-61.
106. Gall SA, Hill GB. High-dose cefamandole therapy in obstetric and gynecologic infections. Am J Obstet Gynecol 1980; 137:914-22.
107. Marshall JR, Chow AW, Sorrell TC. Effectiveness of mezlocillin in female genital tract infections. J Antimicrob Chemother Suppl 1982; 9:149-58.
108. Chow AW. Antimicrobial therapy of gynaecological infections: an overview. J Antimicrob Chemother Suppl 1982; 9:139-47.
109. Kunin CM, Perkins RL, Ayers LW, Anderson ED, Iams JD, Svirbely JR, Moore RD, Boman DM. Report of the ad hoc committee on beta lactam antibiotics. Ohio State University Hospital, January 1982, Columbus, Ohio.
110. Hershey DW. Management of the patient with an intrauterine device and a unilateral adnexal mass. J Reprod Med 1980; 25:75-8.
111. Taylor ES. Conservative surgery for pelvic inflammatory disease and endometriosis. Clin Obstet Gynecol 1980; 23:183-9.
112. Rubenstein PR, Mishell Jr. DR, Ledger WJ. Colpotomy drainage of pelvic abscess. Obstet Gynecol 1976; 48:142-5.
113. Fraser AC. Surgical treatment of acute pelvic sepsis. J Obstet Gynaecol Br Commonw 1972; 79-560-4.
114. Volkin LB, Thompson DS, Sheperd GG. Epidemiologic follow-up study of patients with gonococcal pelvic inflammatory disease. Sex Transm Dis 1979; 6:267-9.
115. Potterat JJ, Phillips L, Rothenberg RB, Darrow WW. Gonococcal pelvic inflammatory disease: case-finding observations. Am J Obstet Gynecol 1980; 138:1101-4.
116. Curran JW, Schrader MV, Moyer JK, Kramer MA, Lossick JG, Brown WE. Gonorrhea in the emergency department: management, case follow-up, and contact tracing of cases in women. Am J Obstet Gynecol 1980; 138: 1105-8.
117. Meheus AZ. Surveillance, prevention, and control of sexually transmitted agents associated with pelvic inflammatory disease. Am J Obstet Gynecol 1980; 138:1064-70.
118. Hagenfeldt K, Szanto E. Sacroiliitis in women—a late sequela to acute salpingitis. Am J Obstet Gynecol 1980; 138:1039-41.
119. Weiner S, Wallach EE. Ovarian histology in pelvic inflammatory disease. Obstet Gynecol 1974; 43:431-7.
120. van Nagell JR, Parker Jr. JC, Maruyama Y, Utley J, Hager WD, Donaldson ES, Wood EG. The effect of pelvic inflammatory disease on enteric complications following radiation therapy for cervical cancer. Am J Obster Gynecol 1977; 128:767-71.

EIGHT

Nongenital Gonococcal Syndromes

Thomas M. File, Jr. and James S. Tan
Northeastern Ohio Universities
College of Medicine
Rootstown, Ohio
and Akron City Hospital
Akron, Ohio

INTRODUCTION

Gonococcal infections localized to the genitalia (urethra and cervix) are generally not serious health problems for the individual patient. However, serious complications may occur when infection spreads to extragenital sites. Nongenital gonococcal syndromes may present diagnostic problems to the health care professional, expecially when genital infections are asymptomatic.

Nongenital gonococcal syndromes usually result from the spread to extragenital sites by one of two pathways: (1) direct or contiguous spread and (2) by dissemination during bacteremia. Accordingly, this presentation is subdivided to include those complications occurring by direct or contiguous spread (epididymitis, prostatitis, pharyngeal infection, anorectal infection, perihepatitis, adult conjunctivitis, primary skin infection) and those occurring secondary to bacteremia (disseminated disease, dermatitis-arthritis syndrome, arthritis, meningitis, endocarditis). The most common manifestations associated with the complications

Table 1 Nongenital Gonococcal Syndrome Manifestations (Pathogenesis by Direct or Contiguous Spread)

Syndrome	Characteristic syndrome	Findings	Differential considerations
Epididymitis	Dysuria, epididymal swelling and pain	Tender epididymis (100%),[a] purulent discharge (100%)[a]	Chlamydial infection (<35 years), gram-negative bacilli (>35 years), testicular torsion, tumor
Anorectal infection[b] (proctitis)	Pain, discharge, tenesmus	Edema, friability (occasionally ulcers) of anal crypts, discharge	Herpes simplex virus, *Chlamydia trachomatis*, syphilis, amebiasis, enteric pathogen
Pharyngeal infection[b]	Mild sore throat (rarely severe)	Mild erythema (rarely ulcers, exudate)	Viral pharyngitis, streptococcal pharyngitis

Perihepatitis (Fitz-Hugh-Curtis syndrome)	Fever, right upper quadrant pain (rarely left upper quadrant pain)	Fever, right upper quadrant tenderness, Murphy's sign (66%),[c] liver rub (50%),[c] elevated transaminase (20%),[c]	Cholecystitis, appendicitis, pyelonephritis, RLL pneumonia
Conjunctivitis	Painful and swollen eyelids, purulent discharge	extensive inflammatory reaction	Other bacterial conjunctivitis
Disseminated infection, bacteremic stage	Chills, fever, multiple joint aches, rash	Rash–petechial, vesiculopustular; extremity and periarticular	Differential diagnosis: meningococcemia, staphylococcal infection, vasculitis
Septic joint	Monoarticular (knee most common) swelling and pain	Monoarticular arthritis	Pyogenic arthritis

[a]Ref. 2.
[b]The majority of patients are asymptomatic
[c]Ref. 41.

Table 2 Therapy for Common Nongenital Gonococcal Syndromes[a]

Syndrome	Penicillin therapy	Alternative therapy	PPNG[b]
Epididymitis	Amoxicillin 500 mg three times daily (ampicillin 500 mg four times daily) for 10 days	Tetracycline[c] 500 mg four times daily (doxycycline 100 mg twice daily) for 10 days	10-day course of oral trimethoprim/sulfamethoxazole or parenteral cefotaxime, cefoxitin, or spectinomycin
Anorectal	Procaine penicillin G 4.8 million units plus probenicid[d]	Spectinomycin	Spectinomycin 2 g intramuscularly
Pharyngeal	Procaine penicillin G 4.8 million units plus probenicid[d]	Tetracycline 500 mg four times daily for 7 days	Trimethoprim/sulfamethoxazole (80 mg/400 mg), 9 tablets for 5 days
Perihepatitis (peritonitis, pelvic inflammatory disease)	Cefoxitin 2 g intravenously every 6 hr[e] plus doxycycline 100 mg orally every 12 hr (both for at least 4 days, then doxycycline to complete 10 to 14 days)	Clindamycin plus gentamicin/tobramycin or doxycyline plus metronidazole	Cefoxitin plus doxycycline
Ophthalmia (conjunctivitis)	Aqueous penicillin G 10 million units for at least 5 days plus local irrigation	Same as PPNG	Cefoxitin, cefotaxime, spectinomycin
Disseminated infection (dermatitis, arthritis)	Aqueous penicillin G 10 million units intravenously every day until improvement (or oral amoxicillin 3.0 g (ampicillin 3.5 g) plus probenicid)[d], then amoxicillin (or ampicillin) orally to complete at least 7 days	Tetracycline 500 mg four times daily for at least 7 days	Cefoxitin (1.0 g) or cefotaxime (500 mg) intravenously every 6 hr for at least 7 days

[a]Based on recommendations of Sexually transmitted diseases treatment guidelines 1982. Morbid Mortal Week Rep (Suppl) 1982; 31:37S-46S.
[b]Penicillinase-producing *Neisseria gonorrhoeae*.
[c]Preferred therapy if *Chlamydia trachomatis* also suspected.
[d]Probenicid dosage: 1 g orally.
[e]Since the etiology is often mixed (including *C. trachomatis*) and unconfirmed, recommendations for pelvic inflammatory disease are included.

are indicated in Table 1 and a summary of antimicrobial therapy is provided in Table 2.

SYNDROMES SECONDARY TO DIRECT OR CONTIGUOUS SPREAD

Gonococcal Epididymitis and Prostatitis

Although the epididymis and prostate are components of the reproductive tract, gonococcal epididymitis and prostatitis are briefly discussed since they are complications of urethritis, occurring secondary to spread of infection from the urethra. *Neisseria gonorrhoeae* is a relatively common cause of epididymitis in patients less than 35 years of age [1]. Berger et al. found that *N. gonorrhoeae* accounted for 20% of cases of acute epididymitis in this age group [2]. *Chlamydia trachomatis* was the cause in 50% of cases. In the same study *N. gonorrhoeae* was not an etiological agent of epididymitis in patients over age 35 years (in this group epididymitis was associated with urinary tract infections caused by Enterobacteriaceae or *Pseudomonas*). While similar studies documenting the etiology of prostatitis are not available, it appears that the gonococcus is an uncommon cause of acute symptomatic prostatitis [3]. However, Thin reported that prostatitis (defined as excess leukocytes in expressed prostatic fluid, even in the absence of symptoms) was evident in 36.8% of military personnel with preceding gonococcal urethritis [4].

Acute gonococcal epididymitis presents as scrotal pain associated with tenderness and swelling of the epididymis. In Berger's study every gonococcal patient had epididymal tenderness and swelling, spontaneous urethral discharge, scrotal swelling, erythema, and dysuria. In contrast, 65% of patients with *C. trachomatis* epididymitis had urethral discharge (only 41% being spontaneous discharge), and only 43% had dysuria [1]. Some relief of pain may be obtained by elevation of the involved epididymis and testes (Phren's sign) [5].

The diagnosis of epididymitis is suggested by the above clinical findings. Other conditions which may present with similar findings include torsion of the spermatic cord (a surgical emergency), hematocele, or testicular tumor. Since torsion is a relatively common acute scrotal condition in boys, one must always consider this diagnosis in the younger patient. The demonstration of decreased blood flow to the twisted testis by ultrasound or radionuclide scan can be diagnostic [1]. The presence of white blood cells on a urethral smear is evidence of epididymitis. Diagnosis of gonococcal epididymitis can usually be confirmed by culture of material obtained from the urethra or expressed prostatic secretions [5]. Rarely, epididymal aspiration is required.

Acute symptomatic prostatitis is characterized by fever, chills, perineal pain, and symptoms of urinary tract infection associated with difficulty in urinating. On examination the prostate is swollen and usually very tender [3]. The gonococcus can usually be isolated from urethral swabs; however, purulent urethral discharge may not be evident unless prostatic massage is performed [3].

Since acute epididymitis in sexually active adults is more likely to be chlamydial than gonococcal, the U.S. Public Health Service recommends intial therapy with tetracycline hydrochloride 500 mg four times a day or doxycycline 100 mg twice a day for at least 10 days [6]. The following regimens can also be considered: amoxicillin 500 mg three times a day or erythromycin 500 mg four times a day for at least 10 days [6]. For epididymitis caused by penicillinase-producing *N. gonorrhoeae* (PPNG), experience is limited, but a 10-day course of therapy with oral trimethoprim/sulfamethoxazole or parenteral cefotaxime, cefoxitin, or spectinomycin can be used [6]. Bed rest and scrotal elevation are recommended to promote adequate lymphatic drainage of the infected epididymis. Failure to improve within 3 days requires a diagnostic reevaluation.

Patients with acute bacterial prostatitis often respond favorably to antibiotics, regardless of their "penetrability" into the prostate [3]. This is probably due to the intense inflammatory reaction which allows for passage of the antibiotics from plasma into the gland. Accordingly, a course of amoxicillin (ampicillin) or tetracycline (doxycycline) should be effective for penicillin-sensitive infections. Therapy for PPNG prostatitis would logically include trimethoprim/sulfamethoxazole, since trimethoprim does readily diffuse into the prostate [7].

Anorectal Gonococcal Infection

Anorectal gonococcal infection is relatively common among women and homosexual men. A total of 44% of women with cervical gonococcal infection will also have positive anorectal cultures, and the anorectal culture is the only positive culture in approximately 4% of women with gonorrhea [8]. Penile-anal contact probably represents the most significant mode of infection in the female. Pariser and Marino [9] reported that 75% of women with anorectal gonorrhea admit to having such contact. Extension of infection to the anorectum from infected vaginal secretions is another possible mechanism of anorectal involvement.

Anorectal infection in men occurs mostly among the homosexual population. A total of 90% of males with anorectal involvement are admitted to be homosexual [8]. The estimated prevalence of anorectal gonorrhea among homosexual men attending sexually transmitted disease clinics ranges from 28 to 55% [8]. Recent studies have indicated that homosexual men are susceptible to a number of agents which cause enteral or anorectal infection. Goodell et al. determined the etiology of proctitis and enteritis in homosexual men and found *Giardia lamblia* and *Campylobacter jejuni* as the most common causes of enteritis (gonococci were isolated from 4%), whereas gonorrhea was most commonly associated with proctitis, isolated in 41% of cases [10]. Multiple pathogens, herpes simplex virus

(HSV), *C. jejuni*, and *C. trachomatis* were isolated in 32, 27, 24, and 11%, respectively, of cases of proctitis.

Most patients with anorectal gonococcal infection are asymptomatic. Clements and Hughes reported that only 3% of their female patients with anorectal gonorrhea complained of any local discomfort and only 12% had signs of purulent discharge [11]. However, in a more recent study, one-third of homosexual males with anorectal infection had symptoms referable to the anorectum [12]. The actual probability of symptomatic proctitis among homosexual men with newly acquired rectal gonorrhea is presently unknown. Symptoms associated with anorectal gonococcal infection include anorectal pain, purulent discharge, change in bowel habits (constipation or diarrhea), tenesmus, and hematochezia [8]. Such symptoms are not specific for gonococcal infection, however, and may also be associated with other causes of proctitis. Gonococcal proctitis in homosexual men is generally associated with less pain than that associated with either HSV or *C. trachomatis* [13]. Symptomatic anorectal gonorrhea may be confused with a variety of other disorders, including ulcerative or granulomatis colitis, ischemic colitis, radiation- or drug-induced proctitis, early neoplasm, amebiasis, syphilis, granuloma inguinale, chancroid, or lymphogranuloma venereum [8,14].

Anoscopic findings of gonococcal proctitis are nonspecific and include inflammation with mucopurulent discharge, edema, friability, and occasionally ulceration of the anal crypts [14]. A Gram stain of the anorectal secretions done without anoscopic visualization has been reported to be positive in 30 to 50% of cases [15]; however, the Gram stain is positive in approximately 79% of anoscopically directed swab specimens [15]. Cultures are best obtained by moving the swab from side to side in the anal canal to sample crypts; allow 10 to 30 sec for absorption of organisms onto the swab [16]. Radiographic findings (barium enema) associated with gonococcal proctitis include mucosal granularity or diffuse ulceration, spasm, loss of distensibility, and a widened presacral space [17]. These radiographic findings resolve quite rapidly with therapy.

Awareness of the wide spectrum of sexually transmitted diseases that may cause anorectal disease (proctitis) in the homosexual male is extremely important to the health professional. A careful history is required to determine sexual activity and recent illness among sexual contacts. An examination should include anoscopy of all patients with symptoms already described. Laboratory tests should include a Gram stain of rectal exudate, syphilis serology, and culture for *N. gonorrhoeae*. A dark-field examination and cultures for HSV (especially if ulcers are present), *C. trachomatis*, and even *Shigella* sp., *Salmonella* sp., and *C. jejuni* should also be considered. Therapy should be directed specifically to identified pathogens.

The therapy of choice for anorectal gonorrhea is procaine penicillin G, 4.8 million units intramuscularly, plus 1 g of probenicid orally [6]. Alternative therapy for a patient who is allergic to penicillin or when PPNG is suspected or isolated is spectinomycin, 2 g intramuscularly. Both regimens are highly effective, with cure rates of 95 to 97% [18,19]; however, penicillin has the advantage of being effective therapy for concurrent pharyngeal gonorrhea. Efficacy of oral ampicillin is questionable. Lebedeff and Hochman [20] found cure rates using 3.5 g of ampicillin plus 1 g of probenicid orally similar to intramuscular procaine penicillin; however, Sands and Sellers [19] found that a second dose given 8 to 14 hr after the first was required to reduce the failure rate from 11 to 2%. Treatment with tetracycline has been found to be less effective for anorectal infection [20]. In addition, both oral ampicillin and tetracycline are less effective for anorectal infection in homosexual men [14]. The gonococcal auxotypes involved in homosexual infections tend to be different than in heterosexuals and are also less sensitive to penicillin [14]. Careful follow-up with culture 7 to 10 days after therapy is essential. Evaluation for other etiological agents (see Chap. 10) is also required, especially if symptoms do not resolve with therapy.

Possible complications of anorectal gonorrhea include anal fistulas, fissures, perianal abscess, and anorectal vaginal fistula.

Pharyngeal Gonococcal Infection

The prevalence of pharyngeal gonococcal infection depends upon the sexual activity of the population evaluated. Among gonococcal patients evaluated at a sexually transmitted disease clinic the prevalence of pharyngeal gonorrhea was 7% for heterosexual men, 10% for women, and 25% for homosexual men [21]. Approximately half of those patients with positive pharyngeal cultures have the pharyngeal site as the only positive culture for gonorrhea [22].

The mode of infection of the pharynx is usually associated with the practice of fellatio. Wiesner found pharyngeal gonococcal infections in 20% of patients with genital infection who practiced fellatio, but in only 3.1% of infected patients who denied fellatio [23]. Sackel et al. reported that 16.7% of women and 7.1% of men who had genital gonococcal infection and who practiced fellatio had concurrent pharyngeal infection [24]. Association of cunnilingus with pharyngeal gonorrhea has not been well established. Neither Wiesner [23] nor Sackel et al. [24] observed a significant difference among patients who admitted to the practice of cunnilingus versus those who did not; however, Bro-Jorgensen and Jensen found a greater frequency of pharyngeal gonorrhea among heterosexual men who admitted to the practice of cunnilingus than among those who did not [21]. It is reasonable to postulate that cunnilingus may contribute to pharyngeal gonorrhea, but it is less a risk facter than fellatio. In addition, oral-oral contact may be a method of spread, but it is probably very rare. The prerequisite for pharyngeal infection is possibly related to traumatic injury to the pharynx associated with fellatio, as opposed to cunnilingus or kissing.

The vast majority of patients with pharyngeal gonococcal infection are asymptomatic. Bro-Jorgensen and Jensen found 79% of patients with pharyngeal gonococcal infection to be asymptomatic [21]. Komaroff et al. found that only 1%

of patients with sore throat seen at a general medical clinic had positive pharyngeal cultures for *N. gonorrhoeae* [25]. A patient with symptomatic infection usually has a mild sore throat and examination reveals only mild erythema; however, oral ulcerative lesions as well as exudate of the pharynx and tonsils have been described [26,27].

Because the vast majority of infections are asymptomatic, some investigators doubt that gonococci produce significant pharyngeal disease. Wallin and Siegel followed 19 patients with untreated pharyngeal gonorrhea and noted spontaneous loss of gonococci from the pharynx in all patients without evidence of symptomatic disease [28]. Other investigators have reported generalized gonococcemia in conjunction with pharyngeal colonization [29]. The possibility that organisms in the pharynx may serve as a potential source of gonococcemia is still unclear. Another unsettling issue is the significance of pharyngeal infection as a source of spread to the genitalia during oral-genital sexual activity [30,31]. Wallin and Siegel found no spread to sexual partners of the 19 patients with untreated infection [28]; however, Tice and Rodriquez reported the transmission of *N. gonorrhoeae* via oral to genital spread in 46 of 2695 cases of gonococcal urethritis seen in the Philippines [32].

The asymptomatic nature and uncertain significance of pharyngeal gonorrhea has raised questions as to who should have pharyngeal cultures. It would seem appropriate to culture the pharynx in the following situations: (1) male homosexuals; (2) patients with signs or symptoms of pharyngitis who have evidence of genital gonococcal infection; (3) patients with sore throats who are sexual contacts of established gonorrhea cases; (4) the occasional patient with pharyngitis refractory to conventional therapy for streptococcal infection, since these regimens may fail to eradicate pharyngeal gonococcal infection; and (5) patients being evaluated for a sexually transmitted disease who admit to the practice of fellatio.

Procaine penicillin, 4.8 million units intramuscularly, plus 1 g of probenicid orally or tetracycline, 500 mg orally four times a day for 7 days, is the preferred therapy for pharyngeal gonococcal infection [6]. Pharyngeal infection is not effectively treated by either amoxicillin/ampicillin regimens or spectinomycin. Patients with pharyngeal infection caused by PPNG should receive trimethoprim/sulfamethoxazole [nine tablets (80 mg/400 mg) each day for 5 days] [6,33].

Gonococcal Perihepatitis-Peritonitis (Fitz-Hugh-Curtis Syndrome)

The clinical picture of gonococcal peritonitis of the upper part of the abdomen was first described by Stajano in 1920 [34]. Curtis reported an association of violin string or band adhesions between the anterior surface of the liver and the parietal peritoneum with coexisting evidence of gonococcal pelvic inflammatory disease [35]. In 1934 Fitz-Hugh characterized the clinical presentation and popularized the term "gonococcal perihepatitis" [36].

This syndrome classically involves women and the proposed pathophysiology involves bacterial spread from the fallopian tubes into the paracolic gutters, through the subphrenic space, and infection of the surface of the liver or peritoneum [37]. Rarely, this syndrome has been described in men, with proposed mechanisms being bacteremic seeding or bacterial migration through retroperitoneal lymphatics from an anorectal source [38,39].

The incidence of gonococcal perihepatitis-peritonitis is unknown because many cases go unrecognized and many are diagnosed clinically without bacteriological confirmation. The recent recognition that perihepatitis is a consequence of chlamydial infection as well as gonococcal infection demands a reevaluation of previous reports of the syndrome [40]. In one prospective study of 124 patients with pelvic inflammatory disease, 12% were felt to have perihepatitis [41]. Approximately one-half of these patients had gonococcal cervicitis. Litt and Cohen showed by a retrospective analysis of clinical findings that this syndrome may occur in up to 21% of cases of salpingitis [42].

The clinical presentation may vary from a mildly symptomatic to an acutely ill individual. A typical history would include genitourinary symptoms, such as menorrhagia or vague lower abdominal pain, occurring days to weeks preceding the onset of acute upper abdominal pain. Symptoms may be dramatic, with fever, excruciating pain in the right upper quadrant, and pleuritic pain referred to the shoulder or axilla. The pain may be bilateral and has been reported localized to the left upper quadrant (secondary to localized subphrenic peritonitis) [43]. Hiccups, nausea, chills, sweating, and headaches may be present.

Upper quadrant tenderness (usually on the right side) is invariably present. A positive Murphy's sign may be present and was found in 10 of 15 (66%) patients described by Semchyshyn [41]. A rub over the liver (often described as crunching to and fro or "new snow creeking") was found in 50% of the cases [41].

Routine laboratory studies usually demonstrate an elevated white blood count and possibly an elevated amylase [41]. Liver function tests are usually normal; however, elevated transaminases were reported in 4 of 15 cases [41]. During the acute phase of illness, there may be failure to visualize the gallbladder by cholecystogram probably secondary to dense pericholecystic adhesions which interfere with normal flow through the cystic duct [37].

The most difficult clinical problem is the differentiation of perihepatitis from other intra-abdominal inflammatory processes, especially acute cholecystitis. Other disease processes such as appendicitis, perforated peptic ulcer, subphrenic abscess, and other forms of localized peritonitis must be included within the differential diagnosis. Pyelonephritis, perinephric abscess, and lower lobe pneumonia may also be considered if the pain is localized posteriorly.

The diagnosis of Fitz-Hugh-Curtis syndrome requires a high index of suspicion and is based on the combination of clinical findings and exclusion of other mentioned causes. Gonorrhea cultures of cervical or urethral secretions are positive in 50 to 85% of the cases during the acute episode [41,42]. The diagnosis should be entertained in any sexually active patient with hepatic or upper quadrant tenderness. Rapid resolution of symptoms usually follows antibiotic therapy. Untreated, pain persists for 1 to 4 weeks, with an eventual change in character to a dull ache which eventually abates [37].

Perihepatitis in the acute stage is actually an acute peritonitis. In the chronic stage the violin string-like adhesions are noted. These may persist for many years, causing intermittent attacks of right upper quadrant pain (occasionally worsening during menstruation), or remain asymptomatic [41]. The formation of subphrenic abscesses is rare.

The therapy of gonococcal Fitz-Hugh-Curtis syndrome is the same as that for gonococcal pelvic inflammatory disease. If symptoms do not resolve following medical therapy, one must consider other diagnoses or the exacerbation of chronic perihepatitis due to adhesions. In the case of chronic right upper quadrant pain secondary to adhesions, laparoscopy has offered immediate relief of symptoms by lysis of adhesions [44].

Gonococcal Ophthalmia

Gonococcal infection of the eye is most commonly a neonatal disease (see Chap. 15). Rarely, *N. gonorrhoeae* causes adult conjunctivitis [45]. This usually occurs via direct sexual contact or indirectly via contaminated hands. Laboratory-acquired gonococcal conjunctivitis by accidental inoculation with clinical isolates has also been reported [46,47].

Gonococcal conjunctivitis may occasionally present as a mild inflammation [47]; however, the typical reaction is the acute onset of purulent conjunctivitis. This may be potentially sight threatening and is characterized by an extensive inflammation with copious purulent secretions, edema of the eyelids, and corneal ulceration if untreated. The affected eye is very tender, and associated signs can include preauricular suppurative adenopathy and fever.

The diagnosis may be suspected on the basis of Gram-stained conjunctival scrapings showing gram-negative intracellular diplococci; however, similar Gram stain findings apply to *Moraxella* sp., a noted conjunctival pathogen. Diagnosis can be confirmed by culture isolation. Anogenital and pharyngeal specimens should also be obtained in patients with suspected gonococcal conjunctivitis.

Treatment of gonococcal conjunctivitis involves the use of systemic antimicrobial agents plus frequent local irrigations and should be started as soon as the diagnosis is suspected.

Optimal treatment regimens for adults have not been established; however, high doses of intravenous penicillin G (10 million units each day for at least 5 days) are recommended [6]. If PPNG is suspected or confirmed, appropriate antibiotics would include cefoxitin, 1 g, or cefotaxime, 0.5 g, intravenously four times a day [6].

Primary Skin Infection and Suppurative Lymphadenopathy

Primary skin infections (those occurring by direct inoculation rather than secondary to bacteremia) are uncommon, since the squamous epithelium is relatively impenetrable to the gonococcus; however, pyogenic skin infections from direct digital-genital contact have been reported, particularly in patients with abrasions or areas of skin abnormalities (i.e., abrasions) [48]. These lesions have been described as pyogenic granulomas, cellulitis, or vesicular (resembling herpes infection) [48]. The diagnosis of such lesions may be missed, since routine culture techniques may not readily support growth of *N. gonorrhoeae*.

Inguinal adenopathy secondary to gonococcal urethritis has been described [49], and this organism must be considered in the differential of inguinal adenitis in sexually active persons.

SYNDROMES SECONDARY TO BACTEREMIA

Disseminated Infection

Transient bacteremia is probably quite common in patients with localized gonococcal infections. Disseminated gonococcal infection (DGI) occurs when bacteremia results in extragenital manifestations. Disseminated gonococcal infection may present clinically as dermatitis, arthritis, tenosynovitis, endocarditis, myopericarditis, or meningitis.

In the preantibiotic era, DGI occured in 1 to 3% of all cases of gonococcal infection, with a preponderance in males [50]. Since the introduction of antibiotics, the frequency of DGI has ranged between 0.1 and 0.3% of the total cases, with females outnumbering males by a ratio of 4 to 1 [51-54].

The majority of women develop symptoms during pregnancy, especially the third trimester, or within 7 days of the start of their menstrual period [52,53,55, 56]. Disseminated gonococcal infection has been reported in neonates and elderly patients, but the highest incidence is in the sexually active age group.

Sites of infection which serve as the portals of entry include the endocervix, pelvic organs, urethra, pharynx, anorectum, and in rare occasions skin and other mucous membranes. Since a significant number of patients have asymptomatic local infection [52,57,58], the source of initial infection may not be detected unless careful culturing of multiple sites is performed.

It appears that only certain gonococcal strains have a predisposition to disseminate. Weisner et al. [59] have demonstrated that only highly antibiotic-sensitive gonococcal strains are associated with DGI. Resistance to antibiotics descreases the ability of the organism to disseminate. Schooknik et al. [60] have shown that DGI strains are resistant to the bactericidal activity of human serum. This resistance may be due to IgG-binding receptors found on the surface of the gonococcus [61]. Investigators have also shown that DGI and asymptomatic strains have a unique requirement for arginine, hypoxanthine, and uracil, also known as the $Arg^- Hyx^- Ura^-$ auxotype [62,63]. This auxotype has also been found to be associated with a β-lactamase-producing strain isolated from a patient with DGI [64].

In normal hosts DGI strains are generally resistant to human serum and complement [60]. Rice and Goldenberg have shown that the clinical manifestations of the disease may be related to differences in serum resistance [65]. Strains of *N. gonorrhoeae* isolated in disseminated disease are more serum resistant than strains isolated in suppurative arthritis.

Complement deficiencies have been demonstrated to be associated with an increased predisposition to DGI [66-68]. Specifically, patients with C5, C6, C7, or C8 deficiency are at significant risk for DGI [69].

Disseminated gonococcal infection has been reviewed extensively [52,57, 70,71]. Clinically, patients with DGI may be divided into two major presentations as described by Keiser et al. [54]. The bacteremic form is characterized by chills, fever, typical skin lesions, and asymmetrical polyarticular involvement. The septic joint form presents with monoarthritis and joint effusion, but without systemic manifestations. An indeterminate presentation is characterized by asymmetrical manifestations, monoarthritis, and joint effusion. This form appears to bridge the bacteremic and the septic joint forms.

The incubation period is not well established, since a great number of cases are asymtomatic carriers. Patients in the bacteremic stage present with an acute onset of chills and fever, asymmetrical polyarthralgia, polyarthritis, tenosynovitis, and/or typical skin lesions. The joint involvement in this form is characterized by multiple articular involvement ranging from migratory or sustained painful joints to arthritis, but with minimal effusion. Immune complexes have been found in the sera [72,73] and joint fluids [74]. One series reported involvement of 2 to 9 joints, with a mean of 4.4, in each patient [54]. Joint manifestations are frequently accompanied by tenosynovitis. The most frequent locations are the tendons proximal and distal to the wrist and ankles [75]. Skin lesions associated with gonococcal arthritis were first recognized by Vidal in 1893, and their association with gonococcemia was reported in 1903 by Silvestrini [76]. About half of the patients with DGI have skin manifestations. The lesions are found predominantly on the extremities, especially the pariarticular region, and are usually fewer than 10 in number. The tiny papules or petechiae may progress to vesiculopustular, hemorrhagic, or bullous lesions surrounded by a wide erythematous base and may develop a dark center resembling a hemorrhagic infarct. Lesions appear at different stages of development and they usually measure about 5 mm or less, although sizes greater than 2 cm have been observed [76-78]. The pathophysiology of these lesions is unsettled. Scherer and Braun-Falco suggested that gonococcal skin lesions were the results of complement activation [79]. Kahn and Danielsson have demonstrated gonococci around the blood vessels in tissue sections [80]. Some believe that skin lesions represent septic infarcts [81,82]. These lesions reverse spontaneously within 4 days.

The patient with the septic joint form presents with a mono- or oligoarthritis. Skin lesions and other systemic symptoms are generally absent. The most common joint involved is the knee. Other commonly involved joints include the elbow, wrist, hand, and ankle. Less commonly involved are the shoulder, hip, foot, spine, and sternoclavicular, temporomandibular, and sacroiliac joints. Culture from the joint produces a high yield of the organism.

Although DGI is principally seen in the sexually active population, it has also been described in newborns, children, and the elderly [83-87]. In the case of the newborn the conjunctiva may be the portal of entry. Other entry sites include the mouth, upper respiratory tract, umbilicus, anus, and genital tract. The majority of cases have the septic joint form and have been associated with fever and/or irritability. Skin lesions have been found, but gonococci have not been isolated from these lesions. In older children and adolescents gonococcal arthritis is also more common than the bacteremic form.

A rare complication associated with bacteremia is pyomyositis [88,89]. Diagnosis may be difficult, since there is no typical clinical picture.

The diagnosis of DGI should be considered in any sexually active person who presents with arthritis or dermatitis with arthralgia. The disease is less likely when these manifestations appear in the very young or the elderly; however, age should not be used as an exclusion factor. Tenosynovitis, although suggestive of gonococcal infection, may be caused by trauma, rheumatoid arthritis, gout, tuberculosis, coccidioidomycosis, histoplasmosis, syphilis, and *Haemophilus influenzae*.

Laboratory diagnosis is based on culture. Positive blood, joint, or skin cultures for *N. gonorrhoeae* provide unequivocal proof of DGI. However, the yield from blood cultures has not been exceptionally high. This may be due to low-grade bacteremia or the inability of some culture media to adequately support growth of this fastidious organism [52,90,91]. Therefore more than six blood cultures may be necessary and cultures should be observed for at least 4 weeks. Both joint and pustule aspirates should be inoculated immediately onto chocolate agar without antibiotics. Care should be taken that the media used are warm (ideally 35 to 37°C) and are placed into a carbon dioxide-enriched (3 to 10% CO_2) environment as soon as possible.

A presumptive diagnosis is made when clinical manifestations are compatible with DGI and blood, skin, and joint cultures are negative but a mucous membrane culture is positive. Every effort should be made to culture the endocervix, urethra, throat, and rectum. If conjunctivitis is present, an eye culture should also be obtained.

Penicillin is the therapy of choice for non-PPNG strains. Table 2 lists the Centers for Disease Control recommendations and alternate drugs. Although high-dose penicillin is suggested, low-dose procaine penicillin (600,000 units every 12 hr intramuscularly) was shown in one study to be just as effective [92]. Cefoxitin or cefotaxime is effective against PPNG strains. Other cephalosporins are active against PPNG, but have not been officially approved for use. Patients generally have a rapid clinical response (24 to 48 hr) to antibiotics, with reduction in joint discomfort, and total resolution is usually observed within 5 days [93]. Pregnant patients should not be given tetracycline as an alternate to penicillin. Spectinomycin, 2.0 g intramuscularly twice daily for 3 days, or erythromycin, 500 mg four times daily for 7 days, may be given.

Most patients with DGI are not "septic" and need not be hospitalized as long as compliance can be assured. The contacts should be traced and treated. If the patient looks toxic or if endocarditis or meningitis is suspected, hospitalization is mandatory.

Endocarditis and Meningitis

Since the introduction of penicillin, these two complications of DGI have rarely been reported. In Masi and Eisenstein's review in 1981 [70,71] only 18 culture-proven cases in the English literature had been reported. Since then only isolated cases have been reported [94-98]. Most patients have had no previous heart disease. The aortic valve is by far the most commonly involved. When the valve is affected, rapid destruction is observed. Skin lesions are found in a third of cases. Deteriorating renal function has been attributed to immune complex nephritis [99]. Gonococcal meningitis has also been rarely reported in the Engligh literature [52,100]. Gonococcal meningitis may be mistaken for meningococcal meningitis.

Myocarditis and pericarditis have been reported as complications of gonococcemia. Findings include tachycardia, ST-T wave changes, premature ventricular beats, and heart block [101,102].

Meningitis and endocarditis caused by the gonococcus require high-dose intravenous penicillin therapy. Optimal duration of therapy is unknown, but most authorities treat endocarditis for a month. Therapy of penicillin-allergic patients must be individualized.

REFERENCES

1. Berger RE. Acute epididymitis. Sex Transm Dis 1981; 8:286-289.
2. Berger RE, Alexander ER, Harnisch JP, Paulsen CA, Monda GD, Ansell J, Holmes KK. Etiology manifestations and therapy of acute epididymitis: prospective study of 50 cases. J Urol 1979; 121:650-754.
3. Meares EM. Prostatitis: a review. Urol Clin North Am 1975; 2:3-27.
4. Thin RNT. Prostatitis after urethritis in Singapore. Br J Vener Dis 1974; 50: 370-372.
5. Sufrin G. Acute epididymitis. Sex Transm Dis Suppl 1981; 8:132-139.
6. Sexually transmitted disease treatment guidelines. Morbid Mortal Week Rep Suppl 1982; 31:37S-46S.

7. Vandenbroucke-Grauls CMJE, Rozenberg-Arska M, den Hengst CW, Verhoef J. Prostatitis due to penicillinase-producing *Neisseria gonorrhoeae*. Br J Vener Dis 1982; 58:311-313.
8. Klein EJ, Fisher LS, Chow AW, Guze LB. Anorectal gonococcal infection. Ann Intern Med 1977; 86:340-346.
9. Pariser H, Marino AF. Gonorrhea—frequently unrecognized reservoirs. South Med J 1970; 63:198-201.
10. Goodell SE, Quinn TC, Mkrtichian EE. The infectious etiology and histopathology of proctitis and enteritis in homosexual men. Gastroenterology 1981; 80:1159.
11. Clements PA, Hughes KEA. The incidence of proctitis in gonorrhoeae of females. Lancet 1935; 2:18-19.
12. Owen RL, Hill JL. Rectal and pharyngeal gonorrhea in homosexual men. JAMA 1972; 220:1315-1318.
13. Hook III EW, Stamm WE. Sexually transmitted diseases in men. Med Clin North Am 1983; 67:235-251.
14. Quinn TC, Corey L, Chaffee RG, Schuffler MD, Brancato FP, Holmes KK. The etiology of anorectal infections in homosexual men. Am J Med 1981; 71:395-406.
15. William DC, Felman YM, Riccardi NB. The utility of anoscopy in the rapid diagnosis of symptomatic anorectal gonorrhea in men. Sex Transm Dis 1981; 8:16-17.
16. Centers for Disease Control. Criteria and techniques for the diagnosis of gonorrhea. Center for Disease Control, Atlanta, Ga., 1974.
17. Sider L, Mintzer RA, Mendelson EB, Rogers LF, Degesys GE. Radiographic findings of infectious proctitis in homosexual men. Am J Radio 1982; 139: 667-671.
18. Fluker JL, Deherogoda P, Platt DJ, Gerken A. Rectal gonorrhoea in male homosexuals: presentation and therapy. Br J Vener Dis 1980; 56:397-399.
19. Sands M, Sellers T. Therapy of anorectal gonorrhea in men. Efficacy of oral antibiotic regimens. West J Med 1980; 133:469-471.
20. Lebedeff DA, Hochman EB. Rectal gonorrhea in men: diagnosis and treatment. Ann Intern Med 1980; 92:463-466.
21. Bro-Jorgensen A, Jensen T. Gonococcal pharyngeal infections. Report of 110 cases. Br J Vener Dis 1973; 49:491-499.
22. Osborne NG, Grubin L. Colonization of the pharynx with *Neisseria gonorrhoeae*: experience in a clinic for sexually transmitted diseases. Sex Transm Dis 1979; 6:253-256.
23. Wiesner PJ. Gonococcal pharyngeal infection. Clin Obstet Gynecol 1975; 18:212-219.
24. Sackel SG, Alpert S, Fiumara FN, Donner A, Laughlin CA, McCormack WM. Orogenital contact and the isolation of *Neisseria gonorrhoeae, Mycoplasma hominis,* and *Ureaplasma urealyticum* from the pharynx. Sex Transm Dis 1979; 6:64-68.
25. Komaroff AL, Aronson MD, Pass TH, Ervin CT. Prevalence of pharyngeal gonorrhea in general medical patients with sore throats. Sex Transm Dis 1980; 7:116-119.

26. Van Overbeek JJM. Gonorrheal infections in the oropharynx. Arch Otolaryngol 1976; 102:94-96.
27. Jamsky RJ, Christen AG. Oral gonococcal infections. Oral Surg 1982; 53: 358-362.
28. Wallin J. Siegel MS. Pharyngeal *Neisseria gonorrhoeae*: coloniser or pathogen? Br Med J 1979; June 1462-1463.
29. Cramolini GM, Litt IR. The pharynx as the only positive culture site in an adolescent with disseminated gonorrhea. J Pediatr 1982; 100:644-646.
30. Harrison WO. Pharyngeal gonorrhea. JAMA 1981; 246:2726-2727.
31. Braff EH. Pharyngeal gonorrhea. JAMA 1982; 248:427-428.
32. Tice AW, Rodriquez VL. Pharyngeal gonorrhea. JAMA 1981; 246:2717-2719.
33. Lindberg M. Ringertz O, Sandstrom E. Treatment of pharyngeal gonorrhoea due to beta-lactamase-producing gonococci. Br J Vener Dis 1982; 58:101-104.
34. Stajano C. La reaccion frencia en ginecologia. Sem Med Buenos Aires 1920; 27:243.
35. Curtis AH. Adhesions of the anterior surface of the liver. JAMA 1932; 99: 2010.
36. Fitz-Hugh T. Acute gonococcic peritonitis of the right upper quadrant in women. JAMA 1934; 102:2094.
37. Rutkow IM. Gonococcal perihepatitis (the Fitz-Hugh-Curtis syndrome): a diagnostic dilemma. Am Surg 1979; 45:369-373.
38. Davidson AC, Hawkins DA. Pleuritic pain: Fitz-Hugh-Curtis syndrome in a man. Br Med J 1982; 284:808.
39. Fung GL, Silpa M. Fitz-Hugh and Curtis syndrome in a man. JAMA 1981; 245:128.
40. Wang SP, Eschenbach DA, Holmes KK, Wager G, Grayston JT. *Chlamydia* trachomatis infection in Fitz-Hugh-Curtis syndrome. Am J Obstet Gynecol 1980; 138:1034-1038.
41. Semchyshyn S. Fitz-Hugh and Curtis syndrome. J Reprod Med 1979; 22:45-48.
42. Litt IF, Cohen MI. Perihepatitis associated with salpingitis in adolescents. JAMA 1978; 240:1253-1254.
43. Smith MS. Left upper quadrant presentation of Fitz-Hugh-Curtis syndrome in an adolescent. West J Med 1979; 130:70-72.
44. Feichert JA, Valle RF. Fitz-Hugh-Curtis syndrome: a laparoscopic approach. JAMA 1976; 236:266-268.
45. Gonococcal eye infections in adults–California, Texas, Germany. Morbid Mortal Week Rep 1981; 30:341-343.
46. Bruins SC, Tight RR. Laboratory-acquired gonococcal conjunctivitis. JAMA 1979; 241:274.
47. Podgore JK, Holmes KK. Ocular gonococcal infection with minimal or no inflammatory response. JAMA 1981; 246:242-243.
48. Scott Jr. MJ, Scott Sr., MJ. Primary cutaneous *Neisseria gonorrhoeae* infections. Arch Dermatol 1982; 118:351-352.
49. Dahl R, Dans PE. Gonococcal lymphadenitis. Arch Intern Med 1974; 134: 1116-1117.

50. Wehrbein HL. Gonococcus arthritis–a study of 610 cases. Surg Gynecol Obstet 1929; 49:105-113.
51. Goobar JE, Clark GM. Rheumatological manifestations of gonorrhea. Arch Interam Rheumatol 1964; 7:1-24.
52. Holmes KK, Counts GW, Beaty HN. Disseminated gonococcal infection. Ann Intern Med 1971; 74:979-993.
53. Suleiman SA, Grimes EM, Jones HS. Disseminated gonococcal infections. Obstet Gynecol 1983; 61:48-51.
54. Keiser H, Ruben FL, Wolinsky E, Kushner I. Clinical forms of gonococcal arthritis. N Engl J Med 1968; 279:234-240.
55. Garcia-Kutzbach A, Dismuke SE, Masi AT. Gonococcal arthritis: clinical features and results of penicillin therapy. J. Rheumatol 1974; 1:210-221.
56. Taylor HA, Brandford SA, Patterson SP. Gonococcal arthritis in pregnancy. Obstet Gynecol 1966; 27:776-782.
57. Handsfield HH. Disseminated gonococcal infection. Clin Obstet Gynecol 1975; 18:131-142.
58. Colin MJ, Weissman G. Disseminated gonococcal infection and tenosynovitis from an asymptomatically infected intrauterine contraceptive device. N Engl J Med 1976; 294:598-599.
59. Weisner PH, Handsfield HH, Holmes KK. Antibiotic resistance of gonococci causing disseminated infection. N Engl J Med 1973; 288:1221-1222.
60. Schooknik GK, Buchanan TM, Holmes KK. Gonococci causing disseminated gonococcal infection are resistant to bactericidal action of normal human sera. J Clin Invest 1976; 58:1163-1173.
61. McCutchan JH, Katzenstein D, Norquist D, Chikami G, Wunderlich A, Braude A. Role of blocking antibody in disseminated gonococcal infection. J Immunol 1978; 121:1884-1888.
62. Knapp JS, Holmes KK. Disseminated gonococcal infections caused by *Neisseria gonorrhoeae* with unique nutritional requirements. J Infect Dis 1975; 132:204-208.
63. Crawford G, Knapp JS, Hale J, Holmes KK. Asymptomatic gonorrhea in men: caused by gonococci with unique nutritional requirement. Science 1977; 196:1352-1353.
64. Thompson J, Dunbar JM, van Gent A, van Furth R. Disseminated gonococcal infection due to a beta-lactamase producing strain of *Neisseria gonorrhoeae*. A case report. Br J Vener Dis 1981; 57:325-326.
65. Rice PA, Goldenberg DL. Clinical manifestations of disseminated infection caused by *Neisseria gonorrhoeae* are linked to differences in bactericidal reactivity of infectious strains. Ann Intern Med 1981; 95:175-178.
66. Leddy JP, Frank MM, Gaither T, Baum J, Klemperer MH. Hereditary deficiency of the sixth component of complement in man. I. Immunochemical, biologic and family studies. J Clin Invest 1974; 53:544-553.
67. Peterson BH, Graham JA, Brooks GF. Human deficiency of the eighth component of complement: the requirement of C8 for serum *Neisseria gonorrhoeae* bactericidal activity. J Clin Invest 1976; 57:283-290.
68. Lee TJ, Utsinger PD, Snyderman R, Young WJ, Sparling PF. Familiar deficiency of the seventh component of complement associated with recurrent bacteremia infections due to *Neisseria*. J Infect Dis 1978; 138:359-368.

69. Petersen BH, Lee TJ, Snyderman R, Brooks GF. *Neisseria meningitidis* and *Neisseria gonorrhoeae* bacteremia associated with C6, C7, C8 deficiency. Ann Intern Med 1979; 90:917-920.
70. Eisenstein BI, Masi AT. Disseminated gonococcal infection (DGI) and gonococcal arthritis (GCA): I. Bacteriology, epidemiology, host factors, pathogen factors, and pathology. Semin Arthritis Rheum 1981; 10:155-172.
71. Masi AT, Eisenstein BL. Disseminated gonococcal infection (DGI) and gonococcal arthritis (GCA): II. Clinical manifestations, diagnosis, complications, treatment, and prevention. Semin Arthritis Rheum 1981; 10:173-197.
72. Goldman J, Thompson III S, Jacobs N. Circulating immune complexes in disseminated gonococcal syndrome. Arthritis Rheum. 1975; 18:402.
73. Walker LC, Ahlin TD, Tung KSK, Williams RC. Circulating immune complexes in disseminated gonorrheal infection. Ann Intern Med 1978; 89:28-33.
74. Manicourt DH, Orloff S. Gonococcal arthritis–dermatitis syndrome. Arthritis Rheum. 1982; 25:574-578.
75. Brofadir SP, Schimmer BM, Myers AR. Spectrum of the gonococcal arthritis-dermatitis syndrome. Semin Arthritis Rheum 1979; 8:177-183.
76. Barr J, Danielsson D. Septic gonococcal dermatitis. Br Med J 1971; 1:482-485.
77. Ackerman AB, Miller RC, Shapiro L. Gonococcemia and its cutaneous manifestations. Arch Dermatol 1965; 91:227-232.
78. Abu-Nassar H, Hill N, Fred HL, Yow E. Cutaneous manifestations of gonococcemia. Arch Intern Med 1963; 112:731-737.
79. Scherer R, Braun-Falco O. Alternative pathway complement activation: a possible mechanism inducing skin lesions in benign gonococcal sepsis. Br J Dermatol 1976; 95:303-309.
80. Kahn G, Danielsson D. Septic gonococcal dermatitis. Arch Dermatol 1969; 99:421-425.
81. Shapiro L, Teisch JA, Brownstein MH. Dermatohistopathology of chronic gonococcal sepsis. Arch Dermatol 1973; 107:403-406.
82. Seifert MH, Warin AP, Miller A. Articular and cutaneous manifestations of gonorrhea. Review of sixteen cases. Ann Rheum Dis 1974; 33:140-146.
83. Kohen DP. Neonatal gonococcal arthritis. Three cases and review of the literature. Pediatrics 1974; 53:436-440.
84. Cooperman MB. Gonococcus arthritis in infancy. Am J Dis Child 1927; 33:932-948.
85. Litt IF, Edberg SC, Finberg L. Gonorrhea in children and adolescents: a current review. J Pediatr 1974; 85:595-607.
86. Partain JO, Cathcart ES, Cohen AS. Arthritis associated with gonorrhea. Ann Rheum Dis 1968; 27:156-162.
87. Straus SE, Vest JV, Glew RH. Gonococcal arthritis in the elderly. South Med J 1978; 71:214-215.
88. Swarts RL, Martinez LA, Robson HG. Gonococcal pyomyositis. JAMA 1981; 246:246-247.
89. Owino SO, Goldmeier D, Wall RA. Gonococcal septicemia presenting as subcutaneous abscess. Br J Vener Dis 1981; 57:143-144.
90. Cooke HB, Arensberg D, Felner JM, Rimland D, Lesser L. Gonococcal endocarditis in the antibiotic era. Arch Intern Med 1979; 139:1247-1250.

91. Kraus SJ. Complications of gonococcal infection. Med Clin North Am 1972; 56:1115-1125.
92. Trenthan DE, McGravey JW, Masi AT. Low dose penicillin for gonococcal arthritis. JAMA 1976; 236:2410-2412.
93. Handsfield HH, Weisner PJ, Holmes KK. Treatment of gonococcal arthritis-dermatitis syndrome. Ann Intern Med 1976; 84:661-667.
94. Mansheim BJ. Gonococcal endocarditis. South Med J 1980; 73:1645-1646.
95. Rubin B, Dratch M. Gonococcal endocarditis in a male homosexual. Report of a case. J Am Osteopathol Assoc 1981; 80:534-537.
96. Timmis AD, Crofts MA, Metcalfe J, Monaghan MJ, Sharp J, Jackim G. Gonococcal endocarditis with penicillin-induced bone marrow hypoplasia. JAMA 1981; 246:672-673.
97. Hopkins CB, Postic B, Killiam H. Gonococcal endocarditis: cross-sectional echocardiographic diagnosis of aortic ring abscess. J Clin Ultrasound 1982; 10:279-281.
98. Sugar AM, Utsinger PD, Sanfaro J. Gonococcal endocarditis in a patient with mitral valve prolapse: study of host immunology and organism characteristics. Am J Med Sci 1982; 283:165-168.
99. Ebright JR, Komorowski R. Gonococcal endocarditis associated with immune complex glomerulonephritis. Am J Med 1980; 68:793-796.
100. Sayeed ZA, Bhaduri U, Howell E, Meyers HL. Gonococcal meningitis. A review. JAMA 1972; 219:1730-1731.
101. Fraser HS, Liburd AL, Figueroa JP, Nicholson GA, James OB, Whitbourne F, Alleyne BA. Gonoccemia with arthritis dermatitis and myocarditis. Postgrad Med J 1974; 50:759-764.
102. Vietzke WM. Gonococcal arthritis with pericarditis. Arch Intern Med 1966; 117:270-272.

NINE

The Urethral Syndrome

William G. Gardner
Northeastern Ohio Universities
College of Medicine
Rootstown, Ohio
and Akron General Medical Center
Akron, Ohio

INTRODUCTION

The term "urethral syndrome" refers to the occurrence of symptoms of dysuria and frequent urination in women. These symptoms can occur in any age group, but are particularly common in young, sexually active women and suggest the diagnosis of lower urinary tract infection. The importance of this syndrome is illustrated by a study suggesting that 20% of women develop these symptoms each year [1]. Other studies have shown that 30 to 50% of women with dysuria and frequency will have negative urine cultures using the traditional criteria established by Kass, who defined significant bacteriuria as a colony count of at least 10^5 organisms per milliliter of a single bacterial species in a clean-voided midstream urine specimen [2-4]. Those women with dysuria and frequency without evidence of bacterial urinary tract infection by traditional criteria are considered to have urethral syndrome.

ETIOLOGY

There are several possible etiologies for the urethral syndrome. These can be divided into noninfectious and infectious causes. Of the infectious causes, some are due to sexually transmissible agents. The major etiologies that have been proposed for the urethral syndrome are listed in Table 1. These will be discussed briefly, since each must be considered in the evaluation of the woman with dysuria and frequency.

Noninfectious Causes of Urethral Syndrome

Several reviews in the urological literature have addressed the possible noninfectious causes of urethral syndrome [5-8]. Obstruction to outflow of urine from the bladder as a result of external sphincter spasm and hyperactivity of the pelvic floor has been postulated as a cause of dysuria and frequency in some women [9,10]. In one uncontrolled study this hypothesis was supported by relief of symptoms after administration of diazepam. Other studies suggesting that urethral dilatation or urethrotomy will relieve symptoms further support outflow obstruction as a cause of dysuria [11,12]; however, in one study showing a benefit from urethral dilatation, the patients were also treated with long-term antibiotics, making it difficult to definitely attribute the response to the procedure [11]. In another controlled study there was no significant benefit of urethral dilatation over medical treatment alone in preventing recurrent infections [13]. In a study of young women with dysuria and frequency, urodynamic

Table 1 Etiology of Dysuria-Frequency (Urethral Syndrome)

Noninfectious
Outflow obstruction
Urethral trauma
Interstitial cystitis
Chemical irritation
Allergic reactions
Psychological factors
Miscellaneous
Infectious
Cystitis
Vaginitis
Low colony count bacterial cystitis
Gonococcal infection
Chlamydial infection
Genital herpes infection
Viral cystitis
Cystitis-urethritis due to fastidious bacteria

measurements failed to show evidence of outflow obstruction in a significant number, suggesting that outflow obstruction was not a cause of the symptoms and that urethral dilatation or urethrotomy was not indicated for treatment [14]. Thus the data available do not support urethral obstruction as a significant cause of urethral syndrome in young women.

Transvaginal traumatic cystourethritis has been postulated as a cause for urethral syndrome with negative urine cultures [15]. Certain women may be predisposed because of anatomical factors to developing inflammation of the urethra and trigone as a result of coital trauma. Furthermore, urethral trauma has been shown to predispose to ascending urinary tract infection [16]. These data suggest that in certain women urethral syndrome may result from anatomical abnormalities such as an incompliant vagina resulting in excessive urethral trauma during intercourse. In such patients surgical correction might alleviate the symptoms.

Investigators have suggested that women with persistent lower urinary tract irritative symptoms, repeatedly sterile urine cultures, and negative urine cytologies should be suspected of having interstitial cystitis, an entity characterized by nonspecific submucosal edema, vasodilatation, and chronic inflammation of the bladder wall [17]. The symptoms are very similar to the acute urethral syndrome, but the onset is less acute and the duration longer. The differentiation from acute urethral syndrome is made by cystoscopy demonstrating a reduced bladder capacity, the presence of a Hunner's ulcer, and pinpoint petechial hemorrhages of the bladder mucosa on second filling. The characteristic Hunner's ulcer, however, may be absent in the early stages and the diagnosis is made based on the other criteria. Antibiotics have not been shown to be of benefit in the treatment of interstitial cystitis.

Several other factors have been suggested as potential causes of dysuria and frequency. These include chemical or allergic irritation to one of the commonly used vaginal or perineal preparations such as contraceptive foams or creams, vaginal douches, and deodorants, or reactions to rubber contraceptive devices. In postmenopausal women estrogen deficiency may cause vaginal irritation, but this is unlikely in the young, sexually active population. Psychological factors may play a role, as suggested by studies in which the Minnesota Multiphasic Personality Inventory evaluation was done on women with urethral syndrome [18,19]. These studies showed that women with urethral syndrome scored significantly higher on the hypochondriasis, hysteria, and schizophrenia scales than did the control patients. Urethral irritation from nylon clothing, excessive perineal cleansing, poor personal hygiene, and self-induced trauma are all noninfectious factors that should be considered in the patient with dysuria and frequency.

Infectious Causes of Urethral Syndrome

When considering the infectious causes of dysuria and frequency in women, a major consideration is an acute bacterial cystitis. Bacterial cystitis can usually be excluded by doing a routine urinalysis, a Gram stain of the urinary sediment, and, when necessary, a quantitative culture of a clean-voided urine specimen revealing at least 10^5 bacteria per milliliter of urine [4].

Vaginitis can produce dysuria and frequency by contiguous involvement of the periurethral area in women. The dysuria that occurs with vaginitis differs from the dysuria that occurs with cystitis or urethritis in that the pain is felt in the inflamed vaginal labia as a stream of urine is passed. This has been referred to as "external dysuria" [20]. The diagnosis of vaginitis can usually be established by a good medical history, pelvic examination, and examination of the vaginal secretions. Establishing the diagnosis of vaginitis, however, does not exclude the other causes of urethral syndrome, since multiple sexually transmitted diseases may occur in the same individual [21]. The problem of differentiating cystitis and vaginitis from acute urethral syndrome will be discussed further in Section III.

A recent study by Stamm and colleagues showed that many cases of acute urethral syndrome are due to common urinary tract pathogens such as coliform bacteria and *Staphylococcus saprophyticus*, a novobiocin-resistant, coagulase-negative staphylococcus, but with colony counts lower than the traditional 10^5 bacteria per milliliter needed for diagnosis of bacterial urinary infection [22]. They studied 59 women with acute urethral syndrome: 32 had sterile routine urine cultures and the remaining 27 had bacteria present in colony counts of up to 34,000 per milliliter; 42 of the 59 women had significant pyuria ($\geq$8 white blood cells per cubic millimeter) on routine urinalysis. The 27 women with bladder bacteriuria all had significant pyuria, whereas none of the women without pyuria had bacteriuria. The other significant pathogen isolated from women with "sterile" pyuria was *Chlamydia trachomatis*, which will be discussed later. Their data suggest that many women with urethral syndrome will actually have bacterial infection, but that the usual criterium of 10^5 bacteria per milliliter is not sensitive enough to detect these on routine culture. Furthermore, the presence of pyuria in women with urethral syndrome is helpful in predicting the presence of a pathogen.

The pathogenesis of urethral syndrome due to staphylococcus or coliform bacteria is probably similar to that for bacterial cystitis. Studies have shown that periurethral or vaginal colonization with coliform bacteria frequently precedes symptomatic bacterial cystitis [23,24]. In the study of Stamm et al. colonization of the vagina or urethra with *Escherichia coli* occurred frequently in women with urethral syndrome and bladder bacteriuria, but was uncommon in women with sterile bladder urine with or without pyuria [22]. In another study no difference was found in the rate of introital colonization with coliform bacteria in women with urethral syndrome compared to an asymptomatic control group [25]; however, many of those women with urethral syndrome and introital colonization subsequently developed bacterial urinary tract infection, suggesting that some women with urethral syndrome may actually be between episodes of bacterial urinary infection.

Chlamydia trachomatis has been implicated as a common cause of nongonococcal urethritis in men [26,27]. The increased frequency of isolation of *C. trachomatis* from female sexual partners of men with nongonococcal urethritis suggests a sexually transmissible role for this agent [28]. There have been several case reports of the isolation of *C. trachomatis* from sexually active women with dysuria and frequency, suggesting that *Chlamydia* may be a cause of female urethral syndrome [29,30]. In a study of 22 women with acute urethral syndrome *C. trachomatis* was isolated from 59% compared to only 13% in an asymptomatic control group [31]. In the study of Stamm et al. *C. trachomatis* was isolated from 10 of 16 women with acute urethral syndrome and "sterile" pyuria, but in only 1 of 16 without pyuria [22]. These data support the role of *Chlamydia* as a sexually transmissible cause of female urethral syndrome, much the same as in nongonococcal urethritis in men. However, in a study of female partners of men with nongonococcal urethritis, only 53% of women with *C. trachomatis* isolated from the urethra had symptoms of urethritis, suggesting that *Chlamydia* may often be present in the female urethra in the absence of symptoms [32].

Another sexually transmissible pathogen implicated as a cause of female urethral syndrome is *Neisseria gonorrhoeae* [33]. In a study of 35 women presenting to a large city hospital emergency room for treatment of urinary tract symptoms, 13 were found to have sterile urine cultures [34]. *Neisseria gonorrhoeae* was cultured from 8 of the 13 women, and in 5 cases was cultured from a catheterized urine specimen. Six of the eight culture-positive women had significant pyuria noted on routine urinalysis. The results of this study suggest that infection with *N. gonorrhoeae* is a common cause of dysuria and frequency in women. This is in sharp contrast to the study of Stamm et al., in which *N. gonorrhoeae* was not isolated from any patient with urethral syndrome [22]. Another study failed to show any increased frequency of infection with *N. gonorrhoeae* in women with urethral syndrome when compared to those with bacterial urinary tract infection [35]. The reasons for these differing results are probably related to the prevalence of gonorrhea in the population of women studied and the culture techniques utilized. Certainly in sexually active women with urethral syndrome, infection with *N. gonorrhoeae* should be considered as a possible cause, especially in populations with a high prevalence of gonococcal infection such as sexually transmitted disease clinics or inner city emergency rooms.

Sexually transmissible pathogens that have not been proven to cause female urethral syndrome include *Ureaplasma urealyticum*, *Mycoplasma hominis*, and *Gardnerella vaginalis*. *Ureaplasma urealyticum* has been implicated as a cause of nongonococcal urethritis in men [36,37]; however, studies of women with urethral syndrome have not shown an increase in frequency of *U. urealyticum* isolates when compared to women with bacterial urinary infections [22,35]. One study did demonstrate an increase in *M. hominis* isolates in the urine of women with urethral syndrome, but the numbers of patients were small [37]. In another study *G. vaginalis* was isolated more frequently from the urine of pregnant women with pyuria, negative routine urine cultures, and known or suspected renal disease when compared with healthy pregnant women [38]. *Ureaplasma urealyticum* was also found more frequently in this group, but was usually present with another organism, such as *G. vaginalis*. Whether either of these organisms alone can cause symptomatic urinary infection remains unclear, and there is insufficient evidence to implicate them as a cause of urethral syndrome.

Several investigators have proposed that the urethral syndrome may be due to infection with anaerobic or fastidious bacteria that have special growth requirements making them difficult to isolate on routine urine culture [39-42]. In one study *Lactobacillus* species, *Corynebacterium* species, or *Streptococcus milleri* were isolated from urine in pure culture with colony counts of 10^4 or more organisms per milliliter in 73 women, 68 of whom had urinary symptoms at the time of isolation [39]. Many of these women appeared to respond symptomatically to antibacterial therapy directed against these pathogens, supporting the role of fastidious bacteria in causing urethral syndrome. Other studies, however, have pointed out the high spontaneous remission rate of urethral syndrome, making evaluation of any antimicrobial agent difficult without appropriate controls [43]. Furthermore, fastidious organisms have not been found in some studies, even when specific isolation techniques were employed [44,45].

Primary genital herpes simplex infection causes dysuria in up to 83% of cases and should be considered in the differential diagnosis of acute urethral syndrome, especially if the dysuria is external [46,47]. Cytomegalovirus has also been postulated as a cause, but in prospective studies is rarely isolated [22].

In summary, the leading infectious causes of acute urethral syndrome are *C. trachomatis, N. gonorrhoeae* and low colony counts of coliform bacteria, and *S. saprophyticus*. The role of *Ureaplasma, Mycoplasma,* anaerobic or fastidious bacteria, *G. vaginalis*, herpes simplex, and other viruses remains unproven. Of the noninfectious causes, urethral trauma probably accounts for some cases, perhaps by predisposing to infection. Other causes such as outflow obstruction, interstitial cystitis, chemical irritation, hormonal factors, and psychological factors remain unproven.

DIAGNOSIS

There are two major questions to consider in the diagnosis of women with dysuria and frequency: (1) Where is the site of origin of the dysuria and (2) what is the pathogen responsible for the dysuria? It is important to note that dysuria can be due to disease in the upper urinary tract, urinary bladder, urethra, or periurethral area. The diagnostic approach should include a medical history, sexual history, physical examination, pelvic examination, routine urinalysis, and appropriate smears and cultures when indicated. This approach will often provide the answers needed to choose appropriate therapy.

The diagnosis of acute urethral syndrome requires that the presence of vaginitis and acute bacterial cystitis or pyelonephritis first be excluded. The diagnosis of vaginitis is supported by a history of new onset of vaginal discharge or an increase in discharge, the presence of vaginal irritation, and the relative absence of urinary tract symptoms of dysuria, frequency, and suprapubic pain. Women with vaginitis may complain of "external" dysuria, referring to a burning sensation in the periurethral area as urine passes over the inflamed labia. However, there is usually no urgency or frequency unless there is a concomitant urinary tract infection. Labial or perineal itching is frequently present with monilia vaginitis, and a disagreeable vaginal odor may be present with nonspecific vaginitis due to *G. vaginalis*.

The pelvic examination is helpful in establishing the specific etiological diagnosis of vaginitis, as well as excluding cervical and upper genital tract disease. Vaginitis due to *Trichomonas vaginalis* or *Candida albicans* can be diagnosed in many cases with a wet preparation of the vaginal secretions. The presence of clue cells is suggestive of *G. vaginalis* infection, but clue cells may be present in the absence of vaginitis [48].

In a study of 821 women with urinary or vaginal complaints, a vaginal infection was rarely present if vaginal irritation and discharge were denied and symptoms of dysuria and frequency were present [20]. These data suggest that a detailed history can be very helpful and often of greater value than the physical examination in excluding the diagnosis of vaginitis.

Bacterial cystitis must also be excluded before making the diagnosis of urethral syndrome. Bacterial cystitis is suggested by symptoms of dysuria, urgency, frequency, and suprapubic discomfort. The presence of significant pyuria on routine urinalysis and bacteria on a Gram stain of unspun urine are also helpful, but a definitive diagnosis is made by a quantitative culture revealing 10^5 or more organisms per milliliter of urine.

Women with dysuria and frequency without clinical signs of vaginitis or significant bacteriuria on quantitative culture are considered to have the urethral syndrome. Therefore clinical diagnosis of urethral syndrome is not difficult; however, determining the specific etiology accounting for the symptoms is often a problem.

It is helpful from a diagnostic aspect to categorize women with urethral syndrome into those with and those without significant pyuria. Significant pyuria is considered to be at least 8 white blood cells per cubic millimeter, or over 10 white blood cells per 400X field on microscopic examination of the urine. Women without significant pyuria are less likely to have an identifiable infectious etiology for their symptoms [20]. In women with pyuria and negative routine urine cultures the major diagnostic considerations are infections with (1) coliform bacteria or *S. saprophyticus* with low colony counts ($<10^5$ bacteria per milliliter), (2) *N. gonorrhoeae*, or (3) *C. trachomatis*.

Several factors should suggest the possibility of a low colony count bacterial cystitis as a cause for the symptoms. These include a relatively abrupt onset of dysuria and frequency, hematuria, suprapubic pain, a history of previous urinary tract infection, and no recent change in sexual partner. In this setting a urine culture yielding less than 10^5 bacteria per milliliter of a coliform or *S. saprophyticus* may represent a true pathogen [22]; however, the problem is in determining whether small numbers of coagulase-negative staphylococci or coliform bacteria represent true infection or urethral contamination. The diagnosis of infection can be supported by obtaining a urine culture by urethral catheterization or suprapubic aspiration, but such measures are usually not indicated in patients with only lower tract symptoms. Instead, if the midstream urine culture yields a pure growth of one of these bacteria and the patient is symptomatic, the bacteria should be considered a potential pathogen. In this situation a coagulase-negative staphylococcus should be speciated to determine if it is *S. saprophyticus*.

If the history is one of a more gradual onset of symptoms without hematuria or suprapubic pain and with a recent change in sexual partner or exposure to a sexual partner with a discharge, infection due to the gonococcus or *Chlamydia* should be considered [49].

Attributing urethral syndrome to infection by *N. gonorrhoeae* requires the isolation of the organism from a urogenital site in the absence of other routine urinary pathogens. Curran reported eight cases of urethral syndrome due to *N. gonorrhoeae* [33]. In five cases the gonococcus was cultured from a catheterized urine specimen using Thayer-Martin medium. Because of the special growth requirements of the gonococcus, those cultures would have been negative if only standard urine culture techniques had been used. Urine was the only site from which *N. gonorrhoeae* was cultured in only one case. Other sites that should be cultured for *N. gonorrhoeae* are the endocervix, urethra, and anal canal. The isolation of the gonococcus from one or more of these sites in a woman with dysuria and frequency and a negative routine urine culture should suggest the diagnosis of urethral syndrome due to *N. gonorrhoeae*. Culturing urine on Thayer-Martin medium is indicated for the woman with dysuria and frequency only if there is a high index of suspicion for gonococcal infection based on epidemiological information such as recent exposure.

The clinical presentation of *C. trachomatis* infection can be very similar to *N. gonorrhoeae* in the female. The presence of a mucopurulent cervicitis on pelvic examination should suggest infection by one of these agents. The diagnosis of chlamydia infection is more difficult than for the other organisms, because isolation of this organism requires tissue culture techniques generally not available in most hospitals [50]. As a result, the diagnosis of chlamydia cervicitis is usually made on clinical grounds and a negative culture for *N. gonorrhoeae*. Serological techniques have not been useful in the diagnosis of *C. trachomatis* infection because of the high prevalence of antichlamydial antibodies in the sexually active population [28]. In addition, since many chlamydia infections tend to be chronic, the necessary rise in antibody titer required for serological diagnosis is difficult to demonstrate. Therefore the diagnosis of *C. trachomatis* urethritis is suggested by a compatible clinical history in a woman with dysuria and frequency, pyuria on urinalysis, negative routine urine culture, and negative cultures for *N. gonorrhoeae*.

An etiology is rarely found for the urethral syndrome in women without significant pyuria on routine urinalysis. A few of these may be due to mechanical factors such as chemical irritants or trauma related to intercourse. Some may proceed to develop pyuria and bacterial cystitis in the near future. However, the woman without pyuria should not have an extensive diagnostic workup, since this will fail to demonstrate a treatable pathogen in the majority of such cases [22]. Instead, she should be reevaluated in 24 to 48 hr if the symptoms persist. A more extensive evaluation should be reserved for the woman with persistent or recurrent dysuria.

The role of cystoscopy in the diagnosis of the woman with urethral syndrome is controversial. Cystoscopy is not indicated for every patient with urethral syndrome. It should be reserved for those with unexplained hematuria or pyuria persisting after treatment of infection [51]. Cystoscopy is helpful in excluding primary bladder disease such as interstitital cystitis as a cause of urethral syndrome [17].

The diagnostic approach to the woman with dysuria-frequency syndrome is outlined in Figure 1. In summary, bacterial cystitis ($\geqslant 10^5$ organisms per milliliter)

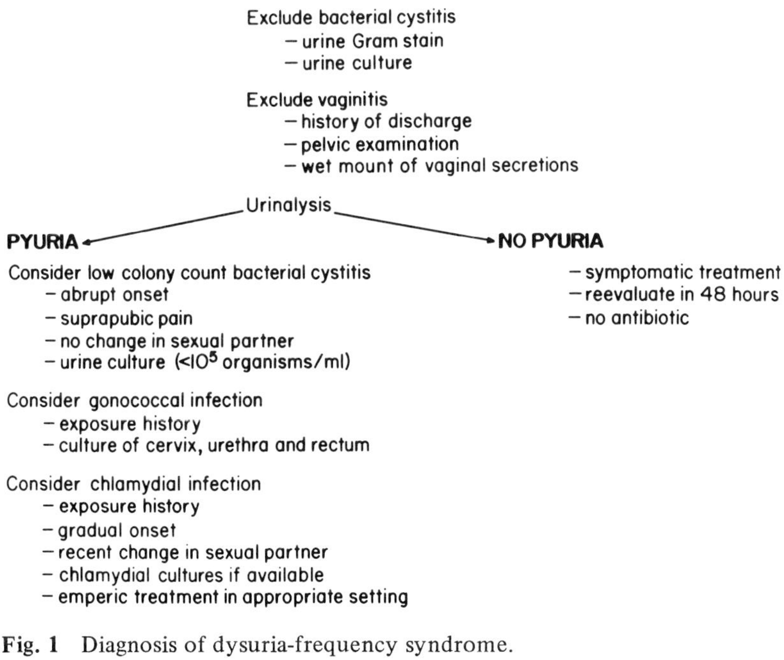

Fig. 1 Diagnosis of dysuria-frequency syndrome.

and vaginitis must be excluded. If no pyuria is noted on urinalysis, the patient should be treated symptomatically and reevaluated in 48 hr if symptoms persist. Most will spontaneously resolve, but a few will develop bacterial infection. If pyuria is noted, cultures should be obtained for *N. gonorrhoeae*. If the symptoms are of gradual onset and if there is a history of exposure to a male with nongonococcal urethritis or a recent change in sexual partner, chlamydial infection should be considered. Chlamydial cultures are not routinely indicated, but in the proper clinical setting a therapeutic course of an antimicrobial agent active against chlamydia is warranted.

TREATMENT

Successful treatment of women with dysuria and frequency is dependent on an accurate diagnosis. Therefore vaginitis and acute bacterial cystitis must first be excluded by the procedures discussed previously before attributing the symptoms to urethral syndrome.

There have been few studies on the treatment of urethral syndrome. In a double-blind, placebo-controlled study, Stamm and colleagues found doxycycline, 100 mg twice a day, to be effective therapy [52]. Clinical cure was noted in 11 of 12 women with low colony count bacteriuria and all 10 women with "sterile" pyuria treated with doxcycline. In the placebo-treated group clinical cure was noted in only 4 of the 10 women with bacteriuria and 3 of 9 with "sterile" pyuria. Of the 19 women with "sterile" pyuria, 11 were infected with *C. trachomatis*. Another significant finding of this study was a clinical cure rate of 70% in women without pyuria, whether treated with antibiotic or placebo, suggesting that antibiotics are not indicated for treatment of urethral syndrome in the absence of pyuria.

Several studies have pointed out the efficacy of treating lower urinary tract infections with a single dose of antimicrobial agent [53-57]. While such studies are not available in women with urethral syndrome, it seems likely that those with low colony count bacteriuria would respond to single-dose antimicrobial therapy. Therefore either a single dose of ampicillin (3.5 g), a single dose of trimethoprim-sulfamethoxazole (four single-strength tablets), or a multiple-dose regimen of tetracycline (500 mg four times a day for 7 days) is appropriate therapy for urethral syndrome due to low colony count bacteriuria [49]. A follow-up urine culture should be obtained 1 week after completion of therapy and, if positive, a 7-day course of an appropriate antimicrobial agent should be given. A single daily dose of trimethoprim-sulfamethoxazole has been shown to be effective prophylaxis for recurrent urinary tract infections [58]. A similar prophylactic regimen should be considered in women with recurrent urethral syndrome due to low colony count bacteriuria.

In women with urethral syndrome and sterile pyuria, the common pathogens are *C. trachomatis* and *N. gonorrhoeae*. In this setting cultures for *N. gon-*

orrhoeae should be obtained prior to therapy. If chlamydia infection is suspected, treatment with tetracycline (500 mg orally four times a day for 7 days) or doxycycline (100 mg orally twice a day for 10 days) is appropriate [52,59]. For those patients who cannot take tetracyclines, erythromycin (250 mg four times a day for 7 days) has been shown to be an effective regimen for chlamydia infections of the female cervix and male urethra [60-62]. These regimens should be effective treatment for urethral syndrome due to chlamydia, but controlled studies are not available.

If *N. gonorrhoeae* is isolated from the cervix, urethra, or rectum, one of the standard treatment regimens recommended by the Centers for Disease Control should be used [63]. Test of cure cultures should be performed on all women treated for gonorrhea 1 week after therapy. This is particularly important because of the increased incidence of penicillinase-producing *N. gonorrhoeae* which may not be eradicated by the standard treatment regimens [64].

Examination and treatment of sexual partners of women with gonococcal or chlamydia infections is important in preventing reinfection. Because of the difficulty in establishing the diagnosis of *C. trachomatis* infection with certainty in the woman with urethral syndrome, it may be necessary to empirically treat the sexual partner, especially in cases of recurrent disease. In women with urethral syndrome due to low colony count bacteriuria, examination and treatment of the sexual partner are unnecessary.

It is possible that some women with urethral syndrome and "sterile" pyuria who do not respond to one of the antimicrobial regimens listed previously may have fastidious organisms such as lactobacilli or anaerobes causing their symptoms [39,40]. Therefore, in those cases not responding to one agent such as tetracycline, it might be appropriate to try another such as ampicillin or erythromycin [65]. Studies to support this practice, however, are not available.

In those women with urethral syndrome without pyuria, antimicrobial therapy is not indicated [52]. They should be treated symptomatically with a urinary analgesic and reevaluated in 24 to 48 hr if symptoms persist [47].

The efficacy of urethral dilatation and urethrotomy in treatment of urethral syndrome has not been established [11,13]. These two procedures are contraindicated in women with acute infection and their role in chronic or recurrent dysuria is unclear.

REFERENCES

1. Waters WE, Elwood PC, Asscher AW, Abernethy M. Clinical significance of dysuria in women. Br Med J 1970; 2:754-7.
2. Tapsall JW, Taylor PC, Bell SM, Smith DD. Relevance of significant bacteriuria to etiology and diagnosis of urinary-tract infection. Lancet 1975; 2: 637-40.
3. Stamm WE, Counts GW, Running KR, Fihn S, Turck M, Holmes KK. Diagnosis of coliform infection in acutely dysuric women. N Engl J Med 1982; 307:463-8.

4. Kass EH. Bacteriuria and the diagnosis of infections of the urinary tract. Arch Intern Med 1957; 100:709-14.
5. Charlton CAC. The urethral syndrome. Practitioner 1979; 223:333-7.
6. Smith P. The urethral syndrome. Clin Obstet Gynecol 1981; 8:161-72.
7. Graham JB. The female urethral syndrome? Urol Clin North Am 1980; 7: 59-62.
8. Smith PJB. The management of the urethral syndrome. Br J Hosp Med 1979; 578-87.
9. Kaplan WE, Firlit CF, Schoenberg HW. The female urethral syndrome: external sphincter spasm as etiology. J Urol 1980; 124:48-9.
10. Schmidt RA, Tanagho EA. Urethral syndrome or urinary tract infection? Urology 1981; 18:424-7.
11. Hendry WF, Stanton SL, Williams DI. Recurrent urinary infections in girls: effects of urethral dilatation. Br J Urol 1973; 45:72-83.
12. McLean P, Emmett JL. Internal urethrotomy in women for recurrent infection and chronic urethritis. J Urol 1970; 101:724-8.
13. Kaplan GW, Sammons TA, King LR. A blind comparison of dilatation, urethrotomy and medication alone in the treatment of urinary tract infection in girls. J Urol 1973; 190:917-9.
14. Rees DLP, Whitfield HN, Islam AKMS, Doyle PT, Mayo ME, Wickham JEA. Urodynamic findings in adult females with frequency and dysuria. Br J Urol 1976; 47:853-60.
15. O'Donnell RP. Acute urethral syndrome in women. N Engl J Med 1980; 303:1531.
16. Jaffe JW, Persky L. Effect of transvaginal trauma on induction of bladder infection. J Urol 1967; 98:353-5.
17. Messing EM, Stamey TA. Interstitial cystitis. Urology 1978; 12:381-92.
18. Carson CC, Osborne D, Segura JW. Psychological characteristics of patients with female urethral syndrome. J Clin Psychol 1979; 35:312-3.
19. Carson CC, Segura JW, Osborne DM. Evaluation and treatment of the female urethral syndrome. J Urol 1980; 124:609-10.
20. Komaroff AL, Pass TM, McCue JD, Cohen AB, Hendricks TM, Friedland G. Management strategies for urinary and vaginal infections. Arch Intern Med 1978; 138:1069-73.
21. Fiumara NJ, Calhoun J. Multiple sexually transmitted diseases. Sex Transm Dis 1982; 9:98-9.
22. Stamm WE, Wagner KF, Amsel R, Alexander ER, Turck M, Counts GW, Holmes KK. Causes of the acute urethral syndrome in women. N Engl J Med 1980; 303:409-15.
23. Gruneberg RN. Relationship of infecting urinary organism to the faecal flora in patients with symptomatic urinary infection. Lancet 1969; 2:766-8.
24. Stamey TA, Sexton CC. The role of vaginal colonization with Enterobacteriaceae in recurrent urinary infections. J Urol 1975; 113:214-7.
25. O'Grady FW, McSherry MA, Richards B, O'Farrell SM, Cattell WR. Introital enterobacteria urinary infection, and the urethral syndrome. Lancet 1970; 2:1208-10.

26. Schachter J. Chlamydial infections. N Engl J Med 1978; 298:428-34.
27. Holmes KK, Stamm WE. Chlamydial genital infections: a growing problem. Hosp Pract 1979; 14:105-17.
28. Schachter J, Grossman M. Chlamydial infections. Annu Rev Med 1981; 32: 45-61.
29. Tait A, Rees E, Jameson RM. Urethral syndrome associated with chlamydial infection of the urethra and cervix. Br J Urol 1978; 50:425.
30. Dunlop EMC, Darougar S, Hare MJ, Treharne JD, Dwyer RSC. Isolation of *Chlamydia* from the urethra of a women. Br Med J 1972; 1:386.
31. Weil A, Gaudenz R, Burgener L, Schultz B. Isolation of *Chlamydia trachomatis* from women with urethral syndrome. Arch Gynecol 1981; 230:329-33.
32. Paavonen J. *Chlamydia trachomatis*-induced urethritis in female partners of men with nongonococcal urethritis. Sex Transm Dis 1979; 6:69-71.
33. Curran JW. Gonorrhea and the urethral syndrome. Sex Transm Dis 1977; 4:119-21.
34. Curran JW, Rendtorff RC, Chandler RW, Wiser WL, Robinson H. Female gonorrhea. Its relation to abnormal uterine bleeding, urinary tract symptoms, and cervicitis. Obstet Gynecol 1975; 45:195-8.
35. Greenberg RN, Rein MF, Saunders CV, Stamm WE. Urethral syndrome in women. JAMA 1981; 245:923.
36. Bowie WR, Wang SP, Alexander ER, Floyd J, Forsythe PS, Pollock HM, Lin JSL, Buchanan TM, Holmes KK. Etiology of nongonococcal urethritis. J Clin Invest 1977; 59:735-42.
37. Stimson JB, Hale J, Bowie WR, Holmes KK. Tetracycline-resistant *Ureaplasma urealyticum*: a cause of persistent nongonococcal urethritis. Ann Intern Med 1981; 94:192-4.
38. McDowall DRM, Buchanan JD, Fairley KF, Gilbert GL. Anaerobic and other fastidious microorganisms in asymptomatic bacteriuria in pregnant women. J Infect Dis 1981; 144:114-22.
39. Maskell R, Pead L, Allen J. The puzzle of "urethral syndrome": a possible answer? Lancet 1979; 1:1058-9.
40. Maskell R, Pead L. Microbiology of the urethral syndrome. Lancet 1982; 1:343.
41. Gragan RA, Brumfitt W, Hamilton-Miller JMT. Do anaerobes cause urinary infection? Lancet 1980; 1:37.
42. Drabu YL, Sanderson PJ. Urine culture in urethral syndrome. Lancet 1980; 1:37-8.
43. Brumfitt W, Ludlam H, Hamilton-Miller JMT, Gooding A. Lactobacilli do not cause frequency and dysuria syndrome. Lancet 1981; 2:393-5.
44. Seal DV, Cuthbert EH. Doubtful significance of fastidious bacteriuria in the urethral syndrome. Lancet 1982; 1:115.
45. Brumfitt W, Hamilton-Miller JMT. Urethral syndrome or dysuria/frequency syndrome: a terminological and microbiological dilemma. Lancet 1982; 1:1066-7.
46. Corey L, Adams HG, Brown ZA, Holmes KK. Genital *Herpes simplex* virus infections: clinical manifestations, course, and complications. Ann Intern Med 1983; 98:958-72.

47. Stamm WE. Management of the acute urethral syndrome. Drug Ther 1982; 12:155-65.
48. Amsel R, Totten PA, Spiegel CA, Chen KSC, Eschenbach D, Holmes KK. Nonspecific vaginitis. Am J Med 1983; 74:14-21.
49. Stamm WE. Etiology and management of the acute urethral syndrome. Sex Transm Dis 1981; 8:235-8.
50. Mardh P, Westrom L, Colleen S, Wolner-Hanssen W. Sampling, specimen handling, and isolation techniques in the diagnosis of chlamydial and other genital infections. Sex Transm Dis 1981; 8:280-5.
51. Asscher AW. Use of antibiotics. Management of frequency and dysuria. Br Med J 1978; 1:1531-3.
52. Stamm WE, Running K, McKevitt M, Counts GW, Turck M, Holmes KK. Treatment of the acute urethral syndrome. N Engl J Med 1981; 304:956-8.
53. Fang LS, Tolkoff-Rubin NE, Rubin RH. Efficacy of single-dose and conventional amoxicillin therapy in urinary tract infection localized by the antibody-coated bacteria technic. N Engl J Med 1978; 298:413-6.
54. Bailey RR, Abbott GD. Treatment of urinary tract infection with single dose of trimethoprim-sulfamethoxazole. Can Med Assoc J 1978; 118:551-2.
55. Greenberg RN, Sanders CV, Lewis AC, Marier RL. Single-dose cefaclor therapy of urinary tract infection. Am J Med 1981; 71:841-5.
56. Savard-Fenton M, Fenton BW, Reller LB, Lauer BA, Byyny RL. Single-dose amoxicillin therapy with follow-up urine culture. Am J Med 1982;73:808-13.
57. Stamm WE. Single-dose treatment of cystitis. JAMA 1980; 244:591-2.
58. Stamm WE, Counts GW, Wagner KF, Martin D, Gregory D, McKevitt M, Turck M, Holmes KK. Antimicrobial prophylaxis or recurrent urinary tract infections. Ann Intern Med 1980; 92:770-5.
59. Brunham RC, Kuo CC, Stevens CE, Holmes KK. Therapy of cervical chlamydial infection. Ann Intern Med 1982; 97:216-9.
60. Scheibel JH, Kristensen JK, Hentzer B, Secher L, Ullman S, Verdich J, Weismann K. Treatment of chlamydial urethritis in men and *Chlamydia trachomatis*-positive female partners: comparison of erythromycin and tetracycline in treatment courses of one week. Sex Transm Dis 1982; 9:128-31.
61. Bowie WE, Manzon LM, Borrie-Hume CJ, Fawcett A, Jones HD. Efficacy of treatment regimens for lower urogenital *Chlamydia trachomatis* infection in women. Am J Obstet Gynecol 1982; 142:125-9.
62. Johannisson G, Lowhagen GB, Lycke E. Genital *Chlamydia trachomatis* infection in women. Obstet Gynecol 1980; 56:671-5.
63. U.S. Department of Health, Education, and Welfare, Public Health Service, Centers for Disease Control. Sexually transmitted diseases treatment guidelines 1982. Morbid Mortal Week Rep 1982; 31:37S-42S.
64. McCormack WM. Penicillinase-producing *Neisseria gonorrhoeae*—a retrospective. N Engl J Med 1982; 307:438-9.
65. Maskell R. Should fastidious organisms alter our approach to the treatment of urinary symptoms? J Antimicrob Chemother 1981; 7:315-7.

TEN

The "Gay Bowel" Syndrome

James H. Caldwell
The Ohio State University
College of Medicine
Columbus, Ohio

INTRODUCTION

The term "gay bowel syndrome" was coined less than 10 years ago in a paper describing the variety of anal, rectal, and colon diseases found in homosexual males [1]. In this report only 15.7% of the cases had proven infectious etiologies, and many nonvenereal lesions were included, for example, polyps, hemorrhoids, fissures, and fistulas. The case chosen as an example, however, was a man in whom syphilis, amebiasis, and hepatitis coexisted. This emphasis on multiple concurrent, recurrent, or sequential enteric infections has become what is generally meant by "gay bowel syndrome" [2]. The purpose of this chapter is to review the typical clinical syndromes, pathogens incriminated, and the differential diagnostic approach to the patient.

Transmission of enteric infection may occur through anal intercourse, analingus, or fellatio following anal intercourse. Different pathogens are transmitted and different clinical syndromes are produced by different sexual practices. Both case-finding studies and evaluation of individual patients depend on interview techniques that include inquiry about specific sexual practices. It is apparent that homosexuals are not uniquely at risk for venereal transmission of enteric organisms. Heterosexual anal intercourse or analingus may transmit infection if one of the partners harbors a pathogen. On the other hand, lesbians have no higher rate of enteric infection than the heterosexual population [3]. The emphasis on gay men as carriers and patients at risk of gay bowel syndrome is largely due to sexual practices involving the digestive tract among multiple, anonymous sexual partners, a characteristic of some gay males.

CLINICAL SYNDROMES

Enteric infections can be broadly grouped into two categories: proctitis and enteritis. With some overlap, the syndromes are historically distinguishable and tend to be caused by separate groups of pathogens [4].

Proctitis

Symptoms of proctitis include rectal discharge, rectal bleeding, rectal aching or discomfort, painful or ineffective straining at stool (tenesmus), urgent defecation, and changes in stool consistency and frequency. Constipation is characteristic with some infections (e.g., herpes), while increased frequency of passage of small stools is more typical of other infections. Large-volume diarrhea is not characteristic of purely rectal inflammation. Symptoms of proctitis, with the exception of urgency and increased frequency, may be caused by purely anal infections or by noninfectious anal conditions such as fissures. When proctitis is not accompanied by more proximal bowel involvement, it is usually caused by anal intercourse, and the infections found are those transmitted by penile or urethral infection, that is, gonorrhea, syphilis, herpes, and chlamydia. Anoscopy and sigmoidoscopy are often abnormal in symptomatic anorectal infections. Specific findings, when described, are included below in the discussion of individual infections.

Enteritis

Abdominal pain, bloating, nausea, cramping, and diarrhea, occasionally bloody, are seen with infections of the small intestine or colon. These occur as a result of infection with pathogens that are usually transmitted by the fecal-oral route, and are the consequence of analingus or of fellatio following anal intercourse with an infected partner. Most of the major enteric bacterial pathogens (*Shigella* sp., *Campylobacter* sp.) and protozoa (amebae, *Giardia lamblia*) have been found in this form of gay bowel syndrome. Some of these infections also involve the rectum, so that patients may have symptoms of proctitis as well as enteritis. Patients with either syndrome may have fever or other constitutional symptoms of less discriminating value. Specific features that are hallmarks of particular pathogens are described below.

CAUSES OF PROCTITIS

Herpes Simplex Virus

Proctitis caused by herpes simplex virus (HSV) is the most common nongonococcal anorectal infection in gay men [5]. Jacobs observed as recently as 1976 that anal HSV was described 240 years ago but ignored in standard proctological texts [6]. His clinical observations of 16 cases, 14 of them homosexual males who practiced anal intercourse, led him to predict that screening large numbers of homosexuals would yield a significant incidence of HSV infection. Nearly all symptomatic patients have anal pain, sometimes severe, and half have pruritus. Serous, purulent, or bloody rectal discharge is common, and most patients are also constipated. Other clinical features significantly more common in HSV proctitis than in that due to other organisms are fever, tenesmus, and inguinal lymphadenopathy [7].

On physical examination, 30 to 70% will have perianal or anal vesicular or ulcerative lesions [6,7]. Small vesicles with perivesicular erythema occur first and within a few days become ulcerated following rupture of the vesicle roof. Confluent ulceration in the anal canal produces an ulcerative cryptitis with an erythematous, edematous border and a foul-smelling discharge [6]. Nearly all patients have abnormal rectal mucosa by sigmoidoscopy, with diffuse or focal friability and ulceration in the distal 10 cm. Rectal biopsies show nonspecific acute colitis in most cases, but about 40% have findings suggestive of HSV infection, including perivascular cuffing with lymphocytes, multinucleated cells, and intranuclear inclusions [7]. A syndrome apparently unique to herpes infection is sacral root paresthesias and dysfunction [8]. Urinary retention, posterior thigh pain, and paresthesias in the buttock and perineum were found in half of the Seattle patients with HSV proctitis, while none with proctitis of other etiology had the full constellation of symptoms. The clinical diagnosis of HSV proctitis is likely when severe pain, diffuse distal rectal ulceration, urinary retention, and paresthesias are present. Confirmation can be achieved by viral culture and by seroconversion or fourfold rise in titer of HSV-2 neutralizing antibody [7]. A more severe, chronic form of perianal HSV infection complicates AIDS [9].

Chlamydia Proctitis and Lymphogranuloma Venereum

In the landmark paper cited earlier in this chapter, lymphogranuloma venereum was found in only 3 of 260 cases of "gay bowel" [1]. One case had a long-standing rectal stricture, two had rectal masses, and Frei tests were positive in all three.

With the isolation of *Chlamydia trachomatis* in many cases of nongonococcal urethritis, it was expected that this agent might be found in the rectum of men who experienced anal intercourse, as was reported in two cases without symptoms in 1977 [10]. Three symptomatic cases were reported subsequently, all homosexual men with bloody mucoid rectal discharge and painful defecation, who had other diagnoses made on first examination because of the discovery of giardiasis in one and gonorrhea in the other two patients. Following appropriate initial therapy, symptoms persisted and sigmoidoscopy revealed edematous, friable mucosa with multiple large ulcers and dense infiltration of biopsies with acute and chronic inflammatory cells. Seropositivity by complement fixation tests for chlamydia group infection led to different antimicrobial therapy and cure [11].

The prospective and comprehensive studies of the etiology of proctitis in gay men from Seattle have further characterized both lymphogranuloma venereum (LGV) and non-LGV chlamydial proctitis in this population [12]. Symptomatic men and asymptomatic controls were evaluated with rectal smears, rectal swab, and stool specimens for all possible pathogens and serological study. Proctitis patients had sigmoidoscopy and biopsy. Serum specimens and rectal isolates from *C. trachomatis*-positive patients were immunotyped for LGV and non-LGV strains. A total of 11 patients (8 of 96 symptomatic and 3 of 75 control) had non-LGV stains cultured from rectal material. These were associated with fecal leukocytes on smear and mild mucosal abnormalities on inspection and biopsy of the mucosa. Symptoms were comparatively mild or absent. Acute phase antibody was present in four of eight, and seroconversion or a fourfold rise in titer in six of eight. In contrast, three patients with LGV strains of *C. trachomatis* had more severe symptoms, including abdominal pain, fever, and diarrhea, and ulcerations were found on sigmoidoscopy. Two of these had crypt abscesses and granulomata on biopsy mimicking Crohn's disease. Only these patients had antibody titers of 1:512 or greater. All patients had symptomatic and histological cure after 2 to 3 weeks of tetracycline. A later report of three additional cases of LGV-positive proctitis confirmed that a severe acute ulcerative proctitis results from infection with LGV strains of chlamydia and that microimmunofluorescence antibody titers are more sensitive serological tests than complement fixation [13]. In these acute cases of LGV, anal strictures, suppurative inguinal adenopathy, and other complications of the disease described in older literature [14] do not occur. The Frei test is insensitive, and growth of the organism is the best way to confirm the diagnosis pending the wide availability of new serological tests [15]. It is likely that many cases of "nonspecific proctitis," negative for traditional pathogens and relatively mild, are due to infection with strains of *C. trachomatis* more commonly associated with ocular or genital infection.

Anorectal Syphilis

Syphilis is a common venereal disease among homosexual men, but until recently primary syphilis of the rectum without extragenital anal chancres was considered rare [15]. Several reports of cases in homosexual males appeared in the 1970s [16-18] and 12% of a group of gay men with anorectal symptoms had positive serological tests for syphilis [19]. Interpretation of findings is difficult in this group, since only two of six had positive dark-field examination and four of six had coexisting rectal herpes or gonorrhea.

Most patients have been symptomatic, with anorectal pain, altered bowel habit, rectal discharge, bleeding, and tenesmus [15]. Physical findings include inguinal adenopathy, tender anterior rectal indurated lesions which may be hyperplastic or ulcerated, and a variety of anoscopic and sigmoidoscopic appearances mimicking polyps, carcinoma, fissures, Crohn's disease, cryptitis, and idiopathic proctitis. Condyloma latum and the skin rash of secondary syphilis may be present. Solitary or multiple circular masses, indurated or ulcerated and 2 cm or more in diameter and extending several centimeters above the anal verge, may be the most specific sigmoidoscopic findings but are by no means invariable [20]. All patients who may harbor rectal syphilis should have serological tests for syphilis, and asymptomatic patients with positive serologies should have proctoscopy. Any visible lesions should be examined by dark field, and by biopsy as well if they are not typical chancres. Histology, silver staining, and immunofluorescence studies of biopsy material may be of additional diagnostic aid [20]. Other criteria supportive of the diagnosis include a Jarisch-Herxheimer reaction to therapy and resolution of the proctoscopic abnormalities with appropriate therapy.

The likely coexistence of other infections and the absence of methods for diagnosis of HSV, chlamydial, and *Campylobacter* infections in older reports makes assessment of the clinical picture of isolated primary rectal syphilis difficult at this time. It is more important to recognize the great variability of clinical presentations and the possibility of both genital and extragenital syphilis in every homosexual male being examined for any sexually related illness.

Rectal Gonorrhea

Extragenital gonococcal infections are considered in detail in Chapter 8. Anorectal infection with *Neisseria gonorrhoeae* in homosexual men is briefly mentioned here for completeness. It is established that gay men have a greater risk of classic venereal disease than heterosexuals [21,22]. Much of the older literature on rectal gonorrhea in men does not include systematic searches for other pathogens, so attribution of any specific signs or symptoms to gonorrhea in the rectum may be invalid, since multiple pathogen infection is so common in gay bowel. Recovery of gonococci from the rectum is the most common microbiological finding in both symptomatic and asymptomatic homosexual men [5]. Most rectal infections with *N. gonorrhoeae* are asymptomatic or associated only with complaints of mucus in the stool and perianal itching or irritation [23].

In studies of patients that concentrate on symptoms or interpret minimal complaints as positive for symptoms, mucosal hyperemia and exudate are frequently seen at anoscopy [24]. The squamous mucosa of the anal canal is spared, in contrast with HSV proctitis [25]. Where studies include all patients with rectal culture positive for *N. gonorrhoeae*, only 2 to 5% of newly infected cases will have symptoms of proctitis [25] and less than 1% will have bloody discharge in the stool [26]. The treatment of rectal gonorrhea in gay men has been the subject of several recent studies [24,26-29]. Standard therapy of aqueous procaine penicillin G, 4.8 million units intramuscularly, plus 1 g of probenecid orally cures 96 to 97% of cases [24,29]. Spectinomycin, 2 to 4 g intramuscularly, may have a higher cure rate [22,29] but is not the treatment of choice, except for penicillin-allergic patients, since it is not effective against incubating syphilis [15]. Treatment failure may be related to interactions between gonococci and other organisms in the bowel [26] or to differences in antibiotic susceptibility of isolates of gonococci found in homosexuals [30].

Because of the frequent coexistence of other pathogens and the risk of sequential infections with new pathogens, treatment failure of rectal gonorrhea should be culture proven rather than assumed in cases where symptoms persist after specific therapy for gonorrhea. If circumstances do not allow for comprehensive microbiological study of rectal material in all gay patients found to have rectal gonorrhea, a thorough evaluation is recommended for those who return unimproved after therapy, since they are more likely to harbor additional nongonococcal pathogens than to merely represent treatment failures.

CAUSES OF ENTERITIS

Campylobacter

Campylobacter sp. were once considered strictly veterinary pathogens, rarely causing human infection, and then only in immunocompromised hosts. Improved culture methods established their existence in fecal isolates from cases of diarrhea in 1969. Since the early 1970s *Campylobacter jejuni* has been found more often than salmonella or shigella as a cause of bacterial diarrhea [31]. The typical features of food- or water-borne *Campylobacter* enteritis in the general population are the sudden onset of abdominal pain and fever after a 1- to 7-day incubation period, followed within 24 hr by diarrhea. Although the illness may be as mild as viral gastroenteritis, two-thirds have more than eight loose stools daily at the peak of the illness, and 50 to 60% have bloody stools. Many patients have malaise, anorexia, and other constitutional symptoms such as headache, arthralgias, and myalgias. The majority of cases last 1 week or less without treatment, but 20 to 25% of untreated cases relapse [32]. The jejunum, ileum, and colon are equally involved with an exudative enteritis, and the histopathology resembles acute idiopathic ulcerative colitis or infectious colitis due to shigella or salmonella [31].

Early studies for *Campylobacter* sp. in homosexual men were negative [33] and the first case report in 1979 described only pus in the stools with no other features of enteritis or proctitis [34]. In 1980 the first complete description of a well-documented case in which other etiologies of enteric infection were excluded was published [35]. Since this report, prospective studies in Seattle have established the importance and frequency of *Campylobacter* infections in homosexual men. *Campylobacter jejuni* was found in 6% of those with proctitis or colitis and in 3% of asymptomatic gay control subjects [5]. Thus in gay men *Campylobacter* sp. is a common bacterial cause of nongonococcal proctitis and may exist in an asymptomatic carrier state. Although *C. jejuni* infection is usually self-limited, the frequency of multiple pathogens in enteric infections of gay men, the potential for infecting others, and the high relapse rate in untreated cases all argue for treatment of identified symptomatic cases and asymptomatic homosexual carriers. The treatment of choice is erythromycin 500 mg four times a day for 7 days [32].

Shigella

Surveillance by the San Francisco Department of Public Health identified an outbreak of shigellosis in the city in early 1974, predominantly in young gay men [36]. By 1976, 70% of 545 cases in that city occurred in men aged 20 to 39 years, a 10-fold increase in the attack rate for that group [37]. Shigellosis was reported about five times more frequently than amebiasis during this period in San Francisco, and attack rates per 100,000 population for shigellosis approached those for amebiasis in New York City during this period. Homosexual men were also found disproportionately often among shigellosis cases in other cities [38]. According to Dritz and Back [36], this epidemic was associated with a two- to threefold expansion of the homosexual population of San Francisco, beginning in 1974, to a 1979 estimate of about 100,000. Shigellosis incidence began to fall in 1977, at least partly owing to publicity among the gay community and heightened physician awareness [23]. In the most recent studies shigellosis was found in 3% of symptomatic patients [5].

Shigellosis may be mild and self-limited or a systemic life-threatening illness. After a 24- to 48-hr incubation period, it begins insidiously or acutely with fever, abdominal distress, and nonspecific diarrhea, and may resolve completely or progress to dysentery with severe cramps, tenesmus, urgency, and bloody mucoid rectal discharges. This biphasic behavior may reflect two properties of *Shigella*: the production of an enterotoxin and mucosal invasion. When proctocolitis is established, the sigmoidoscopic appearance resembles that of acute idiopathic ulcerative colitis. Systemic complications are uncommon in adults, but may occur in severe infections. Treatment for mild illness is correction of fluid and electrolyte losses and avoidance of opiate or anticholinergic antidiarrheals, which may prolong symptoms and delay clearance of the organism. Antibiotic therapy should be individualized, weighing risk of evolving antibiotic resistance against benefit from shortening the symptomatic period and duration of carriage of organisms. In homosexual cases, because of the high infectivity of *Shigella* sp. and the likelihood of spread in the community, specific therapy is probably advisable for all such cases. Ampicillin was the former drug of choice, but in sexually transmitted shigellosis, the Centers for Disease Control (CDC) recommend trimethoprim-sulfamethoxazole at this time [4]. The effectiveness of single-dose tetracycline therapy has been reported and might have specific application in venereal disease clinic situations, but experience with such therapy in the gay population has not been reported [39].

Entamoeba histolytica

In the 1967 Presidential Address to The American Society of Tropical Medicine and Hygiene, Most alluded to a quartet of homosexuals who shared infection with amebae and other intestinal parasites, and suggested they had infected one another and others via their sexual practices [40]. Although this phenomenon was already familiar to public health workers [41], it was another decade before substantial literature on the subject developed as case reports [1,2,42,43] and epidemiological studies [37,38,44]. A 5-year review of experience at New York Hospital revealed that 40% of the cases of amebiasis occurred in gay men who had not traveled outside of the New York area [44]. A history of previous venereal enteric infection was reported by 45% of these men. This concentration of amebic infection in gay men was confirmed as a recent phenomenon by studies in San Francisco showing a sharp increase in annual incidence beginning in 1975. Unlike shigellosis, cases of amebiasis have continued to increase annually to more than 700 per year since 1980 [45].

Analysis of a 20-year experience from the New York City Department of Health illuminated the magnitude of the problem [46]. Before 1965 there were about 1000 cases of amebiasis annually in New York, about half of these in Manhattan. In 1978 there were 1875 cases in the city, with virtually the entire increase occuring in Manhattan. The cases in New York City represented more than 40% of the cases reported for the entire United States [38]. Before 1965 the male/female attack ratio was about 1:1 and in 1978 was 2.1:1 for the entire city. In certain areas of Manhattan's Lower West Side health district, the attack rate among men is more than 25 times that of the overall city rate [46], suggesting that amebiasis is "hyperendemic" in this population [47]. These retrospective reports have prompted prospective studies designed to characterize and quantitate the frequency of amebic infection in the homosexual populations. Studies of gay volunteers in Toronto [48] and of consecutive patients attending a clinic for sexually transmitted diseases in Manhattan [47] documented carriage rates of 27 and 19.6%, respectively, for *Entamoeba histolytica*. In both studies symptoms were correlated with homosexuality and with analingus, but not with *E. histolytica* isolation. It has been suggested that many of the identified infections are with nonpathogenic amebae, since isoenzyme electrophoresis is required to separate pathogenic *E. histolytica* from morphologically similar commensal organisms [49].

The frequency of symptoms with venereal amebiasis is unclear. The cited prospective studies of carriage did not evaluate infection with other potential pathogens or address the issue of treatment response, nor did they distinguish between cyst passers (who are asymptomatic but infectious for others) and those whose stool specimens contained trophozoites [47,48]. Since a substantial minority of symptomatic infections are due to multiple pathogens [4], ascribing symptoms to a single agent is difficult if there is no well-defined clinical syndrome or treatment response to a single agent. In the clinical cases reported from Seattle, *E. histolytica* was identified in 29% of the symptomatic group and 25% of the asymptomatic control homosexual men [5]; 60% of the symptomatic cases had one or more additional pathogens isolated.

Infections with *E. histolytica* are often asymptomatic. Cysts excreted in the stool of asymptomatic carriers are resistant to gastric acid and are infectious when swallowed. Symptomatic amebiasis ranges from mild diarrhea to severe dysentery with prostration and bloody mucoid diarrhea. Ischemic or idiopathic inflammatory bowel disease may be mimicked by the x-ray findings of pseudopolyps, thumbprinting, or toxic megacolon. Extraintestinal infection may occur, most commonly as liver abscess, which may spread to involve the lungs, pleura, or pericardium. Diagnosis depends on demonstration of *E. histolytica* in stool exudate or rectal biopsy by an experienced observer. Serological tests are most useful in patients with active intestinal and extraintestinal infection, and not helpful in the asymptomatic cyst passer. The treatment of amebiasis is complex and depends on the nature of the infection and the potential toxicity of some of the available drugs. Cyst passers may be treated with diiodohydroxyquin or diloxanide furoate. High-dose metronidazole (750 mg three times a day for 5 to 10 days) has been used successfully for symptomatic intestinal infection and for extraintestinal infection. A number of other regimens have also been advocated [50].

Giardia lamblia

The history of *G. lamblia* infection in the gay bowel syndrome parallels that of amebiasis. Simultaneous or sequential detection of both parasites is common in symptomatic infection [42]. This was often attributed to resistance to treatment until the role of analingus in transmitting infection was appreciated [43]. Evidence for sexual transmission was further strengthened by the observation of six cases over a 2-month period in Seattle attributable to sexual contact with an index case [51]. A 5-year retrospective review of 146 cases from New York Hospital revealed three patient groups: those who had traveled to endemic areas, those with immunodeficiency, and homosexual males. Homosexuals with a past history of sexually transmitted disease constituted 22% of men with giardiasis [52]. Prospective studies of prevalence disclosed giardiasis in 3.9 and 13% of gay volunteers in Manhattan [47] and Toronto [48], respectively. There was no correlation between symptoms and infection in these groups. By contrast, the study of infectious etiologies of symptomatic homosexual men found *G. lamblia* in 14% of those with enteritis and in 4% of the asymptomatic controls [5]. Although coinfection was found in 50% of those with giardiasis, infection with *G. lamblia* was significantly associated with the enteritis syndrome.

Because the proximal small intestine is the principal site of infection, proctitis is absent and stools are negative for blood and leukocytes. For the same reason, upper gastrointestinal symptoms, including epigastric pain, vomiting, foul sulfuric eructation and nausea, may be prominent. These symptoms in a patient with diarrhea should immediately suggest giardiasis. The natural history of giardiasis is the abrupt onset of explosive diarrhea, distention, and flatulence, and in a few days the acute untreated illness may settle into a more subacute or chronic illness. Patients with giardiasis may then have low-grade symptoms for months, with malabsorption and weight loss [53]. Reports of prevalence [5, 47,48] based on fecal recovery of the organism may underestimate the actual rate of infection with *G. lamblia*. Although Wolfe claims that the diagnosis can be made by stool examination in the great majority of cases [53], others claim that up to 50% of proven cases have persistently negative examinations of stool for cysts or trophozoites [54]. Jejunal biopsy and aspiration for histological examination and microscopy of mucus are necessary in these cases [55]. Many authorities agree that a therapeutic trial is justified in clinically suspect cases in which diagnosis cannot be established by available methods [53]. The standard therapy is quinacrine hydrochloride 100 mg three times a day for 7 days. A frequently used alternative (not approved for giardiasis in the United States) is metronidazole 250 mg three times a day for 7 days [4].

OTHER PROBLEMS

Less Important Infections

Salmonella

Unlike shigellosis, salmonella infection has been documented infrequently as a result of venereal transmission. Two cases of typhoid fever in gay men whose sexual partners were carriers of the same strain have been reported [56]. Both cases were food handlers, suggesting a public health component of venereal enteric infection rarely considered in the literature. The lack of an outbreak of salmonellosis in the gay community may be related to the large inoculum required to produce clinical illness compared to that required with shigellosis [23].

Neisseria meningitidis

Meningococcal infections of the anorectum or genitourinary tract are thought to be rare. A Denver study speciated all anogenital isolates of *Neisseria* sp. from

731 consecutive homosexual men attending a venereal disease clinic, regardless of the presenting complaint [57]. Of 100 neisserial isolates, 15 were *Neisseria meningitidis*, demonstrating a statistically higher prevalence of *N. meningitidis* among gays compared to heterosexuals. Of the 15 gay men, 3 had anal symptoms of mild pain and burning. Treatment with recommended antigonococcal regimens resulted in symptom resolution in these three cases and negative post-treatment cultures in all patients. It is currently unresolved whether differentiating meningococcal from gonococcal infections of the rectum is necessary or if other meningococcal infections are common in the gay community [15].

Helminths and Nonpathogenic Protozoa

Enterobiasis has been found frequently in limited studies of homosexual men [58,59], although there is some question whether it is transmitted by sexual contact [58]. *Strongyloides* and *Trichuris*, although infrequent, were significantly correlated with analingus in a recent study [47]. Several nonpathogenic protozoa, including *Endolimax nana, Entamoeba hartmanni* and *Entamoeba coli, Iodamoeba buetschlii,* and *Dientamoeba fragilis*, have been reported frequently in studies of gay men [47,48]. The simultaneous finding of multiple pathogenic and nonpathogenic protozoa in stools of gay men was previously reported [40], and it was proposed that transmission was via fecal-oral spread rather than environmental or food contamination [41]. The finding of nonpathogenic protozoa in single specimens should prompt examination of additional stools, since *E. histolytica* may be discovered by more vigorous search in these circumstances [15,47].

Intestinal Spirochetosis

This phenomenon was described in 36% of a group of 100 consecutive homosexual male patients in whom the histopathology and microbiology of the rectum were well characterized [60]. It was seen as often in those with no diagnosable lesion as in those with syphilis or gonorrhea, and was not clearly responsible for symptoms or inflammatory changes in tissue. Although matched control groups were not investigated, it was claimed that homosexuals exhibit intestinal spirochetosis significantly more often than other populations. Nielsen et al. found histological evidence of spirochetosis in only 5% of 300 rectal biopsies done for a variety of reasons. Neomycin and bacitracin therapy eliminated the spirochetes without an effect on symptoms [61]. The clinical significance of intestinal spirochetosis as a prevalent condition in homosexuals is unknown.

Anorectal Carcinoma

Sohn and Robilotti mentioned two anorectal cancers in their group of 260 homosexual men, but thought the association might be fortuitous [1]. Eight additional cases of transitional (cloacogenic) or squamous carcinoma have been reported in male homosexuals, with a mean age of onset of 39 years [62-64]. This epithelium is similiar in embryological origin to that of the cervix, in which carcinogenesis is related to multiple sexual partners [62]. An epidemiological study of anal cancer showed that a history of syphilis and single marital status is found more often among men with anal cancer than expected, suggesting anal intercourse as a risk factor [65]. It may be that anal cancer, like Kaposi's sarcoma, is a neoplasm to which homosexuality is a major contributing cause.

Anorectal Trauma

Not all anorectal complaints in gay men result from infections. Proctological conditions such as hemorrhoids and fissures are said to be common [1]. Traumatic rectal and genital erosion may result from anal intercourse, and secondary infection may result in impetiginous lesions [4]. Noninfectious proctitis may result from contact or allergic reactions to the ingredients in perfumes, soaps, and other agents used as lubricants [23]. Foreign objects such as bottles, billiard balls, and beverage glasses may be inserted for a variety of reasons and may cause rectal laceration or become impacted, requiring ingenious methods for removal [23]. Peritonitis resulting from colon perforation following insertion of the fist, occasionally to the forearm, has been reported [66]. The management of foreign bodies, lacerations of the mucosa, anal sphincter disruption, and rectosigmoid perforations has been discussed in a recent review [67]. Willcox has provided a graphic glimpse at the variety of penile adornments and prostheses available and apparently used for additional sexual stimulation by some homosexual men [68]. The traumatic potential of these rings, balls, rods, studded leather penile collars, and so on, has not been described in detail but seems considerable.

The Intestine in Acquired Immune Deficiency Syndrome

The present outbreak of acquired immune deficiency syndrome (AIDS) among male homosexuals and others has focused awareness on Kaposi's sarcoma and opportunistic infection, usually of the lung, esophagus, or central nervous system, as part of the illness. Although gay bowel per se does not enter into the differential diagnosis of this condition, a few observations seem relevant to this chapter. Men with histories of enteric pathogen infection are at increased risk for AIDS [45]. A few cases of severe chronic diarrhea with malabsorption due to cryptosporidiosis have been reported in immunosuppressed humans, including some with AIDS [69]. This disease is difficult to diagnose, usually requiring examination of jejunal biopsies by experienced pathologists. The recent report of a successful method for detection of cryptosporidiosis in stools suggests that it is more sensitive than biopsy for detection of this infection [70]. The duration of the illness and its systemic features should prevent confusion with the usually brief illnesses that are common in sexually transmitted enteric infection.

Kaposi's sarcoma in AIDS, unlike the originally described classic dermatological form of the disease, often involves the digestive tract and may do so in the absence of characteristic skin lesions. The radiographic findings in this disease include a variety of abnormalities in the distal rectum, ranging from subtle nodularity to diffuse narrowing and irregular rigidity [71]. The possibility of confusing this appearance with some of the findings described in infectious proctitis exists, especially with LGV proctitis [72]. Appropriate microbiological and histological studies are necessary to resolve these potential diagnostic conflicts.

A recent report of ulcerative pancolitis with electron-microscopic evidence of HSV infection suggests that viral colitis may cause diarrhea in immunosuppressed patients [73]. One of two similar cases in homosexual men with evidence of HSV and/or cytomegalovirus infection died with evidence of immune deficiency and other opportunistic infections [74].

Antibiotic-Associated Diarrhea

With growing awareness and concern about infections among the gay community, it is likely that some individuals will attempt self-treatment with antibiotics. Others may experience gastrointestinal reactions to antibiotics prescribed for venereal infection. It is necessary to include a history of recent antibiotic use in the evaluation of all patients with diarrhea, including homosexuals. Pseudomembranous colitis, due to the overgrowth of toxin-producing *Clostridium difficile* in the bowel, accounts for a significant number of cases of antibiotic-associated diarrhea [75]. Since anoscopy and sigmoidoscopy may not reveal pseudomembranes in all such patients [76], stool culture and assay for *C. difficile* toxin are the most sensitive diagnostic tools. Although some cases resolve with cessation of antimicrobials, this potentially serious disease should be treated specifically when the diagnosis is established. The most common advocated therapy is oral vancomycin [75].

APPROACH TO THE PATIENT

Physicians and other medical personnel experienced in dealing with venereal disease and those who work in clinics established for the gay community will not have difficulty in asking about sexual practices and in accepting their gay patients. Individuals working in emergency rooms, offices, and hospitals in those communities where gay health concerns are inapparent may find themselves uncomfortable with the issue of homosexuality in patient care. Similarly, gay patients may be more or less open about their sexual preference, depending on the community and the attitudes of its health professionals. Some physicians will choose to avoid or ignore the issue, assuming all patients are heterosexual unless the patients volunteer otherwise. Before the detailed history, physical examination, and laboratory indices of venereal enteric infection can be applied appropriately, it is necessary to find out if the patient is, in fact, at risk of infection transmitted via homosexual practices. Such patients are more comfortable when asked about being "gay" rather than homosexual, and the use of the term connotes a degree of familiarity on the examiner's part. Those who are concerned about offending heterosexuals by direct questions or who prefer to explore the patient's self-awareness of the situation are advised to ask, "Is there anything about your life-style, such as recent travel, sexual practices, or use of drugs that might help me to diagnose your medical problem?" [77] This nonaccusatory, completely open-ended question allows the patient several options and, in my experience, is not offensive to heterosexual patients.

Further examination of the gay male patient depends on the symptoms, circumstances (e.g., a request for examination because of illness in a sexual contact), and resources available. Suggested evaluation schemes appropriate for the office [4], emergency department [78], and referral hospitals [5,15] have been described. As gay patients become more health conscious and are provided informed and sympathetic medical care [79], the demand for more sophisticated diagnostic testing will increase. This concluding section is an attempt to summarize options concerning evaluation at different levels of care. Asymptomatic patients requesting evaluation for infection should be questioned about travel, drug use, and sexual practices, including possible exposure to an infected partner, as well as past history of sexually transmitted disease. Physical examination should include inspection of the mouth and throat, genitalia and perianal skin, and palpation of inguinal and femoral nodes. Laboratory screening should include serological tests for syphilis and hepatitis B and gonorrheal cultures of anus, urethra, and pharynx [4, 15]. When feasible, stool cultures and stool examination for ova and parasites are recommended for the asymptomatic patient [15].

The evaluation of the symptomatic patient is based on the principles outlined in the section on causes of proctitis and enteritis. Since all identifiable infections have specific therapeutic approaches and pose risks for sexual contacts, a specific microbiological diagnosis should be attempted. Detailed history may provide clues to the likely route of infection and may direct attention to careful inspection of the rectum in cases of proctitis. Complete physical examination, including a search for metastatic infection and cutaneous evidence of primary and secondary syphilis, is indicated. Because of the frequency of mixed infections and symptomatic overlap between proctitis and enteritis, all symptomatic patients should be evaluated for the pathogens capable of causing either syndrome, and all should have sigmoidoscopy or anoscopy [19]. The examination of a Gram-stained smear of rectal exudate will allow the immediate diagnosis of gonorrhea [26] and *Campylobacter* infection [80] in about 50% of cases, and may suggest giardiasis if leukocytes are absent. Leukocytes will also be absent in diarrhea due to simple viral gastroenteritis, irritable bowel, laxative drugs, infections causing intestinal secretion without mucosal invasion, and so on. If fecal leukocytes are present, any of the other enteric infections described, including pseudomembranous colitis, are likely [4,5].

In the past, the isolation of *N. gonorrhoeae* was considered sufficient evidence to explain rectal complaints, and further studies were deferred pending the response to antigonococcal therapy. Since asymptomatic rectal carriage of gonorrhea is so common, a case can be made for suspecting at least one other organism in every symptomatic patient [4]. Therefore, when the appropriate facilities are available, multiple stool examinations for ova and parasites; stool cultures for *Shigella* sp., *C. jejuni*, and other enteric pathogens; dark-field examination of visible anal or distal rectal lesions; and culture of mucosal exudate and rectal biopsy for HSV and chlamydia are all recommended. In cases of proctitis, histological findings in the rectal biopsy may support the diagnosis of syphilis [16], HSV [7], chlamydial infection [12], or amebiasis [50]. Anoscopy or sigmoidoscopy should be done without preparation, since enemas may obscure the subsequent identification of parasites. Other substances that may interfere with microscopy of stool include antibiotics, laxatives, nonspecific antidiarrheal medications, and barium sulfate [50]. The future availability of an enzyme-linked immunosorbent assay for *E. histolytica* antigen in stool may simplify the diagnosis of amebiasis [77].

There are two circumstances in which limited diagnostic resources may justify empirical therapy. A trial of metronidazole has been advocated for suspected giardiasis where stools are negative and jejunal biopsy and aspiration are not possible. The other situation is the "nongonococcal proctitis syndrome," where there are no features of HSV infection or syphilis, studies for enteric pathogens and parasites are negative, and chlamydial testing is not available or substantially delayed. An empirical trial of tetracycline, as prescribed for "nonspecific urethritis," seems reasonable in this situation.

Post-treatment follow-up of all infections should include assessment of symptomatic response, documentation of cure for infections where asymptomatic carriage or treatment resistance is common, and education of the patient as to the mode of transmission of infection. The latter affords an opportunity for case-finding those sexual contacts who have not been examined in the interval between beginning treatment and follow-up. Dritz has pointed out that the incidence of some infections has decreased in areas where intensive community awareness programs have been successful [23]. Emphasis on the interruption of disease transmission has implications for the sake of the general public health as well as the health of the gay community. In calling attention to the need for improved means of diagnosis, treatment, and prevention of sexually transmitted infection, Dritz has reported that about 10% of the positive samples for enteric infection in San Francisco are from people employed as food handlers, and the majority of these people are homosexual [81]. The obvious conclusion is that the problems addressed herein are of potential concern to all health care personnel and all communities.

REFERENCES

1. Sohn N, Robilotti JG. The gay bowel syndrome. A review of colonic and rectal conditions in 200 male homosexuals. Am J Gastroenterol 1977; 67:478-484.

2. Kang JY, Stiel D, Doe WF. Proctocolitis caused by concurrent amoebiasis and gonococcal infection. The "gay bowel" syndrome. Med J Aust 1979; 2:496-497.
3. William DC. Hepatitis and other sexually transmitted diseases in gay men and in lesbians. Sex Transm Dis 1981; 8:330-332.
4. Hook EW, Stamm WE. Sexually transmitted diseases in men. Med Clin North Am 1983; 67:235-251.
5. Quinn TC, Stamm WE, Goodell SE, Mkrtichian E, Benedetti J, Corey L, Schuffler MD, Holmes KK. The polymicrobial origin of intestinal infections in homosexual men. N Engl J Med 1983; 309:576-582.
6. Jacobs E. Anal infections caused by herpes simplex virus. Dis Colon Rectum 1976; 19:151-157.
7. Goodell SE, Quinn TC, Mkrtichian E, Schuffler MD, Holmes KK, Corey L. Herpes simplex proctitis in homosexual men. Clinical, sigmoidoscopic, and histopathological features. N Engl J Med 1983; 308:868-871.
8. Samarasinghe PL, Oates JK, Maclennan IPB. Herpetic proctitis and sacral radiomyelopathy—a hazard for homosexual men. Br Med J 1979; 2:365-366.
9. Siegal FP, Lopez C, Hammer GS, Brown AE, Kornfeld SJ, Gold J, Hassett J, et al. Severe acquired immunodeficiency in male homosexuals, manifested by chronic perianal ulcerative herpex simplex lesions. N Engl J Med 1981; 305:1439-1444.
10. Goldmeier D, Darougar S. Isolation of *Chlamydia trachomatis* from throat and rectum of homosexual men. Br J Vener Dis 1977; 53:184-185.
11. Levine JS, Smith PD, Brugge WR. Chronic proctitis in male homosexuals due to lymphogranuloma venereum. Gastroenterology 1980; 79:563-565.
12. Quinn TC, Goodell SE, Mkrtichian E, Schuffler MD, Wang SP, Stamm WE, Holmes KK. *Chlamydia trachomatis* proctitis. N Engl J Med 1981; 305:195-200.
13. Bolan RK, Sands M, Schachter J, Miner RC, Drew WL. Lymphogranuloma venereum and acute ulcerative proctitis. Am J Med 1982; 72:703-706.
14. Abrams AJ. Lymphogranuloma venereum. JAMA 1968; 205:199-202.
15. Baker RW, Peppercorn MA. Gastrointestinal ailments of homosexual men. Medicine 1982; 61:390-405.
16. Gluckman JB, Kleinman MS, May AG. Primary syphilis of rectum. NY State J Med 1974; 74:2210-2211.
17. Nazemi MM, Musher DM, Schell RF, Milo S. Syphilitic proctitis in a homosexual. JAMA 1975; 231:389.
18. Akdamar K, Martin RJ, Ichinose H. Syphilitic proctitis. Dig Dis 1977; 22:701-704.
19. Quinn TC, Corey L, Chafee RG, Schuffler MD, Brancato FP, Holmes KK. The etiology of anorectal infections in homosexual men. Am J Med 1981; 71:395-406.
20. Quinn TC, Lukehart SA, Goodell S, Mkrtichian E, Schuffler MD, Holmes KK. Rectal mass caused by *Treponema pallidum*: confirmation by immunofluorescent staining. Gastroenterology 1982; 82:135-139.
21. Fluker JL. A 10-year study of homosexually transmitted infection. Br J Vener Dis 1976; 52:155-160.

22. Judson FN, Penley KA, Robinson ME, Smith JK. Comparative prevalence rates of sexually transmitted diseases in heterosexual and homosexual men. Am J Epidemiol 1980; 112:836-843.
23. Medical Staff Conference, University of California San Francisco. Venereal aspects of gastroenterology. West J Med 1979; 130:236-246.
24. Lebedeff DA, Hochman EB. Rectal gonorrhea in men: diagnosis and treatment. Ann Intern Med 1980; 92:463-466.
25. Klein EJ, Fisher LS, Chow AW, Guze LB. Anorectal gonococcal infection. Ann Intern Med 1977; 86:340-346.
26. Fluker JL, Deherogoda P, Platt DJ, Gerken A. Rectal gonorrhea in male homosexuals. Presentation and therapy. Br J Vener Dis 1980; 56:397-399.
27. Fiumara NJ. The treatment of gonococcal proctitis. JAMA 1978; 239:735-737.
28. Sands M, Sellers T. Therapy of anorectal gonorrhea in men. West J Med 1980; 133:469-471.
29. Sands M. Treatment of anorectal gonorrhea infections in men. JAMA 1980; 243:1143-1144.
30. Bygdeman S. Gonorrhea in men with homosexual contacts. Br J Vener Dis 1981; 57:320-324.
31. Blaser MJ, Reller LB. *Campylobacter* enteritis. N Engl J Med 1981; 305: 1444-1452.
32. Blaser MJ, Berkowitz ID, La Force FM, Cravens J, Reller LB, Wang WL. *Campylobacter* enteritis. Clinical and epidemiological features. Ann Intern Med 1979; 91:179-185.
33. Simmers PD, Tabaqchali S. *Campylobacter* species in male homosexuals. Br J Vener Dis 1979; 55:66.
34. Carey PB, Wright EP. *Campylobacter jejuni* in a male homosexual. Br J Vener Dis 1979; 55:381.
35. Quinn TC, Corey L, Chaffee RG, Schuffler MD, Holmes KK. *Campylobacter* proctitis in a homosexual man. Ann Intern Med 1980; 93:458-459.
36. Dritz SK, Back AF. Shigella enteritis venereally transmitted. N Engl J Med 1974; 291:1194.
37. Dritz SK, Ainsworth TE, Back A, Boucher LA, Garrard WF, Palmer RD, River E. Patterns of sexually transmitted diseases in a city. Lancet 1977; 2:3-4.
38. William DC, Felman TM, Marr JS, Shookhoff HB. Sexually transmitted enteric pathogens in male homosexual population. NY State J Med 1977; 77: 2050-2052.
39. Keusch GT. Shigella infections. Clin Gastroenterol 1979; 8:645-662.
40. Most H. Manhattan: "a tropic isle?" Am J Trop Med Hyg 1968; 222:1309-10.
41. Shookhoff HB. Parasite transmission. JAMA 1972; 222:1310.
42. Mildvan D, Gelb AM, William D. Venereal transmission of enteric pathogens in male homosexuals. JAMA 1977; 238:1387-1389.
43. Hurwitz AL, Owen RL. Venereal transmission of intestinal parasites. West J Med 1978; 128:89-91.
44. Schmerin MH, Gelston A, Jones TC. Amebiasis. An increasing problem among homosexuals in New York City. JAMA 1977; 238:1386-1387.

45. Pearce RB. Intestinal protozoal infections and AIDS. Lancet 1983; 2:51.
46. Pomerantz BM, Marr JS, Goldman WD. Amebiasis in New York City 1958-1978: identification of the male homosexual high risk population. Bull NY Acad Med 1980; 56:232-244.
47. Phillips SC, Mildvan D, William DC, Gelb AM, White MC. Sexual transmission of enteric protozoa and helminths in a venereal-disease-clinic population. N Engl J Med 1981; 305:603-606.
48. Keystone JS, Keystone DL, Proctor EM. Intestinal parasitic infections in homosexual men; prevalence, symptoms and factors in transmission. Can Med Assoc J 1980; 123:512-514.
49. Editorial. Sexual transmission of enteric pathogens. Lancet 1981; 2:1328-1329.
50. Krogstad DJ, Spencer HC, Healy GR. Amebiasis. N Engl J Med 1978; 298: 262-265.
51. Meyers JD, Kamath HA, Holmes KK. *Giardia lamblia* infection in homosexual men. Br J Vener Dis 1977; 53:54-55.
52. Schmerin MJ, Jones TC, Klein H. Giardiasis: association with homosexuality. Ann Intern Med 1978; 88:801-803.
53. Wolfe MS. Giardiasis. N Engl J Med 1978; 298:319-321.
54. Brandborg LL, Owen R, Fogel R, Goldberg H, Garvie J, Grossman S. Giardiasis and traveler's diarrhea. Gastroenterology 1980; 78:1602-1614.
55. Karnath KR, Murugasu R. A comparative study of four methods for detecting *Giardia lamblia* in children with diarrheal disease and malabsorption. Gastroenterology 1974; 66:16-21.
56. Dritz SK, Braff EH. Sexually transmitted typhoid fever. N Engl J Med 1977; 296:1359-1360.
57. Judson FN, Ehret JM, Eickhoff TC. Anogenital infection with *Neisseria meningitidis* in homosexual men. J Infect Dis 1978; 137:458-463.
58. Waugh MA. Sexual transmission of intestinal parasites. Br J Vener Dis 1974; 50:157.
59. McMillan A. Intestinal parasites in homosexual men. Scott Med J 1980; 25: 33-35.
60. McMillan A, Lee FD. Sigmoidoscopic and microscopic appearance of the rectal mucosa in homosexual men. Gut 1981; 22:1035-1041.
61. Nielsen RH, Orholm M, Pedersen JO, Hovind-Hougen K, Teglbjaerg PS, Thaysen EH. Colorectal spirochetosis: clinical significance of the infestation. Gastroenterology 1983; 85:62-67.
62. Cooper HS, Patchefsky AS, Marks G. Cloacogenic carcinoma of the anorectum in homosexual men. Dis Colon Rectum 1979; 22:557-558.
63. Leach RD, Ellis H. Carcinoma of the rectum in male homosexuals. J R Soc Med 1981; 74:490-491.
64. Li FP, Osborn D, Cronin CM. Anorectal squamous carcinoma in two homosexual men. Lancet 1982; 2:391.
65. Daling JR, Weiss NS, Klopfenstein LL, Cochran LE, Chow WH, Daifuku R. Correlates of homosexual behavior and the incidence of anal cancer. JAMA 1982; 247:1988-1990.

66. Owen WF. Sexually transmitted diseases and traumatic problems in homosexual men. Ann Intern Med 1980; 92:805-808.
67. Barone JE, Yee J, Nealon TF. Management of foreign bodies and trauma of the rectum. Surg Gynecol Obstet 1983; 156:453-457.
68. Willcox RR. Sexual behavior and sexually transmitted disease patterns in male homosexuals. Br J Vener Dis 1981; 57:167-169.
69. Petras RE, Carey WD, Alanis A. Cryptosporidial enteritis in a homosexual male with an acquired immunodeficiency syndrome. Cleveland Clin Q 1983; 50:41-45.
70. Ma P, Soave R. Three-step stool examination for cryptosporidiosis in 10 homosexual men with protracted watery diarrhea. J Infect Dis 1983; 147: 824-828.
71. Rose HS, Balthazar EG, Megibow AJ, Horowitz L, Laubenstein LJ. Alimentary tract involvement in Kaposi sarcoma: radiographic and endoscopic findings in 25 homosexual men. AJR 1982; 139:661-666.
72. Sider L, Mintzer RA, Mendelson EB, Roger LF, Degesys GE. Radiographic findings of infectious proctitis in homosexual men. AJR 1982; 139:667-671.
73. Boulton AJM, Slater DN, Hancock BW. Herpesvirus colitis: a new cause of diarrhoea in a patient with Hodgkin's disease. Gut 1982; 23:247-249.
74. Guttman D, Raymond A, Gelb A, Ehya H, Mather U, Mildvan D, Spigland I. Virus-associated colitis in homosexual men: two case reports. Am J Gastroenterol 1983; 78:167-169.
75. Bartlett JG. Antibiotic-associated pseudomembranous colitis. Rev Infect Dis 1979; 1:530-539.
76. Tedesco FJ. Antibiotic associated pseudomembranous colitis with negative proctosigmoidoscopy examination. Gastroenterology 1979; 77:295-297.
77. Owen WF. The clinical approach to the homosexual patient. Ann Intern Med 1980; 93:90-92.
78. Heller M. The gay bowel syndrome: a common problem of homosexual patients in the emergency department. Ann Emerg Med 1980; 9:487-493.
79. Bolan RK. Sexually transmitted diseases in homosexuals: focusing the attack. Sex Transm Dis 1981; 8:293-297.
80. Ho DD, Ault MJ, Ault MA, Murata GH. *Campylobacter* enteritis. Early diagnosis with Gram's stain. Arch Intern Med 1982; 142:1858-1860.
81. Dritz SK. Medical aspects of homosexuality. N Engl J Med 1980; 302:463-464.

ELEVEN

Acquired Immune Deficiency Syndrome

Michael L. Tapper
Lenox Hill Hospital
New York, New York

INTRODUCTION

In the fall of 1980, clinicians in New York and California began to report the occurrence of *Pneumocystis carinii* pneumonia in otherwise healthy young individuals, many of whom were homosexual men or intravenous drug users. The first published report of these unusual cases in the *Morbidity and Mortality Weekly Reports* of the Centers for Disease Control (CDC) in June 1981 [1] alerted physicians to the unprecedented finding of opportunistic infections in individuals lacking the usual history of either antecedent neoplastic disease or immunosuppressive chemotherapy. Simultaneously, dermatologists in New York and California began to report an increased frequency in the occurrence of new cases of Kaposi's sarcoma in young homosexual males [2]. These initial reports heralded a flurry of similar case reports, primarily from urban areas such as New York, San Francisco, Los Angeles, and Miami, and the recognition of a new syndrome of acquired immune deficiency. Since its original description (often referred to as "gay-related immunodeficiency" in the initial months following its recognition), the acquired immune deficiency syndrome (AIDS) has received enormous attention in the medical and popular literature and media.

The case definition currently accepted by the CDC for a case of AIDS requires the presence of a confirmed diagnosis of an illness predictive of a deficit in cell-mediated immunity in an individual with no known cause for such a deficit [3]. Obviously, patients with known prior neoplastic disease or receiving any immunosuppressive therapy are eliminated from inclusion as AIDS cases, even if they should fall into one of the principle risk groups for AIDS. It is equally important to recognize that the current case definition makes no mention of specific risk groups (e.g., homosexual men) in defining a case. Similarly, the documentation of abnormal immunological parameters, as measured in in vitro assays, is neither required nor sufficient to establish a diagnosis of AIDS.

The principle opportunistic infections recognized to date in AIDS have included *P. carinii* pneumonia, disseminated cytomegalovirus infection, disseminated (especially central nervous system) toxoplasmosis, atypical mycobacteriosis, progressive herpes simplex, herpes zoster, disseminated cryptococcosis, and persistent mucosal candidiasis [3]. Smaller numbers of documented cases of cryptosporidium enteritis, histoplasmosis, and progressive multifocal leukoencephalopathy have also been reported. Kaposi's sarcoma remains the principal neoplasm associated with AIDS, although primary central nervous system lymphoma has also been adopted as a criterion for AIDS. Other neoplasms such as non-Hodgkin's lymphoma, Burkitt's lymphoma, and squamous cell carcinoma of the rectum have been recognized with increased frequency in homosexual men but are not currently accepted as sufficient diagnostic criteria for AIDS.

EPIDEMIOLOGY

General

By July 1982 approximately 2000 cases of AIDS had been reported to the CDC [4] and by May 1984 over 4000 cases had been recognized. In retrospect, cases of AIDS were seen as early as 1978, although the initial clusters of cases in New York and California that enabled clinicians to recognize the unusual appearance of a new disease phenomenon did not occur until 1980 to 1981. Approximately 45% of the cases recognized in the United States have come from New York City, with smaller percentages from San Francisco, Los Angeles, and Miami. Although cases have been reported to date from many urban centers, the clustering of cases in certain cities (particularly New York) has remained a striking feature of the disease. Although some of the case clustering may represent heightened awareness, recognition, and reporting in urban areas with large numbers of individuals in recognized risk groups (e.g., homosexual men in San Francisco and Haitians in

Miami), the absence of similar foci of disease in the same groups in other cities is of epidemiological note. Cases have been reported from most states and numerous countries of Western Europe (England, France, Belgium, Switzerland, Denmark, and Germany), Australia, Africa, and the Caribbean [5-11]. Many of these cases have occurred in homosexual men with histories of travel to the United States or sexual contacts with Americans.

Analysis of reported cases of AIDS has identified the principal risk groups for occurrence of the syndrome. Approximately 71% of cases have been reported in men acknowledging a history of homosexual practices, 17% have occurred in individuals with histories of intravenous drug abuse, 5% in Haitian immigrants to the United States, and 1% in patients with hemophilia A receiving factor VIII therapy [12]. Smaller numbers of cases of what is presumably the same syndrome have been reported in recipients of blood transfusions, female sexual contacts of individuals in high-risk groups, and infants born into families with individuals in high-risk groups. Approximately 6% of reported cases do not easily fall into any of the known risk categories. Some of these cases were reported in retrospect or after a patient died, so that it was impossible to assign a risk category; others may represent "background" cases of Kaposi's sarcoma in the general population. Although the vast majority of new cases continue to fall into one of the major risk groups, it is inevitable as the epidemic continues that more cases will occur in individuals not fitting into the principal risk groups.

In addition to clustering of cases within certain populations and the identification of areas of high density of cases such as New York City, more than casual connection has been recognized between certain victims of AIDS. Analysis of one cluster of nine cases of AIDS in homosexual men in California by the CDC revealed a history of sexual contacts and linkages far exceeding that predicted by random chance [13]. Such clusters have given support to the notion of a transmissible agent being responsible for AIDS. Many of the principal groups at risk for AIDS are also known to be at high risk for hepatitis B (homosexual men, intravenous drug abusers, and hemophiliacs), suggesting that the common link between these cases may be an agent, presumably viral or viruslike, that can be transmitted by blood or other infected secretions through shared needles (drug abusers), intimate mucosal contact (homosexual males and female partners of drug users), or through receipt of blood or blood components (hemophiliacs or transfusion recipients). Current concepts of the etiology and transmission of AIDS will be discussed further in the etiology Section III. Despite the epidemiological evidence supporting person-to-person transmission of AIDS, such transmission appears to require intimate contact with blood or other body secretions, and transmission by casual contact has not been reported. Despite the occurrence of clusters of cases in linked individuals, many contacts of AIDS victims (including individuals with prolonged and sustained sexual contact) remain overtly well.

Specific At-Risk Groups for AIDS

Homosexual Men

Homosexual or bisexual men represent 71% of the reported cases of AIDS and have been the most carefully studied group of AIDS victims [14-16]. The detailed case control study reported by the CDC suggested that promiscuity, exposure to feces during sexual contact, recreational drug use, and a prior history of syphilis, non-B hepatitis and enteric infections are independent risk factors in such individuals for the development of AIDS [17]. The frequency of venereal infections and recreational drug use in some homosexual men led to the early theories of "immunological overload" or exhaustion of the immune system as possible etiologies of AIDS. However, cases of AIDS have occurred in nonpromiscuous homosexual men as well as in individuals without histories of nitrite use. Immunological surveys of "healthy" homosexual males in areas of high AIDS occurrence such as New York City have suggested that milder abnormalities of the immune system similar to those associated with AIDS may be widespread throughout the homosexual community [18]. While suggestive of widespread exposure to the presumed etiological agent of AIDS, the significance and natural history of these milder abnormalities of immune function in otherwise healthy individuals are unknown.

One unique feature of AIDS among homosexual men is the increased occurrence of Kaposi's sarcoma, compared with other risk groups. For unknown reasons, the occurrence of Kaposi's sarcoma is higher among homosexual victims of AIDS than among intravenous drug users, hemophiliacs, or Haitian patients. Certain clinical features of AIDS in homosexual men such as the occurrence of progressive ulcerative herpes simplex infection of the perineum and rectum seem clearly to be related to specific homosexual practices such as anal intercourse.

Intravenous Drug Users

Intravenous drug users have long been recognized to be at risk for certain infections, including those transmitted by blood or blood products, presumably related to the use of shared and contaminated injection equipment [19]. The occurrence of AIDS in intravenous drug users supports the etiological notion of a transmissible agent in AIDS. The clinical features of the disease do not differ strikingly from those seen in other high-risk populations, with the notable exception of the decreased incidence of Kaposi's sarcoma compared to the homosexual group [20,21].

A subgroup of the intravenous drug users has emerged with reports of the occurrence of clusters of AIDS cases among prisoners, many of whom give histories of intravenous drug use prior to imprisonment [22].

Haitian Immigrants

The occurrence of AIDS among Haitian immigrants to the United States has been one of the most puzzling aspects of the epidemic [23-25]. Unlike the homosexual, drug user, and hemophiliac/transfusion groups, the Haitian victims of this syndrome appear to have no obvious routes of transmission of a presumed infectious agent. Some clarification of this apparent contradiction may be related to incomplete or inaccurate histories obtained by interviewers from the initial Haitian patients. Cultural and religious taboos against homosexual practices in Haiti, language difficulties with Creole-speaking patients and families, and fears about subsequent deportation from the United States may have led Haitian patients to deny homosexual practices to interviewers. Given the extreme poverty of Haiti, homosexual prostitution by young males is reportedly not uncommon and may have led to the introduction and/or transmission of a possible AIDS agent from or to visiting American or European homosexual men. The sense that Haitian immigrants had been unfairly labeled and stigmatized as an AIDS risk group recently prompted the New York City Department of Health to delete the Haitian category as a specific risk group, although national recognition of the Haitian category by the CDC continues. While most cases of AIDS in Haitians have occurred in males, a significant percentage of cases have also occurred in females who do not appear to fall easily into any other risk category. Medical information from Haiti about the incidence of AIDS within the country is limited, but local physicians apparently feel that there has been an increased incidence of both Kaposi's sarcoma and opportunistic infections in recent years [25]. Although cases of AIDS or AIDS-like illness have also been reported from other Caribbean islands or in immigrants from these islands, the striking concentration in Haitian immigrants to the United States remains an enigma.

The clinical manifestations of AIDS in Haitian patients resemble those of the other risk groups with certain differences. Although not recognized as an AIDS-related diagnosis, severe pulmonary and miliary tuberculosis have occurred in many Haitian patients; disseminated (primarily central nervous system) toxoplasmosis has also been common.

Hemophiliacs and Transfusion Recipients

A limited number of cases of AIDS have been reported in patients with hemophilia A who have received lyophilized factor VIII concentrate therapy [26-30]. Several studies have examined lymphocyte function in healthy recipients of factor VIII concentrates and described immunological abnormalities in a high percentage of otherwise healthy hemophiliacs [31-36]. Such abnormalities do not appear to be present in the hemophiliac patients treated with cryoprecipitate rather than lyophilized factor VIII concentrates, the latter product being derived from a far larger pool of donors. The significance of these abnormalities is unknown, and whether they are secondary to factor VIII therapy itself or to an infectious agent transmitted by such therapy is also uncertain. Although the number of cases of AIDS in hemophiliacs is small, the apparently much wider incidence of immune abnormalities associated with factor VIII therapy has led some hematologists to advocate a return to cryoprecipitate therapy by hemophiliacs [37].

Similar abnormalities have also been described in patients receiving factor IX therapy [38].

Still fewer cases but far more public alarm has been associated with a number of cases of AIDS-like illness occurring in individuals whose only apparent risk factor was the prior receipt of blood transfusions or blood component therapy [39]. Most of these cases occurred following trauma or open-heart surgery requiring relatively massive administration of blood products. At least one case has been reported from France in which a previously healthy tourist developed AIDS following a blood transfusion administered in Haiti after he suffered an automobile accident [40]. The most carefully studied case to date occurred in an infant who underwent exchange transfusion after birth [41]. The child was well until 6 months of age, but subsequently developed numerous opportunistic infections, including recurrent candidiasis and disseminated atypical mycobacteriosis. One of the donors was subsequently found to be a homosexual male who was well at the time of donating platelets to the infant, but who subsequently developed pneumocystis and cytomegalovirus pneumonia and herpes simplex type 2 infection and died 17 months following his platelet donation. Immunological studies in the infant were compatible with the abnormalities associated with AIDS. Understandable public and medical concern with the implications of these apparent transfusion-linked cases has led to initiation of programs calling for voluntary restriction of blood donation by individuals in high-risk categories for AIDS [42,43].

Female Sexual Partners of AIDS Patients or High-Risk Individuals

If AIDS can be transmitted sexually between homosexual patients, it is not surprising that AIDS could also be transmitted between heterosexual couples. Acquired immune deficiency was first reported in women in 1982; many of the women in this report acknowledged use of intravenous drugs, although one patient's only apparent risk factor was regular heterosexual contact with a male intravenous drug user [44]. All five women had pneumocystis pneumonia and combinations of other opportunistic infections, along with immunological abnormalities typical of AIDS. A more recent study noted immunological abnormalities in six of seven female heterosexual contacts of male patients with AIDS [45]. Of the six female sexual partners, one developed clear-cut AIDS manifested by pneumocystis pneumonia and oral candidiasis; a second woman had lymphadenopathy, lymphopenia, and abnormal immunological markers; and four other women had either lymphadenopathy or lymphopenia, with or without immune function abnormalities. All women denied intravenous drug use. These data and the conclusion that female sexual partners of individuals in high-risk AIDS populations are themselves at high risk for AIDS should be interpreted cautiously. Only one bona fide case of AIDS has, in fact, been described in this group, and the significance, incidence, and duration of the immunological abnormalities described in such individuals are entirely unknown. A report of AIDS manifested by pneumocystis pneumonia, oral candidiasis, and herpes simplex infection in a female prostitute who denied intravenous drug use does give support, however, to the notion of heterosexual transmission of AIDS [46]. Similarly, a recent case of AIDS has been reported in a 71-year-old woman whose only risk factor was sexual contact with her 74-year-old hemophiliac husband who died of pneumocystis pneumonia [47].

AIDS in Children

Rubenstein et al. [48], Oleske et al. [49], and Scott et al. [50] have reported on a series of children who have exhibited failure to thrive, lymphadenopathy, hepatosplenomegaly, interstitial pneumonia, and abnormalities of cell-mediated immunity similar to those described in adults with AIDS. Opportunistic infections including pneumocystis pneumonia, oroesophageal candidiasis, and salmonellosis have been present in most of the children described. Many of these children were the offspring of patients (either mother, father, or both) in recognized high-risk groups for AIDS, including intravenous drug users and Haitian immigrants. In one case a nonparental household contact had frank AIDS. Because of the background of many of these infants and the paucity of information regarding their parents in some cases, it is difficult to analyze possible patterns of vertical or horizontal transmission of infection. Pediatric immunologists who have studied these and other similar children feel that these children exhibit a novel type of immunodeficiency. Whether or not this entity represents the same disease as AIDS in adults remains to be clarified. The implication of vertical transmission in utero or of horizontal transmission through intimate household contact would further support the concept of a transmissible agent causing AIDS.

ETIOLOGY

The extensive case control study carried out by the CDC [17] identified promiscuity in homosexual males, use of certain recreational drugs, prior evidence of syphilis, non-B hepatitis and enteric parasitic infections, and fecal contact during sexual relations as risk factors for the development of AIDS. Early theories of causation postulated that "immunological overload" from recurrent infections exhausted the immune system, leaving the patient vulnerable to opportunistic infections and malignancies. Administration of repeated courses of drugs with known mutagenic potential in animals, such as metronidazole for amebiasis, was thought to contribute to immune suppression in homosexual men. Exposure to allogenic sperm [51] or frequent use of amyl or butyl nitrite ("poppers") [52] were also suggested as etiologies of the immune alterations. The continuing recognition of cases in nonhomosexual populations and the more striking relationship between blood and blood component therapy in hemophiliac cases and post-transfusion cases have suggested to most observers that a transmissible agent is likely to be responsible for the AIDS phenomenon.

In addition to the epidemiology of AIDS, which strikingly resembles that of hepatitis B, other evidence has favored the transmissible agent hypothesis: (1) Pathology of lymph nodes in the lymphadenopathy syndrome in homosexual men reveals intensely reactive nodes with marker follicular hyperplasia similar to that seen in certain types of viral-induced lymphadenitis [53]; (2) certain viruses (notably cytomegalovirus and Epstein-Barr virus) are known to produce striking, albeit temporary and reversible, abnormalities of immune function; and (3) the "immune overload" theory does not easily apply to the post-transfusion, pediatric, and Haitian AIDS cases.

Most workers have assumed that the putative AIDS agent will be viral or virus-like, and most speculation has centered about three known agents, although the possibility of a mutated or entirely novel viral agent cannot be dismissed. Epstein-Barr virus (EBV), cytomegalovirus (CMV), and human retroviruses have been the most frequently considered agents. Epstein-Barr virus has been a prime suspect because many AIDS patients have elevated antibody titers to EBV, suggesting recent infection or reactivation of latent infection [21]. Epstein-Barr virus is linked etiologically both with infectious mononucleosis and with Burkitt's lymphoma in Africa and induces transient T-cell abnormalities resembling (although not identical to) those seen in AIDS [54]. Evidence of EBV infection is common in many adults, however, and it is difficult to explain why EBV should suddenly cause an entirely new syndrome in such restricted populations. Evidence of active EBV infection was, however, found in several of the pediatric cases described by Rubenstein et al. [48]. The case for CMV is more compelling although still unconvincing as an etiological candidate for AIDS. Like EBV, CMV can produce profound alterations in immune function in infected individuals, effects that have been documented to last as long as 10 months in one report [55]. Cytomegalovirus can evidently be transmitted sexually, with a high incidence of recovery from semen [56], and CMV infection appears nearly universal in homosexual men [57]. Early studies of Kaposi's sarcoma in Africa revealed tissue antigens reactive with CMV antibody [58], and renal transplant patients who are particularly plagued by severe CMV disease have also been reported to have an increased incidence of Kaposi's sarcoma. Analysis of Kaposi's sarcoma tissue has revealed evidence of CMV antigens and nucleic acids in a number of cases, suggesting the CMV is probably linked etiologically as a cofactor in the genesis of Kaposi's sarcoma, if not the AIDS syndrome itself [59]. Troublesome questions regarding CMV as an etiological agent remain. First, it is not clear why an agent that has long been recognized as a pathogen in both normal and immunocompromised hosts should suddenly cause a devastating new syndrome. Endonuclease restriction analysis of CMV strains recovered from AIDS patients has failed to identify a unique CMV strain in these patients. Although evidence of prior CMV infection appears ubiquitous in homosexual men, evidence of CMV antibody was absent in the California infant transfusion case. Evidence of prior CMV infection is common among healthy adults, although data on its incidence in other high-risk AIDS populations such as intravenous drug users and Haitians are not currently available.

Most interest and excitement has centered around the possible etiological role of a human retrovirus as an etiological agent for AIDS. Interest was initially raised by reports from Gallo and his associates from the National Cancer Institute of identification of proviral DNA sequences of human T-cell leukemia virus (HTLV) in the lymphocytes of two AIDS patients [60]. Peripheral blood lymphocytes of three AIDS victims were also shown to express HTLV antigens, and HTLV-1 was isolated from the lymphocytes of one patient [61]. Montagnier and colleagues from the Pasteur Institute also reported recovery of a novel type of human retrovirus (called lymphadenopathy-associated virus) from a male homosexual with chronic lymphadenopathy [62]. Simultaneously, Essex and co-workers reported that 25% of AIDS patients studied had antibodies to cell membrane antigens of HTLV [63]; similar antibodies were later reported in 26% of asymptomatic hemophiliacs [64].

In April 1984 the Pasteur Institute workers reported that they had again recovered a novel human isolate of retrovirus, this time from one of a pair of identical twins with factor IX deficiency and AIDS [65]. This retrovirus isolate was distinct from previous isolates of human T-cell leukemia virus (HTLV), but similar to the previous isolate of lymphadenopathy-associated virus. One month later a series of papers by Gallo and collaborators [66-69] reported the recovery of a new member of the HTLV group of human retroviruses (called HTLV-3) from 26 of 72 patients with AIDS (35%) and from even a higher number (85%) of individuals in high-risk groups with symptoms designated as "pre-AIDS." Serological analysis of HTLV-3 isolates revealed unique viral antigens, although some overlap existed with antigens of previous human isolates of HTLV (HTLV-1 and HTLV-2). Finally, antibodies to HTLV-3 were reported to be present in nearly 90% of true AIDS victims and in approximately 80% of "pre-AIDS" individuals. Using sera supplied by the CDC, the French workers have detected antibodies to lymphadenopathy-associated virus in 90% of American AIDS and pre-AIDS patients [70]. Studies in progress should clarify whether HTLV-3 and lymphadenopathy-associated virus are identical.

The case for a human retrovirus as the etiological agent of AIDS has therefore become both theoretically and factually compelling. HTLV isolates are intensely T-lymphotrophic and are capable of causing profound immunosuppression in animal models of disease (e.g., feline leukemia virus). It is of interest that a retrovirus has also recently been identified and isolated from rhesus monkeys with "simian AIDS," with successful transmission of disease to healthy animals [71]. This retrovirus, however, is apparently antigenically distinct from human T-cell leukemia virus isolates.

IMMUNOLOGY

A discussion of the complex immunological derangements that accompany AIDS is beyond the scope of this chapter [72-74]. Both in vivo and in vitro parameters of cell-mediated immunity are consistently depressed. Patients are usually anergic to a battery of standard recall antigens, although some delayed hypersensitivity function may be preserved in individual cases. In vitro evaluation of T-cell function using nonspecific mitogens such as phytohemagglutinin (PHA) and concanavalin A (con A) are variably depressed, although the degree of depression varies from patient to patient and for an individual patient as the disease waxes and wanes. Specific mitogen-induced stimulation of lymphocytes by mitogens such as *Candida* or PPD is similarly affected. The patients are frequently and often strikingly lymphopenic: Differentials revealing only 5 to 10% lymphocytes are not uncommon. Superficially, B-cell function appears better preserved than T-cell function, and neutrophil numbers and function do not appear clinically to be significantly impaired. Various degrees of thrombocytopenia are often present, and an ITP-like syndrome which responds favorably to steroids or splenectomy has been described in a number of homosexual patients [75]. Although a polyclonal hypergammaglobulinemia is usually present, antibody responses to opportunistic pathogens are often markedly reduced, suggesting an impairment of T-cell-dependent B-cell function [76].

Most interest has centered about the striking and consistent abnormalities in T-cell subpopulations demonstrated by monoclonal antibodies. Depression of the absolute number and percentage of cells bearing surface markers identifying them as cells of the helper/inducer subset appears to be uniformly present in AIDS and is the most widely accepted immunological "marker" for the syndrome. Cells of the suppressor/cytotoxic subset may be normal or increased in number and percentage, but the ratio of T-helper to T-suppressor cells is characteristically reduced from the normal range of 1.5 to 3.0 to less than 1.0. Ratios as low as 0.2 are not uncommonly found. While consistently present in AIDS cases, it is important for the clinician to recognize that these abnormalities are not pathognomonic or diagnostic of AIDS, and the tendency to use T-cell subsets or the helper/suppressor ratio to diagnose AIDS should be discouraged. Numerous viral infections (including CMV and EBV) may transiently induce such reversal of the normal T-subset ratio, although these changes are usually reversible after a period of weeks to months and are characterized by a marked increase in T-suppressor activity causing a diminished ratio rather than such profound loss of T-helper function. Similar although less striking abnormalities have been described in both healthy homosexual men [18] and in men with unexplained lymphadenopathy in New York City [72], as well as in hemophilia A patients receiving factor VIII concentrates [31-36]. The significance and duration of these T-cell abnormalities as well as the normal variation in T-cell subpopulations in healthy individuals under various conditions of health and illness require additional study.

In AIDS patients individual helper/suppressor ratios may show considerable variation over a period of months with repeated testing, and without clear-cut relation to the patient's clinical status.

Significant derangements have been reported in numerous other immunological parameters, including depression of natural killer cell activity [77] and elevated levels of α_1-thymosin [78], β_2-microglobulin [79], and an abnormal acid-labile α-interferon similar to that described in systemic lupus erythematosus [80,81]. Other defects are likely to be described as the immune system abnormalities are further unraveled. Whether these abnormalities are primary and causational or secondary to a wholly disorganized immune system remains unknown [74]. None of these alterations, apart from the depressed T-helper activity and reversed helper/suppressor ratio, have been found consistently and reproducibly enough to be a useful "marker" or diagnostic test for AIDS. High levels of circulating immune complexes have been described in a number of AIDS patients with opportunistic infections. The origin of these complexes and their pathogenic role, if any, in the symptoms and manifestations of AIDS require further clarification.

CLINICAL MANIFESTATIONS

Kaposi's Sarcoma

Kaposi's sarcoma (KS) diagnoses account for almost 30% of newly reported cases of AIDS. Most of the cases of KS have occurred in homosexual males, with far fewer cases reported among women, intravenous drug users, and Haitians [82-84]. Perhaps the high incidence of concomitant CMV infection in homosexual men with AIDS accounts for this striking preponderance [57,59]. "Classic" KS in the United States is an indolent neoplastic process usually affecting elderly males of Mediterranean background with a propensity to involve the lower extremities [85,86]. In contrast, KS in AIDS tends to begin with multiple sites of cutaneous, mucous membrane and lymphatic and visceral involvement and may be highly aggressive [87]. In this respect, KS in AIDS resembles more closely the disseminated or lymphadenopathic form of the disease seen in Africa. Violaceous papular lesions should be carefully looked for on the skin and mucous membranes, and suspicious lesions biopsied [Fig. 1 (see Plate II, facing p. 296)]. Endoscopy of the upper and lower gastrointestinal tract may reveal a high degree of bowel involvement [Fig. 2 (see Plate II, facing p. 296)]. An excessive percentage of patients bearing HLA type DR-5 has been reported for KS in AIDS as in classic KS [84]. Patients presenting with KS as the sole manifestation of AIDS appear to have a slightly improved prognosis compared to those presenting with opportunistic infections and KS, or opportunistic infections alone, although many patients who present initially with KS alone will develop opportunistic infections in time. Treatment is controversial in these already immunosuppressed patients: Traditional single-drug or combination chemotherapy is often utilized [88], although promising results have been reported recently with recombinant interferon therapy [89].

Opportunistic Infections

Pneumocystis Pneumonia

Pneumonia caused by *P. carinii* is the most common presentation of AIDS, representing almost 50% of initial AIDS diagnoses. Although the disease may begin explosively in some cases, it more commonly presents in an indolent, subacute fashion [90]. Patients often give histories of several weeks or even months of antecedent fatigue, cough, and dyspnea [14-16,20]. Many have received prior courses of antibiotics for presumed bacterial respiratory infections. Chest x-ray usually reveals bilateral interstitial infiltrates (Fig. 3), although in early cases the changes may be minimal and subtle and only careful examination will reveal increased interstitial markings [91-93]. A gallium scan of the lungs may be strikingly positive at a time when x-ray changes are minimal or equivocal, a finding also noted in CMV pneumonitis (Fig. 4). Arterial blood gases usually reveal

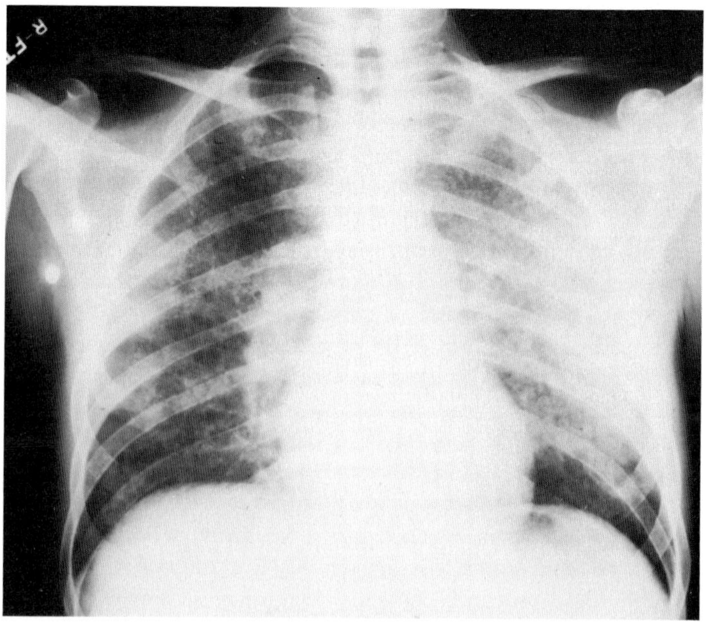

Fig. 3 Admission chest x-ray of a homosexual man with bilateral interstitial infiltrates. Transbronchoscopic biopsy demonstrated *Pneumocystis carinii* pneumonia.

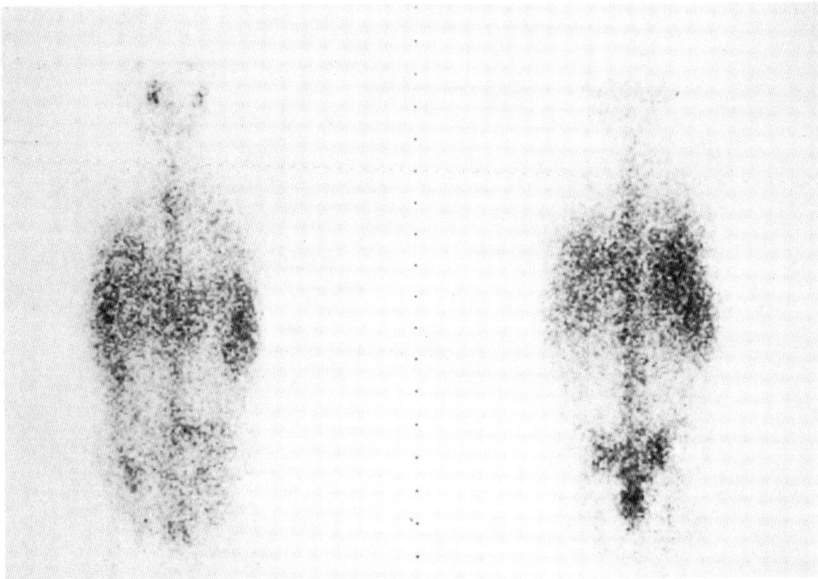

Fig. 4 Gallium scan of the lung in a patient with CMV mononucleosis syndrome. The gallium scan was obtained at a time when the patient had a normal chest x-ray. Two weeks later the patient returned with bilateral interstitial infiltrates; biopsy revealed extensive CMV pneumonitis.

significant hypoxemia early in the disease process. Although the diagnosis can be suspected and appropriate therapy promptly initiated, definitive diagnosis can only be made by transbronchoscopic or open lung biopsy, which should be carried out promptly. Infections with *P. carinii* are often so heavy in untreated AIDS patients that an experienced pathologist will have no trouble recognizing the typical organisms on methenamine silver stains of touch preparations of the biopsy material or on permanent stained sections (Fig. 5). Standard tissue stains (hematoxylin-eosin) will not reveal the parasite, but its presence may be suspected by the characteristic eosinophilic alveolar proteinaceous "foamy" material. Such changes may be reduced or absent in certain patients (particularly those receiving antipneumocystis therapy) and silver staining should be carried out on all suspected cases, regardless of morphology. Because of the high density of organisms present in untreated cases of pneumocystis in AIDS, bronchoalveolar lavage without biopsy may be sufficient for cytological diagnosis.

The current therapy of choice is trimethoprim-sulfamethoxazole (TMP/SMZ) in a dose of 15 to 20 mg/kg per day of the trimethoprim component, given in four divided doses. In acutely ill patients initial therapy should always be intra-

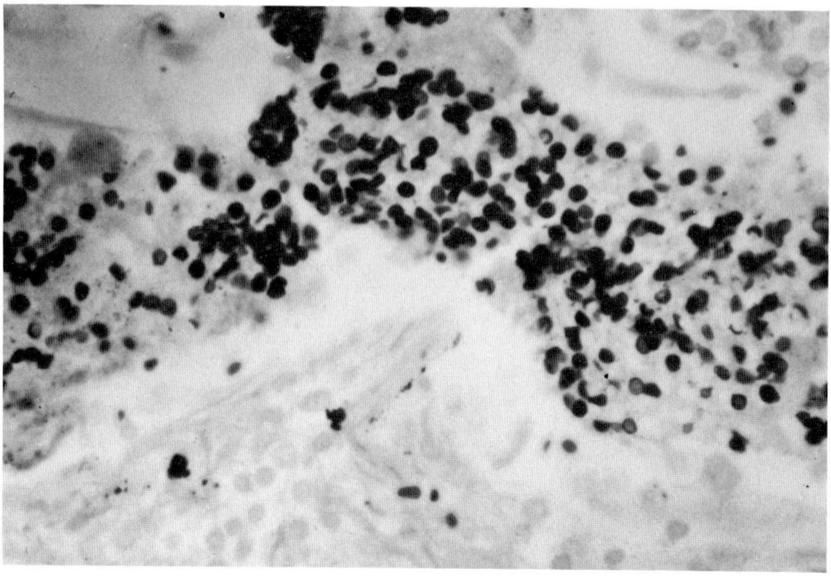

Fig. 5 *Pneumocystis carinii* organisms on transbronchial lung biopsy (Gomori methenamine silver stain 250X). (Photograph courtesy of Dr. R. Snyder, Lenox Hill Hospital, New York, New York.)

venous. Not uncommonly, patients worsen for the first few days, with progressive infiltrates on x-ray and worsening hypoxemia following initiation of therapy, and often require intubation and mechanical ventilation. Improvement is usually apparent between the fourth and fifth day of treatment, although prolonged therapy is usually required. A suggested regimen is 2 weeks of intravenous TMP/SMZ followed by 2 weeks of oral therapy in equivalent doses.

Troubling side effects of TMP/SMZ, including fever, hypersensitivity rashes, and leukopenia are common in AIDS patients for unclear reasons [22,90,94,95]. Folinic acid, 5 to 10 mg, orally, intramuscularly, or intravenously, may be given, but does not uniformly prevent leukopenia in these patients. Many patients can be continued on therapy despite these side reactions, although some may require discontinuation of TMP/SMZ if the leukopenia or rash becomes severe or to differentiate drug fever from drug failure (uncommon in our experience) or a second opportunistic infection. The high incidence of such troubling side effects has made clinicians reluctant to administer prophylactic TMP/SMZ to AIDS patients to prevent pneumocystis infection.

The alternative therapy for pneumocystis pneumonia is pentamidine isethionate given in a daily dosage of 4 mg/kg intramuscularly for 14 days. Pentamidine was approved by the U.S. Food and Drug Administration in October 1984. Most clinicians reserve pentamidine for patients who have relapsed following a course of TMP/SMZ or in whom side effects prohibit use of TMP/SMZ. Persistence of pneumocystis organisms as demonstrated by bronchoscopy following a course of therapy is common in AIDS patients and many patients require repeated courses of one drug or the other. Animal models have suggested that combined therapy with both TMP/SMZ and pentamidine may be antagonistic, although similar data are not available for human disease [96]. The indications for termination of anti-pneumocystis therapy are equally uncertain; in some patients repeat bronchoscopy demonstrates eradication of the pathogen, while in others the load of organisms seems only to be reduced to a level that no longer causes pulmonary symptoms.

Candidiasis

Recurrent oral or oroesophageal candidiasis is frequently present in AIDS patients and may be extremely distressing. Mild cases often respond to high doses of oral nystatin or clotrimazole, although more stubborn or refractory cases may require initiation of oral ketoconazole or intravenous amphotericin B. Mucosal candidiasis frequently recurs when therapy is stopped, and patients may "break through" nystatin or ketoconazole therapy after an initial response. Disseminated candidiasis beyond the gastrointestinal tract, although reported, is less common than in other immunosuppressed hosts such as leukemics.

Herpesvirus Infections

Herpes Simplex. Recurrent herpes simplex infections of the mouth and particularly anogenital herpes simplex in homosexual males may be present in AIDS. In the latter group ulcerative lesions of the perianal area may be particularly troubling and refractory to local care and healing [97]. Such lesions should be cultured both for viruses (many will grow both herpes simplex and CMV) and for secondary bacterial and fungal pathogens. Meticulous local care and topical acyclovir may aid in healing, although intravenous acyclovir should probably be initiated for more severe cases of ulceration.

Herpes Zoster. Patients with subsequent diagnoses of AIDS often give a history of a prior episode of herpes zoster in the months before the diagnosis of AIDS. Clinically, herpes zoster in these patients does not appear to behave differently from the disease in other compromised hosts. Intravenous adenine arabinoside or acyclovir may be of benefit in severe cases or in disseminated varicella-zoster.

Cytomegalovirus. In addition to its possible role as an etiological agent or cofactor in the genesis of Kaposi's sarcoma and of AIDS itself, CMV is an important pathogen in many AIDS cases, and tragically is one of the most untreatable at present. Cytomegalovirus infection in AIDS patients may vary from a prolonged mononucleosis-like illness to a fulminant and lethal syndrome characterized by multiorgan involvement with progressive inanition and death [98]. The propensity of CMV to involve the lungs, adrenal glands, and colon is especially noteworthy. We earlier reported a syndrome of severe CMV colitis accompanied by pneumonitis and multivisceral involvement in two patients [99]. Both had severe and uncontrollable diarrhea as their major complaint, and colonoscopic biopsy revealed diffuse infiltration of the bowel mucosa with CMV inclusions (Fig. 6). Cytomegalovirus pneumonitis may resemble pneumocystis radiographically, and both pathogens may present on the same biopsy specimen. The high propensity for adrenal involvement with CMV suggests that AIDS patients with known CMV infection elsewhere should have their adrenal reserve assessed and should be observed for addisonian crisis late in the disease [100,101]. Isolated rectal or oral ulcerations may be found to be due to CMV if a pathologist painstakingly reviews multiple sections of such ulcers. Cytomegalovirus retinitis has been an inconstant finding in our AIDS patients with CMV infection documented in other organs [Fig. 7 (see Plate II, facing p. 296)] [102]. Although CMV disease may pursue a relentless pattern in some patients, others with evidence of CMV infection seem to have a more indolent course. Despite evidence of overwhelming disease, many

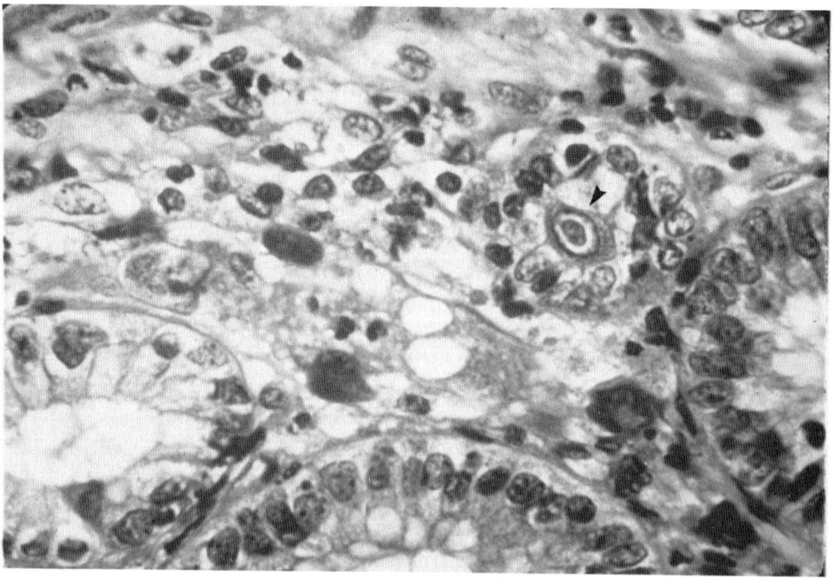

Fig. 6 Colonoscopic biopsy of a bisexual man with a 1-month history of unexplained fever and diarrhea. Cytomegalovirus inclusions (arrow) were present in crypt epithelial and endothelial cells. The patient subsequently died of disseminated CMV (hematoxylin-phloxine-safran stain, 800X). (Photograph courtesy of Dr. H. Z. Rotterdam, Lenox Hill Hospital, New York, New York.)

patients do not appear to mount a marked antibody response to CMV [98]. Evidence of prior exposure to CMV is so common and intermittant viral shedding in urine and semen so frequent in homosexual men in general [57] and in AIDS patients in particular that we have come to rely on tissue biopsies of involved organs in order to diagnose CMV infections. Available antiviral therapy has little effect on CMV, and the development of effective therapy for established CMV infection is one of the most urgent needs of clinicians caring for AIDS patients.

Mycobacterial Infections

Although infections with *Mycobacterium tuberculosis* are not currently recognized as "opportunistic" infections in AIDS, we have seen a number of young homosexual males with unusually severe forms of pulmonary or disseminated human tuberculosis. In one case pulmonary tuberculosis was diagnosed in a homosexual patient 6 months before the initial lesions of Kaposi's sarcoma appeared and 8 months before his death from disseminated toxoplasmosis. Similar reports of severe tuberculosis have come from clinicians caring for Haitian patients. In constrast, disseminated infections with atypical mycobacteria, especially *Mycobacterium avium-intracellulare* (MAI), are now well-recognized manifestations of AIDS [103-105]. Prior to the AIDS epidemic, such infections were extraordinarily unusual, even in immunosuppressed patients. The recognition of such infections is frequently made more difficult by the absence of the usual hallmarks of granulomatous inflammation in mycobacterial infections in many AIDS patients [103]. Close communication between the clinician and the pathologist and performance of acid-fast stains on clinical material even in the absence of the usual criteria for such stains are necessary or the diagnosis will be missed. Once such stains are performed, the number of acid-fast bacilli seen may be rare or overwhelming. Atypical acid-fast infection has been found in the lungs, bone marrow, lymph nodes, spleen, mesentery, and along the gastrointestinal tract [Fig. 8 (see Plate II, facing p. 296)]. A number of patients have been described with a disease that pathologically resembles Whipple's disease, with periodic acid-Schiff and silver-positive acid-fast organisms present in and outside of foamy macrophages of the gastrointestinal tract, lymph nodes, and mesentery [105]. Such pathology has invariably, in our experience, been due to MAI. As with CMV and cryptosporidium, MAI may cause severe chronic diarrhea in AIDS patients; positive stool smears for acid-fast bacilli, colonoscopic biopsy, and culture may confirm this diagnosis.

Myobacterium avium-intracellulare has proven extremely resistant to therapy, and even the most aggressive multidrug regimens have failed to eliminate infections. Most clinicians have utilized regimens combining isoniazid, rifampin, ethambutal, ethionamide, pyrazinamide, or cycloserine. More recently, a rifampin derivative, ansamycin, and an antileprosy agent, clofazamine, have been shown to be more active in vitro against MAI than previously available antituberculous agents [103]. Baron et al. have recently reported that combinations of rifampin and ethambutol in conjunction with either amikacin or N-forminidoyl thienamycin are synergistically active against a number of MAI strains isolated from AIDS patients [106]. If ansamycin is used, it should replace rifampin in the multidrug regimen. The individual and cumulative toxicities of such multidrug regimens are obviously considerable. The appropriate duration of therapy is unknown; most patients have received therapy for months until death from MAI or other opportunistic infections.

Toxoplasmosis

Disseminated infections with *Toxoplasma gondii* usually involve the central nervous system and heart, although other tissues may be involved as well. The most common presentation in AIDS patients has been a single or multiple enhancing lesions (Fig. 9) on axial tomographic scan in a patient presenting with focal neurological defects [107]. As with CMV, serology has often not been helpful in diagnosing toxoplasmosis because of seeming failure to mount an appropriate antibody response [108]. Rising IgG titers or elevated IgM titers, particularly in the cerebrospinal fluid, may suggest the diagnosis, but confirmation usually requires brain biopsy. In patients too ill for brain biopsy or with lesions judged too

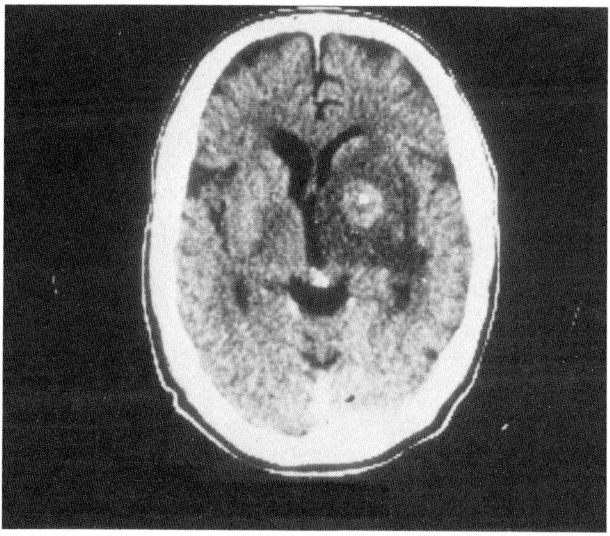

Fig. 9 Computerized axial tomographic scan of the head of a homosexual man admitted with a right basal ganglion lesion. Autopsy revealed multiple tachyzoites and cysts of *Toxoplasma gondii*. (X-ray courtesy of Dr. L. Rothman, Lenox Hill Hospital, New York, New York.)

deep for biopsy, a trial of antitoxoplasma therapy followed by serial axial tomographic examinations can be justified. The therapy of choice is sulfadiazine 100 mg/kg per day in four divided doses with pyrimethamine 25 mg orally daily following a loading dose of 50 to 75 mg. Supplemental folinic acid may ameliorate the marrow-suppressive effects of pyrimethamine without interfering with antiparasitic activity. Anecdotal reports suggest that TMP/SMZ combined with pyrimethamine is also active if an intravenous sulfonamide preparation is required.

As noted in the discussion under pneumocystis, serious side effects of sulfonamide therapy (rash, fever, and leukopenia) are seen with great frequency in AIDS patients and may complicate therapy. Unfortunately, no alternative therapy for toxoplasmosis has been proven to be effective. The duration of therapy is unknown, but probably some therapy should be continued for months in view of the inactivity of the agents used against the encysted forms of *Toxoplasma* and the tendency for relapses to occur once therapy is halted.

Cryptococcosis

Infections with *Cryptococcus neoformans* are well-described in immunocompromised hosts. Meningitis, meningoencephalitis, pneumonitis, and fungemia have all been described in patients with AIDS. Diagnosis is usually facilitated by obtaining a positive cryptococcal antigen from cerebrospinal and/or serum specimens. Therapy and clinical course do not appear substantially different from other compromised patients. Systemic (intravenous) amphotericin B with or without oral 5-fluorocytosine is the therapy of choice. Falling titers and the body fluids or sites may help determine duration of therapy. Prolonged suppressive therapy may be required in some patients.

Cryptosporidiosis

Cryptosporidium represents a newly recognized coccidial protozoan that may cause transient infection and enteritis in healthy humans [109]. The organism is well known as a veterinary pathogen, especially in cattle, and many of the cases of cryptosporidial diarrhea in otherwise healthy humans have occurred in individuals with occupational exposure to cattle. In contrast, a number of cases of severe persistent bowel infections due to *Cryptosporidium* have been reported in AIDS patients [110,111]. Such patients may be either asymptomatic or mildly ill with loose bowel movements, or have a severe cholera-like diarrhea producing profound inanition and fluid and electrolyte disturbances. The small (2 to 6 μm) organisms may be seen along the brush border on bowel biopsies (Fig. 10) or can be identified by their acid-fast staining properties in stool concentrates [112]. Therapy for cryptosporidial diarrhea has been disappointing [113]; numerous agents with activity against other parasites have been tried without success and therapy remains supportive, with fluid and electrolyte replacement and nutritional therapy to prevent or reverse the inevitable cachexia

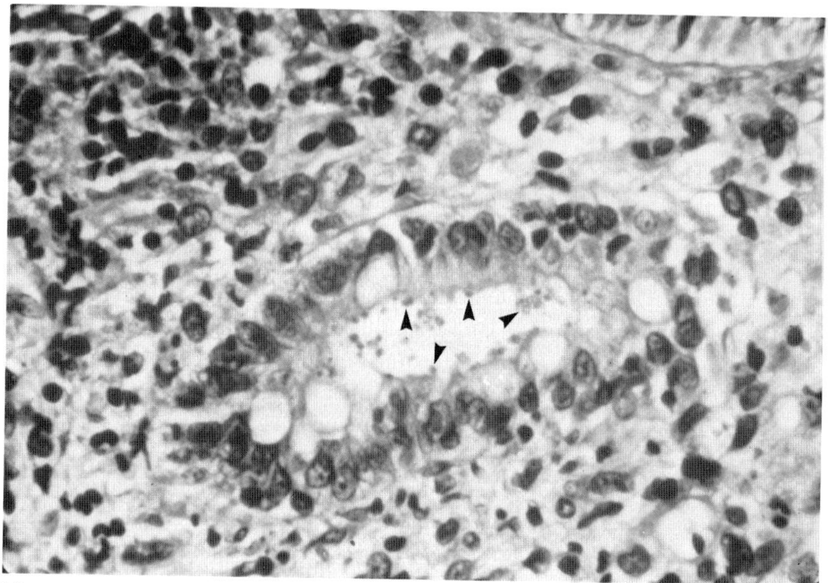

(a)

Fig. 10 (a) Colonoscopic biopsy of a young homosexual man with unexplained diarrhea. The biopsy reveals characteristic 2- to 6-μm cryptosporidia (arrows) along the luminal border of the bowel (hematoxylin-phloxine-safran stain, 400X). (Photograph courtesy of Dr. H. Z. Rotterdam, Lenox Hill Hospital, New York, New York.) (b) Cryptosporidium oocysts (arrow) before sporulation (Sheather's sugar flotation, 1000X). (Photograph courtesy of Dr. C. W. Lerner, Lenox Hill Hospital, New York, New York.) (c) Kinyoun's stain of stool concentrate. Acid-fast staining by traditional or fluorescent techniques readily reveals cryptosporidial organisms and helps differentiate them from yeasts.

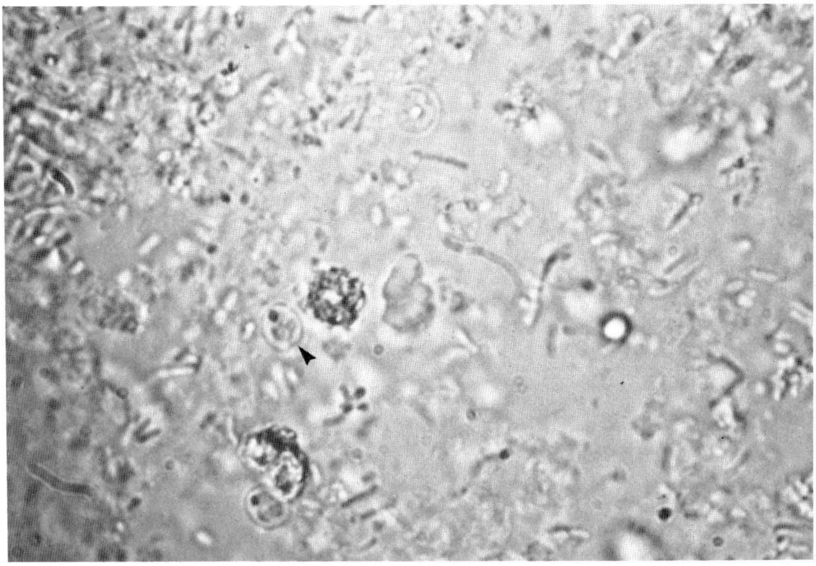

(b)

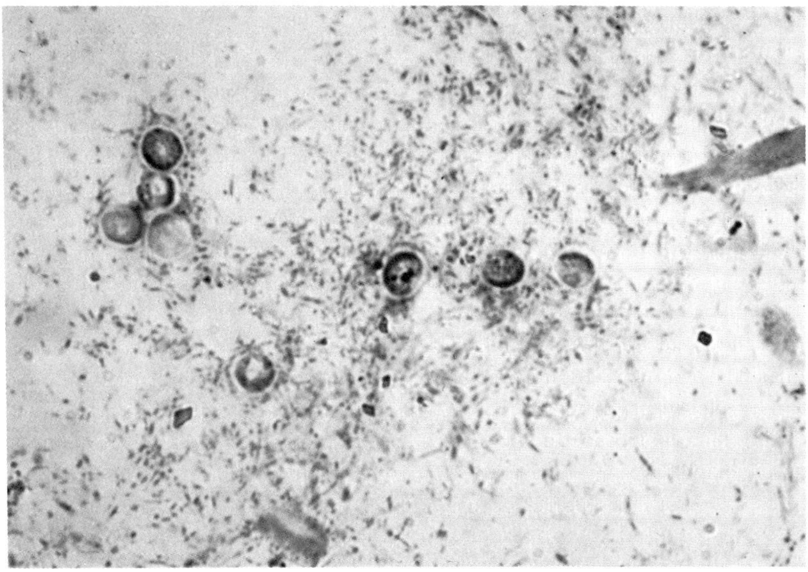

(c)

that accompanies more severe cases. A recent report from the CDC has noted successful therapy for cryptosporidial diarrhea using spiramycin, a macrolide antibiotic related to erythromycin [114].

Miscellaneous Infections

Smaller numbers of cases of infection caused by other pathogens known to affect patients with altered cell-mediated immunity have been reported, including histoplasmosis, progressive multifocal leukoencephalopathy [115], molluscum contagiosum, and enteritis due to *Isospora* species. One of the mysteries of AIDS is the emergence of novel virulent pathogens such as MAI and *Cryptosporidium*, not commonly recognized previously in other immunosuppressed patients, and the relative infrequency or absence of more familiar pathogens such as *Listeria* and *Nocardia* known to afflict other patients with altered cell-mediated immunity.

The Lymphadenopathy Syndrome (AIDS-Related Complex)

Simultaneously with the onset of the AIDS phenomenon, clinicians in several cities began reporting large numbers of homosexual men with unexplained persistent lymphadenopathy [116]. Extensive work-ups for known causes of such diffuse lymphadenopathy were unrevealing in most cases. Apart from the lymphadenopathy, most patients were healthy, although many gave histories of multiple previous venereal infections and most had serological evidence of prior exposure to EBV, CMV, and hepatitis B [53]. Biopsies of lymph nodes reveal a fairly uniform picture of intense reactive hyperplasia, similar to that seen in severe viral disease (Fig. 11). Immunological studies in such patients often show a moderate decrease in T-helper numbers and a reversed T-helper/T-suppressor ratio, similar although not as severe as that noted in AIDS. The precise relation of this "lymphadenopathy syndrome" to AIDS is unclear. In many patients the lymphadenopathy has spontaneously regressed after several months and the patients remain well; others have gone on to develop lymphoma or KS in the involved nodes and have become frank AIDS cases [117]. Many workers speculate that this represents an initial infection by a lymphotrophic viral agent with a varying pattern of subsequent response including progression to AIDS, transformation to lymphoma, or resolution. The concomitant presence of recurrent oral candidiasis or evidence of systemic disease (fever, night sweats, and weight loss) has been associated with a higher incidence of progression to specific AIDS diagnoses in our experience.

Homosexual patients with the lymphadenopathy syndrome should be under close medical surveillance. A period of 2 to 3 months observation is probably justified to allow self-limited lymphadenitis to resolve and to obtain serological studies for known causes of diffuse lymphadenopathy in homosexual men, including EBV, CMV, toxoplasmosis, syphilis, and lymphogranuloma venereum. By the end of this period, biopsy of a node is indicated, and serial biopsies from different sites should be considered if the adenopathy persists particularly if other findings such as oral thrush or fever are also present.

Plate II

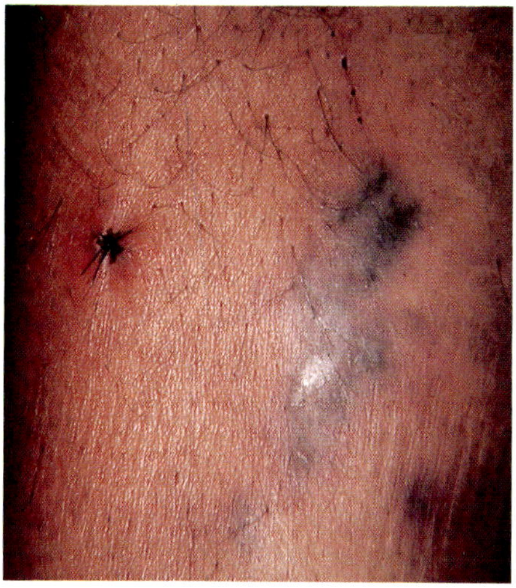

Fig. 1 Kaposi's sarcoma of the lower leg in a young homosexual male. (Photograph courtesy of Dr. H. Hochman, Lenox Hill Hospital, New York, New York.)

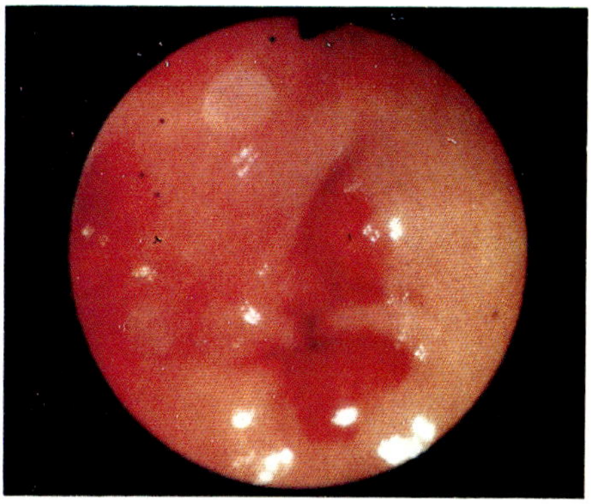

Fig. 2 Kaposi's sarcoma of the stomach found on endoscopic examination of a homosexual patient. (Photograph courtesy of Dr. H. Bornstein, Lenox Hill Hospital, New York, New York.)

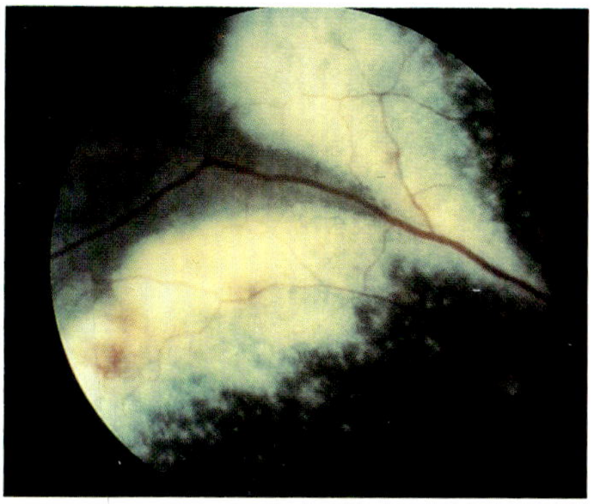

Fig. 7 The ocular fundus of a patient with disseminated CMV; the retinal findings are typical of CMV retinitis (proven at autopsy). (Photograph courtesy of Dr. W. R. Freeman, Lenox Hill Hospital, New York, New York.)

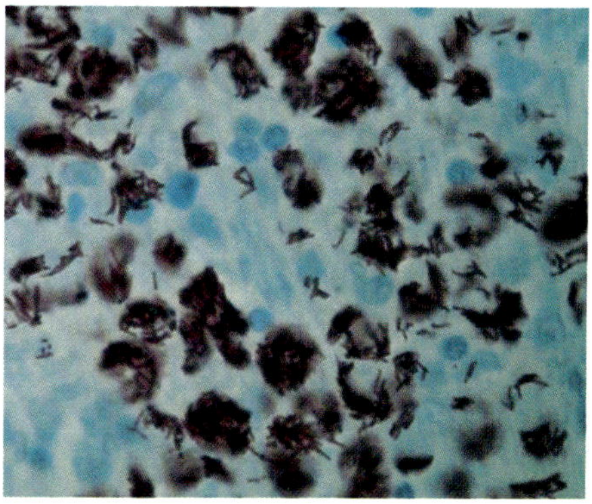

Fig. 8 Acid-fast organisms seen in the para-aortic lymph node of an AIDS patient with disseminated CMV, cryptococcosis, and mycobacteriosis. Bone marrow, sputum, and lymph node cultures grew *Mycobacterium avium-intracellulare* (Kinyoun's acid-fast stain, 400X). (Photograph courtesy of Dr. H. Z. Rotterdam, Lenox Hill Hospital, New York, New York.)

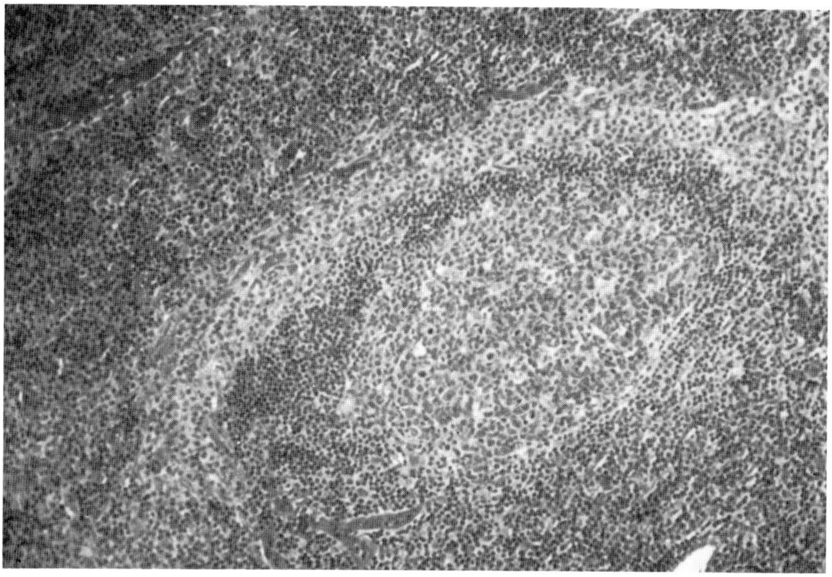

(a)

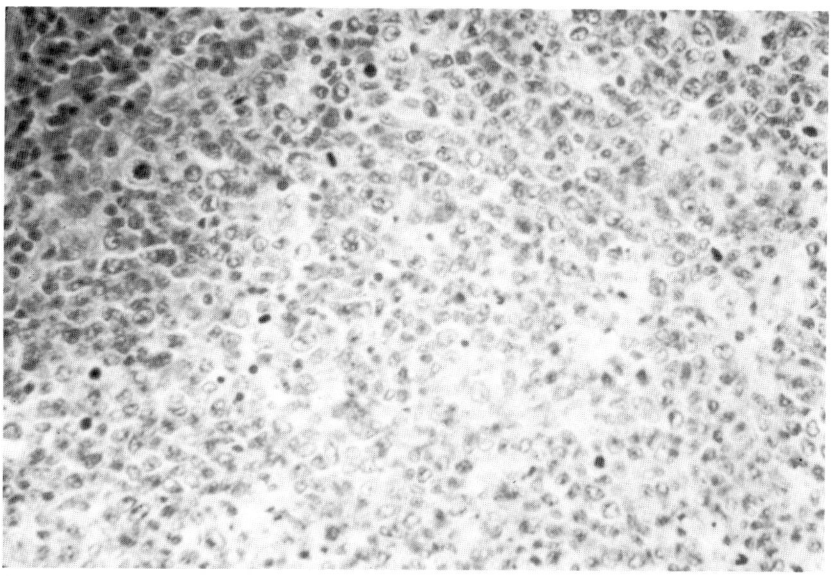

(b)

Fig. 11 (a) Lymph node biopsy from a homosexual man with chronic unexplained lymphadenopathy. Marked germinal center hyperplasia is present (hematoxylin-phloxine-safran stain, 250X). (b) Higher power reveals marked infiltration of lymph node by neutrophils and macrophages ingesting cellular debris (hematoxylin-phloxine-safran stain, 400X). (Photograph courtesy of Dr. H. Ioachim, Lenox Hill Hospital, New York, New York.)

The Wasting Syndrome

Physicians caring for patients with AIDS have noted the frequent presence of weight loss, apathy, depression, and progressive mental and physical deterioration in many patients, even in the absence of proven opportunistic infections or malignancies, a constellation of findings which has been referred to as the "wasting syndrome." While some of these findings may be due to unrecognized infections or malignancies, they do convey the progressive and relentless deterioration that is often seen in these patients. Exclusion of latent infections or malignancies, or borderline adrenal insufficiency [100,101], is obviously important; so too is nutritional therapy and emotional support by family, friends, and health care personnel. The tendency to withdraw from hopelessly ill patients is all too familiar to most health care workers; it is an even more difficult situation when the patient is a member of a high-risk group that may itself be the object of social discrimination, and the victim of a frightening disease of unknown communicability related to individual ethnic background, social habits, or sexual preference. Nutritional support is extremely important in these "wasting" patients. Enteral hyperalimentation may be tried, although patients with bowel inflammation of whatever etiology often find their symptoms exacerbated by enteral feedings. Concern about nosocomial superinfection should not delay the early institution of intravenous hyperalimentation if indicated.

Lymphoma

An increased incidence of diffuse non-Hodgkin's lymphoma [118] and Burkitt's lymphoma [119] in homosexual males has been reported, and isolated central nervous system lymphoma is now accepted as a criterion for the diagnosis of AIDS. In some cases lymphoma appears to have superseded lymphadenitis in chronically enlarged nodes. The relation of these lymphomas to AIDS remains speculative. Many have been unusually aggressive and response to chemotherapy disappointing.

HOSPITAL CARE

Caring for patients with AIDS can impose a considerable physical, financial, and emotional strain on a health care facility and its personnel. Acquired immune deficiency syndrome patients are often chronically ill, severely debilitated, and physically and emotionally dependent. Significant support persons, including family and friends, may withdraw from the patient because of fear about disease transmission or disapproval of life-style. Health care workers may not escape such feelings or fears. The absence of proven transmission of AIDS to any health care worker despite the presence of large numbers of such patients in health care facilities over the past 3 years suggests the low risk of such transmission. Long-term follow-up studies of health care workers with needle stick injuries from AIDS patients are currently in progress to better define this risk [120].

The CDC and the Office of Biosafety of the National Institutes of Health (NIH) have prepared extensive guidelines for the hospital care of AIDS patients and the handling of specimens from such patients. These guidelines have been published in the *Morbidity and Mortality Weekly Reports* and widely reprinted [121]. Recognizing the similarity in epidemiology between AIDS and hepatitis B, the guidelines suggest that all patients be placed on blood and secretion precautions, and body tissues and fluids from such patients be so labeled. Additional forms of isolation appropriate to the patient's condition (e.g., enteric precautions for patients with diarrhea) should also be instituted, but isolation precautions should not be allowed to compromise the patient's physical or emotional care or to ostracize such patients. Ongoing discussion, reassurance, and education by infection control personnel is usually required to assure both protection of staff and other patients and to assure that patient care needs are being met. Disposable equipment should be used preferentially where contamination by a patient's blood or body fluids can be expected; nondisposable instruments such as endoscopes and bronchoscopes should be gas-sterilized after each use. The reader is referred to the CDC and National Institutes of Health guidelines for explicit details.

REFERENCES

1. Centers for Disease Control. Pneumocystis pneumonia—Los Angeles. Morbid Mortal Week Rep 1981; 30:250-2.
2. Centers for Disease Control. Kaposi's sarcoma and pneumocystis pneumonia among homosexual men—New York City and California. Morbid Mortal Week Rep 1981; 30:305-8.
3. Centers for Disease Control. Update on acquired immune deficiency syndrome (AIDS)—United States. Morbid Mortal Week Rep 1982; 31:507-14.
4. Centers for Disease Control. An evaluation of the acquired immune deficiency syndrome (AIDS). Morbid Mortal Week Rep 1983; 32:358-60.
5. Gerstoft J, Malchow-Moller A, Bygbjerg I, Enk C, Halberg P, Haahr S, Jacobsen M, Jensen K, Mejer J, Nielsen JO, Thomsen HK, Sondergaard J, Lorenzen I. Severe acquired immunodeficiency in European homosexual males. Br Med J. 1982; 285:17-9.
6. Rozenbaum W, Klatzmann D, Mayaud C, Brun Vezinet F, Saimot G, Gluckmann JC, Carette MF, Rouzioux C, Couland JP. Syndrome d'immunodépression acquise chez 4 homosexuels. Presse Med 1983; 12:1149-54.
7. Francioli P, Vogt M, Schadelin J, Clément F, Russi E, Belacrétaz F, Perret C, Glauser MP. Syndrome de déficience immunitaire acquise, infections opportunistes et homosexualité. Schweiz Med Wochenschr 1982; 12:1682-7.
8. Offenstadt G, Pinta P, Hericord P, Jagueux M, Jean F, Amstutz P, Valade S, Lesavre P. Multiple opportunistic infection due to AIDS in a previously healthy black woman from Zaire. N Engl J Med 1983; 308:775.

9. O'Connor BH, McEvoy MB, Galbraith NS. Kaposi's sarcoma/AIDS surveillance in the UK. Lancet 1983; 1:872.
10. Sterry W, Marmor M, Konrads A, Steigleder GK. Kaposi's sarcoma, aplastic pancytopenia, and multiple infections in a homosexual (Cologne, 1976). Lancet 1983; 1:924-5.
11. Glauser MP, ed. Acquired immune deficiency syndrome (AIDS) in Europe. Eur J Clin Microbiol 1984; 3:53-67.
12. Centers for Disease Control. Acquired immunodeficiency syndrome (AIDS) update—United States. Morbid Mortal Week Rep 1983; 32:309-10.
13. Centers for Disease Control. A cluster of Kaposi's sarcoma and *Pneumocystis carinii* pneumonia among homosexual male residents of Los Angeles and Orange Counties, California. Morbid Mortal Week Rep 1982; 31:305-7.
14. Gottlieb MS, Schroff R, Schanker HM, Weisman JD, Peng Thim Fan, Wolf RA, Saxon A. *Pneumocystis carinii* pneumonia and mucosal candidiasis in previously healthy homosexual men: evidence of a new acquired cellular immunodeficiency. N Engl J Med 1981; 305:1425-31.
15. Follansbee SE, Busch DF, Wofsy CB, Lewis Coleman D, Gullet J, Aurigemma GP, Ross T, Hadley WK, Drew WL. An outbreak of *Pneumocystis carinii* pneumonia in homosexual men. Ann Intern Med 1982; 96:705-13.
16. Mildvan D, Mathur U, Enlow RW, Romain PL, Winchester RJ, Colp C, Singman H, Adelsberg BR, Spigland I. Opportunistic infections and immune deficiency in homosexual men. Ann Intern Med 1982; 96:700-4.
17. Jaffe HW, Choi K, Thomas PA, Haverkos HW, Auerbach DM, Guinan ME, Rogers MF, Spira TJ, Darrow WW, Kramer MA, Friedman SM, Monroe JM, Friedman-Klein AE, Laubenstein LJ, Marmor M, Safai B, Dritz SK, Crispi SJ, Fannin SL, Orkwis JP, Kelter A, Rushing WR, Thacker SB, Curran JW. National case-control study of Kaposi's sarcome and *Pneumocystis carinii* pneumonia in homosexual men: Part 1, epidemiologic results. Ann Intern Med 1983; 99:145-51.
18. Kornfeld H, Vande Stouwe RA, Lange M, Reddy MM, Grieco MH. T-Lymphocyte subpopulations in homosexual men. N Engl J Med 1982; 307:729-31.
19. Simberkoff MS. Infections in parenteral narcotic and drug abusers. In: Grieco MH, ed. Infections in the abnormal host. New York: Yorke Medical, 1980: 508-20.
20. Masur H, Michelis MA, Greene JB, Onorato I, Vande Stouwe RA, Holzman RS, Wormser G, Brettman L, Lange M, Murray HW, Cunninghan-Rundles S. An outbreak of community-acquired *Pneumocystis carinii* pneumonia: initial manifestation of cellular immune dysfunction. N Engl J Med 1981; 305: 1431-8.
21. Small CB, Klein RS, Friedland GH, Moll B, Emeson EE, Spigland I. Community-acquired opportunistic infections and defective cellular immunity in heterosexual drug abusers and homosexual men. Am J Med 1983; 74:433-41.
22. Wormser GP, Krupp LB, Hanrahan JP, Gavis G, Spira TJ, Cunningham-Rundles S. Acquired immunodeficiency syndrome in male prisoners: new insights into an emerging syndrome. Ann Intern Med 1983; 98:297-303.
23. Vieira J, Frank E, Spira TJ, Landesman SH. Acquired immune deficiency in Haitians: opportunistic infections in previously healthy Haitian immigrants. N Engl J Med 1983; 308:125-9.

24. Pitchenik AE, Fischl MA, Dickinson GM, Becker DM, Fournier AM, O'Connell MT, Colton RM, Spira TJ. Opportunistic infections and Kaposi's sarcoma among Haitians: evidence of a new acquired immunodeficiency state. Ann Intern Med 1983; 98:277-84.
25. Pape JW, Liautaud B, Thomas F, Mathurin JR, St. Amand MMA, Boncy M, Pean V, Pamphile M, Laroche AC, Johnson WD. Characteristics of the acquired immune deficiency syndrome (AIDS) in Haiti. N Engl J Med 1983; 309:945-50.
26. Ragni MV, Lewis JH, Spero JA, Bontempo FA. Acquired-immunodeficiency-like syndrome in two haemophiliacs. Lancet 1983; 1:213-4.
27. Davis KC, Horsburgh CR, Hasiba U, Schocket AL, Kirkpatrick CH. Acquired immunodeficiency syndrome in a patient with hemophilia. Ann Intern Med 1983; 98:284-6.
28. Poon MC, Landay A, Prasthofer EF, Stagno S. Acquired immunodeficiency syndrome with *Pneumocystis carinii* pneumonia and *Mycobacterium avium-intracellulare* infection in a previously healthy patient with classic hemophilia. Ann Intern Med 1983; 98:287-90.
29. Elliott JL, Hoppes WL, Platt MS, Thomas JG, Patel IP, Gansar A. The acquired immunodeficiency syndrome and *Mycobacterium avium-intracellulare* bacteremia in a patient with hemophilia. Ann Intern Med 1983; 98:290-3.
30. Evatt BL, Ramsey RB, Lawrence DN, Zyla LD, Curran JW. The acquired immunodeficiency syndrome in patients with hemophilia. Ann Intern Med 1984; 100:499-504.
31. Menitove JE, Aster RH, Casper JT, Lauer SJ, Gottschall JL, Williams JE, Gill JC, Wheeler DV, Piaskowski V, Kirchner P, Montgomery RR. T-Lymphocyte subpopulations in patients with classic hemophilia treated with cryoprecipitate and lyophilized concentrates. N Engl J Med 1983; 308:83-6.
32. Lederman MM, Ratnoff OD, Scillian JL, Jones PK, Schacter B. Impaired cell-mediated immunity in patients with classic hemophilia. N Engl J Med 1983; 308:79-83.
33. Goldsmith JC, Moseley PL, Monick M, Brady M, Hunninghake GW. T-Lymphocyte subpopulation abnormalities in apparently healthy patients with hemophilia. Ann Intern Med 1983; 98:294-6.
34. Luban NLC, Kelleher Jr. JF, Reaman GH. Altered distribution of T-lymphocyte subpopulations in children and adolescents with haemophilia. Lancet 1983; 1:503-5.
35. DeShazo RD, Andes WA, Nordberg J, Newton J, Daul C, Bozelka B. An immunologic evaluation of hemophiliac patients and their wives: relationships to the acquired immunodeficiency syndrome. Ann Intern Med 1983; 99: 159-64.
36. Kreiss JK, Lawrence DN, Kasper CK, Goldstein AL, Naylor PH, McLane MF, Lee TH, Essex M. Antibody to human T-cell leukemia virus membrane antigens, beta$_2$-microglobulin levels, and thymosin alpha$_1$ levels in hemophiliacs and their spouses. Ann Intern Med 1984; 100:178-82.
37. Desforges JF. AIDS and preventive treatment in hemophilia. N Engl J Med 1983; 308:94-5.
38. DeShazo RD, Andes WA, Nordberg J, Newton J, Daul C, Bozelka B. An immunologic evaluation of hemophiliac patients and their wives: relationships

to the acquired immunodeficiency syndrome. Ann Intern Med 1983; 99: 159-64.

39. Curran JW, Lawrence DN, Jaffe H, Kaplan JE, Zyla LD, Chamberland M, Weinstein R, Lui KJ, Schonberger LB, Spira TJ, Alexander WJ, Swinger G, Ammann A, Solomon S, Averbach D, Mildvan D, Stoneburner R, Jason JM, Haverkos HW, Evatt BL. Acquired immunodeficiency syndrome (AIDS) associated with transfusions. N Engl J Med 1984; 310:69-75.
40. Andreani T, Le Charpentier Y, Brouet JC, Lachance JR, Modigliani R, Galian A, Liance M, Messing B, Vernisse B. Acquired immunodeficiency with intestinal cyrptosporidiosis: possible transmission by Haitian whole blood. Lancet 1983; 1:1187-91.
41. Ammann AJ, Wara DW, Dritz S, Cowan MJ, Weintrub P, Goldman H, Perkins HA. Acquired immunodeficiency in an infant: possible transmission by means of blood products. Lancet 1983; 1:956-8.
42. American Association of Blood Banks, American Red Cross, Council of Community Blood Centers, American Blood Commission, National Gay Task Force, National Hemophilia Foundation, American Blood Resources Association, Centers for Disease Control, Food and Drug Administration. Joint statement on acquired immune deficiency syndrome (AIDS) related to transfusions. Transfusion 1983; 23:87-8.
43. Centers for Disease Control. Prevention of acquired immune deficiency syndrome (AIDS): report of inter-agency recommendations. Morbid Mortal Week Rep 1983; 32:101-3.
44. Masur H, Michelis MA, Wormser GP, Lewin S, Gold J, Tapper ML, Giron J, Lerner CW, Armstrong D, Setia U, Sender J, Siebken RS, Nicholas P, Arlen Z, Maayan S, Ernst JA, Siegal FP, Cunningham-Rundles S. Opportunistic infection in previously healthy women: initial manifestation of a community-acquired cellular immunodeficiency. Ann Intern Med 1982; 97:533-9.
45. Harris C, Small CB, Klein RS, Friedland GH, Moll B, Emeson EE, Spigland I, Steigbigel NH. Immunodeficiency in female sexual partners of men with the acquired immunodeficiency syndrome. N Engl J Med 1983; 308:1181-4.
46. Wallace JI, Downes J, Ott A, Reise R, Monroe J, Jordan D, Thomas Y, Glickman E, Rogozinski L, Chess L. T-Cell ratios in New York City prostitutes. Lancet 1983; 1:58-9.
47. Pitchenik AE, Shafron RD, Glasser RM, Spira TJ. The acquired immunodeficiency syndrome in the wife of a hemophiliac. Ann Intern Med 1984; 100: 62-5.
48. Rubenstein A, Sicklick M, Gupta A, Bernstein L, Klein N, Rubinstein E, Spigland I, Fruchter L, Litman N, Lee H, Hollander M. Acquired immunodeficiency with reversed T_4/T_8 ratios in infants born to promiscuous and drug-addicted mothers. J Am Med Assoc 1983; 249:2350-6.
49. Oleske J, Minnefor A, Cooper Jr. R, Thomas K, dela Cruz A, Ahdieh H, Guerrero I, Joshi VV, Desposito F. Immune deficiency syndrome in children. J Am Med Assoc 1983; 249:2345-9.
50. Scott GB, Buck BE, Leterman JG, Bloom FL, Parks WP. Acquired immunodeficiency syndrome in infants. N Engl J Med 1984; 310:76-81.

51. Shearer GM, Hurtenbach U. Is sperm immunosuppressive in male homosexuals and vasectomized men? Immunol Today 1982; 3:153-4.
52. Goedert JJ, Wallen WC, Mann DL, Strong DM, Neuland CY, Greene MH, Murray C, Fraumeni Jr. JF, Blattner WA. Amyl nitrite may alter T-lymphocytes in homosexual men. Lancet 1982; 1:412-5.
53. Ioachim HL, Lerner CW, Tapper ML. Lymphadenopathies in homosexual men: relationships with the acquired immune deficiency syndrome. J Am Med Assoc 1983; 250:1306-9.
54. Ho M. The lymphocyte in infections with Epstein-Barr virus and cytomegalovirus. J INfect Dis 1981; 143:857-61.
55. Carney WP, Rubin RH, Hoffman RA, Hansen WP, Healey K, Hirsch MS. Analysis of T lymphocyte subsets in cytomegalovirus mononucleosis. J Immunol 1981; 126:2114-6.
56. Lang DJ, Kummer JF, Hartley DP. Cytomegalovirus in semen: persistence and demonstration in extracellular fluids. N Engl J Med 1974; 291:121-3.
57. Drew WL, Mintz L, Miner RC, Sands M, Ketterer B. Prevalence of cytomegalovirus infection in homosexual men. J Infect Dis 1981; 143:188-92.
58. Giraldo G, Beth E, Coeur P, Vogel CL, Dhru DS. Kaposi's sarcome: a new model in the search for viruses associated with human malignancies. J Nat Cancer Inst 1972; 49:1495-507.
59. Drew WL, Miner RC, Ziegler JL, Gullet JH, Abrams DI, Conaut MA, Huang ES, Groundwater JR, Volberding P, Mintz L. Cytomegalovirus and Kaposi's sarcome in young homosexual men. Lancet 1982; 2:125-7.
60. Gelmann EP, Popovic M, Blayney D, Masur H, Sidhu G, Stahl R, Gallot RC. Proviral DNA of a retrovirus, human T-cell leukemia virus, in two patients with AIDS. Science 1983; 220:862-4.
61. Gallo RC, Sarin PS, Gelmann EP, Robert-Guroff M, RIchardson E, Kalyanaraman VS, Mann D, Sidhu GD, Stahl RE, Zolla-Pazner S, Leibowitch J, Popovic M. Isolation of human T-cell leukemia virus in acquired immune deficiency syndrome (AIDS). Science 1983; 220:865-7.
62. Barré-Sinoussi F, Chermann JC, Rey F, Nugeyre MT, Chamaret S, Gruest J, Dauguet C, Axler-Blin C, Vézinet-Brun F, Rouzioux C, Rozenbaum W, Montagnier L. Isolation of a T-lymphotrophic retrovirus from a patient at risk for acquired immune deficiency syndrome (AIDS). Science 1983; 220: 868-70.
63. Essex M, McLane MF, Lee TH, Falk L, Howe CWS, Mullins JI, Cabradilla C, Francis DP. Antibodies to cell membrane antigens associated with human T-cell leukemia virus in patients with AIDS. Science 1983; 220:859-62.
64. Essex M, McLane MF, Lee TH, Tachibana N, Mullins JI, Kreiss J, Kasper CK, Poon MC, Landay A, Stein SF, Francis DP, Cabradilla C, Lawrence DN, Evatt BL. Antibodies to human T-cell leukemia virus membrane antigens (HTLV-MA) in hemophiliacs. Science 1983; 221:1061-4.
65. Vilmer E, Rouzioux C, Vezinet Brun F, Fischer A, Chermann JC, Barre-Sinoussi F, Gazengel C, Dauguet C, Manigne P, Griscelli C, Montagnier I. Isolation of new lymphotrophic retrovirus from two siblings with haemophilia B one with AIDS. Lancet 1984; 1:753-7.

66. Popovic M, Sarngadharan MG, Read E, Gallo RC. Detection, isolation, and continuous production of cytopathic retroviruses (HTLV-III) from patients with AIDS and pre-AIDS. Science 1984; 224:497-500.
67. Gallo RC, Salahuddin SZ, Popovic M. Frequent detection and isolation of cytopathic retroviruses (HTLV-III) from patients with AIDS and at risk for AIDS. Science 1984; 224:500-3.
68. Schupbach J, Popovic M, Gilden RV, Gonda MA, Sarngadharan MG, Gallo RC. Serological analysis of a subgroup of human T-lymphotrophic retroviruses (HTLV-III) associated with AIDS. Science 1984; 224:503-5.
69. Sarngadharan MG, Popovic M, Bruch M, Schupbach J, Gallo RC. Antibodies reactive with human T-lymphotrophic retroviruses (HTLV-III) in the serum of patients with AIDS. Science 1984; 224:506-8.
70. Marx JL. Strong new candidate for AIDS agent: a newly discovered member of the human T-cell leukemia virus family is very closely linked to the immunodeficiency disease. Science 1984; 224:475-7.
71. Marx PA, Haul DH, Osborn KG, Lerche NW, Moody P, Lowenstine LJ, Henrickson RV, Arthur LO, Gilden RV, Gravell M, London WT, Sever JL, Levy JA, Munn RJ, Gardner MB. Simian AIDS: isolation of a type D retrovirus and transmission of the disease. Science 1984; 224:1083-6.
72. Stahl RE, Friedman-Kien A, Dubin R, Marmor M, Zolla-Pazner S. Immunologic abnormalities in homosexual men: relationship to Kaposi's sarcoma. Am J Med 1982; 73:171-8.
73. Rogers MF, Morens DM, Stewart JA, Kaminski RM, Spira TJ, Feorino PM, Larsen SA, Francis DP, Wilson M, Kaufman L, The Task Force on Acquired Immune Deficiency Syndrome. National case-control study of Kaposi's sarcoma and *Pneumocystis carinii* pneumonia in homosexual men: part 2, laboratory results. Ann Intern Med 1983; 99:151-8.
74. Siegal FP. Immune function and dysfunction in AIDS. Semin Oncol 1984; 11:29-39.
75. Morris L, Distinfeld A, Amorosi E, Karpatkin S. Autoimmune thrombocytopenic purpura in homosexual men. Ann Intern Med 1982; 96:714-7.
76. Ammann AJ, Schiffman G, Abrams D, Volverding P, Ziegler J, Conant M. B-Cell immunodeficiency in acquired immune deficiency syndrome. JAMA 1984; 251:1447-9.
77. Cunningham-Rundles S. Analysis of cellular immune deficiency in acquired immunodeficiency disease syndrome. American Society for Microbiology Conference on infections of homosexual men and the acquired immune deficiency syndrome (AIDS), September 1982, Memorial Sloan-Kettering Cancer Center, New York, New York.
78. Reuben JM, Hersh EM, Mansell PW, Rios A, Rossen R, Goldstein AL, McClure JE. Immunological characterization of homosexual males. Cancer Res 1983; 43:897-904.
79. Francioli P, Clément F. Beta$_2$-microglobulin and immunodeficiency in a homosexual man. N Engl J Med 1982; 307:1402-3.
80. DeStefano E, Friedman RM, Friedman-Kien AE, Goedert JJ, Henricksen D, Preble OT, Sonnabend JA, Vilcek J. Acid-labile human leukocyte interferon in homosexual men with Kaposi's sarcoma and lymphadenopathy. J Infect Dis 1982; 146:451-5.

81. Buimovici-Klein E, Lange M, Klein RJ, Cooper LZ, Grieco MH. Is presence of interferon predictive for AIDS? Lancet 1981; 2:598-600.
82. Hymes KB, Greene JB, Marcus A, William DC, Cheung T, Prose NS, Ballard H, Laubenstein LJ. Kaposi's sarcoma in homosexual men—a report of eight cases. Lancet 1981; 2:598-600.
83. Urmacher C, Myskowski P, Ochoa Jr. M, Kris M, Safai B. Outbreak of Kaposi's sarcoma with cytomegalovirus infection in young homosexual men. Am J Med 1982; 72:569-79.
84. Friedman-Kien AE, Laubenstein LJ, Rubenstein P, Buimovici-Klein E, Marmor M, Stahl R, Spigland I, Kim KS, Zolla-Pazner S. Disseminated Kaposi's sarcoma in homosexual men. Ann Intern Med 1982; 96:693-700.
85. Ziegler JL, Templeton AC, Vogel CL. Kaposi's sarcoma: a comparison of classical, endemic, and epidemic forms. Semin Oncol 1984; 11:47-52.
86. Mitsuyasu RT, Groopman JE. Biology and therapy of Kaposi's sarcoma. Semin Oncol 1984; 11:53-9.
87. Rose HS, Balthazar EJ, Megibow AJ, Horowitz L, Laubenstein LJ. Alimentary tract involvement in Kaposi sarcoma: radiographic and endoscopic findings in 25 homosexual men. Am J Roentgenol 1982; 139:661-6.
88. Volberding P. Therapy of Kaposi's sarcoma in AIDS. Semin Oncol 1984; 11:60-7.
89. Krown SE, Real FX, Cunningham-Rundles S, Myskowski PL, Koziner B, Fein S, Mittelman A, Oettgen H, Safai B. Preliminary observations on the effect of recombinant leukocyte A interferon in homosexual men with Kaposi's sarcoma. N Engl J Med 1983; 308:1071-6.
90. Kovacs JA, Hiemenz JW, Macher AM, Stover D, Murray HW, Shelhamer J, Lane HC, Urmacker C, Honig C, Longo DL, Parker MM, Natanson C, Parrillo JE, Fauci AS, Pizzo PA, Masor H. *Pneumocystis carinii* pneumonia: a comparison between patients with the acquired immunodeficiency syndrome and patients with other immunodeficiencies. Ann Intern Med 1984; 100: 663-71.
91. Vanley GT, Huberman R, Lufkin RB. Atypical *Pneumocystis carinii* pneumonia in homosexual men with unusual immunodeficiency. Am J Roentgenol 1982; 138:1037-41.
92. Gamsu G, Hecht ST, Birnberg FA, Coleman DL, Golden JA. *Pneumocystis carinii* pneumonia in homosexual men. Am J Roentgenol 1982; 139:647-51.
93. McCauley DI, Naidich DP, Leitman BS, Reede DL, Laubenstein L. Radiographic patterns of opportunistic lung infections and Kaposi sarcoma in homosexual men. Am J Roentgenol 1982; 139:653-8.
94. Jaffe HS, Ammann AJ, Abrams DI, Lewis BJ, Golden JA. Complications of cotrimoxazole in treatment of AIDS-associated *Pneumocystis carinii* pneumonia in homosexual men. Lancet 1983; 2:1109-11.
95. Gordin FM, Simon GL, Wofsy CB, Mills J. Adverse reations to trimethoprim-sulfamethoxazole in patients with the acquired immunodeficiency syndrome. Ann Intern Med 1984; 100:495-9.
96. Kluge RM, Spaulding DM, Spain AJ. Combination of pentamidine and trimethoprim-sulfamethoxazole in the therapy of *Pneumocystis carinii* pneumonia in rats. Antimicrob Agents Chemother 1978; 13:975-8.

97. Siegal FP, Lopez C, Hammer GS, Brown AE, Kornfeld SJ, Gold J, Hassett J, Hirschman SZ, Cunningham-Rundles C, Adelsberg BR, Parham DM, Siegal M, Cunningham-Rundles S, Armstrong D. Severe acquired immunodefiency in male homosexuals, manifested by chronic perianal ulcerative *Herpes simplex* lesions. N Engl J Med 1981; 305:1439-44.
98. Tapper ML, Lerner CW, Rotterdam HZ. Opportunistic infections complicating acquired immune deficiency syndrome. In: Ma P, Armstrong D, eds. The acquired immune deficiency syndrome and infections of homosexual men, New York: Yorke Medical, 1984:225-39.
99. Tapper ML, Pollock AA, Lerner CW, Bruno MS, Bahr GS, Bruno PJ, Sohn N, Weinstein MA, Robbins R, Wong B, Gold JWM, Armstrong D. Disseminated CMV in immunosuppressed homosexual men presenting as refractory diarrhoea. In: Easmon CSF, Gaya H, eds. Second international symposium on infections in the immunocompromised host. London: Academic, 1983:389-91.
100. Tapper ML, Lerner CW, Seitzman PA, Al'Khafaji K, Rotterdam HZ. Adrenal necrosis and acute adrenal insufficiency in the acquired immune deficiency syndrome. 23rd Interscience Conference on Antimicrobial Agents and Chemotherapy, Las Vegas, Nevada, October 1983.
101. Tapper ML, Rotterdam HZ, Lerner CW, Al'Khafaji K, Seitzman PA. Adrenal necrosis in the acquired immunodeficiency syndrome. Ann Intern Med 1984; 100:239-41.
102. Freeman WR, Lerner CW, Mines JA, Lash RS, Nadel AJ, Starr MB, Tapper ML. A prospective study of the ophthalmologic findings in the acquired immune deficiency syndrome. Am J Ophthalmol 1984; 97:133-42.
103. Greene JB, Sidhu GS, Lewin S, Levine JF, Masur H, Simberkoff MS, Nicholas P, Good RC, Zolla-Pazner SB, Pollock AA, Tapper M, Holzman RS. *Mycobacterium avium-intracellulare*: a cause of disseminated life-threatening infection in homosexuals and drug abusers. Ann Intern Med 1982; 97: 539-46.
104. Zakowski P, Fligiel S, Berlin OGW, Johnson BL. Disseminated *Mycobacterium avium-intracellulare* infection in homosexual men dying of acquired immunodeficiency. J Am Med Assoc 1982; 248:2980-2.
105. Gold JWM, Weikel CL, Tapper ML, Kiehn TE, Lerner CW, Urmacher C, Rotterdam HZ, Armstrong D. Disseminated *Mycobacterium avium-intracellulare* infection in patients with acquired immune deficiency syndrome mimicking Whipple's disease. 23rd Interscience Conference on Antimicrobial Agents and Chemotherapy, Las Vegas, Nevada, October 1983.
106. Baron EJ, Berlin OGW, Bruckner DA, Young LS. Antimicrobial combinations with N-formimidoyl thienamycin and amikacin inhibit *Mycobacterium avium-intracellulare* (MAI). Presented at the 23rd Interscience Conference on Antimicrobial Agents and Chemotherapy, Las Vegas, Nevada, October 1983.
107. Post MJD, Chan JC, Hensley GT, Hoffman T, Moskowitz LB, Lippmann S. Toxoplasma encephalitis in Haitian adults with acquired immunodeficiency syndrome: a clinical-pathologic CT correlation. Am J Neuroradiol 1983; 4:155-62.

108. Wong B, Gold JWM, Brown AE, Lauge M, Fried R, Grieco M, Mildvan D, Giron J, Tapper ML, Lerner CW, Armstrong D. Central nervous system toxoplasmosis in homosexual men and parenteral drug abusers in New York. Ann Intern Med 1984; 100:36-42.
109. Current WL, Reese NC, Ernst JV, Bailey WS, Heyman MB, Weinstein WM. Human cryptosporidiosis in immunocompetent and immunodeficient persons: studies of an outbreak and experimental transmission. N Engl J Med 1983; 308:1252-7.
110. Pitlik SD, Fainstein V, Garza D, Guard L, Bolivar R, Rios A, Hopfer RL, Mansell PA. Human Cryptosporidiosis: spectrum of disease–report of six cases and review of the literature. Arch Intern Med 1983; 143:2269-75.
111. Soave RM, Danner RL, Honig CL, Pearl, Hart CC, Nash T, Roberts RB. Cryptosporidiosis in homosexual men. Ann Intern Med 1984; 100:504-11.
112. Carcia LS, Bruckner DA, Brewer TC, Shimizu RY. Techniques for the recovery and identification of *Cryptosporidium* oocysts from stool specimens. J Clin Microbiol 1983; 18:185-90.
113. Centers for Disease Control. Cryptosporidiosis: assessment of chemotherapy of males with acquired immune deficiency syndrome (AIDS). Morbid Mortal Week Rep 1982; 31:589-92.
114. Centers for Disease Control. Update: treatment of cryptosporidiosis in patients with acquired immunodeficiency syndrome (AIDS). Morbid Mortal Week Rep 1984; 33:117-9.
115. Miller JR, Barrett RE, Britton CB, Tapper ML, Bahr GS, Bruno PJ, Marquardt MD, Hays AP, McMurtry III JG, Weissman JB, Bruno MS. Progressive multifocal leukeoencephalopathy in a male homosexual with T-cell immune deficiency. N Engl J Med 1982; 307:1436-8.
116. Centers for Disease Control. Persistent, generalized lymphadenopathy among homosexual males. Morbid Mortal Week Rep 1982; 31:249-51.
117. Metroka CE, Cunningham-Rundles S, Pollack MS, Sonnabend JA, Davis JM, Gordon B, Fernandez RD, Mouradian J. Generalized lymphadenopathy in homosexual men. Ann Intern Med 1983; 99:585-91.
118. Centers for Disease Control. Diffuse, undifferentiated non-Hodgkin's lymphoma among homosexual males-United States. Morbid Mortal Week Rep 1982; 31:277-9.
119. Ziegler JL, Miner RC, Rosenbaum E, Lennette ET, Shillitoe E, Casavant C, Drew WL, Mintz L, Gershow J, Greenspan J, Beckstead J, Yamamoto K. Outbreak of Burkitt's-like lymphoma in homosexual men. Lancet 1982; 2:631-3.
120. Centers for Disease Control. Prospective evaluation of health-care workers exposed via parenteral or mucous-membrane routes to blood and body fluids of patients with acquired immunodeficiency syndrome. Morbid Mortal Week Rep 1984; 33:181-2.
121. Centers for Disease Control. Acquired immune deficiency syndrome (AIDS): precautions for clinical and laboratory staffs. Morbid Mortal Week Rep 1982; 31:577-80.

TWELVE

Condyloma Acuminatum and Other Human Papillomavirus-Induced Diseases

Charles Camisa
The Ohio State University
College of Medicine
Columbus, Ohio

INTRODUCTION

Condylomata acuminata are benign epithelial tumors of the genitalia, perineum, and anus caused by a type of human papillomavirus. The anatomical sites of predilection and epidemiological considerations suggest that they are sexually transmitted, thus the common synonym genital or venereal warts. Condyloma acuminatum was a well-defined disease in Roman-Hellenistic times. Recorded by Celsus in the beginning of the first century A.D., it was considered to be venereal and mainly transmitted by homosexual intercourse [1]. (The term *condyloma* is derived from Greek and Latin words that mean joint, knuckle, or fist; *acuminata* is a Latin adjective meaning pointed [2].) Evidence that not all genital warts are venereal includes the distinct possibilities of autoinoculation and transmission to children (in utero, during parturition, and by nonsexual contact). An incubation period has never been established (average, 2 to 3 months), and only about 60% of sexual partners of infected individuals develop condylomata acuminata [3].

According to the Centers for Disease Control, the estimated number of consultations for condyloma acuminatum with office-based private physicians in the United States increased 459% in the last 15 years. Moreover, in 1981 condylomata acuminata accounted for more than three times as many consultations as genital herpes [4]. In a limited Centers for Disease Control study of visits to public clinics for sexually transmitted diseases, visits for condyloma acuminatum surpassed those for genital herpes for both sexes [5]. As might be expected, young adults comprise the population at risk: The majority of patients are aged 15 to 29 years. Women are affected about as frequently as men and are most likely to consult a gynecologist or a dermatologist.

This review will cover (1) the etiology of condyloma acuminatum, the human papillomavirus, (2) the role of humoral and cell-mediated immunity, (3) the treatment of condyloma acuminatum by anatomical site, and (4) the relation of human papillomavirus and condyloma acuminatum to other important diseases–juvenile laryngeal papillomatosis, verrucous carcinoma (giant condyloma of Buschke-Lowenstein), bowenoid papulosis, and carcinoma of the cervix.

CLINICAL MANIFESTATIONS

General Considerations

Condylomata acuminata are recognized as pink to gray discrete soft excrescences, single or in clusters, broad based or pedunculated, which may enlarge to form cauliflower-like growths in the anogenital regions. Lesions are usually not symptomatic, but they may be friable and bleed easily on contact. Some patients may complain of pain or pruritus. In clinical practice, the differential diagnosis should include condylomata lata of secondary syphilis and molluscum contagiosum, although these diseases can be easily ruled out with a serological test for syphilis and biopsy, respectively. Patients should also be examined for gonorrhea, since common venereal diseases frequently coexist. They should encourage their sexual partners to be examined and treated if necessary for condyloma acuminatum as well. The same basic clinical morphology obtains whether condyloma acumina-

---

Fig. 1 Perianal condylomata acuminata in a male.

Fig. 2 Condylomata acuminata involving the foreskin and preputial cavity of the penis.

Fig. 3 Vulvar and perianal condylomata acuminata with associated cutaneous candidiasis.

Fig. 6 Clinical photograph demonstrates locally destructive effect of varrucous carcinoma (giant condyloma of Buschke-Loewenstein) arising from the glans penis.

Fig. 7 Bowenoid papulosis is demonstrated by the group of small papules on the shaft of the penis and the violaceous plaque on the glans. The hypopigmented area represents a sequela of liquid nitrogen therapy.

Plate III

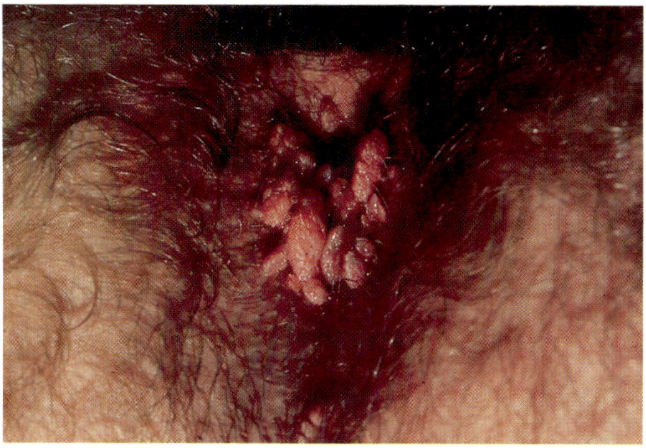

Fig. 1

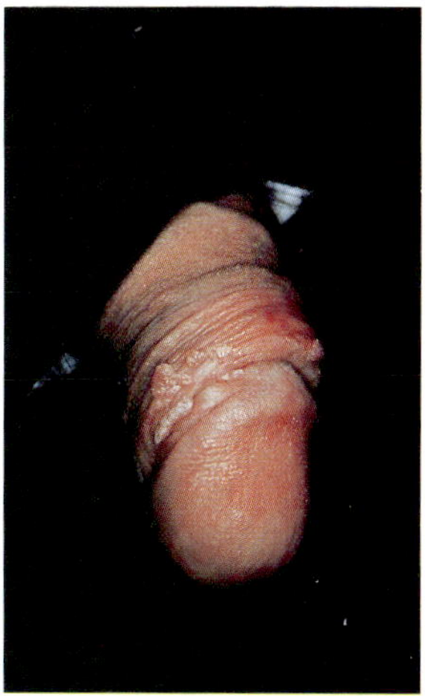

Fig. 2

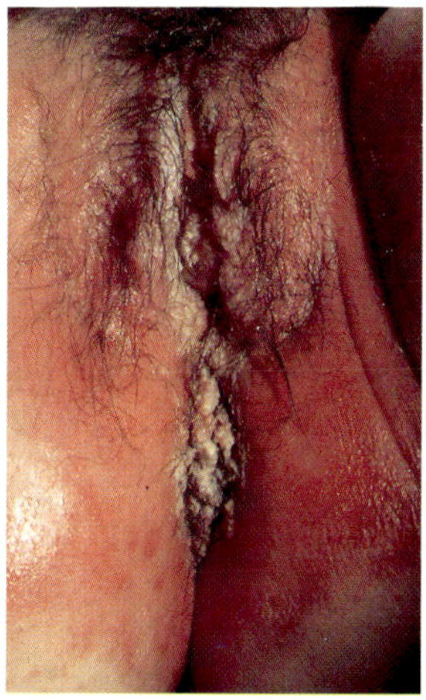

Fig. 3

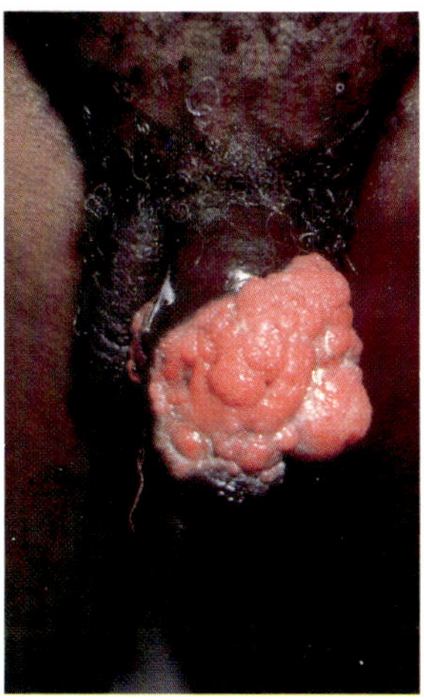

Fig. 6

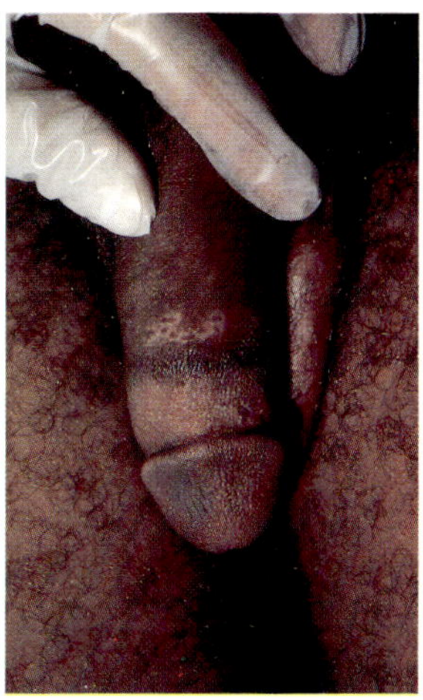

Fig. 7

tum involves the penis, urethra, perineum, anus, rectum, vulva, or vagina [Figs. 1-3 (see Plate III, facing p. 310)]; however, flat and endophytic forms have also recently been recognized in the uterine cervix [6].

Histologically, a typical condyloma acuminatum is characterized by papillated epidermal hyperplasia, parakeratosis, occasional cells with prominent halos around the nuclei in the upper portions of the epidermis (called koilocytes), occasional mitotic figures (none atypical), increased numbers of dilated and tortuous capillaries within the dermal papillae, and sparse perivascular lymphohistiocytic infiltrates (Figs. 4 and 5).

Numerous therapeutic modalities for condyloma acuminatum have been attempted (Tables 1 and 2), attesting to the fact that no one treatment is completely satisfactory for all cases. Table 1 is organized into four categories of treatments, and Table 2 lists treatments of choice for selected lesions by anatomical site.

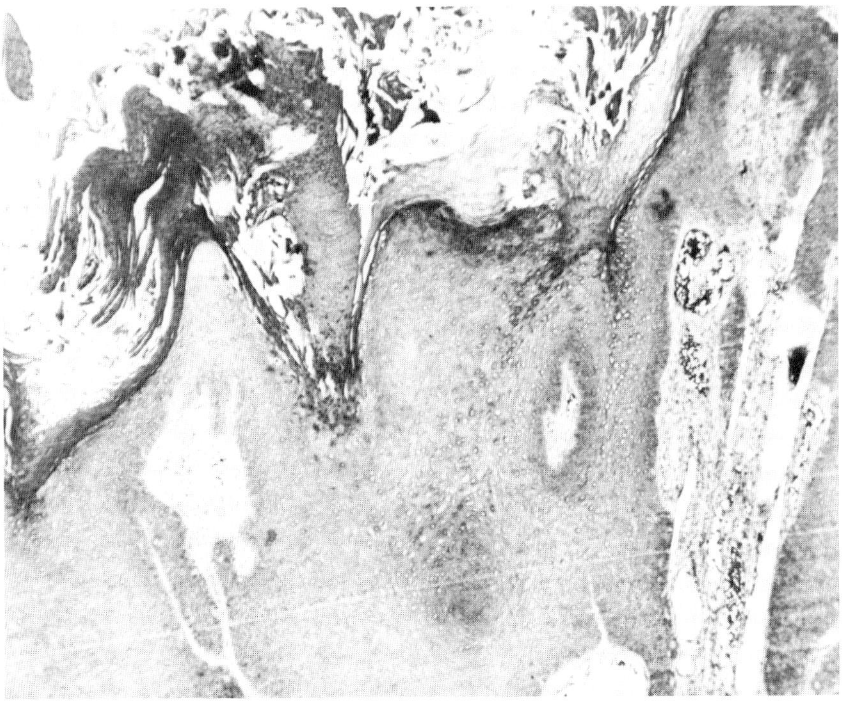

Fig. 4 Biopsy of a large pedunculated condyloma acuminatum demonstrates hyperkeratosis, focal parakeratosis, marked acanthosis, vacuolated keratinocytes in the upper layers of the epidermis, and dilated capillaries in the dermis (hematoxylin-eosin, original magnification 6.3X). (Photograph courtesy of S. Strobel.)

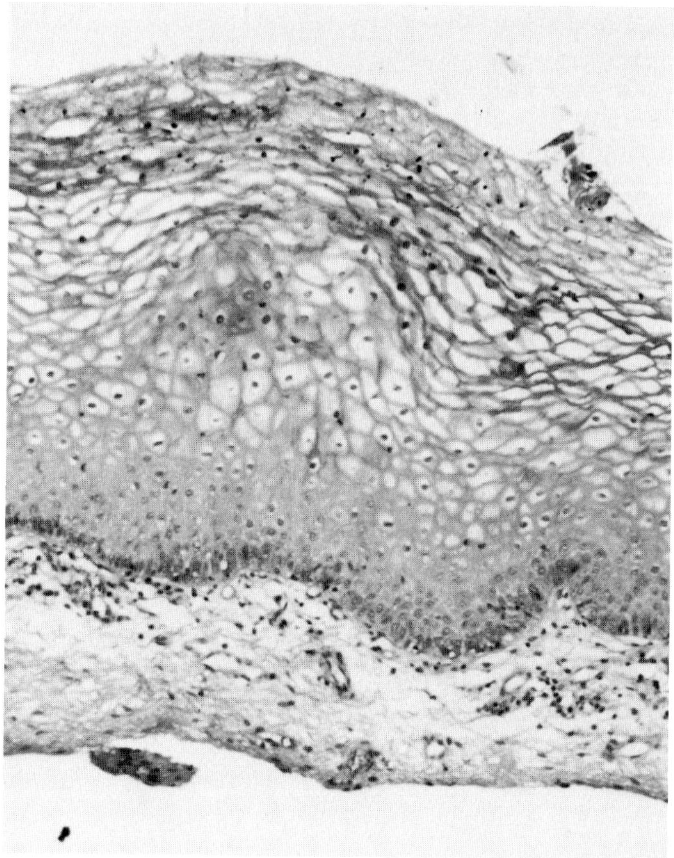

Fig. 5 Biopsy of a small, flat vulvar condyloma acuminatum demonstrates koilocytic changes (hematoxylin-eosin, original magnification 16X). (Photograph courtesy of S. Strobel.)

Human Papillomavirus

As recently as the late 1960s it was believed that the same virus caused all types of warts and that their clinical expression was determined by the infected anatomical site. The human papillomavirus (HPV) is 55 nm in diameter. The genetic information is contained within circular double-stranded DNA with a molecular weight of about 5×10^6 daltons [34]. Research of HPV in general and the cause of condyloma acuminatum in particular has been inhibited by the lack of a successful tissue culture system for the propagation of papillomaviruses and the relative paucity of viral particles in lesions of condylomata acuminata compared to

Table 1 Treatment Modalities for Condyloma Acuminatum

Accepted first choice	Second-line choice	Ineffective or contraindicated	Experimental
Podophyllin [7,8]	Colchicine [19,20]	BCG [25]	Podophyllotoxin [7]
5-Fluorouracil [9-11]	Bleomycin [21,22]	Levamisole [26]	Dinitrochlorobenzene [29]
Halogenated acetic acid [12,13]	Thio-TEPA [23,24]	Cimetidine [27]	Interferon [30]
Cryosurgery (liquid nitrogen) [14]		Radiation therapy [28]	Autogenous vaccine [31-33]
Electrosurgery [15]			
Carbon dioxide laser surgery [16-18]			

Table 2 Treatments of Choice for Condyloma Acuminatum by Anatomical Site

Anatomic site	Treatments of choice
Penis	
Glans	Podophyllin
	Cryosurgery
	Electrosurgery
Shaft	Cryosurgery
	Electrosurgery
	Excision
Urethra	5-Fluorouracil (cream or suppository)
	CO_2 laser surgery
Vulva	Podophyllin[a]
	Cryosurgery
	Electrosurgery
	CO_2 laser surgery
Vagina	Halogenated acetic acid
	Cryosurgery
	Electrosurgery
Cervix	Excision
	CO_2 laser surgery
	Observation
Anus	Podophyllin[a]
	Halogenated acetic acid
	Cryosurgery
	Electrosurgery
	Excision
	CO_2 laser surgery

[a]Podophyllin is contraindicated for use during pregnancy.

skin warts, respectively. Electron-microscopic studies have shown that the number of viral particles in condyloma tissues was about 10,000 times less than in skin warts!

Technical advances in molecular biology made in the 1970s allow for the extraction of viral DNA from wart tissue followed by cesium and/or sucrose density gradient centrifugation, agarose-gel electrophoresis, and ethidium bromide staining. Pooled papillomavirus DNA is then digested with a battery of restriction endonucleases and undergoes electrophoresis. Different papillomavirus DNAs have different fragmentation patterns due to the presence or absence of specific endonuclease restriction sites. Fragments of DNA on the gels are then transferred to nitrocellulose filters using the Southern blot technique. Hybridization with radiolabeled probes of known papillomavirus DNAs can be used to determine the extent of homology. Different types of HPV show less than 50% homology, and subtypes or variants are defined by differences in restriction endonuclease cleavage patterns of their DNA and greater than 50% homology [35].

At least 25 papillomavirus types have now been identified [35], and more will probably be recognized in the future. Their classification is based on the causative HPV rather than the clinical lesion, since some types of HPV may induce more than one type of wart. In 1980 Gissman and zur Hausen [36] characterized the DNA from condylomata acuminata as distinct from the other five types of HPV described up to that time and called it HPV-6. They subsequently cloned the DNA in *Escherichia coli* and confirmed the existence of two DNA subtypes (HPV-6a and 6b) [37]. Staquet et al. [38] found DNA in condylomata acuminata biochemically and immunologically identical to HPV-1, which is usually associated with plantar warts, providing evidence that a single clinical type of wart may also correspond to several types of viruses.

Wart virus-specific IgM, IgG, and IgA antibodies have been found in patients with regressing warts [39]. The cells of regressing warts always contain viral particles. Pass and Maizel [40] demonstrated IgG antibodies directed toward the major structural protein of the viral capsid in 7 of 33 patients with plantar warts. On the other hand, nonregressing warts show very little in the way of immunological activity of the circulating or cell-mediated type. The importance of cell-mediated immunity in wart regression is suggested by the extensive wart development encountered in patients with iatrogenic immunosuppression, for example, renal allograft recipients [41], congenital immunodeficiencies [42], and epidermodysplasia verruciformis [43]. Seski et al. [44] reported that blast transformation of peripheral lymphocytes in response to standard mitogens from 16 women with recalcitrant condylomata acuminata was significantly decreased compared with age-matched controls. Two of their patients were juvenile diabetics, and one had systemic lupus erythematosus. The exuberant proliferation of condylomata acuminata during pregnancy and regression postpartum may be related to a transient depression in cell-mediated immunity [45]. It is also possible that anal condylomata acuminata in homosexual men which are refractory to treatment may represent an early manifestation of the acquired immune deficiency syndrome.

Condyloma Acuminatum in Children

Condyloma acuminatum is rare in prepubertal children; only 34 cases have been reported [46]. It is judicious to suspect sexual abuse [47] and to perform a complete medical and social evaluation. However, in the majority of cases a history of abuse is unobtainable or the mother has had condylomata acuminata prior to or during delivery of the child. Tang et al. [48] reported a case of an infant born with perianal condylomata acuminata to a mother with a single labial lesion. The authors suggested that the child was infected by transplacental hematogenous infections during fetal life. Because of the rising incidence of condylomata acuminata in sexually active adults, it is conceivable that more cases of transmission to children by nonsexual contact with infected family members will be recognized [49].

Penis

In heterosexual men the penis is the anatomical site most often affected by condylomata acuminata. Data from the Denver Metro Health Clinic indicate that genital warts are nearly four times more common in heterosexual compared to homosexual men (6.7 versus 1.7%) [50]. Condylomata acuminata may involve the glans penis and urethral meatus, including the fossa navicularis, preputial cavity (particularly in uncircumcised men), and the skin of the penile shaft. It is estimated that more distal portions of the urethra may be affected in 0.5 to 5% of cases of penile condylomata acuminata.

Topical podophyllin treatment of penile condylomata acuminata was introduced in 1944 and has been considered the drug of choice ever since. The chemically complex powder called podophyllin is extracted from the resin of the plants *Podophyllum peltatum* (May apple or mandrake) and *Podophyllum emodi*, grown in the eastern United States and the Himalayas, respectively. The U.S. Pharmacopeia podophyllin topical solution is 25% podophyllum resin and benzoin in alcohol. The active ingredients are called lignans (e.g., podophyllotoxin), which arrest cell mitosis in metaphase by binding to microtubule proteins. The maximal concentration of podophyllotoxin differs between the American and Himalayan resins, 20 versus 40%, respectively, rendering the latter compound more potent and perhaps more irritating.

Culp and Kaplan [51] reported that 83% of patients with penile condylomata acuminata were cured after one application, and all cases after four applications of 25% podophyllin in mineral oil. Alcohol was subsequently used as a vehicle to limit the application to the warts and prevent spreading of the substance to unaffected tissues.

Studies of the efficacy of podophyllin by von Krogh [7,8] have not been as optimistic. He treated a total of 105 men with weekly applications of alcoholic solutions of 20% podophyllin from *P. peltatum* or *P. emodi* or 8% podophyllotoxin. Only 28% were cured after the first treatment, and an additional 15% after the second. Although the lignan content of the *P. emodi* podophyllin was four times greater than the *P. peltatum* batch, their efficacies were comparable, as shown by cure rates following one to two applications of 40 and 47%, respectively. Patients who had previously been cured of condylomata were more likely to have a complete response than those who had never had the disease. In the podophyllotoxin-treated group, 48% of condylomata acuminata were permanently healed. The three response rates were not statistically different. The time between application and rinsing of the solution was increased as tolerated from

6 to 24 hr. Minor side effects were noted after a fifth of the applications, consisting of itching, burning, or slight tenderness that resolved spontaneously within a few days. Symptoms were more pronounced in cases of multiple condylomata in the preputial cavity.

The cure rate for 8% podophyllotoxin in ethanol was increased to 54% when two applications were separated by 72 hr instead of 1 week. Self-treatment with 0.5 or 1% podophyllotoxin two or three times daily for 3 days resulted in cures in 74 (43%) of 173 patients [8]. The different regimens were equally effective. In general, condylomata in the preputial cavity healed at a higher rate than lesions in the urethral meatus and on the penile skin.

Fisher [52] recently reviewed systemic reactions to podophyllin. Paresthesia, polyneuritis, paralytic ileus, leukopenia, thrombocytopenia, coma, and death have been reported following the topical application of podophyllin. A teratogenic effect has been suggested [53]. The following measures should be taken to avoid systemic reactions:

1. Never use podophyllin during pregnancy.
2. When condylomata acuminata are extensive or cauliflower-like, covering a large surface, or so friable that they bleed with minimal trauma, do not treat all lesions in one visit.
3. Ask the patient to bathe the area 1 hr after the first application. If there are no systemic reactions, increase the time allowed to remain in contact with skin or mucous membranes before washing to 4 to 6 hr.

If podophyllin has failed to eradicate all of the condylomata after the sixth application, it probably should be abandoned for another mode of therapy. Residual lesions may be treated by electrodesiccation (fulguration) and curettage, surgical excision, or cryosurgery. The first two methods are most useful for condylomata acuminata of the penile shaft. The base of the lesion is infiltrated with 1% lidocaine using a 30-gauge needle and deliberately raised above the surface of the normal surrounding tissue. A representative lesion should be biopsied. However, two notes of caution should be observed: First, do not electrodesiccate a lesion prior to biopsy, because the current produces an artifact which distorts the tissue. Second, do not biopsy a podophyllin-treated lesion for at least 1 week after the last application, because podophyllin produces necrotic keratinocytes and a marked increase in the number of mitotic figures in the lower half of the epidermis [54], changes which may suggest a malignancy to the uninformed pathologist. The remaining lesions are carefully electrodesiccated. The base of the lesion (dermis) can be curetted to remove desiccated tissue and any residual wart followed by repeat light electrodesiccation. Discomfort to the patient is minimal, but complete re-epithelialization takes 2 to 3 weeks under optimal conditions (daily 3% hydrogen peroxide cleansing followed by application of polymyxin-bacitracin ointment). Complications such as scarring, infection, and bleeding are rare.

The second method is particularly useful for patients with a few discrete condylomata of less than 0.5 cm in diameter. Following local anesthesia, lesions are excised individually with a gradle scissor by forming an ellipse around the wart including a small margin of normal-appearing skin. Electrodesiccation or the application of a styptic solution such as 25% aluminum chloride tincture or ferric subsulfate may be used for spot coagulation. This technique avoids leaving electrodesiccated debris, which must eventually slough and may also delay healing.

Cryosurgery refers to the application of a cryogen such as carbon dioxide snow, liquidified air, nitrous oxide, or nitrogen to condyloma acuminatum. Liquid nitrogen, the cryogen of choice, is applied by cotton-tipped applicator or by probe or spray if a commercial unit is used (for example, Cryac, Owen Laboratories, Dallas, Texas 75234). Condylomata acuminata are frozen for 5 to 30 sec. Local anesthesia is usually not necessary, and patients complain of discomfort for only minutes after the procedure. Podophyllin may also be applied following cryosurgery. Patients should be warned that erythema followed by blistering and crusting may develop. These changes presage the resolution of the condylomata. Scarring is rare, but darkly pigmented patients should expect the appearance of temporary hypopigmented macules corresponding to treated sites.

Halogenated acetic acid, either 40 to 60% trichloroacetic acid [3] or saturated bichloroacetic acid [13], have been advocated as first- or second-line treatments for condylomata acuminata. These caustic chemicals rapidly coagulate and desiccate tissue. When carefully painted on condylomata with a cotton-tipped applicator or pointed stick, they turn a frosty white within seconds, thus well delineating the treated sites. Mild stinging or burning is experienced by the patient. The discomfort can be alleviated by the application of cool tap water compresses but usually subsides within minutes without it.

Von Krogh [7] treated penile condylomata with 8% colchicine, which presumably has the same mechanism of action as podophyllin. Cures were achieved in 36% of patients after a single application and in an additional 12% after a second application 1 week later. Side effects referable to local irritation appeared after half the applications. Superficial erosions corresponding to the wart site occurred after about 30% of colchicine applications. Von Krogh and Ruden [20] subsequently painted lesions twice at intervals of 48 hr with 2% and 72 hr with 4 and 8% solutions of colchicine. No additional therapeutic advantage over the single application was observed, and the high frequency of intolerable side effects persisted.

The precise incidence of intraurethral condyloma acuminatum in men with genital involvement is unknown but is estimated at 0.5 to 5%. Meatal condylomata respond poorly to podophyllin; only 8 of 31 (26%) patients were cured after one to two applications [7]; topical 8% colchicine solution cleared all lesions in 5 of 9 (56%) cases. Excision or fulguration is complicated by urethral strictures and recurrences. Wallin [55] recommends the use of an otolaryngological speculum to examine the fossa navicularis in such patients. Gigax and Robison [19] reported four cases of intraurethral condylomata which were cured with three to seven weekly instillations of 10 cm^3 of a 0.5% colchicine aqueous solution held in the vertical penis for 20 min before voiding.

5-Fluorouracil (5-FU), a pyrimidine antagonist widely used by dermatologists in the topical treatment of premalignant solar keratoses and superficial basal cell carcinomas, is incorporated into RNA-forming abnormal nucleotides. 5-Fluorouracil inhibits the enzyme thymidylate synthetase and causes disturbances in DNA synthesis. It is therefore selective for the rapidly metabolizing cells of malignant neoplasms and condylomata.

In 1975 Dretler and Klein [9] reported on the use of 5% 5-FU cream for the treatment of intraurethral condylomata acuminata. About 2 cm^3 of the cream was instilled into the meatus with a cone-shaped applicator after each voiding and at bedtime for 3 to 8 days. Contact with scrotal skin was avoided. Five patients with more proximal urethral lesions required larger volumes of the cream to fill the urethra, and two of five (40%) were unable to accomplish this themselves. Of 20 patients (15 of 15 with meatus lesions only), 19 had total eradication of intraurethral condylomata acuminata by this method. The one treatment failure had condylomata in the prostatic urethra and was subsequently treated by fulguration.

Four patients experienced meatal inflammation, adherence of adjacent meatal mucosa, and spraying of the urinary stream, which was corrected with the passage of a sounding device. The one treatment failure developed severe dysuria, urethral irritation, and inability to void following deep instillation of 5-FU.

The results of Dretler and Klein [9] were confirmed by two subsequent studies [56,57], in which 10 of 11 (91%) and 15 of 15 (100%) intraurethral condyloma were completely eradicated after one to three courses of treatment. Side effects (dysuria, edema and erythema of the urethral meatus, and pruritus) were common, but did not cause interruption of therapy. One patient developed urinary retention requiring hospitalization; no permanent strictures were noted. Wallin [55] compared 5-FU and podophyllin in the treatment of penile condylomata. The total cure rates were 10 of 27 (37%) and 14 of 31 (45%), respectively. Treatment with 5-FU was complicated by local irritation and superficial painful ulcerations. In contrast to the previously cited studies, only one of nine (11%) men with meatal condylomata was cured after daily 5% 5-FU cream instillation for 2 weeks.

Von Krogh [10] treated 40 patients with condylomata acuminata in all anatomical locations refractory to podophyllin with 5% 5-FU cream one to two times daily. Cotton swabs were used for the treatment of condylomata involving the meatus. Whereas only 33 to 46% of condylomata involving other sites regressed completely, 13 of 14 (93%) patients with meatal condylomata experienced complete resolution after an average of 3 weeks. Side effects including irritation and ulceration were common in the nonurethral locations, however; only dysuria occurred in 4 of 14 (29%) patients with meatal condylomata. Weimar et al. [11] treated male and female patients with intraurethral condylomata with suppositories formulated from 5-fluorouracil powder (5% by weight) in a polyethylene glycol base. No urethral strictures developed. The suppositories melt within 5 to 10 min; the first voiding after insertion cleanses the urethra of suppository remnants. In summary, 5% 5-FU cream by instillation, topical application, or suppository is the treatment of choice for intraurethral condylomata, particularly of the meatus and fossa navicularis.

Thio-TEPA has been used to treat penile condylomata acuminata. Cheng and Veenema [23] treated three patients with external lesions by bathing the penis in a 0.1% solution for 2 hr one to two times daily; all showed a partial response. Another patient with condylomata of the fossa navicularis was cured after eight daily intraurethral thio-TEPA suppositories (15 mg each). Mild to moderate skin irritation and urethritis developed in all patients. A patient with intraurethral condylomata from the meatus to the external sphincter was treated with weekly thio-TEPA (60 mg in 10 to 15 cm^3 in sterile water) instillations retained for ½ hr by the use of a penile clamp [58]. Slow, steady regression occurred during 3 months of therapy, and a few remaining distal lesions were electrodesiccated without complications. Thio-TEPA instillations or suppositories may be useful adjunctive therapy for intraurethral condylomata acuminata if 5-FU is unsuccessful.

The question of whether panendoscopy should be done before or after treatment of meatal condylomata is somewhat controversial. Dretler and Klein [9] conceded that they may have seeded distal condylomata more proximally with instrumentation and no longer perform endoscopic examination until all meatal lesions have been eradicated. Panendoscopy and biopsy would also be indicated in the event that distal condylomata did not respond to a reasonable course of therapy. On the other hand, Wein and Benson [56] routinely perform a complete endoscopic examination in their patients prior to treatment because they have not observed the development of new condylomata during 5-FU instillations. Follow-up examinations should be made after 6 to 12 months because of the definite risk of recurrence or reinfection.

Fuselier et al. [16] treated 10 patients with genital condylomata acuminata with carbon dioxide laser photocoagulation. Seven patients had lesions in the urethral meatus, and all but two had been treated unsuccessfully with podophyllin or fulguration. All patients were cured without complications. A urethral meatotomy was performed in selected patients for optimal exposure. An additional four patients were treated with rapid superpulsed carbon dioxide laser, followed by complete eradication of condylomata [59]. Dysuria was experienced for a period of 24 to 48 hr postoperatively. There was no evidence of meatal adherence or stricture formation. The authors claimed that the rapid superpulse laser results in less edema and tissue necrosis than the continuous-wave mode. Carbon dioxide laser therapy is a new, safe, fast, and painless method for the eradication of intraurethral condylomata. It may be used as a treatment of first choice or held in reserve for cases that fail to respond to topical 5-FU.

Anus

Perianal and intra-anal condylomata are clinically identical to penile condylomata. They are most commonly seen in patients who engage in anal intercourse. In homosexual men, anal condylomata are five to seven times more common than penile condylomata. The sexual partners of homosexual men with anal condylomata often do not have corresponding penile condylomata, perhaps because the perianal skin and anal and rectal musoca are more easily traumatized during intercourse and the moisture in the region provides a more favorable environment for establishing the infection. Heterosexual men and women who deny anal eroticism may also develop anal condylomata. Nearly every wart treatment available has been attempted for anal condylomata. In this section we describe in detail only those modalities not also widely used for penile condylomata.

Topical podophyllin, 25 to 50%, is the treatment of choice for perianal condylomata [60]. As with penile warts, extensive condylomata should be treated in sections on separate visits and the first application should be washed off in 1 hr. Subsequent weekly applications may remain in contact with lesions for 4 to 6 hr. The rates of treatment failure and recurrence are expected to be as high as 50%. In one study, an average of eight weekly treatments with 50% podophyllin was required to eradicate lesions. During the 6-month follow-up period 42% of the men had recurrences [60]. Residual lesions or recurrences may be treated by electrodesiccation or the scissor excision technique described by Thomson and Grace [61].

Cryosurgery is very effective in the treatment of perianal warts. Local anesthesia is not required, but postoperative sitz baths and oral analgesics are usually needed for a few days. O'Connor [14] treated 936 patients with perianal and anal condylomata with cryosurgery (liquid nitrogen spray or nitrous oxide). An average of 2.4 visits per patient was required to eradicate all lesions. The recurrence rate was 24%. Only 2 of 21 (10%) patients had recurrences when nitrous oxide probes were applied for 30 to 120 sec in an average of three treatments. In our clinics 25% podophyllin is applied to the warts after a light freeze with liquid nitrogen spray (15 to 30 sec). More pronounced postoperative symptoms are accepted to achieve a higher cure rate.

Halogenated acetic acid may be painted on anal condylomata. Swerdlow and Salvati [12] reported "good results" with saturated bichloroacetic acid in 34 patients. An average of four treatments was required, and transient irritation was the only side effect. Permanent scarring and strictures did not develop. Trichloroacetic acid 40 to 60%, may be utilized in a similar fashion.

One might expect topical 5-FU cream to be active against perianal condylomata. Haye [62] treated 10 patients with 5% 5-FU cream to warts once daily for

4 weeks. Only half the patients were cured, but it was noted that lesions of the anal region seemed "particularly susceptible to 5-FU." It may be of practical interest that a patient treated for ovarian cancer with two weekly intravenous doses of 1 g of 5-FU had complete resolution of extensive vulvar, vaginal, and perianal condylomata [63]. In general, local irritation, pruritus, superficial erosions, and low cure rates make topical 5-FU a second- or third-line choice in the treatment of perianal and anal condylomata.

Dinitrochlorobenzene is a potent topical sensitizer. After sensitization, an ointment is applied directly to warts, evoking a delayed hypersensitivity reaction. While this method has been successful in curing 70% of treatment-resistant skin warts in all locations [64], it has not been used extensively for condylomata acuminata [29]. The deliberate evocation of inflammation accompanied by pruritus has limited utility in the perianal region and should be considered experimental.

Another experimental treatment which has been highly efficacious and well tolerated for recalcitrant skin warts is the injection of intralesional bleomycin [65]. A 0.1% solution is injected directly into the substance of the wart. The total volume, 0.2 to 1.0 ml, injected varies according to the size of the lesion. Figueroa and Gennaro [22] cured 7 of 10 (70%) patients with anal condylomata with several injections. Six patients complained of local soreness, but did not require analgesia.

The patient should be examined for internal lesions by proctoscopy or anoscopy. The procedure should be delayed until all perianal (external) condylomata are eradicated to avoid the risk of seeding proximally. It is now recognized that 70 to 80% of homosexual men with perianal condylomata also have lesions in the anal canal and/or rectum [60]. In a large proctological series of homosexual men, more than half the patients had anal condylomata [66]. Internal condylomata must be treated to remove a potential source of autoinoculation and transmission to sexual partners.

All of the treatments listed for perianal condylomata may be employed for anal condylomata. Podophyllin, 25 to 50%, may be applied to discrete lesions in the anal canal via the anoscope. Good lighting, visualization, and allowing the solution to dry before removing the instrument are essential. Extensive condylomata should not be treated in this manner because systemic absorption can occur through the mucous membrane, and the application cannot be "cleansed" except by enema or defecation. Podophyllin should never be painted indiscriminately on the walls of the rectum or anus or applied blindly by inserting a soaked cotton swab into the anal canal! In practice, limited internal applications of podophyllin produce less local irritation than perianal treatments, but the total number of applications required is greater in order to be successful. Cryosurgery may be performed with the use of an extension tube on the spray unit to reach proximal lesions or by the cotton-tipped applicator technique. Podophyllin may be used in conjunction with cryosurgery. An unusual treatment consists of gauze soaked in thio-TEPA (15 mg in 30 ml of water) applied and inserted into the anus for 1 hr four times daily [24]. All lesions resolved in two patients after 1 to 2 months without untoward sequelae or recurrence after 9 months.

If electrodesiccation is employed, anesthesia by caudal or sacral block has been recommended [15]. A clear plastic disposable anoscope which allows visualization and does not conduct electricity should be used to prevent a serious burn.

Billingham and Lewis [17] treated 38 patients with extensive anal condylomata under general anesthesia. All lesions on the right side of the anus were treated with conventional electrodesiccation, while those on the left were cauterized using the laser instrument. Condyloma recurred in all patients at some time during the postoperative period, but 18 were first noted on the laser-treated side. Laser treatment was associated with the same or more pain and was more costly to the patient than electrodesiccation. The authors concluded that the laser provides no advantage and may even be less efficacious than electrodesiccation in the treatment of anal condylomata.

Because cell-mediated and humoral immunity are probably involved in the regression of warts, putative immune adjuvants have been tested against condylomata acuminata. Oral levamisole [26], cimetidine [27], and BCG injections [25] were totally ineffective in the treatment of resistant condylomata and should not be used for this indication. A more controversial method of immunotherapy consists of weekly subcutaneous injections of an autogenous vaccine [31-33]. The vaccine is produced by homogenizing at least 5 g of the patient's own wart tissue, freeze-thawing it to inactivate virus, and heat-treating it (56°C for 1 hr). The suspension is then centrifuged, and the supernate is collected in a sterile tube and tested for bacterial sterility. Abcarian and Sharon [31] reported that 188 (94%) of 200 consecutive patients with treatment-resistant perianal and anal condylomata were cured with this technique. A similar cure rate was found in the series of Eftaiha et al. [32]. Recently, Malison et al. [33] performed a double-blind controlled study of autogenous vaccine in 34 patients. They used a vaccine derived from the patient's own normal skin as a placebo. Patients were randomly selected to receive wart or placebo vaccine. Cure rates were 56% for wart and 25% for placebo vaccine. While the difference was not statistically significant ($p=0.14$), a larger study population may have confirmed the trend toward clinical superiority of autogenous wart vaccine. The mechanism of action of the vaccine is unknown. The use of immunotherapy should probably be reserved for well-controlled clinical trials. The theoretical concern that viral carcinogens, formerly restricted to the outer layer of the skin (epidermis), may be introduced into the circulation should be considered before this form of treatment is used.

Female Genitalia

Genital warts in the female are usually located on the external genitalia and perineal region. They may also be found in the vagina and uterine cervix; however, the typical papillary morphology is usually not apparent in the cervix. Meisels et al. [6] recently described flat and inverted (endophytic) condylomata that can only be recognized with the aid of a colposcope and which are difficult to differentiate from cervical intraepithelial neoplasia (CIN). A high proportion of cervical lesions previously classified as CIN grade 1 or 2 (mild to moderate dysplasia) are now considered to be the flat variant of condyloma acuminatum due to a reinterpretation of cytological, pathological, and colposcopic criteria. Of 97 cases of cervical condyloma studied by transmission electron microscopy and the immunoperoxidase technique, HPV particles and antigen were detected in 24 (25%) and 47 (48%), respectively [67]. All specimens in which viral particles were found were also positive for antigen.

Condylomata of the vulva and perineal region may be treated with all of the conventional treatments recommended for penile and perianal condylomata: podophyllin, cryosurgery, electrodesiccation, and conservative excision. Five percent 5-FU cream and autogenous vaccination have also been used with good results [68]. Recently the carbon dioxide laser was used to vaporize extensive condylomata of the vulva in 43 patients [18]. The recurrence rate after a single treatment was 16%. Interestingly, four of the women in the latter group were immunosuppressed and one was diabetic. Postoperative pain was common; stricture occurred in one patient. Vaginal warts may be treated with cryosurgery and/or podophyllin applied through the speculum, exercising the same cautions that are observed for anal warts. Halogenated acetic acid may be used on a weekly basis, but 5-FU is impractical because daily application is required. While conventional treatment should be reserved for solitary or limited discrete condylomata, the CO_2 laser may be the treatment of choice for recalcitrant or extensive lesions. Once the diagnosis of cervical condyloma is established, periodic follow-up examinations with cytology and colposcopy should be performed because of the risk of progression to CIN (see below). Cervical condylomata may be eradicated by punch biopsy, conization, or laser surgery [70].

The treatment of condyloma acuminatum in pregnant women presents a special problem for the clinician. Obviously, patients must be questioned about the possibility of pregnancy and tested if it is in doubt. The use of podophyllin and 5-FU is contraindicated during pregnancy because of the theoretical risk of absorption and fetal toxicity. If vaginal delivery is contemplated, condylomata acuminata must be eradicated because of the risk of transmission of HPV to the infant during parturition. Trichloroacetic acid application has been used during pregnancy without harmful effects, perhaps because its coagulant effect seals off small blood and lymphatic vessels [13]. Cryosurgery, electrodesiccation, or conservative excision may be adequate for limited lesions, but postoperative bleeding may complicate therapy of extensive condylomata acuminata because of their increased vascularity in pregnancy. For this reason, the nearly bloodless surgery of the CO_2 laser is recommended for extensive condylomata in pregnant women [18,69,71].

Juvenile Laryngeal Papillomatosis

Juvenile laryngeal papillomatosis is considered to be a disease of infancy and early childhood. It may be suspected if hoarseness or an abnormal cry is noted in an infant. Subsequently cough, stridor, and respiratory distress may occur. Multiple papillary lesions most frequently involve the true vocal cords and ventricles, but may extend to the supraglottic endolarynx, subglottic area, trachea, and bronchi [72]. The clinical course is marked by rapid recurrence after surgery. Squamous cell carcinoma has been reported to develop in patients who receive radiation therapy [73].

A viral etiology has long been suspected. Cook et al. [72] studied nine cases and found that the mothers of five children had condylomata at the time of delivery. These five children developed symptoms necessitating surgery much earlier than the other four. Quick et al. [74] determined that 40% of children with the disease were born to mothers who had condylomata during pregnancy or at parturition.

There is molecular evidence indicating that presence of viral DNA in laryngeal papilloma which hybridized with DNA from condylomata [74]. Positive staining by the immunoperoxidase technique for HPV antigens was demonstrated in the most superficial cell layers of the papilloma mucous membrane [73,74]. Types HPV-6 and HPV-11, which are found in association with anogenital and flat cervical condylomata, respectively, may also be associated with juvenile laryngeal papillomatosis [35]. If maternal condylomata are not eradicated by the time of delivery, a cesarean section should be considered.

Verrucous Carcinoma (Giant Condyloma of Buschke-Loewenstein)

In 1925 Buschke and Loewenstein [75] described "carcinoma-like" condyloma of the penis. Clinical-pathological correlation is necessary because the tumors usually appear benign histologically but pursue a locally aggressive course with destruction of underlying tissue [Fig. 6 (see Plate III, facing p. 310)]. Buschke-Loewenstein tumors have subsequently been reported to involve the anus [76], perianal region [77], vulva [78], and vagina. Recently, HPV-6 DNA was found in these tumors [35]. They are best considered a form of low-grade squamous cell carcinoma referred to as verrucous carcinoma [79]. Metastases to regional lymph nodes are rare, but malignant potential is enhanced by x-irradiation [80].

The microscopic appearance of verrucous carcinoma of the anogenital area is very similar to benign condyloma acuminatum, with an undulating keratinized outer layer, papillary fronds, and a sharply circumscribed deep margin. However, deep biopsies usually reveal blunt bullous projections of rete ridges extending into the underlying stroma. Foci of squamous cell carcinoma in situ [81] or anaplastic changes [82] have occasionally been reported.

Verrucous carcinoma does not respond to topical chemotherapy and rapidly recurs after fulguration.The treatment of choice is conservative extirpative surgery.

Regional lymph node dissection is usually not indicated. In the urological literature [80-82] verrucous carcinoma of the penis is treated by penectomy or partial penectomy. Microscopically controlled surgery (Mohs) is now advocated for these tumors, because total ablation is monitored microscopically during the procedure and maximal conservation of tissue is assured [83]. Radiation therapy should not be used.

Bowenoid Papulosis

In 1972 Friedrich [84] reported a case of a 15-year-old pregnant girl with multiple small papules of the vulva following herpetic vulvitis which he called bowenoid vulvar atypia. The lesions regressed spontaneously after delivery. Wade et al. [85] later coined the term "bowenoid papulosis" to describe multiple violaceous papules and plaques of the penis [Fig. 7 (see Plate III, facing p. 310)] which mimicked squamous cell carcinoma in situ histologically. Their clinical differential diagnosis included condylomata acuminata, lichen planus, and psoriasis. One-third of 11 patients gave a history of prior condyloma acuminatum or herpes simplex infection. All lesions responded to conservative management. The same condition was subsequently identified on the female external genitalia.

The following evidence strongly supports the hypothesis that bowenoid papulosis represents condyloma acuminatum with cytologic atypia: (1) There is prior history and subsequent development [86] of condyloma acuminatum in patients with bowenoid papulosis, (2) histological features of condyloma acuminatum and squamous cell carcinoma in situ have been found side-by-side in the same biopsy specimen [85], (3) bowenoid papulosis responds to conservative therapy (5-FU, electrodesiccation and curettage, local excision) [85] or regresses spontaneously [84,86], and (4) the HPV-6 genome has been found in some lesions of bowenoid papulosis [35].

Relation of Cervical Condylomata to Intraepithelial Neoplasia

The recent confirmation of cytological and histological criteria for differentiating condylomata of the uterine cervix from epithelial dysplastic changes or CIN has allowed epidemiological studies to more reliably reflect the relation of these two lesions. Syrjanen [87] studied 169 consecutive biopsies of histologically proved dysplastic lesions. Half of these also demonstrated histological changes meeting the criteria for flat, inverted, or papillomatous condylomata in association with all degrees of epithelial changes, from mild dysplasia to invasive squamous cell carcinoma of the cervix. The mean age of the women with condylomatous lesions was significantly lower than those without these changes. Dysplasia in women under 20 years of age was always associated with condylomatous changes. Walker et al. [88] performed cervical cytology and colposcopy on 50 women attending a sexually transmitted disease clinic for vulvar condylomata acuminata.

Altogether, condylomatous changes were detected in 20 (40%) of the patients; grade 1 or 2 CIN was found alone in 8 (16%) and evidence of papillomavirus infection in 9 (18%). Condylomata and CIN may represent covariables of early age of first intercourse and sexual promiscuity, but evidence is accumulating which suggests that HPV may act alone or in combination with other agents to cause CIN and ultimately cervical cancer. For the physician this possibility means that the young female patient with genital condylomata should have a speculum exam, cervical cytology, and perhaps colposcopy with appropriate gynecological follow-up examination for the early detection of premalignant changes of the cervical epithelium.

CONCLUSIONS AND PROSPECTS FOR THE FUTURE

Condyloma acuminatum is a common sexually transmitted disease caused by a human papillomavirus. The incidence of anogenital condyloma acuminatum in the heterosexual and homosexual populations is rising. The popularity of oral-genital and oral-anal sexual practices is expected to produce an increase in the incidence of oral condylomata [89], which are presently extremely uncommon [90].

The treatment of choice for most forms of condyloma acuminatum has been podophyllin for over four decades, but failure, recurrence, and reinfection rates are unacceptably high. At present the brightest prospect for treatment is the introduction of laser surgery into medical practice. As physicians in the various specialties treating patients with condylomata—dermatologists, gynecologists, urologists, proctologists—become familiar with the operation of the laser instrument, and as its accessibility increases, laser surgery may soon be a routine office procedure.

Interferon, the highly publicized natural glycoprotein with antitumor and antiviral properties, would seem to be a logical choice for the treatment of condyloma acuminatum. Intramuscular injections of α-interferon have been used to treat juvenile laryngeal papillomatosis [91]. Most patients showed a sustained partial response while receiving interferon, but relapse occurred upon discontinuation. Limited trials with intralesional injections of interferon into condyloma acuminatum [30], verruca vulgaris [92], and epidermodysplasia verruciformis [93] have shown that further manipulation of dose and schedule is warranted. Clinical research with interferon has been hindered by the lack of sufficient quantities of pure material and public clamor for a cure for cancer. The recent development of recombinant DNA technology has made unlimited quantities of highly purified interferon of all types available to investigators [94]. Controlled clinical trials of intralesional and systemic administration of recombinant human interferons in the treatment of condyloma acuminatum are currently in progress.

Except for the eradication of existing condylomata and prudent sexual practices during therapy, there is presently no way to prevent the transmission of condyloma acuminatum. It is hoped that the development of a safe and effective polyvalent vaccine administered in early childhood will send human papillomavirus-induced diseases the way of polio, mumps, and measles.

REFERENCES

1. Bafverstedt B. Condylomata acuminata—past and present. Acta Derm Venereol 1967; 47:376-381.
2. Leider M, Bosenblum M. A dictionary of dermatologic words, terms, and phrases. West Haven, Connecticut: Dome Laboratories, 1976.
3. Felman YM, Nikitas JA. Condylomata acuminata. NY State J Med 1979; 79:1747-1749.
4. Centers for Disease Control. Condyloma acuminatum—United States, 1966-1981. Morbid Mortal Week Rep 1983; 32:306-308.
5. Centers for Disease Control. Nonreported sexually transmitted diseases—United States. Morbid Mortal Week Rep 1979; 28:61-63.
6. Meisels A, Fortin R, Roy M. Condylomatous lesions of the cervix. II. Cytologic, colposcopic and histopathologic study. Acta Cytol 1977; 21:379-390.
7. Von Krogh G. Topical treatment of penile condylomata acuminata with podophyllin, podophyllotoxin and colchicine. A comparative study. Acta Derm Venereol 1978; 58:163-168.
8. Von Korgh G. Podophyllotoxin for condylomata acuminate eradication. Clinical and experimental comparative studies on *Podophyllum* lignans, colchicine and 5-fluorouracil. Acta Derm Venereol Suppl 1981; 98:1-48.
9. Dretler SP, Klein LA. The eradication of intraurethral condyloma acuminata with 5 per cent 5-fluorouracil cream. J Urol 1975; 3:195-198.
10. Von Krogh G. 5-Fluorouracil cream in the successful treatment of therapeutically refractory condylomata acuminata of the urinary meatus. Acta Derm Venerol 1976; 56:297-301.
11. Weimar GW, Milleman LA, Reiland TL, Culp DA. 5-Fluorouracil urethral suppositories for the eradication of condyloma acuminata. J Urol 1978; 120:174-175.
12. Swerdlow DB, Salvati EP. Condyloma acuminatum. Dis Colon Rectum 1971; 14:226-231.
13. Kovar WR. Condyloma acuminatum—diagnosis, precautions, treatment. Nebr Med J 1979; 64:306-308.
14. O'Connor JJ. Perianal and anal condylomata acuminata. J Dermatol Surg Oncol 1979; 5:276-277.
15. Robinson JK. Extirpation by electrocautery of the genito-perineo-anal region. J Dermatol Surg Oncol 1980; 6:733-738.
16. Fuselier HA, McBurney EI, Brannan W, Randrup ER. Treatment of condylomata acuminata with carbon dioxide laser. Urology 1980; 15:265-266.

17. Billingham RP, Lewis FG. Laser versus electrical cautery in the treatment of condylomata acuminata of the anus. Surg Gynecol Obstet 1982; 155:865-867.
18. Ferenczy A. Using the laser to treat vulvar condylomata acuminata and intraepidermal neoplasia. Can Med Assoc J 1983; 128:135-137.
19. Gigax JH, Robison JR. The successful treatment of intraurethral condyloma acuminatum with colchicine. J Urol 1976; 105:809-811.
20. Von Krogh G, Ruden AK. Topical treatment of penile condylomata acuminata with colchicine at 48-72 hours intervals. Acta Derm Venereol 1980; 60:87-89.
21. Ichikawa T, Nakano I, Hirokawa I. Bleomycin treatment of the tumors of penis and scrotum. J Urol 1969; 102:699-707.
22. Figueroa S, Gennaro AR. Intralesional bleomycin injection in treatment of condyloma acuminatum. Dis Colon Rectum 1980; 23:550-551.
23. Cheng SF, Veenema RJ. Topical application of thio-tepa to penile and urethral tumors. J Urol 1965; 94:259-262.
24. Kerstein MD. Thio-tepa in the management of anorectal condylomata acuminata: report of two cases. Dis Colon Rectum 1977; 20:625-626.
25. Malison MD, Salkin D. Attempted BCG immunotherapy for condylomata acuminata. Br J Vener Dis 1981; 57:148.
26. Schou M, Helin P. Levamisole in a double-blind study: no effect on warts. Acta Derm Venerol 1977; 57:449-454.
27. Rampen FH, Van Everdingen JJ. Inefficacy of cimetidine in condylomata acuminata. Br J Vener Dis 1982; 58:275.
28. Danoff DS, Holden S, Thompson RW, David R. New treatment for extensive condylomata acuminata: external radiation therapy. Urology 1981; 18:47-49.
29. Moore GE, Norton LW, Meiselbaugh DM. Condyloma. A new epidemic. Arch Surg 1978; 113:630-631.
30. Scott GM, Csonka GW. Effect of injections of small doses of human fibroblast interferon into genital warts. A pilot study. Br J Vener Dis 1979; 55:442-445.
31. Abcarian H, Sharon N. Long-term effectiveness of the immunotherapy of anal condyloma acuminatum. Dis Colon Rectum 1982; 25:648-651.
32. Eftaiha MS, Amshel AL, Shonberg IL, Batshon B. Giant and recurrent condyloma acuminatum: appraisal of immunotherapy. Dis Colon Rectum 1982; 25:136-138.
33. Malison MD, Morris R, Jones LW. Autogenous vaccine therapy for condyloma acuminatum. A double-blind controlled study. Br J Vener Dis 1982; 58:62-65.
34. Coggin JR, zur Hausen H. Workshop on papillomaviruses and cancer. Cancer Res 1979; 39:545-546.
35. Lutzner MA. The human papillomaviruses: a review. Arch Dermatol 1983; 119:631-635.

36. Gissman L, zur Hausen H. Partial characterization of viral DNA from human genital warts (condylomata acuminata). Int J Cancer 1980; 25:605-609.
37. de Villiers EM, Gissman L, zur Hausen H. Molecular cloning of viral DNA from human genital warts. J Virol 1981; 40:932-935.
38. Staquet MJ, Viac J, Bustamante R, Thivolet J. Human papillomavirus type I purified from human genital warts. Dermatologica 1981; 162:213-219.
39. Matthews RS, Shirodaria K. Study of regressing warts by immunofluorescence. Lancet 1973; 1:689-691.
40. Pass F, Maizel JV. Wart-associated antigens. II. Human immunity to viral structural proteins. J Invest Dermatol 1973; 60:307-311.
41. Spencer ES, Anderson HK. Viral infections in renal allograft recipients treated with long-term immunosuppression. Br Med J 1979; 2:829-830.
42. Barnett N, Mak H, Winkelstein JA. Extensive verrucosis in primary immunodeficiency disease. Arch Dermatol 1983; 119:5-7.
43. Lutzner MA. Epidermodysplasia verruciformis: an autosomal recessive disease characterized by viral warts and skin cancer: a model for viral oncogenesis. Bull Cancer 1978; 65:169-182.
44. Seski JC, Reinhalter ER, Silva J. Abnormalities of lymphocyte transformations in women with condylomata acuminata. Obstet Gynecol 1978; 51: 188-192.
45. Purtilo DT, Hallgren HM, Yunis EJ. Depressed maternal lymphocyte response to phytohemagglutinin in human pregnancy. Lancet 1972; 1:769-771.
46. DeJong AR, Weiss JC, Brent RL. Condyloma acuminata in children. Am J Dis Child 1982; 136:704-706.
47. Seidel J, Zonana J, Totten E. Concyloma acuminata as a sign of sexual abuse in children. J Pediatr 1979; 95:553-554.
48. Tang CK, Shermeta DW, Wood C. Congenital condylomata acuminata. Am J Obstet Gynecol 1978; 131:912-913.
49. Stumpf PG. Increasing occurrence of condylomata acuminata in premenarchal children. Obstet Gynecol 1980; 56:262-264.
50. Judson FN, Penley KA, Robinson ME, Smith JK. Comparative prevalence rates of sexually transmitted diseases in heterosexual and homosexual men. Am J Epidemiol 1980; 112:836-843.
51. Culp OS, Kaplan IW. Condylomata acuminata. Two hundred cases treated with podophyllin. Ann Surg 1944; 120:251-255.
52. Fisher AA. Severe systemic and local reactions to topical podophyllum resin. Cutis 1981; 233-266.
53. Karol MD, Conner CS, Watanabe AS, Murphrey KJ. *Podophyllum*: suspected teratogenicity from topical application. Clin Toxicol 1980; 16:283-286.
54. Wade TR, Ackerman AB. The effects of resin of podophyllin on condyloma acuminatum. Am J Dermatopathol 1984; 6:109-122.
55. Wallin J. 5-Fluorouracil in the treatment of penile and urethral condylomata acuminata. Br J Vener Dis 1977; 53:240-243.
56. Wein AJ, Benson GS. Treatment of urethral condyloma acuminatum with 5-fluorouracil cream. Urology 1977; 9:413-415.

57. Bringel PJP, de Andrade, Arruda R. 5-Fluorouracil cream 5% in the treatment of intraurethral condylomata acuminata. Br J Urol 1982; 54:295.
58. Halverstadt DB, Parry WL. Thiotepa in the management of intraurethral condylomata acuminata. J Urol 1969; 101:729-731.
59. Rosenberg SK, Fuller T, Jacobs H. Rapid superpulse carbon dioxide laser treatment of urethral condylomata. Urology 1981; 17:149-151.
60. Schlappner OLA, Shaffer EA. Anorectal condylomata acuminata: a missed part of the condyloma spectrum. Can Med Assoc J 1978; 118:172-173.
61. Thomson JPS, Grace RH. The treatment of perianal and anal condylomata acuminata: a new operative technique. J R Soc Med 1978; 71:180-185.
62. Haye KR. Treatment of condyloma acuminata with 5 per cent 5-fluorouracil (5-FU) cream. Br J Vener Dis 1974; 50:466.
63. Doll DC, Wasserman PI. Anticancer agents in condyloma acuminatum. N Engl J Med 1979; 301:1288-1289.
64. Buckner D, Price NM. Immunotherapy of verrucae vulgares with dinitrochlorobenzene. Br J Dermatol 1978; 98:451-455.
65. Shumer SM, O'Keefe EJ: Bleomycin in the treatment of recalcitrant warts. J Am Acad Dermatol 1983; 9:91-96.
66. Baker RW, Peppercorn MA. Gastrointestinal ailments of homosexual men. Medicine 1982; 61:390-405.
67. Ferenczy A, Braun L, Shah KV. Human papillomavirus (HPV) in condylomatous lesions of cervix. A comparative ultrastructural and immunohistochemical study. Am J Surg Pathol 1981; 5:661-670.
68. Nel WS, Fourie ED. Immunotherapy and 5% topical 5-fluoro-uracil ointment in the treatment of condylomata acuminata. S Afr Med J 1973; 47:45-49.
69. Baggish MS. Treating viral venereal infections with the CO_2 laser. J Reprod Med 1982; 27:737-742.
70. Ropert JF, Marquet M, Mage G, Soualhat C, Bruhat MA. Cervical intraepithelial neoplasia (CIN): the incidence of condylomatous lesions associated with it. The results of treatment using the CO_2 laser. J Gynecol Obstet Biol Reprod 1982; 11:849-854.
71. Calkins JW, Masterson BJ, Magrina JF, Capen CV. Management of condylomata acuminata with the carbon dioxide laser. Obstet Gynecol 1982; 59: 105-108.
72. Cook TA, Brunschwig JP, Butel JS, Cohn AM, Goepfert H, Rawls WE. Laryngeal papilloma: etiologic and therapeutic considerations. Ann Otol 1973; 82:649-655.
73. Costa J, Howley PM, Bowling MC, Howard R, Bauer WC. Presence of human papilloma viral antigens in juvenile multiple laryngeal papilloma. Am J Clin Pathol 1981; 75:194-197.
74. Quick Ca, Krzyzek RA, Watt SL, Faras AJ. Relationship between condylomata and laryngeal papillomata. Clinical and molecular virological evidence. Ann Otol 1980; 89:467-471.
75. Buschke A, Loewenstein L. Uber carcinomahnliche Condylomata Acuminata des Penis. Klin Wochenschr 1925; 4:1726-1728.

76. Alexander RM, Kaminsky DB. Giant condyloma acuminatum (Buschke-Loewenstein tumor) of the anus: case report and review of the literature. Dis Colon Rectum 1979; 22:561-565.
77. Lee SH, McGregor DH, Kuziez MN. Malignant transformation of perianal condyloma acuminatum: a case report with review of the literature. Dis Colon Rectum 1981; 24:462-467.
78. Kovi J, Tillman RL, Lee SM. Malignant transformation of condyloma acuminatum. A light microscopic and ultrastructural study. Am J Clin Pathol 1974; 61:702-710.
79. Headington JT. Verrucous carcinoma. Cutis 1978; 21:207-211.
80. Brums TNC, Lauvetz RJ, Kerr ES, Ross G. Buschke-Loewenstein giant condylomas. Pitfalls in management. Urology 1975; 5:773-776.
81. Rhatigan RM, Jiminex S, Chopskie EJ. Condyloma acuminatum and carcinoma of the penis. South Med J 1972; 65:423-428.
82. Tessler AN, Applebaum SM. The Buschke-Loewenstein tumor. Urology 1982; 20:36-39.
83. Mohs FE, Sahl WJ. Chemosurgery for verrucous carcinoma. J Dermatol Surg Oncol 1979; 5:302-306.
84. Friedrich EG. Reversible vulvar atypia. A case report. Obstet Gynecol 1972; 39:173-181.
85. Wade TR, Kopf AW, Ackerman AB. Bowenoid papulosis of the penis. Cancer 1978; 42:1890-1903.
86. Steffen C. Concurrence of condylomata acuminata and bowenoid papulosis. Confirmation of the hypothesis that they are related conditions. Am J Dermatopathol 1982; 4:5-8.
87. Syrjanen KJ. Condylomatous lesions in dysplastic and neoplastic epithelium of the uterine cervix. Surg Gynecol Obstet 1980; 150:372-376.
88. Walker PG, Colley NV, Grubb C, Tejerina A, Oriel JD. Abnormalities of the uterine cervix in women with vulval warts. A preliminary communication. Br J Vener Dis 1983; 59:120-123.
89. Felman YM, Nikitas JA. Sexually transmitted diseases of the oral cavity: part II. Cutis 1982; 30:181-254.
90. Anneroth G, Anniko M, Romander H. Oral condyloma acuminatum. A light and electron microscopic study. Int J Oral Surg 1982; 11:260-264.
91. Haglund S, Lundquist PG, Cantell K, Strander H. Interferon therapy in juvenile laryngeal papillomatosis. Arch Otolaryngol 1981; 107:327-332.
92. Pazin GH, Ho M, Haverkos HW, et al. Effects of interferon-alpha on human warts. J Interferon Res 1982; 2:235-243.
93. Androphy EJ, Dvoretzky I, Maluish AE, Wallace HJ, Lowy DR. Response of warts in epidermodysplasia verruciformis to treatment with systemic and intralesional alpha interferon. J Am Acad Dermatol 1984; 11:197-202.
94. Merigan TC. Human interferon as a therapeutic agent—current status. N Engl J Med 1983; 308:1530-1531.

THIRTEEN

Ectoparasites and Molluscum Contagiosum

David R. Lambert and Frank W. Yoder
The Ohio State University
College of Medicine
Columbus, Ohio

INTRODUCTION

This chapter is a comprehensive review of what many consider minor venereal disease infections. Although scabies, pediculosis, and molluscum contagiosum are rather benign in that they do not cause mortality or severe morbidity, they are very common infections and therefore are quite important for those interested in sexually transmitted diseases.

SCABIES

Scabies can be a sexually transmitted disease as well as clustering in families, among school children, and in institutionalized populations. It usually presents as intense pruritus, especially nocturnal pruritus. The pathognomonic skin lesion is a linear burrow with or without small vesicles. The lesions are frequently excoriated and may have secondary bacterial infection. Scabies may present with a wide range of skin lesions, including papules, vesicles, bullae, and scaling plaques. A high index of suspicion is essential. The diagnosis of scabies should be considered in any patient with itching and rash.

Etiology

Human scabies is caused by infestation of the skin by a tiny insect, the itch mite, *Sarcoptes scabiei* var. *hominis*. This disease is common, rising in incidence, and contagious. Human scabies live and complete their life cycle only on humans and are not vectors for other diseases [1]. Many varieties of animal scabies are transmissible to humans but are self-limited conditions.

The mites measure 0.2 to 0.4 mm in length. The female mites are larger and are most commonly seen. Tiny white or translucent creatures, they are marked by transverse wrinkles and brown spines and bristles on the dorsal surface. The adults have four pairs of legs and the larvae have three pairs. The adult female can move up to 2.5 cm/min across the skin surface. After mating on the skin, the female soon burrows just beneath the stratum corneum. The burrowing mite feeds on intercellular fluid and deposits fecal pellets along its way [2].

Within days of mating, the female mite begins laying two or three large eggs per day as it extends the burrow up to 5 mm per day [2,3]. The eggs hatch and larvae move to the surface of the skin in 3 or 4 days, undergo three moltings, and then as adults mate and the females repeat the burrowing process. This maturation takes 14 to 17 days to complete and the adult female lives approximately 30 days, long enough to lay 10 to 25 eggs [3,4]. The infested patient has an average of 11 female mites present [5].

Pathogenesis

The burrowing mite and its by-products induce an intense pruritus in the patient. Initial infestation is asymptomatic for 4 to 6 weeks. Subsequent contact with the scabies mite induces itching and rash as soon as 24 hr. Many people may be immune to reinfestation, but the mechanism of this immunity is uncertain [6].

Histopathological studies have shown the primary skin lesion in scabies to be curving linear burrows with vesicles containing female mite, eggs, larvae, and fecal material. Secondary lesions include papular, nodular, and crusted psoriasiform lesions [7]. All of these may be excoriated and secondarily infected, inducing pyoderma. The lesion sites are not limited to areas where mites are lodged.

Immunological studies suggest the scabies mite induces a hypersensitivity response to uncharacterized antigenic stimuli. A combined cellular and humoral immune reaction is likely. Both primary and secondary lesions have been shown to include prominent lymphocytic infiltration as well as immunoglobulins and complement [7-9]. Persistence of the lesions following eradication of the mite may be caused by continuing antigenic stimulation.

Epidemiology

Incidence and Prevalence

Scabies has a worldwide distribution and has been observed to have a cyclic variation. Approximately every 30 years a peak of cases has been seen, with epidemics lasting about 15 years [10]. Since 1973 substantially more cases have been diagnosed in the United States [1]. Scabies has recently accounted for 2.6% of visits to dermatologists [11]. In the United States scabies is significantly less common among blacks than among whites [12].

Epidemics of scabies in the past have been attributed to conditions of poverty, overcrowding, uncleanliness, sexual promiscuity, and wartime conditions. While these may contribute, scabies is not limited to any socioeconomic group and the disease may be seen in those with good personal hygiene. Epidemics may represent new generations of susceptible hosts in whom an acquired immunity gradually develops, decreasing the incidence of scabies [13].

Transmission

The scabies mite is acquired by close personal contact. Skin-to-skin contact is necessary, since the mite does not "jump" between people [2]. Often scabies shows a familial pattern, and school children are likely to be the first cases. An epidemiological study in England [14] concluded that schools were not a major source of scabies, but the most frequently reported sources of familial scabies were friends and relatives (90%). Because of the long incubation period, it may be difficult to trace the source in any particular case. Outbreaks of scabies are not unusual in nursing homes and other institutions [15].

The role of fomites in scabies is unlikely but possible. Studies of transmission via shared clothing and linen have shown the risk to be small [13,16]. Some treatment of potential fomites in the home continues to be advised as a precaution.

Scabies as a Sexually Transmitted Disease

Scabies can be transmitted by sexual contact, and this is a major source of scabies among young adults in the United States. As many as 60 to 80% of patients acquired scabies through sexual relations or sleeping in the same bed with an infested person [15]. While many venereal diseases may frequently be spread by brief sexual relations, scabies is more likely to be contracted by sharing a night in bed [5]. Since infestation may be subclinical for weeks, tracing contacts is difficult.

The diagnosis of scabies should prompt the search for coexisting venereal diseases. Scabies and gonorrhea occurring together is well known. In a series of 946 patients with scabies examined for other venereal diseases, 8% of women and 1.4% of men had asymptomatic gonorrhea [17].

Scabies has also been reported with pediculosis pubis and syphilis [18]. Nodular penile lesions of scabies look like chancres and may coexist with them. Seconday syphilis, with its faint red-brown maculopapular rash, could be confused with scabies.

Clinical Features

Scabies can be recognized by a pruritic, pleomorphic rash of insidious onset in a characteristic distribution, often occurring in clusters of cases.

Pruritus

Itching is the most prominent symptom and it may be intense. The severity of itching typically is worst at night. The patient may report being awakened by itching. This could represent a higher activity level of the mite due to temperature or light sensitivities. Other dermatoses may present with nocturnal pruritus, but scabies should be considered likely. This is especially true with a history of blood found on sheets, pajamas, or underwear due to vigorous scratching [19].

Insidious Onset

Since initial infestations are clinically latent for up to 4 to 6 weeks, patients report a gradual awareness of rash and pruritus. Reinfestation may produce prompt symptoms, making a history of transmission of the mite more easy to elicit.

Pattern of Spread

The scabies mite is spread by close contact. This includes families, sexual partners, school-aged children, and the institutionalized. Holding hands has been cited as an example of such contact. In young adults living alone, venereal transmission is probable [5]. A history of pruritic dermatitis in close contacts of the patient is helpful diagnostically and essential to good treatment. Family members and others close to the patient may be asymptomatic owing to the latency of the disease, and their examination may be helpful.

Pleomorphic Lesions

The scabies burrow is unique, but scabies has been called a "great imitator." Typically patients present with a variety of lesions, including vesicles, bullae, scales, crusts, pustules, nodules, and excoriations. Vesicles appear with burrows and also away from them. Bullous lesions are mainly seen in infants.

Characteristic Distribution

In classic cases of scabies, the lesions are generally symmetrical. The hands are most commonly involved, especially the interdigital webs, sides of digits, and flexor aspects of the wrists. As many as 85% of patients have burrows on the hands [4]. The extensor surfaces of the elbows show dry, eczematous, or occasionally nodular lesions. This can be better appreciated by wetting them with water or mineral oil [2].

The anterior axillary folds are sites of papules and nodules, as is the abdomen, especially the periumbilical area. The female breasts may show papular or eczematous changes. The genitals are affected, particularly the penis and scrotum

Plate IV

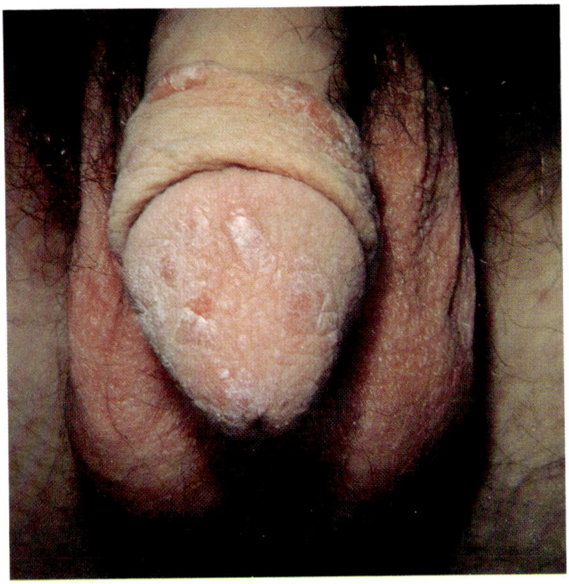

Fig. 1 Scabies infestation of the glans penis and foreskin.

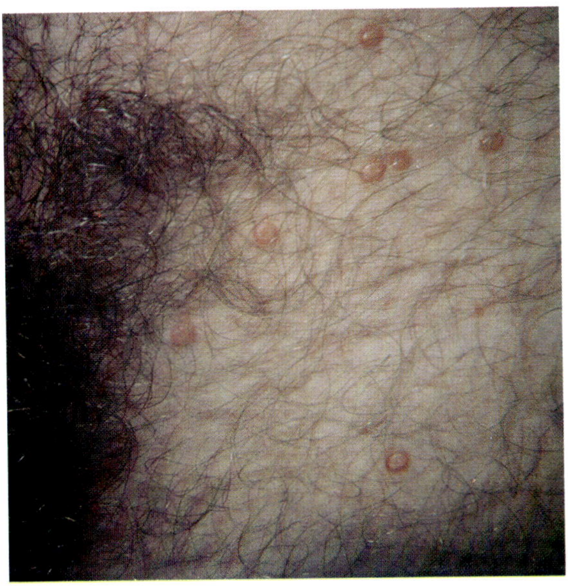

Fig. 2 Papular lesions of molluscum contagiosum in the pubic area.

[Fig. 1 (see Plate IV, facing p. 336)]. Penile lesions may be nodular or resemble chancres. The gluteal folds, buttocks, upper thighs, extensor areas of the knees, ankles, and toes may all show scabies rash.

In children the palms and soles are more likely to be affected than in adults. Also, in children, the face and head may be involved, which is distinctly unusual in adults.

Persistent Lesions

It is characteristic of scabies to have continuing rash and pruritus, even after effective elimination of living mites. This represents a hypersensitivity reaction and the continued presence of mite antigen in the skin. Dermatitis and pruritus are common and urticaria may occur [2]. Nodular lesions which are reddish brown, pruritic, and irritable can be particularly bothersome. They can measure up to 12 mm in diameter and can persist for several months. They are present in only about 7% of cases [4]. Common sites for nodules are areas covered by clothing: axillary areas, chest, abdomen, groin, penis, or scrotum.

Diagnosis

The diagnosis of scabies may often rest on clinical characteristics, but visualization of a burrow and the mite or its products is preferable.

The Burrow

The burrow of scabies is pathognomonic. It is seen as a curving linear lesion as small as a few millimeters long. It can appear as a dark line, a scaly line, or a linear erythematous lesion, slightly elevated from the skin surface. It can best be found in the interdigital areas, wrists, elbows, feet, and ankles [19]. Asymptomatic burrows may be felt with the fingertips, since they may not appear inflamed. A careful, thorough search with good lighting and a magnifying lens may be required.

Several techniques are available to improve the yield of burrows. Applying mineral oil to areas of the skin may improve visualization of the burrows [2]. The burrow ink test method is to saturate a likely area with liquid ink or cover it with ink from a felt-tipped pen. Excess ink is washed away with alcohol, leaving residual ink in the burrow [20]. In a similar technique, tetracycline in alcohol solution (e.g., Topicycline) is used to cover an area of skin. The solution is allowed to dry for a few minutes and then well removed with alcohol wiping. Scabies burrows may be seen as fluorescent yellow or green lines under a Wood's light where the solution has been retained in the lesion [21].

The Mite

Seeing the mite, larvae, eggs, and fecal pellets is the next diagnostic step. Selection of fresh, unexcoriated burrows will make identification most likely. An early papule or vesicle may also be used.

A very superficial shaving of the skin with a #15 scalpel blade will remove a thin piece of epidermis containing the lesion [2]. Mineral oil is applied to the skin prior to shaving. Examination under 25th to 50th power through the microscope should reveal mites, eggs, or fecal pellets, all of which are diagnostic.

A variation on this technique uses a sharp (18 to 22 gauge) needle to unroof the burrow and remove the mite at its blind end. Following this, microscopic examination confirms the finding of a mite.

Scraping the skin has been recommended as a rapid method of collecting the specimen [22]. The skin is moistened with mineral oil in an area of an early burrow or papule. By scraping the skin tangentially with the edge of a #15 scalpel blade, the roof of the lesion and its contents can be removed and collected on the blade. Repeating this procedure for several lesions will increase the likelihood of positive findings. The skin debris is placed on a microscope slide and examined for mites, eggs, and feces.

Skin biopsy is another technique for revealing mite infestation. A small piece of anesthetized skin is removed by scalpel excision or punch technique. Thin sections must be prepared to ensure seeing the mite and its by-products. This is the most traumatic method.

Each method is only as good as the lesions selected. Older lesions may not contain mites.

Differential Diagnosis

Many skin conditions may simulate scabies because of its great variability. Nocturnal pruritus, pleomorphic lesions, insidious onset, and characteristic distribution lead to the diagnosis of scabies.

Eczema

The hypersensitivity dermatitis of scabies may be confused with contact dermatitis or atopic dermatitis. In contact dermatitis onset is often sudden, with a history of irritant or allergen exposure hours or days earlier. The rash shows much vesiculation and edema and is prominent in exposed areas. Excoriation and lichenification may be present, but the rash usually spares the axillae and groin.

Atopic dermatitis is a chronic and recurrent problem. It may be associated with asthma, hay fever, and a family history of atopic disease. Severe, frequent itching leads to lichenified areas of skin. The rash is characteristically found in flexor folds of the neck, elbows, wrists, and knees, and occasionally on the face and scalp.

Acute Urticaria

The various causes of urticaria produce characteristic wheals which are erythematous and edematous. Intense pruritus often occurs. The individual lesions are quite changeable, lasting 8 to 12 hr each, as new lesions appear. The appearance of all lesions are similar, with blanched edematous centers surrounded by erythema. Chronic urticaria represents a rash of more than 6 weeks duration.

Scabies has been reported to present as acute urticaria [23]. A history of intense itching preceding the onset of hives up to several weeks is suggestive. A search for scabietic lesions should be made.

Pyoderma

Impetigo presents with pustules, papules, erosions, and a characteristic thick yellow crust. Bullae may be present. The disease is usually pruritic and very contagious among infants and children, but less so in adults. Involvement of the face and other exposed areas is typical. Streptococci and less commonly staphylococci are the causative agents.

Scabies and impetigo may coexist. The excoriations of scabies can lead to secondary bacterial infection, especially in children. Cases of poststreptococcal glomerulonephritis have been reported with scabies and impetigo.

Folliculitis is infection of the hair follicles, producing pustules. Frequently they are painful. The follicular location of the lesions distinguishes it from scabies.

Erythrasma is a mild, chronic bacterial infection of intertriginous areas of the skin such as the inguinal, axillary, and inframammary folds. The sharp-edged plaques show a smooth or scaly surface. Scaling or fissuring in the toe webs may be seen. Erythrasma is most often confused with fungal skin infections.

Insect Bites

Insect bites present as acute onset of pruritic or painful lesions. Usually these are papules or vesicles with a central punctum and are uniform in appearance. Face, scalp, ears, neck, and other exposed areas are typically involved. Severe local reactions include localized edema, pustules, and nodules.

Neurodermatitis

Neurodermatitis presents with fixed, chronic areas of lichenified skin. The rash is perpetuated by a lower itch threshold due to repeated excoriation leading to chronic thickening of the skin. The areas involved are usually those easily accessible to scratching. Nodules may develop which are similar to the persistent pruritic nodule of scabies.

Dermatitis Herpetiformis

This disease is chronic, recurrent, and autoimmune. Very pruritic eruptions of erythematous papules and vesicles appear in clusters. The lesions are usually on extensor surfaces of the extremities, shoulder, scalp, back, buttocks, and pelvic areas. Irritation and itching of the skin often precede the onset of the rash by several hours. Face and scalp involvement and sparing of scabietic areas serve to distinguish the conditions.

Treatment

Treatment of patients with scabies must be extended to include family members and sexual partners who may be asymptomatic for 4 to 6 weeks. Treatment failures have been observed in cases where all family members were not treated simultaneously. The most frequently recommended agents are lindane, crotamiton, and sulfur.

The Centers for Disease Control state that lindane (1%) cream or lotion is the primary treatment for adults and children over the age of 10 [24]. Alternative therapies are recommended for pregnant or lactating women, young children less than 10 years old, and infants. For these patients crotamiton (10%) or sulfur (6%) in petrolatum are advised. Controversy exists regarding the hazards of lindane [25,26]. Recent reviews have emphasized the safety of proper use of lindane in patients of all ages [27-29].

Lindane Therapy

Lindane (1%) lotion or cream (Kwell) is generally considered the most effective scabicide. The medication is applied thinly to the entire skin surface from the neck down, including the umbilicus and soles of the feet. One ounce (about 30 g) is enough to cover the average adult. Bathing prior to application is unnecessary and may increase systemic absorption [30]. Lindane should be left on the skin for 8 to 12 hr and then washed off. In children and infants a 6-hr application has been advised [28]. The medication must be applied to normal as well as affected skin. If hands are washed during the treatment period, the solution should be reapplied. Lindane should be used on the face and scalp only if scabies has been diagnosed there.

One proper application of the medication is sufficient to achieve a 96 to 98% cure rate [31]. Continued lesions and pruritus may be expected even though the mites and eggs have been killed and the patient is no longer contagious. If patients are not informed of this, they may be tempted to overuse the medication and risk side effects and toxicity.

Lindane Toxicity

Repeated applications of lindane may occur if patients believe mite infestation is continuing. Resistance to lindane, if properly used, has not been reported [29]. Overuse of lindane solutions can induce an irritant dermatitis.

Central nervous system toxicity, including seizures in children, has been reported following use of lindane [32]. A review of reported cases of adverse drug reactions to lindane has revealed no instances of toxicity when the medication was used properly [28]. It is recognized that excessive topical application or ingestion may induce central nervous system toxicity [25,26]. Percutaneous absorption of lindane has been demonstrated [33].

The data on carcinogenicity of lindane in animals have been inconclusive. Teratogenicity or mutagenicity has not been demonstrated. Cases of aplastic anemia have been seen following exposure to industrial pesticides containing lindane, but not following medicinal use [26].

Overall, the safety and efficacy of properly administered lindane is well accepted. Good medical care should include careful instructions to patients regarding application method and duration of treatment and warning about overuse. Children and infants should be covered with clothing and even mittens to minimize the possibility of ingestion by licking the skin. The amount of lindane prescribed and dispensed should be carefully controlled by physicians and pharmacists. Reapplication of lindane should be at least 7 days after initial use and then only with demonstrated treatment failures.

Crotamiton

Crotamiton (10%) cream or lotion (Eurax) is an effective scabicide and may have antipruritic properties also. After a bath or shower it is applied to the entire body from the neck down. It is massaged well into the skin. After 24 hr the application is repeated, and 48 hr after the first treatment crotamiton is washed off. Some physicians prefer crotamiton for use in young children, infants, and lactating and pregnant women. It may be used on the face and scalp if they are involved. It is contraindicated on raw, weeping skin.

Crotamiton is generally held to be less effective then lindane as a scabicide. Limited comparative studies indicate a lower cure rate [34]. Most clinical studies have shown crotamiton to be effective but have used repeated applications from 3 to 5 consecutive nights [35,36]. Possible resistance to therapy has been reported [37]. Major toxic reactions to crotamiton have not been reported, but good studies in this area have not been done [26].

Sulfur

Sulfur (6%) in petrolatum is the third line of therapy for scabies and has been used for centuries. For use in both adults and children, it is applied to the entire body from the neck down for 3 nights. Patients may bathe before each application and should leave the final treatment on the skin for 24 hr. Compliance may be a problem because of the odor and messiness of the preparation.

A recent comparative trial showed a 4-day regimen of sulfur to be an effective scabicide in infants, but with a lower cure rate than lindane [34]. Good modern studies of sulfur toxicity are lacking. Irritant dermatitis and adverse central nervous system reactions have been reported [26,38].

Other Measures

In order to minimize reinfestation, the small possibility of fomite transmission should be eliminated. After the completion of scabicide treatment all clothing which has come in contact with the skin is washed through a hot cycle in a washing machine or is dry-cleaned. The patient should also be instructed to wash towels and bed linen in the same way. Other family members should not use clothing or linen that the patient has come in contact with until it is cleaned. Outerwear such as hats and overcoats and clothing which has already been cleaned need not be washed.

Persistent pruritus and rash may be helped by prescribing an oral antihistamine antipruritic medication. Since most of the body will show continuing symptoms for about 2 weeks, patients should be told that this does not mean infestation is still present. In the hands and feet continuing irritation can be seen for 1 month or longer.

For pruritus and rash which is more bothersome topical corticosteroids may be prescribed. In rare, severe cases of intense pruritus after adequate scabicide treatment, a tapering dose of oral corticosteroid may be given.

Other Forms of Scabies

Scabies in Clean Persons

In patients with good hygiene findings may be minimal in scabies. Frequent bathing removes mites and lesions are slight. Burrows may be difficult to find. Papules containing larvae may be seen [5].

Scabies Incognito

If a patient has been using topical or systemic corticosteroids prior to the diagnosis of scabies, the morphology of the disease will be changed. Also, scabies may be confused with or coexist with a number of other skin disorders [10].

Nodular Scabies

The reddish brown pruritic nodules seen in some patients can persist for many months after scabicide treatment. They may simulate lymphoma and histiocytosis X. The nodules may clear spontaneously. Treatment can include topical tar gel applications nightly for 2 to 3 weeks (Estar). Also intralesional steroid injection is helpful (triamcinolone acetonide, 5 mg/ml) [5].

Norwegian Scabies

Norwegian or crusted scabies is comparatively rare. It is mainly seen in institutionalized patients who are immunocompromised or mentally handicapped. Cases of Norwegian scabies may be the nidus of mini-epidemics among hospitalized or institutionalized patients.

Patients with Norwegian scabies may have minimal pruritus or intense pruritus. Their skin is host to tremendous infestation of scabies mites, producing a crusted, scaling rash. The rash can affect hands, feet, scalp, neck, and trunk and may become generalized. Lesions of the ears, palms, and soles are seen. Generalized superficial lymphadenopathy and blood eosinophilia may be seen.

Norwegian scabies may be undiagnosed for some time and mimic other skin conditions such as exfoliative dermatitis, psoriasis, and Darier's disease. The usual scabicide treatment should be doubled in these cases, and the face and scalp treated. Contacts should also be treated, including staff, and care taken to disinfect the patients' environment [2,4,39].

PEDICULOSIS PUBIS

Pediculosis pubis has been increasingly diagnosed. This infestation by the pubic louse, *Phthirus pubis*, should be suspected in any patient complaining of groin irritation or pruritus. A search should be made for crab lice and their eggs, or nits, in the pubic hair. They may also infest chest hair, axillae, eyebrows, eyelashes, and, on rare occasions, scalp hair. Other sexually transmitted diseases may also be present.

Etiology

Phthirus pubis, the pubic louse, may be distinguished from *Pediculus humanis* var. *capitis*, the head louse, and *Pediculus humanis* var. *corporis*, the body louse. The head and body lice share a species and differ mainly in size, the body louse being the largest. Pubic lice measure less than 2 mm in length, while the head and body lice are 2 to 4 mm in length and have an elongated triple-segmented body. Pubic lice have a rounded, short body with two pairs of prominent, claw-like legs giving the resemblance to crabs connoted by their popular name, crab lice. These clawlike legs give the lice a means to firmly grip the rather widely spaced hairs in their favorite body areas.

The lice are pale brown to pale gray in color. They move rather slowly compared with body lice, about 10 cm a day. The insects' heads are specialized sucking apparatus which are inserted into the skin capillary, sucking blood frequently. They can only survive apart from a host less than 48 hr [40].

The typical crab louse lives about 30 to 35 days as an adult, following a nymph stage of 13 to 17 days, during which the insect molts three times [40]. One or two days after mating, the female begins laying eggs, about three per day, to a total average of 26 [41]. Each egg is attached firmly to the base of a single hair by a cement which the female secretes. These eggs (nits) are pale gray, translucent, and ovoid, measuring 0.5 mm long. They have a pointed cap, the operculum, which dislodges when the nymphs hatch in 7 to 8 days [41,42]. From egg to egg the life cycle is about 25 days [40].

Pathology

The average infested patient carries about six adult lice and innumerable nits [43]. The distribution of the insects is related to hair density, with hairs spaced approximately 2 mm apart being favored [41]. Usually only the pubic hairs are involved, but spread to perianal hairs is common. Widespread lice can be found in the hair of the trunk, thighs, axillae, eyelashes, eyebrows, beard, mustache, and, on rare occasions, scalp. About 1% of louse involvement in the hair of children are crab lice [44]. *Phthirus pubis* may also infest the eyebrows and eyelashes of children.

Unique cutaneous macules, the maculae caeruleae, may accompany public lice. These blue-gray lesions, 0.5 to 1.0 cm in diameter, may be seen on the lower abdomen and upper thighs. They do not blanch with pressure. The maculae may result from altered blood pigments at the site of bites [45] or a substance secreted by the salivary glands of the louse [41].

No known disease is transmitted by the pubic louse as a vector. Body lice are known to transmit louse-borne typhus fever, trench fever, and epidemic relapsing fever [42].

Epidemiology

Pediculosis pubis is spread by close personal contact. It is more contagious than any other sexually transmitted disease. The chance of contracting pediculosis pubis following one sexual encounter is 95% as compared with the 33% chance of contracting syphilis or gonorrhea [40].

Pediculosis pubis is most commonly encountered during adolescence and young adulthood [43]. From ages 15 to 19 years, pediculosis pubis is more common in females. After age 20, males more commonly are seen with pubic lice [41]. There is no racial preference for the disease [40]; all social groups are affected [43].

Humans are the only host for the pubic louse. Transmission of lice and nits by fomites is possible when sharing the same bed, blanket, clothing, or towels with infested persons [40,45]. The likelihood of fomite transmission is much less than that of bodily contact. Those pubic lice which are dislodged from the host without transfer to another host have a low rate of infectivity [44]. Body lice, by contrast, live mainly on the clothing and can be spread readily by linen and apparel. They are correlated with poor hygiene and crowded living conditions. The crab louse is seen in persons of good hygiene, and its increasing diagnosis has been attributed to either greater sexual promiscuity or more forthright patients [44].

Clinical Features

The patient with pubic lice may be asymptomatic or complain of intense pruritus or irritation. The time from exposure to the onset of symptoms has been estimated at 30 days [41]. The itching is thought to result from sensitization and involves not only the groin, but also the trunk and thighs [40]. Widespread excoriations can result, and secondary infection and eczematization can be seen. Severe cases are associated with fever, malaise, lymphadenopathy, leukocytosis, and headache. Bullous lesions may result from bites in very sensitive patients [45].

In some cases the patient may report seeing the crab lice or nits, or relate the recent treatment for pediculosis of a sexual partner or roommate.

Diagnosis

A high index of suspicion is important in pediculosis pubis. Visualization of lice, larvae, and nits can be aided by use of a magnifying lens. Also seen are rust-colored specks of lice feces on the skin. Maculae caeruleae are also diagnostic. The groin should be examined, and the axillae, trunk, and thighs as well.

Microscopic examination of a louse will reveal the typical crablike morphology. If the lice are not seen, diagnosis can be made by plucking a hair and examining it with mineral oil under a cover slip. The typical nit may be seen close to the root. They adhere strongly to the hair.

Differential Diagnosis

Other conditions may be considered in pubic lice infestation. These include impetigo, pyoderma, seborrheic dermatitis, infectious eczema, contact dermatitis, psoriasis, neurodermatitis, and factitial dermatitis [40].

Complications

The presence of *P. pubis* should be considered a sexually transmitted disease and a search made for coexisting venereal diseases. In one series 46% of pediculosis patients had another venereal infection [41]. In a 5-year investigation of all patients with crab lice, 15.3% of women and 7.2% of men also had gonorrhea [46]. Syphilis, nongonococcal urethritis, trichomoniasis, candidiasis, genital warts, and scabies have also been reported [41,46].

Crab lice infesting the eyelashes, *P. pubis* palpebrae, has been observed. In infants, spread from the breast hair of the mother has been suspected [45]. Generally, hand contact from genital area to eye is the mode of transmission. Eyelash infestation is usually by the crab louse rather than the head or body louse, which may be due to the spacing of the hairs [42].

Phthiriasis palpebrae may simulate seborrheic or infectious eczematous blepharitis [40]. Clinical manifestations include pruritic lids and inflamed conjunctivae. Preauricular lymphadenopathy and secondary infection of the lids may result, and maculae caeruleae can be seen. Close examination of the lid margins should reveal lice, nits, or feces.

Pediculosis patients who are misdiagnosed or self-medicated may be treated with topical steroids. While the pruritus may partially respond, the infestation continues. Generalized infestation by *P. pubis* has been reported in a patient treated for 2 months with steroid cream [47].

Treatment

The treatment of choice for pediculosis pubis is gamma-benzene hexachloride (1%) or lindane. Lindane shampoo is the most convenient form and should be massaged into the genital and anal regions, the axillae, and any other affected areas. Lindane is contraindicated around the eyes. The shampoo is lathered and left on for at least 4 min and then rinsed off thoroughly. An alternative approach is to apply a thin layer of lindane lotion or cream to the body, leave it on for 12 hr, and then wash it off thoroughly. This may be useful in widespread cases [40,48].

Lindane has been associated with central nervous system and blood toxicities and is percutaneously absorbed. Pretreatment bathing and leaving the medication on the skin longer than 12 hr are not recommended. Lindane should be used with caution in infants, children, and pregnant women [25]. Resistance to lindane is probably rare, but its ovicidal action is unproven [25,49]. To minimize possible toxicity, reapplication after 1 week should be reserved for cases of proven continuing infestation and is usually unnecessary [25].

Topical medications containing pyrethrins are an alternative medication and are available over the counter. They are applied to dry hairy areas, left on for 10 min, and then washed off thoroughly. In two studies they were shown to be safe and as effective as lindane [48,50]. They are not to be used near the eyes.

Following either treatment, combing the affected areas with a fine-toothed comb is useful to remove remaining lice and nits. Mild pruritus may persist for several days and can be treated with topical steroids. A feeling of continuing infestation, parasitophobia, is sometimes seen in patients. A search for continuing infestation and reassurance of cure is indicated. Since the pediculocides are potentially irritating, people who are sensitive to them or overuse them may develop a dermatitis requiring topical steroid treatment.

Infestation of the eyelashes may be treated with yellow mercuric oxide 1% ophthalmic ointment, physostigmine 0.25% ophthalmic ointment, or plain petrolatum thickly applied twice daily for 1 week. Mechanical removal by the professional of lice and nits with fine tweezers is helpful [42].

It is usually recommended that clothing and linen be washed and dried by machine using a hot cycle to eliminate fomite transmission. Alternatives include dry-cleaning or just machine-drying on the hot setting [40,44].

It is essential to treat all sexual partners of patients at the same time to prevent reinfestation. Family members, roommates, and others need not be routinely treated if asymptomatic. The patient presenting with pubic lice needs to be screened for coexistent disease by serological test for syphilis and culture for gonorrhea.

MOLLUSCUM CONTAGIOSUM

Molluscum contagiosum is a viral skin infection of children and young adults. The small, firm, umbilicated papules may be seen on the extremities or the trunk, and in sexually transmitted cases the lesions are in the genital area. The papules are usually asymptomatic, but may be inflamed or pruritic. The condition is benign and self-limited, but it is contagious via skin contact and fomites.

Etiology

Molluscum contagiosum virus has a worldwide distribution. It is a poxvirus containing double-stranded DNA. Serologically it is distinguished from all other poxviruses, including smallpox and cowpox [51,52]. Its life cycle is similar to other poxviruses, with cytoplasmic replication, prominent inclusion bodies, and cytopathic hyperplasia [53]. Serial propagation in tissue culture has been accomplished, but the virus is rather inert in vitro [54,55].

Ultrastructural studies reveal a large, brick-shaped virion measuring 300 by 200 by 100 nm. The DNA is contained in a central dumbell-shaped nucleoid [53]. Studies of infected cells show viral proliferation in the cytoplasm produces ovoid accumulations of numerous maturing virions. These are the molluscum bodies, which are pathognomonic. Eventually they enlarge to nearly fill the swollen cells, leaving remnants of the cell nuclei compressed at the margin [56].

Pathology

The typical skin lesion of molluscum contagiosum is a smooth papule, white to flesh-colored, measuring 2 to 5 mm. It can slowly increase to a nodule as big as 10 mm. The lesions are dome shaped and can be identified by their characteristic central umbilication [Fig. 2 (see Plate IV, facing p. 336)]. This is an opening from which caseouslike material can be expressed [52]. Molluscum contagiosum lesions usually are discrete, but have been seen in conjunction with epidermal inclusion cysts, hair follicles, and intradermal nevi [56].

Infection by the virus occurs externally. The papules are formed by epidermal proliferation which invaginates the dermis below and projects above the adjacent skin superficially [53]. The central umbilication projects deeply into the lesion, forming a canal containing desquamated cell debris and molluscum bodies. The epithelial lining cells of the canal appear normal [57].

At the bottom of this epidermal cylinder cytopathic changes reveal molluscum contagiosum involvement of all epidermal layers. The stratum basale and deep portion of the stratum spinosum show enlarged cells with large nuclei. The upper portion of the stratum spinosum and the stratum granulosum show cytoplasmic vacuolization and eosinophilic condensations progressing to large spherical molluscum bodies. These measure up to 35 μm in diameter and nearly fill the cells. The nuclei appear crescent shaped and pyknotic and are pushed to the side of cells that desquamate in the central zone [56,57].

Subadjacent dermal changes have been reported, but the basement membrane remains intact. Collagen proliferation and vascular ectasia have been seen [56]. Inflamed molluscum contagiosum lesions show dermal infiltration by lymphocytes, histiocytes, leukocytes, and giant cells [53].

Immunofluorescent studies of molluscum contagiosum virus have shown viral antigens detectable in the stratum spinosum, stratum granulosum, and the keratin matrix. Virus-specific antibodies have been demonstrated in 69% of patients. The predominant antibodies were IgG, with IgM being rare. Those patients without detectable virus-specific antibodies may have had lesions in which viral antigen remained isolated from the immune system owing to lack of skin trauma [51]. Serological testing for molluscum contagiosum has been inconsistent and is not clinically useful [53].

Epidemiology

Molluscum contagiosum is generally held to be a disease of humans only. Transmission is by skin-to-skin contact, fomites, and autoinoculation. Numerous studies have shown local outbreaks occur among children playing together [53,58]. Contacts among wrestlers, patients of a surgeon with a hand lesion, and clients sharing a masseur have acquired the lesions. Fomite transmission has been reported among people sharing bathing facilities, swimming pools, towels, gym equipment, and benches [52,53].

The incubation period of molluscum contagiosum is 2 to 7 weeks, based upon experimental inoculation studies. A review of the epidemiological studies indicates two forms of molluscum contagiosum. The childhood disease affects the face, trunk, and limbs and is transmitted by skin contact and fomites. The disease of young adults affects the genital area and is acquired by skin contact during sexual relations [53].

Clinical Features

Clinical Course

The dome-shaped papules of molluscum contagiosum develop slowly and remain stable for long periods. Usually less than 5 mm in diameter, they occasionally coalesce or expand to form plaques up to ½ in. in diameter [59]. The number of lesions is usually less than 20, but many hundreds of lesions have been reported in some cases [53,60].

Molluscum contagiosum is usually asymptomatic, but may be accompanied by pruritus or an eczematous reaction. Lesions may be seen in a linear distribution, presumably from scratching [52,53]. Following trauma, or spontaneously after several months, the lesions may become inflamed. Tenderness, suppuration, crusting, and eventually complete healing may then be seen [61]. Usually the life of a lesion is less than 2 months, but it can last several years. A crop of molluscum contagiosum is typically self-limited to 6 to 9 months duration [55].

Disease in Children

Lesions in children are mainly seen on the trunk, neck, face, and limbs. Lesions on the palms and soles are rare [53,55]. In a study of affected children in Alaska, child-to-child transmission by playing together was shown [58]. The range in age was 10 months to 13 years in the 13 cases studied. Multiple cases occurred in only one-fourth of families. The outbreak was not related to poor hygiene.

Venereal Molluscum Contagiosum

Sexually transmitted molluscum contagiosum is seen among adolescents and adults presenting with genital lesions [62,63]. The papules may be seen on the lower abdomen, pubic area, penis, vulva, perineum, anus, buttocks, and thighs. Molluscum contagiosum affects mainly normal skin rather than mucous membranes, but has been seen on the borders of the lips [53,63]. The lesions are typically multiple.

Venereal warts (condylomata acuminata) are verrucous papules rather than smooth, umbilicated ones. As compared with molluscum contagiosum, veneral warts more commonly affect the penis, vulva, and anus, showing a predilection for mucous membranes, including the mouth [52]. They may be stalked, sessile, and have satellite lesions. A similar appearance may be shown by condyloma lata, genital lesions of secondary syphilis. These tend to be flatter, grayish papules, positive for spirochetes on dark-field examination [64].

Other papular genital lesions include pearly penile papules, which occur near the corona. They are multiple, gray, white, or pink in appearance, and of no pathological importance. Genital infections of *Candida* sp. produce papular lesions, usually pruritic and erythematous and often pustular. Early, transient papular lesions are seen in syphilis, scabies, lymphogranuloma venereum, and chancroid [64].

Venereal molluscum contagiosum may be increasing in frequency. New cases reported in English hospital clinics increased 40% from 1974 to 1978. The incidence of the disease per 100,000 population was 2.01 in 1978. This represented 1 new case of molluscum contagiosum for every 62 new cases of gonorrhea [65]. In the United States a group of sexually transmitted disease clinics have reported one case of molluscum contagiosum for every 42 cases of gonorrhea during 1976 to 1980, comprising 1 patient in 190 consulting these clinics [66].

Because the incubation period of molluscum contagiosum may be as long as 7 weeks, tracing case contacts is difficult. Molluscum contagiosum may be an incidental finding in a patient with other sexually transmitted diseases. It has been reported with gonorrhea and herpes genitalis. Serological testing for syphilis and culture for the gonococcus is indicated in patients with genital molluscum contagiosum [67].

Molluscum Dermatitis

Typical asymptomatic papules of molluscum contagiosum may become pruritic and inflamed, developing a painful localized eczema. Molluscum dermatitis has been reported in 10% of cases [53,68]. This is generally held to be a delayed hypersensitivity reaction and may be followed by spontaneous clearing of the lesions. Dermal infiltration is predominantly lymphocytes and histiocytes [61]. The condition may resemble furunculosis or secondary bacterial infection [69]. Treatment of the molluscum will clear the dermatitis.

Diagnosis

Examination of the patient should reveal smooth, light-colored papules with an umbilicated center. Usually multiple, they will be seen in the characteristic distribution of children or young adults. If the diagnosis is in doubt clinically, microscopic examination can be done.

A lesion may be squeezed, expressing the white caseous material from the core. This can be facilitated by nicking the lesion with a #11 scalpel blade. Alternatively, the lesion may be curetted off, with or without anesthesia. The material obtained should be crushed on a slide and stained with Wright, Giemsa, or Gram stain. The cells will reveal the large intracytoplasmic molluscum bodies which are pathognomonic [52,53].

A punch biopsy may be performed to reveal the characteristic histopathology of molluscum contagiosum. The eosinophilic inclusion bodies will be seen throughout the cells of the stratum malpighii of the epidermis.

Differential Diagnosis

Multiple lesions of molluscum contagiosum are usually distinctive, but solitary lesions may present diagnostic questions. Small, multiple lesions may suggest flat warts. Single or multiple keratoacanthomas usually occur in patients over 40 years, an older group than usually seen with molluscum contagiosum [52]. Syringomas and hydrocytomas may be considered, especially with lesions around the eye [70]. Large lesions and secondarily infected ones simulate furuncles. Other possibilities include epidermal inclusion cysts, basal cell epitheliomas, eruptive xanthomas, pyogenic granulomas, and rarely many other lesions [52,53]. Biopsy may be useful.

Complications

Aside from molluscum dermatitis, most complications are unusual. If lesions are excoriated, they may become secondarily infected by streptococci or staphylococci. This can mimic molluscum dermatitis.

Lesions have been described near the eyelids [55,63]. A mild or severe chronic conjunctivitis may result. Superficial punctate keratitis has also been seen. The ocular sequelae are thought to result from a hypersensitivity reaction or a toxic effect of the caseous material of the lesions [55,71].

Very extensive molluscum contagiosum lesions can occur in normal individuals, but have been associated with a variety of other conditions [53]. Atopic dermatitis may predispose to extensive lesions due to deficient cell-mediated immunity or other defective host defense mechanisms [72]. Impaired cellular immunity and extensive molluscum contagiosum has been observed with acquired T-cell deficiency and other disorders [53,73].

Immunosuppressive therapy has been implicated in extensive molluscum contagiosum. Treatment with prednisone and methotrexate led to generalized lesions in two cases [60]. Multiple facial eruptions of molluscum contagiosum have been associated with the use of topical corticosteroids [74].

Treatment

Molluscum contagiosum is a benign and self-limited disease. Treatment is to prevent spread and for cosmetic reasons. Since the lesions may heal spontaneously without scarring, any therapy should be fairly innocuous.

An efficient surgical approach is to make a tiny superficial incision of the top of the lesion, using a #11 blade. The contents may then be extruded using a comedo extractor. Healing without scarring may then be expected [75]. The base of the lesion may be touched with a caustic agent such as 1% tincture of iodine, podophyllin, or trichloroacetic acid. Light electrodessication is an alternative [76].

Curetting off the lesions is another approach. Superficial scraping with a sharp dermal curet is followed by cautery of bleeding points by chemical or electrical means. This may be done without anesthesia, or with larger lesions ethyl chloride spray or injection of lidocaine hydrochloride is a preliminary step [59,76].

A popular therapy for multiple lesions is cryosurgery with liquid nitrogen. A wide variety of topical preparations have been applied to lesions. A 5% tincture of iodine may be applied twice daily for 1 to 2 weeks [76]. Office application of cantharidin, which may be repeated on new or persistent lesions at weekly intervals, has been utilized [77].

If lesions become secondarily infected, they may first be treated with Burow's solution compresses and systemic antibiotics. This is followed by removal of the papules as above [76].

Patients should be seen for follow-up examination in about 6 weeks for treatment of any new lesions which may have arisen. Sexual partners of patients with genital molluscum contagiosum should also be examined and treated to prevent reinfection.

REFERENCES

1. Weary PB. Scabies. In: Mandell GL, Douglas PG, Bennet JE, eds. Principles and practice of infectious diseases. New York: Wiley, 1979:2203-2204.
2. Estes SA. The diagnosis and management of scabies. Piscataway, N.J.: Reed and Carnrick, 1981.
3. Blecka LJ. Concise medical parasitology. Menlo Park, Calif.: Addison-Wesley, 1980:182-184.
4. Rook A. Scabies. In: Rook A, Wilkinson DS, Ebling FJ, eds. Textbook of dermatology. Oxford: Blackwell Scientific, 1979:927-941.
5. Orkin M, Maibach H. Scabies, a current pandemic. Postgrad Med 1979; 66: 53-65.
6. Baer RL. Current views on the management of pediculosis and scabies: introduction. Cutis Suppl Sept 1981; 5-6.

7. Falk ES, Eide TJ. Histologic and clinical findings in human scabies. Int J Dermatol 1981; 20:600-605.
8. Hoeffling KK, Schroeter AL. Dermatoimmunopathology of scabies. J Am Acad Dermatol 1980; 3:237-240.
9. Van Neste D. Immunologic studies in scabies. Int J Dermatol 1981; 20:264-269.
10. Orkin M. Today's scabies. Arch Dermatol 1975; 111:1431-1432.
11. Shaw P, Juranek D. Recent trends in scabies in the United States. J Infect Dis 1976; 134:414-416.
12. Knox D, Yoder F, Kramer M. Incidence of scabies in white and black populations. Arch Dermatol 1979; 115:1286.
13. Cohen, HB. Scabies continues. Int J Dermatol 1982; 21:134-135.
14. Church RE, Knowelden J. Scabies in Sheffield: a family infestation. Br Med J 1978; 1:761-763.
15. Tschen E. What treatment for skin infestations in the elderly? Geriatrics 1982; 37:38-44.
16. Mellanby K. The development of symptoms, parasitic infection, and immunity in human scabies. Parasitology 1944; 35:197-206.
17. Munkvad JM, Nielsen AO, Secher L. Venereal disease in patients with scabies: a five-year survey. Acta Derm Venereol 1982; 62:274-275.
18. Fiumara NJ, Calhoun J. Multiple sexually transmitted diseases. Sex Transm Dis 1982; 9:98-99.
19. Estes SA. Diagnosis and management of scabies. Med Clin North Am 1982; 66:955-963.
20. Woodley D, Saurat J. The burrow ink test and the scabies mite. J Am Acad Dermatol 1981; 4:715-722.
21. Cullen S, Childers R. Oral Levamisole "safe, effective" against scabies. Dermatol Pract Jan-Feb 1978; 274-275.
22. Muller G, Jacobs P, Moore N. Scraping for human scabies. Arch Dermatol 1973; 107:70.
23. Chapel TA, Krugel L, Chapel J, Segal A. Scabies presenting as urticaria. JAMA 1981; 246:1440-1441.
24. Guidelines for sexually transmitted diseases. J Am Acad Dermatol 1983; 8: 589-605.
25. Shacter B. Treatment of scabies and pediculosis with lindane preparations: an evaluation. J Am Acad Dermatol 1981; 5:517-527.
26. Rasmussen JE. The problem of lindane. J Am Acad Dermatol 1981; 5:507-516.
27. Ginsburg CM. Scabies in infants and children: a pediatrician's view. Cutis Suppl Sept 1981:10-14.
28. Kramer MS. Toxicity of 1% gamma benzene hexachloride (GBH): an operational assessment. Cutis Suppl Sept 1981:20-25.
29. Baer RL. Roundtable discussion scabies and pediculosis: clinical guidelines. Cutis Suppl Sept 1981:26-31.
30. Solomon LM, Fahrner L, West DP. Gamma benzene hexachloride toxicity. Arch Dermatol 1977; 113:353-357.

76. Olansky S
1970; 47:
77. Funt TR,
contagiosi

31. Talpin, quoted in Rasmussen JE. The problem of lindane. J Am Acad Dermatol 1981; 5:507-516.
32. Pramanik AK, Hansen RC. Transcutaneous gamma benzene hexachloride absorption and toxicity in infants and children. Arch Dermatol 1979; 115: 1224-1225.
33. Feldman RJ, Maibach HI. Percutaneous penetration of some pesticides and herbicides in man. Toxical Appl Pharmacol 1974; 28:126-132.
34. Amer M, El-Bayoum M, Rizk M. Treatment of scabies: preliminary report. Int J Dermatol 1981; 20:289-290.
35. Cubela V, Yawalkar SJ. Clinical experience with crotamiton cream and lotion in treatment of infants with scabies. Br J Clin Pract 1978; 32:229-231.
36. Konstantinov D, Stanoeva L, Yawalkar SJ. Crotamiton creme and lotion in the treatment of infants and young children with scabies. J Int Med Res 1979; 7:443-448.
37. Coskey RJ. Scabies-resistance to treatment with crotamiton. Arch Dermatol 1979; 115:109.
38. Rasmussen JE. Percutaneous absorption in children. In: Dobson RL, ed. Yearbook of dermatology. Chicago: Yearbook Medical, 1979:15-38.
39. Moschella SL. Parasitology and tropical dermatology. In: Moschella SL, et al., eds. Dermatology. Philadelphia: Saunders, 1975:1517-1522.
40. Felman YM, Nikitas JA. Pediculosis pubis. Cutis 1980; 25:482, 487-489, 559.
41. Fisher I, Morton RS. *Phthirus pubis* infestation. Br J Vener Dis 1970; 46: 326-329.
42. Bonivk MM, Friedman AH. Diagnosing and treating *Phthirus pubis* palpebrarum. Surv Opthalmol 1982; 26:219-225.
43. Altchek A. Epidemic pediculosis and gonorrhea. Obstet Gynecol 1970; 35: 638-641.
44. Maunder JW. Human lice—biology and control. R Soc Health J 1977: 97: 29-32.
45. Rook A. Skin diseases caused by arthropods and other venomous or noxious animals. In: Rook A, et al., eds. Textbook of dermatology. 3rd ed. Oxford: Blackwell Scientific, 1979:925-928.
46. Munkvad IM, Klemp P. Co-existence of venereal infection and pediculosis pubis. Acta Derm Venereol 1982; 62:366-367.
47. Nielsen AO, Secher L. Pediculosis pubis in a patient treated with topical steroids. Cutis 1980; 25:655, 658.
48. Smith DE, Walsh J. Treatment of pubic lice infestation: a comparison of two agents. Cutis 1980; 26:618-619.
49. Orkin M. Treatment of today's scabies and pediculosis. JAMA 1976; 236: 1136-1139.
50. Newsome JH. Treatment of infestation with *Phthirus pubis*: comparative efficacies of synerginized pyrethrins and gamma-benzene hexachloride. Sex Transm Dis 1979; 6:203.
51. Shirodaria PV, Matthews RS. Observations on the antibody responses in molluscum contagiosum. Br J Dermatol 1977; 96:29-34.
52. Felman YM, Nikitas JA. Genital molluscum contagiosum. Cutis 1980; 26:28, 30, 32.

53. Brc
198
54. Fra
lusc
388
55. Nag
Tex
656,
56. Kwi
Sina
57. Veh
Path
58. Over
in Ar
59. Calve
60. Roser
ment
61. Steffe
sum.
62. Cobb
diseas
63. Jacob
64. Rein
Princi
65. Chief
tract f
Br J V
66. Johnsc
quoted
8:227-
67. Wilkin
a vener
68. Kippin
69. Lynfiel
Cutis 1
70. Janis B
2nd ed.
71. Thomas
tice of i
72. Pauly C
ity, and
73. Peachy
Br J Der
74. Hellier F
oids. Br
75. Resnik S
molluscu

FOURTEEN

Miscellaneous Infections

Cytomegalovirus, Hepatitis B, and Group B Streptococcus

Joseph F. Plouffe
The Ohio State University
College of Medicine
Columbus, Ohio

INTRODUCTION

Infections by cytomegalovirus, hepatitis B virus, and group B streptococcus previously would not have been discussed in a textbook of sexually transmitted diseases (STD), but recently these have been recognized to be more prevalent in populations attending STD clinics. These organisms cause a diverse spectrum of clinical illnesses involving multiple organ systems, but usually cause no specific disease of the genital tract that would bring a patient to the STD clinic.

CYTOMEGALOVIRUS

Introduction

Cytomegalovirus (CMV) is associated with a number of clinical syndromes involving neonates, healthy adults, and immunosuppressed individuals [1]. Cytomegalovirus is a member of the herpesvirus family, which includes herpes simplex virus types 1 and 2, varicella zoster virus, and Epstein-Barr virus. The viruses are DNA viruses and have the capability of interacting with human DNA to produce chronic, recurrent, or latent infections.

Cytomegalovirus was initially recognized as a human pathogen in rare instances of fulminant congenital infection [2]. It is now known that infection with CMV is common both in the perinatal period and in young adult life, with most infections being asymptomatic [3,4]. The role of sexual transmission of CMV was suggested by the finding of CMV in semen and cervical secretions [5-7]. Cytomegalovirus was successfully cultured less than 30 years ago [8-10]. The syndrome of mononucleosis in young adults caused by CMV was described 20 years ago [11].

Biological Characteristics

The CMV genome consists of double-stranded DNA which is approximately 50% larger than the herpes simplex virus genome. After the virus infects a human cell, several conditions are possible. The virus can replicate and destroy the infected cell or it can become incorporated into the host cell DNA. At this stage the viral DNA may or may not initiate viral protein synthesis. Incorporation of the viral DNA into the host genome established the latent infection. The details of the structure and function of the CMV genome are discussed by Stinski et al. [12].

Isolation of CMV is the most definitive diagnostic test [1]. Cytomegalovirus can be grown in human fibroblast cell culture, and typical cytopathic effects are seen from several days to several weeks, depending on the inoculum of virus. After the initial isolation from salivary glands, CMV has been cultured from multiple sites, including urine, semen, cervical secretions, buffy coats, and multiple organs at autopsy [13].

Several methods for measuring antibodies to CMV are available, including the complement fixation assay [1,14], fluorescence antibody, [15] and the anticomplement immunofluorescent test. Antibody studies have shown the presence of several serotypes of CMV. The clinical importance of the different serotypes is not well defined [1].

Epidemiology

Prevalence of antibody to CMV varies worldwide, depending on the population studied, with rates ranging from 40 to 100% [16]. The higher prevalence rates were seen in the populations of underdeveloped countries and lower socioeconomic groups. Several studies have shown higher prevalence of antibodies in females [17,18]. Studies [7,19] examining the association of CMV and venereal disease have demonstrated higher prevalence rates of antibody in women being evaluated for venereal diseases (83%) compared to a control population (50%). Also, the rate of isolation of CMV from cervical secretion was higher (13.3%) in the suspected STD population versus control (0%). Most of the CMV isolates (88%) were from women aged 15 to 24 years. Knox et al. studied 1101 indigent women and found that CMV cervical shedding was 15% in the 11- to 14-year age group and positive cultures declined with age until it was undetectable over the age of 30 years [20].

Handsfield et al. [21] reported that 57% of women attending STD clinics had a positive titer to CMV, compared to 35.9% of controls ($p < 0.001$). Cytomegalovirus was isolated from the cervix of 24.7% of STD clinic women. Shedding of virus and antibody titers were positively correlated with number of sex partners and with current or past STD. They followed 86 women who were initially seronegative and culture negative, and 7 of these subjects seroconverted and developed positive cervical cultures for CMV to give a 28% annual incidence of primary infection in this population, a 10-fold increase compared to control women aged 15 to 34 years. Cytomegalovirus was isolated from 3 of 6 sex partners of women who had positive CMV cultures, as compared to 0 of 16 partners of women with negative cultures.

Studies of homosexual men have shown an antibody prevalence rate of 94%, compared to 54% in the heterosexual men attending the STD clinic. Cytomegalovirus was cultured from the urethra of 14 of 190 homosexual men and 0 of 101 heterosexual men [22].

Clinical Syndromes

Congenital Infections

Initially it was thought that congenital infections were rare events, the classic presentation being a small, microcephalic neonate with hepatosplenomegaly, chorioretinitis, jaundice, and purpura [23]. Stagno et al. [24] found that 3.4% of neonates born to a group of women (82% seropositive) were congenitally infected. In three prospective studies primary CMV infection developed in 0.5% of pregnancies. Over half of the neonates were infected and a fourth were symptomatic [25-27]. The congenitally infected neonate, even if asymptomatic at birth, may subsequently develop hearing difficulties [28].

Perinatal Infection

Cytomegalovirus can be isolated from cervical secretions in pregnant females. The rate of isolation increased throughout pregnancy. Reynolds et al. [29] reported that 37% of neonates born to mothers who had a positive cervical culture during the third trimester became infected. A total of 57% of those born to mothers who had positive cultures postpartum became infected. The neonates were asymptomatic and cultures of urine were negative at birth. Urine cultures became positive at 1 to 2 months of age. The long-term effects of perinatal infection are unknown [30].

Mononucleosis

A syndrome similar to Epstein-Barr virus mononucleosis is caused by CMV in healthy young adults [11,31-33]. Fever, mild adenopathy, and fatigue are frequent. Pharyngitis is unusual. Lymphocytosis with atypical lymphocytes is frequent and the heterophile antibody is absent. Approximately half of heterophile-negative cases of mononucleosis are due to CMV. There have been several reports of sexual contacts of patients with CMV mononucleosis becoming infected with CMV [31,34].

Immunosuppressed Patients

Cytomegalovirus can be a major problem in the immunosuppressed population such as renal and cardiac transplants [35-37]. The patient may have febrile illnesses, interstitial pneumonitis, retinitis, and hepatitis. The infections can be either primary or a reactivation of a latent infection [35]. Seronegative recipients of organs from a seropositive donor are at risk of developing primary disease [36-38]. Blood products from seropositive donors are also a risk factor [39]. Patients with acquired immunodeficiency syndrome are also at risk of developing severe CMV infections [40,41].

Therapy

Treatment of severe CMV infections has been attempted with antiviral drugs (adenosine arabinoside) [42] and immunomodulating agents (interferon [43, 44], transfer factor [45]) with little success. Preliminary studies with acyclovir have shown some promise in a small number of cases [46].

Trials with attenuated vaccines are in progress [47-49]. Initial results seem promising with the development of humoral and cellular immunity [50]. There is still some concern that the attenuated strain may be capable of causing disease in the immunosuppressed individual. Production of subunit vaccines capable of eliciting an immune response without causing a latent infection offers the most promise.

Passive immunization with cytomegalovirus immune globulin has some effect in the bone marrow transplant population [51,52].

Newer techniques are becoming available for rapid diagnosis of CMV infection [53] and for use in sorting out the complex epidemiology [54] of CMV infections.

HEPATITIS B VIRUS

Introduction

In the past 20 years vast strides have been made toward understanding hepatitis B and preventing its occurrence. Many years ago clinicians recognized two types of hepatitis: a short incubation type with suspected fecal-oral spread and a longer incubation type with suspected parenteral transmission [55]. In 1964 Blumberg reported the presence of the Australia antigen [56], which was subsequently shown to be hepatitis B surface antigen (HB_sAg) [57,58]. This discovery led to screening of blood donors and decreased the rate of transfusion hepatitis [59]. The next step at disease prevention was taken with postexposure passive immunization with hyperimmune gammaglobulin. Most recently, active immunization has been accomplished with a safe and effective vaccine. The Centers for Disease Control [60] estimate that 200,000 people in the United States are infected with hepatitis B virus (HBV) each year. A total of 25% become icteric and 5% are hospitalized each year. The Centers for Disease Control estimate that there are currently 400,000 to 800,000 carriers of HB_sAg, with 25% of that group developing chronic active hepatitis which often progresses to cirrhosis. A small number of patients die from hepatitis B-related liver cancer [60].

Biological Characteristics

Hepatitis B (serum hepatitis) is caused by HBV, a complex DNA virus which contains hepatitis B surface antigen (HB_sAg) on its surface and is coated with a lipid envelope and has a nuclear core with hepatitis core antigen (HB_cAg). Hepatitis B virus infects liver cells, where it multiplies [61]. Most patients are able to mount an immune response which clears the infection. Antibodies are produced to the core antigen (anti-HB_c) and surface antigen (anti-HB_s); however, 6 to 10% of patients are unable to eradicate the virus and have HB_sAg persistently in their blood (chronic carriers) [60]. Another antigen, hepatitis B e antigen, was correlated with high levels of HB_sAg, infectivity, and chronic liver disease.

Epidemiology

It was suggested 10 years ago that HBV may be sexually transmitted [62]. Researchers at STD clinics recognized that a higher percentage of patients attending clinics had exposure to hepatitis B compared to controls [63-67]. Homosexual men (40 to 75%) had markers of prior exposure to HBV [68-70]. Studies in prostitutes also suggested that sexual exposure may be a route of transmission, since levels of anti-HB_s were higher in prostitutes than in controls and also were correlated with length of time in service [71,72]. Reiner et al. [73] studied 27 homosexual men with HB_sAg in their blood. On proctoscopic examination, 13 of 22 had multiple punctate bleeding sites; HB_sAg was demonstrated from 10 of the 13 lesions, as well as in 10 of 16 fecal specimens and 13 of 22 rectal swabs. These data indicate that asymptomatic bleeding rectal lesions are common and may be a source of HBV for those engaging in rectal intercourse. Also, HB_sAg has been found in saliva [74] and semen [73].

Although clinical hepatitis is unusual in homosexual men, elevated liver enzyme tests have been found in 17 to 52% of those with HB_sAg. Liver biopsy specimens have shown some discrepancy with either mild changes or evidence of chronic active hepatitis [75-77]. Another population with high prevalence of exposure to HBV is the drug addict population, and this is believed to be due to sharing of contaminated needles [78].

Passive Immunization

Two preparations are available for passive immunization. Recent lots of immune globulin (IG) have measurable titers of anti-HB_s, while hepatitis B immune globulin (HBIG) has approximately 100- to 1000-fold more antibody. The cost of HBIG is approximately 20 times that of IG. Recommendations of the Immunization Practices Advisory Committee [79] suggest giving HBIG (0.06 mg/kg) to susceptible subjects exposed to HB_sAg-positive blood. The exposure may be a needle stick or mucous membrane exposure. One dose should be given immediately and a second dose 1 month later. It is more difficult to know what to do when the HB_sAg status is not known. In the hospital setting exposure to blood containing HB_sAg carries a risk of clinical hepatitis of 1 in 20. If the blood is of unknown status, the risk is 100 times lower. If the source is known and potentially high risk, IG (0.06 mg/kg) can be given immediately. If the source tests positive for HB_sAg, then HBIG (0.06 mg/kg) can be given at that point and 1 month later. Low-risk exposure requires a judgment as whether to withhold therapy or IG (0.06 mg/kg). Sexual exposure to HB_sAg has not been well studied. One study suggests a protective effect of HBIG for sexual contacts [80]. Problems of repeated exposure of a susceptible individual to a HB_sAg consort is better handled with active immunization.

Active Immunization

Initial studies by Krugman suggested that active immunization to HBV is possible [81]. Recently HBV vaccine has been licensed by the U.S. Food and Drug Administration for use. It is a suspension of inactivated, alum-adsorbed antigen particles purified from human plasma. Three doses (20 μg/1.0 ml) are required for immunization at 0, 1, and 6 months. The vaccine has been shown to be effective in a male homosexual population with a reduction of clinical or subclinical hepatitis from 18 to 27% in the placebo group to 1.4 to 3.4% in the vaccine group in an 18-month period [82]. The incidence of side effects was minimal. Other studies have also shown efficacy of the vaccine in high-risk populations, including a multicenter study of homosexuals [83], hemodialysis staff [84], and infants in an endemic area [85]. Unfortunately, the vaccine was ineffective in eradicating the chronic carrier state [86].

The Advisory Committee for Immunization Practices [60] published guidelines for vaccine use which are summarized below. Currently the vaccine is expensive ($100 for a three-dose regimen). Vaccinating those at high risk for exposure to HB_sAg would be most cost effective. High-risk groups include immigrants from areas of high HBV endemicity, clients in institutions for the mentally retarded, parenteral drug abusers, homosexually active males, household contacts of HB_sAg carriers, and patients in hemodialysis units. Intermediate-risk groups include prisoners, staff of institutions for the mentally retarded, and health care workers with frequent blood contact.

Mulley et al. [87] performed a cost-effective analysis and concluded that screening homosexual males and vaccinating susceptible males and vaccinating surgical residents without prior screening were both cost effective. Neither screening nor vaccination was cost effective for the general population. These analyses were based on current costs of vaccine. With reductions in the cost of vaccine, it should become cost effective to immunize the general population.

GROUP B STREPTOCOCCUS

Introduction

In the past 20 years group B streptococci (GBS) (*Streptococcus agalactiae*) have been recognized to cause sepsis, pneumonia, and meningitis in neonates [88]. More recently serious disease in the adult population has been recognized, especially in the elderly, diabetics, and those with genitourinary disorders [89-92].

Biological Characteristics

The GBS are differentiated from other streptococci on the basis of their polysaccharide antigens [93]. The organisms are typically pigmented and are β-hemolytic. The GBS can be identified by the CAMP test [94] in which lysis occurs with GBS grown in a zone of staphylococcal β toxin activity on sheep blood agar [95]. The GBS can be subdivided into five serotypes by characterization of the polysaccharide and protein antigens [96,97].

Baker and Kasper [98,99] have shown that development of type-specific antibody in pregnant women protected the neonate, while neonates born to mothers colonized with GBS without antibody were at high risk of infections.

Epidemiology

Group B streptococci have been cultured from the pharynx [100], gastrointestinal tract, and genital tract [101-104]. Badri et al. [101] found almost twice as many rectal carriers (18%) as vaginal carriers (10%) in a pregnant population and suggested that the gastrointestinal tract was the primary site of colonization. Easmon et al. [102] were able to culture GBS from 6% of fecal specimens, compared to 25% of rectal mucosa and perianal skin samples in a male homosexual population. Anthony et al. [103] found no difference between gastrointestinal and genital carriage of GBS. Sexual transmission may be a route of acquisition. Baker et al. [104] surveyed college women and discovered that only 7% of virgins were colonized with GBS, compared to 20% of sexually experienced women. However, there was no correlation with the number of partners.

The STD clinic populations have a higher rate of GBS carriage than other populations. Christensen et al. [105] cultured GBS from the urethra of 2.4% of male medical students, 10.6% of males without gonorrhea attending STD clinics, and 22% of those with gonorrhea. Manuel et al. [106] also found a higher rate of GBS urethral colonization in males with gonorrhea (10.7%) versus 6.7% in those without gonorrhea. Wallin and Forsgren [107], however, did not find a correlation with gonorrhea, as 17% of males without gonorrhea attending the STD clinic had GBS colonization of the urethra compared to 11% of males with gonorrhea.

Persson et al. [108] found 41% of females attending STD clinics have colonization with GBS, compared to 28% of controls. They found positive correlation with intrauterine device use and tampon use. They found no correlation with active gonococcal infections. Franciosi et al. [109] cultured the husbands of women with GBS colonization and found that 45% were colonized, compared to 5.6% of males in prison. Chretien et al. [110] cultured GBS from 4.4% of patients with acute pharyngitis; 43% of these patients admitted to recent oral-genital sex. Christensen et al. [111] were also able to measure higher antibody levels to GBS in a STD clinic population compared to controls.

Studies of neonates have demonstrated that colonization with GBS is relatively common (20 to 30%) [112]. If the mother is colonized at the time of delivery, the neonatal colonization rate is 70% [109]. The most common method of transmission appears to be passage through an infected birth canal, although reports of GBS sepsis in neonates delivered by cesarean section have been recorded [113] and GBS have been isolated from cultures of amnionic fluid [114].

Infants also appear to be at risk for nosocomial acquisition of GBS in the nursery [115].

Clinical Manifestations

Severe infections in neonates associated with low birth weight, sepsis, pneumonia, and meningitis occur both early ($\leqslant$ 5 days) and late, with a mean onset of 4 weeks [88,109,116]. The mortality rate is approximately 50% for early onset and 20% for late onset GBS disease [117]. Most of the late onset disease is caused by type III GBS [117].

In women undergoing cesarean section, those with GBS colonization had more fever (66.6 versus 30.5%), endomyometritis (61.1 versus 12.5%), and use of antibiotics (61.1 versus 26.3%) than women without GBS colonization [118]. Although GBS is present in vaginal and urethral flora, there has been no correlation with symptoms of vaginitis or urethritis [119]. Brook reported a case of balanitis due to GBS which was successfully treated with ampicillin [120]. Serious infections in adults caused by GBS have been reported, including sepsis, endocarditis, meningitis, pneumonia, pyelonephritis, osteomyelitis, and endometritis

[89-92]. Possibly pharyngitis may be caused by GBS, as they were isolated from 4.4% of pharyngitis patients who had negative cultures for *Streptococcus pyogenes* [110]. Risk factors in the adult were urinary tract abnormalities, diabetes mellitus and old age [89-92].

Therapy

In neonatal GBS sepsis the mortality approaches 50% [121]. Penicillin is frequently used. The GBS are sensitive to penicillins using standard methods (minimal inhibitory concentration, 0.02 μg/ml). However, testing higher inocula, the minimal inhibitory concentrations increased to 2 to 4 μg/ml. No clinical studies have been performed which demonstrate a better antibiotic regimen. Prevention of neonatal GBS disease has been attempted by administration of antibiotics to the mother during labor [122] and to the neonate in a small number of studies [123]. No large controlled studies have shown efficacy in disease prevention. In a recent study over 1000 neonates weighing less than 2000 g were randomized to receive penicillin or a placebo within 1 hr of birth [124]. Bacteremia with GBS and mortality were similar in both groups. Since maternal antibodies appear to be protective, a vaccine seems to be a logical approach. Strict infection control measures in the nursery may help prevent some of the late onset cases of neonatal sepsis, as the neonates may acquire GBS in the hospital [115].

REFERENCES

1. Weller TH. The cytomegaloviruses: ubiquitous agents with protean clinical manifestations. N Engl J Med 1971; 285:203-214, 267-274.
2. Cappell DF, McFarlane MN. Inclusion bodies (protozoan-like cells) in the organs of infants. J Pathol Bacteriol 1947; 59:385-398.
3. Hanshaw JB. Congenital cytomegalovirus infection: a fifteen year perspective. J Infect Dis 1971; 123:555-561.
4. Starr JG, Bart RD, Gold E. Inapparent congenital cytomegalovirus infection. Clinical and epidemiological characteristics in early infancy. N Engl J Med 1970; 282:1075-1077.
5. Lang DJ, Kummer JF. Demonstration of cytomegalovirus in semen. N Engl J Med 1972; 287:756-758.
6. Lang DJ, Kummer JF, Hartley DP. Cytomegalovirus in semen: persistence and demonstration in extracellular fluid. N Engl J Med 1971; 291:121-123.
7. Jordan MC, Rousseau WE, Noble GR, Stewart JA, Chin TDY. Association of cervical cytomegalovirus with venereal disease. N Engl J Med 1973; 288:923-934.
8. Smith MG. Propagation in tissue culture of a cytopathic virus from human salivary gland virus (SGV). Proc Soc Exp Biol Med 1956; 92:424-430.
9. Rowe WP, Hartley JW, Waterman S, Turner HC, Huebner RJ. Cytopathic agent resembling human salivary gland virus recovered from tissue cultures of human adenoids. Proc Soc Exp Biol Med 1956; 92:418-424.

10. Weller TH, Macauley JC, Craig JM, Wirth P. Isolation of intranuclear inclusion producing agents from infants with illnesses resembling cytomegalic inclusion disease. Proc Soc Exp Biol Med 1957; 94:4-12.
11. Klemola E, Kaariainen L. Cytomegalovirus as a possible cause of a disease resembling infectious mononucleosis. Br Med J 1965; 2:1099-1102.
12. Stinski MF, Thomsen DR, Wathen MW. Structure and function of the cytomegalovirus genome. In: Nahmias AJ, Dowdle WR, Schinazi RF, eds. The human herpes-viruses. New York: Elsevier, 1981; 72-84.
13. Stagno S, Pass RF, Reynolds DW, Moore M, Nahmias AJ, Alford CA. Comparative study of diagnostic procedures for congenital cytomegalovirus infection. Pediatrics 1980; 65:251-257.
14. Reynolds DW, Stagno S, Alford CA. Laboratory diagnosis of cytomegalovirus infections. In: Lenette EH, Schmidt NJ, eds. Diagnostic procedures for viral, richettsial and chlamydial infections. 5th ed. Washington DC: American Public Health Association 1979; 299-439.
15. Hanshaw JB, Steinfeld HJ, White CJ. Fluorescent-antibody test for cytomegalovirus macroglobulin. N Engl J Med 1968; 279:566-570.
16. Krech U. Complement-fixing antibodies against cytomegalovirus in different parts of the world. Bull WHO 1973; 49:103-106.
17. Luby JP, Shasby DM. A sex difference in the prevalence of antibodies to cytomegalovirus, JAMA 1972; 222:1290-1291.
18. Haldane EV, Embil JA, Wall AD. A serologic study of cytomegalovirus in the population of Easter Island. Bull WHO 1969; 40:969-973.
19. Willmott FE. Cytomegalovirus in female patients attending a VD clinic. Br J Vener Dis 1975; 51:278-280.
20. Knox GE, Pass RF, Reynolds DW, Stagno S, Alford CA. Comparative prevalence of subclinical cytomegalovirus and herpes simplex virus infections in the genital and urinary tracts of low-income urban women. J Infect Dis 1979; 140:419-422.
21. Hansfield HH, Chandler SC, Caine VA, Wiesner PJ, Gutman L, Wentworth BB, Alexander ER, Holmes KK. Sexual transmission of cytomegalovirus. Presented at the First Sexually Transmitted Diseases World Congress, November 15-21, 1981, Puerto Rico.
22. Drew WL, Mintz L, Miner RC, Sands M, Ketterer B. Prevalence of cytomegalovirus infections in homosexual men. J Infect Dis 1981; 143:188-192.
23. Hanshaw JB. Cytomegalovirus. In: Remmington JS, Klein JO, eds. Infectious diseases of the fetus and newborn infant. Philadelphia: Saunders, 1976:107-155.
24. Stagno S, Reynolds DW, Huang ES, Thames SD, Smith RJ, Alford CA. Congenital cytomegalovirus infection: occurrence in an immune population. N Engl J Med 1977; 296:1254-1258.
25. Monif GRG, Egan EA, Held B, Eitzman DV. The correlation of maternal cytomegalovirus infection during varying stages in gestation with neonatal involvement. J Pediatr 1972; 80:17-20.
26. Stern H, Tucker SM. Prospective study of cytomegalovirus infections in pregnancy. Br Med J 1973; 2:268-270.
27. Gold E, Nankervis GA. Cytomegalovirus. In: Evans AS, ed. Viral infections of humans. New York: Plenum, 1976:143-161.

28. Reynolds DW, Stagno S, Stubbs G, Dahle AJ, Livingston MM, Saxon SS, Alford CA. Inapparent congenital cytomegalovirus infections with elevated cord IgM levels. N Engl J Med 1974; 290:291-296.
29. Reynolds DW, Stagno S, Hosty TS, Tiller M, Alford C. Maternal CMV excretion and perinatal infection. N Engl J Med 1973; 289:1-5.
30. Hanshaw JB, Scheiner AP, Moxley AW, Goev L, Abel V, Scheiner B. School failure and deafness after "silent" congenital cytomegalovirus infection. N Engl J Med 1976; 295:468-470.
31. Klemola E, von Essen R, Henle G, Henle W. Infectious mononucleosis-like disease with negative heterophil agglutination test. Clinical features in relation to Epstein-Barr virus and cytomegalovirus and antibodies. J Infect Dis 1970; 121:608-614.
32. Jordan MC, Rousseau WE, Stewart JA, Noble GR, Chin TDJ. Spontaneous cytomegalovirus mononucleosis. Ann Intern Med 1973; 79:153-160.
33. Klemola E. Cytomegalovirus infection in previously healthy adults. Ann Intern Med 1973; 79:267-268.
34. Chretien JH, McGinniss CG, Muller A. Venereal causes of cytomegalovirus mononucleosis. JAMA 1977; 238:1644-1645.
35. Suwansirikul S, Rao N, Dowling J, Ho M. Primary and secondary cytomegalovirus infection–clinical manifestations after renal transplantation. Arch Intern Med 1977; 137:1026-1029.
36. Betts RF, Freeman RB, Douglas RG, Talley TE. Clinical manifestations of renal allograft derived primary cytomegalovirus infection. Am J Dis Child 1977; 131(7):759-763.
37. Pollard RB, Arvin AM, Gamberg P, Rand KH, Gallagher JG, Merigan TC. Specific cell-mediated immunity and infections with herpesviruses in cardiac transplant recipients. Am J Med 1982; 73:679-687.
38. Henle W, Henle G, Scriba M, Joyner CR, Harrison FS, von Essen R, Paloheimo J, Klemola E. Antibody responses to the Epstein-Barr virus and cytomegaloviruses after open-heart and other surgery. N Engl J Med 1970; 282: 1068-1074.
39. Kane RC, Rousseau WE, Noble GR, Tegtmeier GE, Wulff H, Herndon HB, Chin TDY, Bayer WL. Cytomegalovirus infections in a volunteer blood donor population. Infect Immun 1975; 11:719-723.
40. Urmacher C, Myskowski P, Ochoa M, Kris M, Safai B. Outbreak of Kaposi's sarcoma with cytomegalovirus infection in young homosexual males. Am J Med 1982; 72:569-575.
41. Centers for Disease Control. Kaposi's sarcoma and pneumocystis pneumonia among homosexual men–New York City and California. Morbid Mortal Week Rep 1981; 30:305-307.
42. Ch'ien LT, Cannon NJ, Whitley RJ, Diethelm AG, Dismukes WE, Scott CW, Buchanan RA, Alford CA. Effect of adenine-arabinoside on cytomegalovirus infections. J Infect Dis 1974; 130:32-39.
43. Arvin AM, Yeager AS, Merigan TC. Effect of leukocyte interferon on urinary excretion of cytomegalovirus by infants. J Infect Dis 1976; 133S:A205-A210.
44. Emodi G, O'Reilly R, Muller A, Everson LK, Binswanger U, Just M. Effect of human exogenous interferon in cytomegalovirus infection. J Infect Dis 1976; 133S:A199-A204.

45. Thomas IT, Svothill JF, Hawkins GT, Marshall WC. Transfer-factor treatment in congenital cytomegalovirus infection. Lancet 1977; 2:1056-1057.
46. Balfour HH, Bean B, Mitchell CD, Sachs GW, Boen JR, Edelman CK. Acyclovir in immunocompromised patients with cytomegalovirus disease:a controlled trial in one institution. Am J Med 1982; 73:241-248.
47. Plotkin SA, Farquhar J, Hornberger E. Clinical trials of immunization with the Towne 125 strain of human cytomegalovirus. J Infect Dis 1976; 134: 470-475.
48. Osborn JE. Cytomegalovirus: pathogenicity, immunology, and vaccine initiatives. J Infect Dis 1981; 143:618-630.
49. Glazer JG, Freidman HM, Grossman RA, Starr SE, Barker CF, Perloff LJ, Huang ES, Plotkin SA. Live cytomegalovirus vaccination of renal transplant candidates: a preliminary trial. Ann Intern Med 1979; 91:676-683.
50. Starr SE, Glazer JP, Freidman HM, Farquhar JD, Plotkin SA. Specific cellular and humoral immunity after immunization with live Towne strain cytomegalovirus. J Infect Dis 1981; 143:585-589.
51. Myers JD, Leszczynski J, Zaia JA, Flournoy N, Newton B, Syndman DR, Wright GG, Levin MJ, Thomas ED. Prevention of cytomegalovirus infection by cytomegalovirus immune globulin after marrow transplantation. Ann Intern Med 1983; 98:442-446.
52. Winston DJ, Pollard RB, Ho WG, Gallagher JG, Rasmussen LE, Huang SN, Lin CH, Gossett TG, Merigan TC, Gale RP. Cytomegalovirus immune plasma in bone marrow transplant recipients. Ann Intern Med 1982; 97:11-18.
53. Chou S, Merigan TC. Rapid detection and quantitation of human cytomegalovirus in urine through DNA hybridization. N Engl J Med 1983; 308:921-925.
54. Spector SA. Transmission of cytomegalovirus among infants in hospital documented by restriction-endonuclease-digestion analyses. Lancet 1983; 1:378-381.
55. Krugman S, Giles JP, Hammond J. Infectious hepatitis, evidence for two distinctive clinical, epidemiological and immunological types of infection. JAMA 1967; 200:365-373.
56. Blumberg BS. Polymophisms of the serum proteins and the development of isoprecipitins in transfused patients. Bull NY Acad Med 1964; 40:377-386.
57. Giles JP, McCollum RW, Berndtson LW, Krugman S. Viral hepatitis: relation of Australia/SH antigen to the Willowbrook MS-2 strain. N Engl J Med 1969; 281-119-122.
58. Blumberg BS, Gerstley BJS, Hungerford DA, London WT, Sutnick AI. A serum antigen (Australia antigen) in Down's syndrome, leukemia and hepatitis. Ann Intern Med 1967; 66:924-931.
59. Dodd RY, Holland PV, Ni LY, Smith HM, Greenwalt TJ. Hepatitis B antigen: regional variation in incidence and subtype ratio in the American Red Cross donor population. Am J Epidemiol 1973; 97:111-115.
60. Centers for Disease Control. Inactivated hepatitis B virus vaccine. Recommendations of the Immunization Practices Advisory Committee. Ann Intern Med 1982; 97:379-383.
61. McCollum RW. Viral hepatitis. In: Evans AS, ed. Viral infections of humans. New York: Plenum, 1976; 235-252.

62. Fass RJ. Sexual transmission of viral hepatitis? JAMA 1974; 230:861-862.
63. Ostrow DG, Shaskey DM. The experience of the Howard Brown Memorial Clinic of Chicago with sexually transmitted diseases. Sex Transm Dis 1977; 4:53-55.
64. Hentzer B, Skinhoj P, Høybye G, Nielsen AO, Kvorningsa SA, Faber V. Viral hepatitis in a venereal clinic population. Scand J Infect Dis 1980; 12:245-249.
65. Fulford KWM, Dane DJ, Catterall RD, Woof R, Deuning JV. Australia antigen and antibody among patients attending a clinic for sexually transmitted disease. Lancet 1973; 1:1470-1473.
66. Wright RA. Hepatitis B and the hepatitis B surface antigen carrier, an outbreak related to sexual contact. JAMA 1975; 232:717-721.
67. Szmuness W, Much MI, Prince AM, Hoofnagle JH, Cherubin CE, Harley EJ, Block GH. On the role of sexual behavior in the spread of hepatitis B infection. Ann Intern Med 1975; 83:489-495.
68. Dietzman DE, Harnisch JP, Ray CG, Alexander ER, Holmes KK. Hepatitis B surface antigen (HB_sAg) and antibody to HB_sAg. Prevalence in homosexual and heterosexual men. JAMA 1977; 238:2625-2626.
69. Murphy BL, Schreeder MJ, Maynard JE, Hadler SC, Sheller M. Serologic testing for hepatitis B in male homosexuals. Special emphasis on hepatitis B e antigen and antibody by radioimmunoassay. J Clin Microbiol 1980; 11:301-303.
70. Høybye G, Skinoj P, Hentzer B, Faber V, Mathiesen L. An epidemic of acute viral hepatitis in male homosexuals. Scand J Infect Dis 1980; 12:241-444.
71. Frosner GG, Buchholz HM, Gerth HJ. Prevalence of hepatitis B antibody in prostitutes. Am J Epidemiol 1975; 102:241-250.
72. Papaevangelou G, Trichopoulos D, Kremastinou T, Papoutsakis G. Prevalence of hepatitis B antigen and antibody in prostitutes. Br Med J 1974; 2:256-258.
73. Reiner NE, Judson FN, Bond WW, Francis DP, Petersen NH. Asymptomatic rectal mucosal lesions and hepatitis B surface antigen at sites of sexual contact in homosexual men with persistent hepatitis B virus infection. Ann Intern Med 1982; 96:170-173.
74. Villarejos VM, Visona KA, Gutiérrez A, Rodriquez A. Role of saliva, urine and feces in the transmission of type B hepatitis. N Engl J Med 1974; 291: 1375-1378.
75. Baker AL. Chronic type B hepatitis in gay men, experience with patients referred from Howard Brown Memorial Clinic to University of Chicago. J Homosex 1980; 5:311-315.
76. Shah N, Ostrow D, Baker A. Frequency and spectrum of chronic hepatitis B in homosexual males. Gastroenterology 1981; 80:1348.
77. Ellis WR, Coleman JC, Fluker IL, Keeling PWN, Banatvala JE, Murray-Long IM, Evans BA, Bull J, Simmons PD, Willcox JR, Thompson RPH. Liver disease among homosexual men. Lancet 1979; 1:903-904.
78. Seeff LB, Kierman T, Zimmerman HJ, et al. Hepatitis disease in asymptomatic parenteral narcotic drug abusers—a Veterans Administration collaborative study. Am J Med Sci 1975; 270:41-47.
79. Centers for Disease Control. Immune globulins for protection against viral hepatitis. Morbid Mortal Week Rep 1981; 30:423-425.

80. Redecker AG, Mosley JW, Gocke DJ, McKee AP, Pollack W. Hepatitis B immune globulin as a prophylactic measure for spouses exposed to acute type B hepatitis. N Engl J Med 1975; 293:1055-1059.
81. Krugman S, Giles JP. Viral hepatitis, type B (MS-2 strain): further observations on natural history and prevention. N Engl J Med 1975;293:1063-1067.
82. Szmuness W, Stevens CE, Harley EJ, Zang EA, Oleszko WR, William DC, Sadovsky R, Morrison JM, Kellner A. Hepatitis B vaccine. Demonstration of efficacy in a controlled clinical trial in a high-risk population in the United States. N Engl J Med 1980; 303:833-841.
83. Francis DP, Hadler SC, Thompson SE, et al. The prevention of hepatitis B with vaccine. Report of the Centers for Disease Control. Multicenter efficacy trial among homosexual men. Ann Intern Med 1982; 97:362-366.
84. Szmuness W, Stevens CE, Harley EJ, Zang E, Alter HJ, Taylor PE, DeVera A, Chen GTS, Kellner A. Hepatitis B vaccine in medical staff of hemodialysis units. N Engl J Med 1982; 307:1481-1486.
85. Maupas P, Barin F, Chiron JP, Coursaget P, Goudeau A, Perrin J, Denis F, Diop Mar I. Efficacy of hepatitis B vaccine in prevention of early HB_sAg carrier state in children. Lancet 1981; 1:289-292.
86. Dienstag JL, Stevens CE, Bhan AK, Szmuness W. Hepatitis B vaccine administered to chronic carriers of hepatitis B surface antigen. Ann Intern Med 1982; 96:565-579.
87. Mulley AG, Silverstein MD, Dienstag JL. Indications for use of hepatitis B vaccine based on cost-effectiveness analysis. N Engl J Med 1982; 307:644-652.
88. Eickoff TC, Klein JO, Daly AK, Ingall D, Finland M. Neonatal sepsis and other infections due to group B beta-hemolytic streptococci. N Engl J Med 1964; 271:1221-1228.
89. Bayer AS, Chow AW, Anthony BF, Guze LB. Serious infections in adults due to group B streptococci. Am J Med 1976; 61:498-503.
90. Verghese A, Beck JL, Boelen LJ, Smith JK. Group B streptococcal pneumonia in the elderly. Arch Intern Med 1982; 142:1642-1645.
91. Dworzack DL, Hodges GR, Barnes WG, Rosett W. Group B streptococcal infections in adult males. Am J Med Sci 1979; 277:67-73.
92. Lerner PI, Gopalakrishna KV, Wolinsky E, McHenry ML, Tan JS, Rosenthal M. Group B streptococcus (*S. agalactiae*) bacteremia in adults: analysis of 32 cases and review of the literature. Medicine 1977; 56:457-473.
93. Lancefield RC. A serologic differentiation of specific types of bovine hemolytic streptococci (group B). J Exp Med 1934; 59:441-459.
94. Christie R, Atkins NE, Munch-Petersen E. A note on a lytic phenomenon shown by group B streptococci. Aust J Exp Biol Med Sci 1944; 22:197-200.
95. Darling CL. Standardization and evaluation of CAMP reaction for the prompt, presumptive identification of *Streptococcus agalactiae* (Lancefield group B) in clinical materials. J Clin Microbiol 1975; 1:171-174.
96. Lancefield RC. Two serological types of group B hemolytic streptococci with related, but not identical, type specific substances. J Exp Med 1938; 63:25-40.

97. Pattison IH, Matthews PRJ, Maxted WR. Type classification by Lancefield's precipitin method of human and bovine group B streptococci isolated in Britain. J Pathol Bacteriol 1955; 69:43-50.
98. Baker CJ, Kasper DL. Correlation of maternal antibody deficiency with susceptibility to neonatal group B streptococcal infection. N Engl J Med 1976; 294:753-756.
99. Baker CJ, Kasper DL. Immunological investigation of infants with septicemia or meningitis due to group B streptococcus. J Infect Dis 1977; 136S: S98-S104.
100. Duma RJ, Weinberg AN, Medrek TF, Kunz LJ. Streptococcal infections–a bacteriologic and clinical study of streptococcal bacteremia. Medicine 1969; 48:87-127.
101. Badri MS, Zawaneh S, Cruz AC, Mantilla G, Baer H, Spellacy WN, Ayoub EN. Rectal colonization with group B streptococcus: relation to vaginal colonization of pregnant women. J Infect Dis 1977; 135:308-312.
102. Easmon CSF, Tanna A, Munday P, Dawson S. Group B streptococci–gastrointestinal organisms? J Clin Pathol 1981; 34:921-923.
103. Anthony BF, Eisenstadt R, Carter J, Kim KS, Hobel CJ. Genital and intestinal carriage of group B streptococci during pregnancy. J Infect Dis 1981; 143:761-766.
104. Baker CJ, Goroff DK, Alpert S, Corckett VA, Zinner SH, Eurard JR, Rosner B, McCormack WM. Vaginal colonization with group B streptococcus–a study in college women. J Infect Dis 1977; 135:392-397.
105. Christensen KK, Christensen P, Flamholc L, Ripa T. Frequencies of streptococci of groups A, B, C, D, and G in urethra and cervix swab specimens from patients with suspected gonococcal infections. Acta Pathol Microbiol Scand B 1974; 82:470-474.
106. Manuel FR, Macdonald SW, Ernbil JA. Prevalence of group B beta-hemolytic streptococci in the male urethra. Scand J Infect Dis 1980; 12:33-35.
107. Wallin J, Forsgren A. Group B streptococci in venereal disease clinic patients. Br J Vener Dis 1975; 51:401-404.
108. Persson K, Bjerre B, Hansson H, Forsgren A. Several factors influencing the colonization of group B streptococci–rectum probably the main reservoir. Scand J Infect Dis 1981; 13:171-175.
109. Franciosi RA, Knostman JD, Zimmerman R. Group B streptococcal neonatal and infant infections. J Pediatr 1973; 82:707-718.
110. Chretien JH, McGinniss CG, Thompson J, Delaha E, Garagusi VF. Group B beta-hemolytic streptococci causing pharyngitis. J Clin Microbiol 1979; 10:263-266.
111. Christensen KK, Christensen P, Juldorf F, Dahlander K. Quantitation of antibodies against group B streptococci, types Ia, Ib, and III in sera from different groups of individuals: high antibody level in sera from venereal disease clinic patients. Scand J Infect Dis 1981; 13:165-169.
112. Baker CJ, Barrett FF. Transmission of group B streptococci among parturient women and their neonates. J Pediatr 1973; 83:919-925.

113. Pass MA, Gray BM, Dillin HC. Puerperal and perinatal infections with group B streptococci. Am J Obstet Gynecol 1982; 143:147-152.
114. Gravett MG, Eschenbach DA, Speigel-Brown C, Holmes KK. Rapid diagnosis of amniotic-fluid infection by gas-liquid chromatography. N Engl J Med 1982; 306:725-728.
115. Aber RC, Allen N, Howell JT, Wilkinson HW, Facklam RR. Nosocomial transmission of group B streptococci. Pediatrics 1976; 58:346-353.
116. Baker CJ, Barrett FF, Gordan RC, You MD. Suppurative meningitis due to streptococci of Lancefield group B: A study in 33 infants. J Pediatr 1973; 82:724-729.
117. Baker CJ, Barrett FF. Group B streptococcal infections in infants: the importance of various serotypes. JAMA 1974; 230:1158-1160.
118. Minkoff HL, Sierra MF, Pringle GF, Schwarz RH. Vaginal colonization with group B beta-hemolytic streptococcus as a risk factor for post-cesarean section febrile morbidity. Am J Obstet Gynecol 1982; 142:992-995.
119. Osborne NG, Grubin L, Pratson L. Vaginitis in sexually active women: relationship to nine sexually transmitted organisms. Am J Obstet Gynecol 1982; 142:962-967.
120. Brook I. Balanitis caused by group B β-hemolytic streptococci. Sex Transm Dis 1980; 7:195-196.
121. Baker CJ. Summary of the workshop on perinatal infections due to group B streptococcus. J Infect Dis 1977; 136:137-152.
122. Yow MD, Mason EO, Leeds LJ, Thompson PK, Clark DJ, Gardner SE. Ampicillin prevents intrapartum transmission of group B streptococcus. JAMA 1979; 241:1245-1247.
123. Lloyd DJ, Scott KE, Aterman K, Belgaumkar TK, Wort AJ, Krause VW. Prevention of group B beta-hemolytic streptococcal septicemia in low-birth-weight neonates by penicillin administered within two hours of birth. Lancet 1979; 1:713-715.
124. Pyati SP, Pildes RS, Jacobs NM, Ramamurthy RS, Yeh TF, Raval DS, Lillien LD, Amma P, Mutzger WI. Penicillin in infants weighing two kilograms or less with early onset group B streptococcal disease. N Engl J Med 1983; 308:1383-1389.

FIFTEEN

Congenital, Perinatal, and Prepubertal Infections

An Overview

Blaise L. Congeni
Northeastern Ohio Universities
College of Medicine
Rootstown, Ohio

INTRODUCTION

Children are exposed to a variety of sexually transmissible agents. Among those agents that pose a significant threat are cytomegalovirus, herpes simplex virus, hepatitis B virus, group B streptococcus, *Chlamydia trachomatis* and *Neisseria gonorrhoeae*.

CYTOMEGALOVIRUS

The neonate may become infected with cytomegalovirus (CMV) either in utero or perinatally (acquired). The epidemiology, clinical manifestations, and pathogenesis are markedly different for these two types of infection.

The possibility of in utero acquisition has been recognized for over 20 years. Over half the women in the United States of child-bearing age have immunity to

CMV [1,2]. Most individuals have acquired immunity following subclinical infections. Approximately 1% of those mothers without preceding immunity will experience a primary infection with CMV during pregnancy [3]. In 10% of all pregnancies, though, the mother will excrete CMV. Therefore most CMV infections that occur during pregnancy occur in the face of preceding immunity, that is, secondary infections.

Relative to congenital infection, the neonate is at the greatest risk for damage when the maternal infection is a primary infection [2,3]. After a primary infection the risk of intrauterine infection is about 50% [3]. The risk of intrauterine infection appears greatest if the infection occurred during the third trimester, but the risk of fetal damage is greatest if the infection occurred early in pregnancy during the period of organogenesis.

During a secondary maternal infection, CMV can also be transmitted to the fetus. It has generally been accepted that fetal damage does not occur following such infections [4]. Recently, Ahlfors et al. have described a newborn with hepatosplenomegaly and deafness in association with a secondary CMV infection in the mother [5].

To summarize the epidemiology of CMV infections, approximately 10% of pregnant women will excrete CMV during pregnancy, 10% of their infants might be congenitally infected, and 10% of those infants might demonstrate significant neurological handicaps. In other words, approximately 1 in 100 neonates will be congenitally infected with CMV and 1 in 1000 infants would have significant hearing loss or retardation as a result of a congenital cytomegalovirus infection [6,7].

Most infants tend to have subclinical or unrecognized disease, whether infected congenitally or perinatally. Those congenitally infected infants who are symptomatic demonstrate a variety of manifestations as can be seen in Figure 1. Only the minority demonstrate classic cytomegalic inclusion disease characterized by hepatosplenomegaly, petechiae, chorioretinitis, cerebral calcifications, and microcephaly [6,8].

The possibility of perinatally acquired disease was first recognized by Kumar et al. [9] when they found that 7 of 21 infants had symptoms which appeared at the time of viruria. Those affected infants demonstrated various combinations of pneumonitis, rash, organomegaly, and/or hepatitis. It has subsequently been shown that postnatally acquired CMV is not an uncommon event and is unusually asymptomatic [7]. The major manifestation of postnatally acquired cytomegalovirus infection is pneumonitis [10]. The Alabama group was able to implicate cytomegalovirus as the etiology in approximately 20% of infants with pneumonitis who presented under 3 months of age [11]. This type of pneumonitis shares similarities with that caused by *C. trachomatis* or *Ureaplasma urealyticum* and will be discussed in greater detail.

Laboratory diagnosis of CMV infection in the neonate is accomplished primarily by viral isolation. In either congenital or perinatally acquired infection, the virus is readily recoverable from throat or urine. To distinguish congenital from

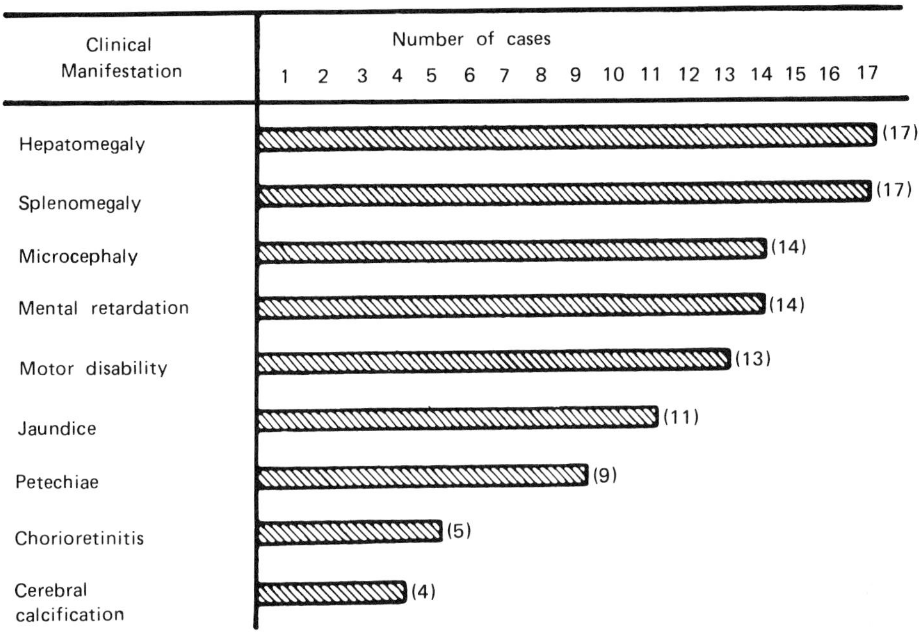

Fig. 1 Clinical features of 17 infants with cytomegalic inclusion disease. (From Ref. 8.)

perinatally acquired infection, a urine culture should be obtained within the first week of life, before perinatally infected infants become viruric [12]. In a congenitally infected infant, virus is present in high titer during the first week of life, with cultures usually positive in 2 to 7 days. Sufficient quantities of virus are present, so that urine stored at 4°C can be shipped to a virology laboratory without significant loss in sensitivity.

Immunoserological procedures are not as helpful in establishing a diagnosis of cytomegalovirus infections [12]. The usual fourfold change between acute and convelescent titers does not apply to congenital CMV infections. A major reason why serology is not useful is the fact that maternal antibody to CMV crosses the placenta. One way to distinguish neonatal from maternal antibody would be to assay for IgM antibodies specific for CMV. Unfortunately, IgM-specific tests are not routinely available, and false positive and negative results are frequently encountered [12].

Frequently infants who present with the "TORCH syndrome" (those suspected of having *to*xoplasmosis, *r*ubella, *c*ytomegalovirus, or *h*erpes) have "TORCH titers" drawn. Under these circumstances, antibody levels to the four TORCH agents are determined. The National Institutes of Health has recently evaluated

TORCH package antibody tests [13]. The results of these tests were frequently erroneous, whether evaluating the mother or the neonate.

No specific antiviral agent is available for the treatment of CMV infections. For the congenitally infected neonate, accurate diagnosis is important so that handicaps may be identified and specific remediation offered. Obviously, disease prevention is preferable and preliminary trials of the immunization of seronegative women have been reported. In these studies the investigators have demonstrated seroconversion after immunization [14,15]. Unfortunately, a clinically useful vaccine does not appear feasible at this time. However, the prevention of some CMV infections can be accomplished utilizing other strategies. For example, a major vehicle by which CMV is transmitted to neonates is parenteral blood products. The screening of blood products used in neonatal nurseries and the use of seronegative blood can reduce the incidence of the postnatally acquired infection that is frequently seen after administration of blood products [16,17].

HERPES SIMPLEX VIRUS

Clinical illness produced by herpes simplex virus (HSV) in the neonate differs significantly from that due to CMV. Asymptomatic disease in the neonate is unusual and efforts at treatment and prevention have shown significant progress in the last decade.

The incidence of disease in the neonate is approximately 1 in 7500 live births [18]. Clinical disease may be acquired by the newborn via the transplacental, intrapartum, or postpartum route. In contrast to CMV, transplacental transmission is rare. Although a primary genital infection in the mother would pose the greatest threat to the offspring, transmission of infection to neonates has also been documented in association with nongenital maternal infections and infections in fathers, other patients, and nursing personnel [19-21].

The characteristics of 56 mothers and their infants with neonatal HSV infections were recently examined [22]. A total of 70% of such infants were born to mothers who were asymptomatic, although several of these asymptomatic mothers had a history of previous genital infection with herpes or a history of exposure to a sex partner with an HSV infection. The presence of antibody to HSV in the neonate or mother did not help in predicting outcome. Approximately two-thirds of these infections were due to HSV-2 and the remainder due to HSV-1.

Clinical disease seen in the newborn remains localized to the central nervous system (CNS), eye, skin, or oral cavity in about half the cases or may be disseminated, as can be seen in Table 1 [23,24]. Rarely is the disease asymptomatic. Those infants with disseminated disease or with CNS involvement are at much greater risk for sequelae.

The infant with disseminated disease usually presents with some combination of temperature instability, lethargy, skin lesions, or feeding difficulty. The

Table 1 Clinical Spectrum and Outcome in 266 Cases of Neonatal Herpetic Infection[a]

Clinical groups	Number of patients	Outcome in infant: Died	Survived: With sequelae	Survived: Without apparent sequelae
Disseminated				
Without CNS involvement	91 (4)[b]	84 (2)	1 (1)	6 (1)
With CNS involvement	89 (16)	64 (6)	14 (6)	11 (4)
Localized[c]				
CNS	43 (8)	17 (2)	18 (4)	8 (2)
Eye	10 (2)	0	5 (1)	5 (1)
Skin	28 (3)	0	8	20 (3)
Oral cavity	3 (1)	0	0	3 (1)
Asymptomatic	2	0	0	2
Total	266 (34)	165 (10)	46 (12)	55 (12)

[a]An additional 12 cases could not be classified owing to insufficient data.
[b]Numbers in parentheses refer to patients treated systemically with antiviral agents.
[c]Classified according to major site of involvement if more than one site is infected.
Source: Ref. 24.

skin lesions seen are usually vesicles, but rarely the infant may present with diffuse erythema. Those infants with a vesicular rash who recover may be troubled with recurrences of the vesicular rash during the first year of life. The presence of skin, eye, or oral cavity lesions aids the physician in the early diagnosis of an HSV infection in the newborn [Fig. 2 (see Plate V, facing p. 378)]. Unfortunately, 14 of 20 infants with disseminated disease or HSV encephalitis had no such lesions in a recent study [25].

Given the importance of intrapartum and postpartum transmission, disease prevention in the newborn is a consideration when HSV infection is documented or suspected not only in the mother, but also in others who have direct contact with the infant. The risk of infection in the offspring born to a mother with a genital infection depends on both the mode of delivery and whether or not the membranes have been ruptured for more than 4 hr (Table 2). Those infants born by cesarean section with membranes ruptured less than 4 hr appeared to have a lower risk of developing disease [24].

If the infant is to be delivered vaginally, it should be done as rapidly as possible after membranes have ruptured to minimize the risk of ascending infection. Kibrick has proposed guidelines for handling infants born to mothers with primary or secondary genital and nongenital infections (Table 3) [26].

Table 2 Risk of Neonatal Herpetic Infection from Mother with Genital Infection at Delivery[a]

Type of delivery	Number of infants infected per total number of cases
Vaginal	10/20 (50%)
Cesarean section	
After membrane rupture over 6 hr	6/7 (86%)
Before or within 4 hrs of membrane rupture	1/16 (6%)

[a]Based on virological or cytological diagnosis.
Source: Ref. 24.

Fathers and nursing personnel with herpetic lesions on exposed surfaces should be advised to avoid contact with neonates until the lesions have crusted.

Several of the antiviral agents effective against HSV have been employed in neonatal infections. In the largest study to date, adenine arabinoside given intravenously decreased mortality in the severest form of the disease (CNS or disseminated disease) from 74% in a placebo group to 38% in the group treated with the adenine arabinoside [27,28]; nevertheless, the outcome of survivors with disseminated disease was poor even with therapy. Those infants examined at 1-year follow-up were rarely "normal." Early institution of therapy appears to be crucial.

Acyclovir has been shown to be more effective than adenine arabinoside in vitro against HSV [29]. One neonate with progressive disease being treated with adenine arabinoside was noted to improve coincidental with a change in therapy to intravenous acyclovir [30].

HEPATITIS B VIRUS

On a global basis, hepatitis B virus (HBV) is a major factor in the development of chronic liver disease and hepatocellular carcinoma. Significant advances in the diagnosis and prevention of HBV infection have been made during the last decade. The neonate has benefited, since it is now increasingly possible to interrupt transmission of HBV.

Hepatitis B virus, previously referred to as the "Dane particle," is 42 nm in diameter and has several distinct antigenic components, including hepatitis B surface antigen (HB_sAg), hepatitis B core antigen (HB_cAg), and hepatitis B e antigen (HB_eAg). The presence of HB_eAg is associated with a greater risk of developing chronic liver disease [31,32] and a greater capacity for HBV transmission [33]. This relates to the neonate, since infants born to HB_eAg-positive mothers are at greater risk of becoming infected and becoming chronic HBV carriers [34].

Transmission of HBV may occur from mother to infant in four possible ways: (1) transplacentally, (2) perinatally, (3) postpartum, or (4) transcolostrally [35,36].

Plate V

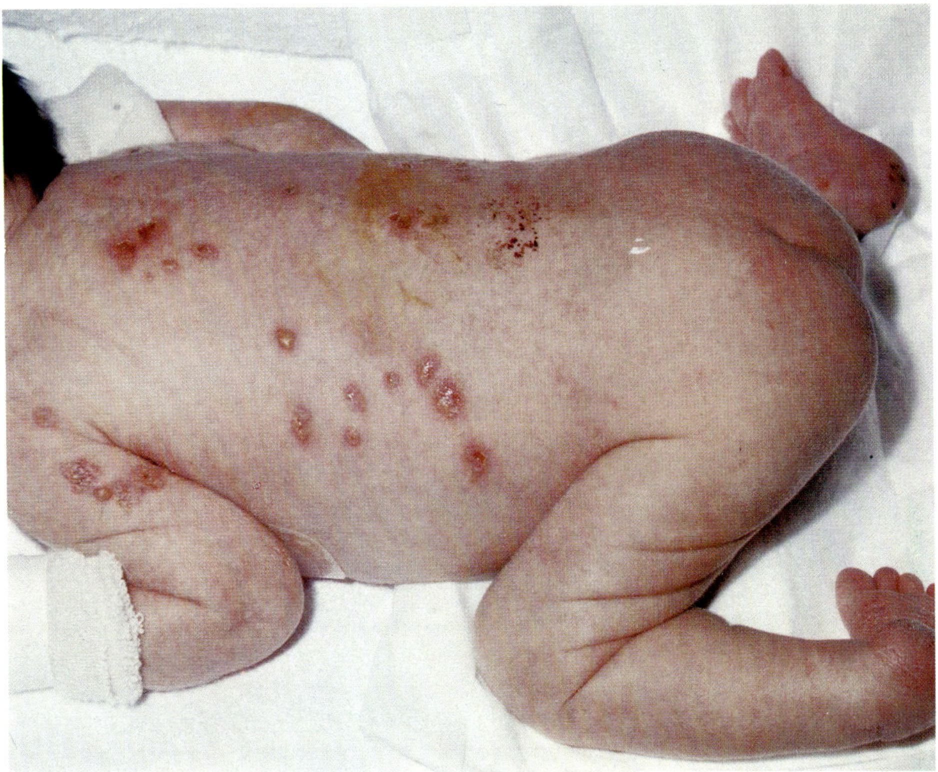

Fig. 2 Skin lesions in a neonate with HSV infection.

Table 3 Recommendations for Cesarean Section at Term in Women with Prior or Concurrent Herpes

Genital herpetic lesions present at term	Group	Primary genital lesions	Recurrent genital lesions (or genital reinfection)	Status of membranes[a]	Recommended route of delivery[b]	Isolation of mother	Isolation of newborn
Yes	1	+	–	Intact or ruptured <4-6 hr	Cesarean section	Yes	Yes
	2	+	–	Ruptured >4-6 hr	Per vaginam	Yes	Yes
	3	+	or +	Baby has been delivered per vaginam	–	Yes	Yes
	4	–	+	Intact or ruptured <4-6 hr	Cesarean section	Yes	Yes
	5	–	+	Ruptured >4-6 hr	Per vaginam	Yes	Yes
No, but cervicovaginal culture or cytology is positive for herpes	6	–	–	Intact or ruptured <4-6 hr	Cesarean section	Yes	Yes
	7	–	–	Ruptured >4-6 hr	Per vaginam	Yes	Yes
No, but there is past history of genital herpes, presently inactive or status unknown	8	–	–	Intact or ruptured	Per vaginam	No	No
No, but nongenital herpes is present at term	9	–	–	Intact or ruptured	Per vaginam	Yes	No at birth (yes, after newborn goes out to mother)
No, but there is past history of nongenital herpes	10	–	–	Intact or ruptured	Per vaginam	No	No

[a]The shorter the interval between rupture of the membranes and cesarean section, the less the risk of fetal infection. The critical period appears to be 4 to 6 hr.
[b]Dependent on evaluation of individual risks and benefits. *Source*: Ref. 26.

Nonmaternal transmission is also possible in the postpartum period. Mothers with HBV disease in the third trimester or during the first two postpartum months seem highly capable of transmitting the virus to their offspring (75% HB_sAg positive). Infants born to mothers with HBV disease during the first two trimesters are at a much lower risk (10% HB_sAg positive) [35]. The efficacy with which carriers transmit the virus to offspring is much greater in France, Southeast Asia, and tropical Africa [37-41].

Most infected infants remain anicteric and asymptomatic [35]. Unfortunately, HB_sAg may persist indefinitely in their sera and, despite a normal physical exam, chronic hepatitis is a common development in these infants. In the studies of Schweitzer et al., a high incidence of low birth weight and prematurity was seen in infants born to mothers with HB_sAg-positive disease [35]. Hepatitis B virus disease in the neonate was rarely fulminant or overt. Only 2 of 17 infants developed icteric disease, and they recovered without persistent antigenemia. Some investigators have reported a higher incidence of overt disease. Dupuy et al. found overt disease with termination of antigenemia was the rule rather than the exception in 80 French children [40,41].

Since infected neonates are at great risk for chronic liver disease and peristent antigenemia, prevention is highly desirable. Two types of immune globulins are available for postexposure HBV prophylaxis, regular immune serum globulin, as well as high-titered immune serum globulin, hepatitis B immune globulin (HBIG). When 0.5 ml of HBIG was given at birth and at 3 and 6 months to a group of 40 infants born to HB_eAg-positive mothers, the HB_sAg carrier rate was decreased from 91 to 23% [42].

Good results have been obtained using active immunization in the neonate. The recently licensed inactivated hepatitis B vaccine Heptavax-B has been found to be highly immunogenic when given to infants born to mothers who had anti-HB_c, anti-HB_s, or HB_sAg present [43] Studies using both vaccine and HBIG are ongoing. Both passive and active immunity are desirable, since infants passively protected at birth are likely to be repeatedly exposed when the mother is a chronic HBV carrier. Currently HBIG appears to be the treatment of choice for infants born to HB_sAg-positive mothers. Infants born to chronic carrier mothers should probably also receive the vaccine [44].

GROUP B STREPTOCOCCUS

Although rarely encountered as a neonatal pathogen before 1960, group B streptococcus (GBS) (*Streptococcus agalactiae*) is now recognized as the major cause of neonatal meningitis and sepsis. In addition, since the 1960s GBS has been found to cause a variety of other illnesses, including osteomyelitis, septic arthritis, and pneumonia [45]. Recently invasive disease due to this organism has been reported in adults, especially diabetics [46,47].

Early studies underestimated the prevalence of maternal genital colonization with GBS [48,49], but those studies utilizing selective culture media found approximately one-quarter of the mothers to be colonized [50,51]. Most infants born to colonized mothers will rapidly acquire the same GBS serotype. Early colonization of the neonate is one of the major risk factors associated with the subsequent development of early onset invasive disease. About 25% of all neonates are found to be colonized and 1 to 2% of colonized infants subsequently developed invasive disease. The prevalence of childhood colonization outside the newborn period remains fairly constant, between 3.7 and 25%, depending on the site cultured and age [52,53].

Two distinct GBS syndromes are recognized in the neonate (Table 4). Early onset disease occurs before 7 days of age and usually presents with respiratory distress or a clinical picture suggesting sepsis. This syndrome is difficult to distinguish from hyaline membrane disease [54-56], is acquired in utero or perinatally, and is associated with a high incidence of maternal obstetric complications. Prematurity and low birth weight are frequently encountered in these infants.

Late onset disease occurs after 7 days of life, and the method by which the neonate acquires the organism is not clear. The clinical presentation most often encountered is meningitis and the prognosis is better than the early onset form.

The presence of maternal GBS colonization appears to be a major risk factor for the development of early disease, while the absence of maternal GBS antibody is a major risk factor for both early and late onset disease, especially due to GBS serotype III [57]. Since the mode of transmission for GBS in early onset disease is vertical (mother to infant), the serotypes responsible for early onset disease mirror those found in the female genital tract (Ia, Ib, Ic, II, III). Meningitis, whether early or late in onset, is usually due to type III [58].

Diagnosis requires the standard bacteriological techniques of Gram stain and culture of infected body fluids. Latex particle agglutination is a rapid technique in which GBS antigen is detected in the cerebrospinal fluid, blood, and concen-

Table 4 Syndromes of Neonatal Group B Streptococcus Disease

	Early onset ($<$7 days)	Late onset ($>$7 days)
Risk factors	Maternal colonization Absence of maternal antibody	 Absence of maternal antibody
Neonatal characteristics	Prematurity Low birth weight	
Clinical syndrome	Respiratory distress Shock	Meningitis
Serotypes	Ia, Ib, Ic, II, III	Primarily III
Mortality	50-60%	15-20%

trated urine [59.60]. Group B streptococcus antigen is detected in the cerebrospinal fluid of 92% of meningitis patients and in the concentrated urine of 89% of bacteremic infants utilizing a commercially available kit, Streptogen [61].

Empiric therapy for ill neonates prior to culture results usually includes a penicillin, frequently ampicillin, and an aminoglycoside. When modest doses of penicillin have been used for GBS disease, relapses and recurrences have been reported [62-65]. Consequently the dose of aqueous penicillin G now recommended is 250,000 to 400,000 units/kg per day for meningitis and 250,000 units/kg per day for nonmeningitic disease [66,67]. Once the diagnosis of GBS infection is established, many investigators have suggested continuing the aminoglycoside, at least until sterilization has been achieved, because of the possibility of synergism with this combination [67]. In vitro synergism has been reported with ampicillin and gentamicin for GBS [68]. The duration of therapy is 2 to 3 weeks for meningitis and 10 days for the nonmeningitic early onset disease.

A serendipitous finding reported by Seighman et al. suggested that the prevention of early onset disease due to GBS was possible [69]. Since 1952 all infants born at New York's Mt. Sinai Hospital have received 50,000 units of aqueous penicillin G intramuscularly for the prevention of gonococcal ophthalmia neonatorum. To date, no case of early onset GBS disease has occurred.

Several studies have evaluated injectable penicillin for the prophylaxis of GBS disease. In a retrospective study, 11 cases of early onset disease were seen in 1208 low birth weight infants during a 4½-year period, which contrasted with the 1 case of GBS sepsis seen during the subsequent 2½ years, when all infants under 2500 g received injectable penicillin [70].

In a larger prospective study of over 30,000 infants, Siegel et al. demonstrated a significant decrease in early onset GBS disease in infants who received parenteral aqueous penicillin G at birth instead of tetracycline ophthalmic ointment [71, 72]. The incidence of infection with penicillin-resistant organisms was not significantly increased. Unfortunately, injectable penicillin does little to prevent late onset disease or early onset disease acquired in utero. Baker found that over half the infants with early onset disease become clinically evident before 6 hours of age [73]. These infants probably acquired their disease in utero and the infection progressed despite the fact that many received large doses of antibiotics during the first 6 hr of life. More recently Pyati et al. evaluated 1187 neonates weighing less than 2000 g [74]. Prophylactic penicillin did not appear to exert a protective effect. These investigators noted that blood cultures obtained at 1 hr of age were positive in 21 of 24 of the infants with early onset disease, suggesting that the infection was already established. Currently prophylactic penicillin is not routinely recommended.

CHLAMYDIA TRACHOMATIS

The relation between neonatal inclusion conjunctivitis and maternal genital infections has been appreciated for over 40 years [75]. Renewed interest in the etiological agent, *C. trachomatis*, has occurred during the last decade. *Chlamydia trachomatis* is an obligate intracellular parasite with 15 recognized serotypes, 3 that cause lymphogranuloma venereum and 12 that cause ocular and genital infections.

Chlamydia trachomatis has been isolated from 2 to 18% of cervical specimens collected during pregnancy. The risk of inclusion conjunctivitis in the newborn of infected women is 50% [76-80]. Those characteristics that distinguish inclusion conjunctivitis from gonococcal ophthalmia neonatorum are listed in Table 5.

Inclusion conjunctivitis usually appears after 5 days, and discharge is either absent or mucopurulent. Chlamydial inclusion conjunctivitis is unilateral in two-thirds of cases, but clinically there is considerable overlap between chalmydial and gonococcal conjunctivitis [81]. Definitive diagnosis for inclusion conjunctivitis rests on demonstration of intracytoplasmic inclusions in a conjunctival scraping or recovering *C. trachomatis* from the eye. Infants with inclusion conjunctivitis occasionally suffer recurrences with subsequent scarring, although complications are rare with appropriate early therapy [82].

In 1977 Beem and Saxon reported the association between *C. trachomatis* and a distinctive pneumonitis syndrome [83]. Infants with chlamydial pneumonitis are felt to acquire their infection at birth and the usual portal of entry is the conjunctiva or nasopharynx [76]. In another study *C. trachomatis* was implicated as the etiology in 25% of infants presenting with pneumonitis before 3 months of age [11]. The infant typically presents with a history of congestion and a stacatto cough reminiscent of pertussis. The patient is afebrile, in no acute distress, and diffuse rales may be noted. Eosinophilia and significant increases in IgG and IgM antibodies may suggest the diagnosis before *C. trachomatis* culture

Table 5 Ophthalmia Neonatorum

	Gonococcal	Chlamydial
Clinical manifestations	Frequently bilateral	Usually unilateral
Onset (mean)	Less than 1 week	Over 1 week
Eye discharge	Thick, purulent	Mucopurulent or absent
Diagnosis		
Rapid	Gram stain	Conjunctival scraping-Geimsa stain
Culture	Thayer-Martin media	McCoy cells
Treatment		
Topical	Chloramphenicol, tetracycline, or penicillin (optional)	Erythromycin, tetracycline, or sulfonamide
Systemic	Penicillin G, intramuscularly, 10 days	Erythromycin, orally, 2 weeks

results are available. The diagnosis is confirmed by isolation of the organism from the respiratory tract. A history of conjunctivitis is obtained in approximately half of these infants.

The following case report illustrates the clinical pattern of chlamydial pneumonia.

> K. H., a 6-week-old black female, presented with a 2-week history of "chest congestion." This youngster had a 1-week history of a worsening cough which occasionally occurred in paroxysms. One episode of vomiting was noted.
>
> On physical examination, the vital signs were as follows: temperature, 37.4°C rectally; pulse, 150; respiration, 90. Thoracic exam revealed tachypnea with intercostal retractions and diffuse inspiratory rales in all lung fields. Laboratory data were as follows:

CBC: WBC, 17,400 cells per mm^3	Capillary blood gases
Bands, 6%	*pH, 7.26
Segs, 19%	*pCO_2, 49 mmHg
Lymphs, 42%	PO_2, 49 mmHg
Atypical lymphs, 2%	HCO_3, 21 mmol/liter
*Monos, 26%	
Eos, 5%	
*Hgb, 11.1 g/dl	
IgE, <5 IU/ml	Urinalysis, normal
IgA, 23.6 mg/dl	
*IgM, 76 mg/dl	
*IgG, 1206 mg/dl	

> *Chlamydia trachomatis* was isolated from nasopharyngeal secretions.
> Chest x-ray, see Figure 3.

Chlamydia trachomatis has also been recovered from the middle ear, vagina, and rectum of infants [84]. Its role in disease production at these sites is unclear. A relationship between maternal infection and prematurity and increased perinatal mortality has also been suggested [85].

The infants with inclusion conjunctivitis should be treated with a topical sulfonamide or erythromycin for 2 to 3 weeks. Recently Beem et al. have demonstrated that oral erythromycin was an effective adjunct in terminating chlamydial shedding in conjunctivitis patients [86]. Consequently, both a topical preparation and oral erythromycin for 2 weeks would seem to be prudent. Infants with chlamydial pneumonitis are treated systemically with erythromycin or a sulfonamide for a minimum of 2 weeks.

---

*Abnormal values.

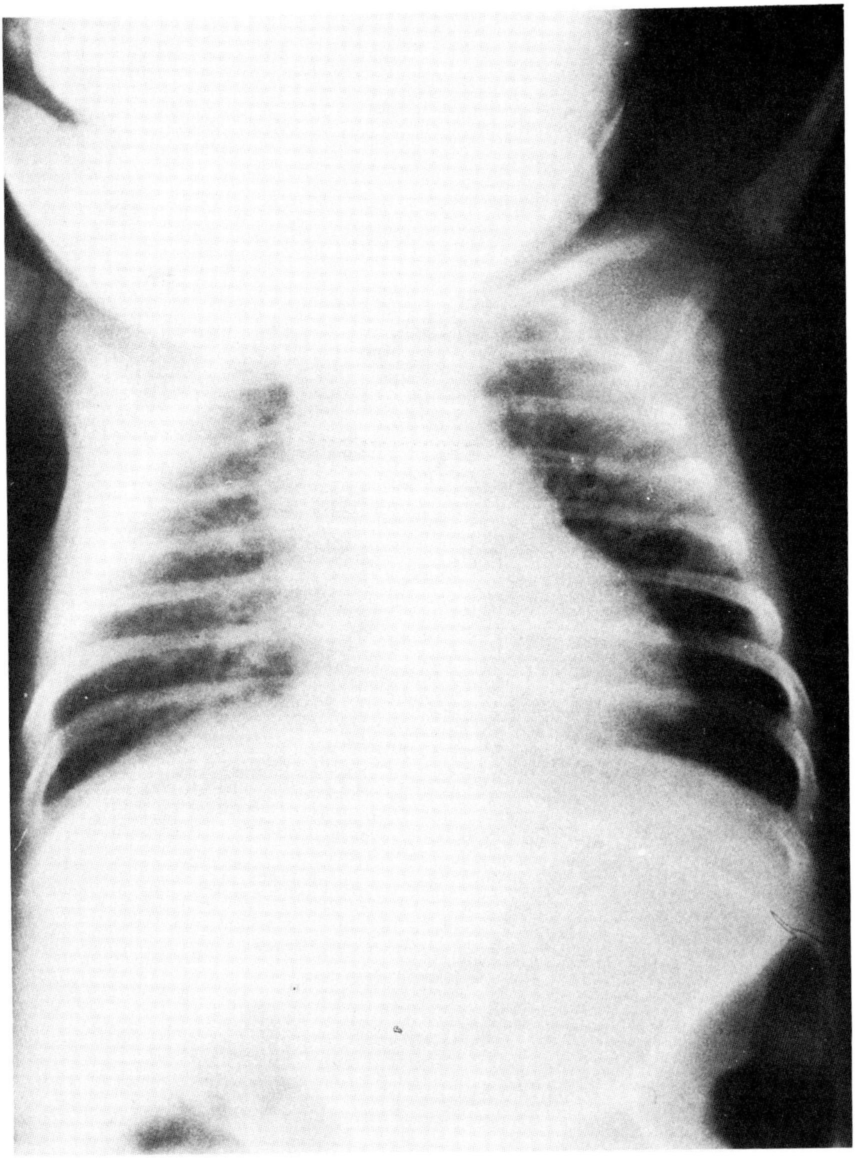

Fig. 3 Chest x-ray from a youngster with *C. trachomatis* pneumonitis.

NEISSERIA GONORRHOEAE

Neonatal Disease

The major clinical form of gonococcal disease acquired perinatally is conjunctivitis. The manifestations that differentiate chlamydial inclusion conjunctivitis from gonococcal conjunctivitis are listed in Table 5. The impact of gonococcal ophthalmia neonatorum is realized when it is noted that, prior to routine prophylaxis, 25% of children entering a school for the blind had a history of gonococcal conjunctivitis [87]. In addition to conjunctivitis, the infant born to a mother with gonorrhea may develop vaginitis, sepsis, or arthritis [88-90]. Gonococcal scalp abscesses have also been reported in infants traumatized by intrauterine monitoring devices [91].

Any mucous membrane can serve as the portal of entry and, although conjunctival cultures have the greatest yield, positive cultures have also been obtained from the umbilicus and rectum. All newborn receive either topical or parenteral therapy to prevent gonococcal ophthalmia neonatorum. A recent study found that approximately 80% of hospitals in the United States use silver nitrate drops for this purpose [92]. Over 90% of infants receiving silver nitrate develop a "chemical conjunctivitis." This condition is mild and self-limited and resolves within 24 hr. Discharge is absent or minimal. To minimize the chemical conjunctivitis, the eyes are frequently rinsed with saline. The efficacy of this procedure is not clearly established, while excessive rinsing may diminish the effectiveness of silver nitrate. When properly used, silver nitrate is not totally effective and the newborn of a culture-positive mother should also receive 50,000 units of procaine penicillin intramuscularly (20,000 units if the infant weighs less than 2000 g).

Disease During Infancy and Prepubescence

The mode of acquisition of gonococcal disease outside the newborn period varies with age (Table 6). In all age groups beyond infancy, the possibility of nonvenereal transmission either via fomites or infected individuals is suggested by several pieces of information. In 1927 an outbreak of gonococcal arthritis was reported in 44 children from a single ward in a hospital [97]. Although the mode of trans-

Table 6 Major Modes of Acquisition of Gonorrhea in Children

Age	Route
Neonate	Birth canal
1 month to 1 year	Transmission from infected parents
1 to 10 years	Nonvoluntary sexual contact
Over 10 years	Voluntary sexual contact

Source: Modified from Refs. 95 and 96.

mission was not defined, a caretaker and/or various fomites, such as thermometers, were implicated. Other information suggesting nonvenereal transmission includes reports of children with conjunctivitis in the absence of genital disease. Shore and Winkelstein found that five of seven children with various gonococcal infections shared an infected parent's bed [98]. The exact mode of transmission is unclear and any possible role for fomites, such as bedding, is usually circumstantial.

Most children under age 10 years have become infected via involuntary sexual contact. In a recent study 85% of cases were females and the median age was 4 years [99]. Positive anal cultures were obtained in 52% of females and 25% of males, and positive throat cultures in 18% of females and 13% of males. On several occasions anal cultures were positive in the absence of positive genital cultures. When a youngster less than 10 years of age is found to have gonorrhea, hospitalization is indicated. Rarely is the source of infection elicited during the initial history. A multidisciplinary approach and sufficient time are usually necessary to identify the source of infection [100]. When culturing of family members is possible, a significant percentage of positive cultures are found. Folland et al. reported a 27% positive culture rate from 203 family contacts of 73 preadolescent children with gonorrhea [101].

Disease in prepubertal children over 10 years of age is usually secondary to voluntary sexual contact [95]. Frequently these youngsters are misinformed and confuse protection from pregnancy with protection from sexually transmitted diseases [102].

The clinical diseases usually seen in the prepubertal period are vaginitis and male urethritis. Gonorrhea in the prepubertal female differs significantly from the clinical presentation in the adult. The alkaline pH and thin wall of the immature vagina encourage a diffuse vaginitis with dysuria as opposed to the localization of disease to the cervix [102,103]. Although salpingitis, perihepatitis, and peritonitis have been reported, these complications are distinctly unusual in the prepubertal female [104-106]. Other causes of vaginitis in the prepubertal female include shigella [107] and other gram-negative enterics, along with group A streptococcus, *Staphylococcus aureus, Streptococcus pneumoniae,* and pinworms [103]. A foreign body should always be considered when the discharge is bloody. *Candida* sp. and trichomonads are less common causes of prepubertal vaginitis, in contrast to the postpubertal female [104].

Gonococcal pharyngitis and proctitis are usually asymptomatic [108]. Among sexually active asymptomatic adolescents in an urban area, 1.9% of males and 7% of females were found to have positive genital cultures for *N. gonorrhoeae* [109].

The diagnosis of gonococcal disease in children is similar to that in adults and is discussed in Chapters 3 and 4. One possible difference is the observation that the Gram-stained smear of vaginal secretions of a prepubertal female is more specific than that of postpubertal females. Wald found that two or more polymorphonuclear leukocytes having eight or more gram-negative intracellular diplococci was associated with a 96% culture positivity rate [110].

Treatment of the neonate with a gonococcal eye infection is found in Table 5. The treatment of the prepubertal youngster with uncomplicated genital gonorrhea is similar to that in an adult. Either single-dose oral therapy with ampicillin or amoxicillin or parenteral therapy with procaine penicillin is highly effective. Children weighing over 45 kg (100 lb) are treated with adult regimens. Recommended treatment schedules from the Centers for Disease Control have recently been updated [111]. A multiple-day regimen using tetracycline hydrocholoride can be used in the youngster over 8 years of age. Penicillinase-producing gonococci have been isolated from a prepubertal youngster with vaginitis [112]. Rettig et al. [113] administered spectinomycin to 24 prepubertal children, which was well tolerated and produced a 96% cure rate but did not prevent postgonococcal chlamydial infections. Spectinomycin therapy should be considered for the youngster with an allergy to penicillin or a penicillinase-producing strain of *N. gonorrhoeae*.

REFERENCES

1. Lang DJ. The epidemiology of cytomegalovirus infections: interpretation of recent observation. In: Krugman S, Gershon AA, eds. Infection of the fetus and the newborn infant. Vol. 3. New York: Alan R. Liss, 1975.
2. Stagno S, Pass RF, Dworsky ME, Henderson RE, Moore EG, Walton PD, Alford CA. Congenital cytomegalovirus infection. The relative importance of primary and recurrent maternal infection. N Engl J Med 1982;306:945-949.
3. Kumar ML, Gold E, Jacobs IB, Ernhart CB, Nankervis GA. Primary cytomegalovirus infection in pregnancy. Pediatrics (in press).
4. Stagno S, Reynolds DW, Huang ES, Thames SD, Smith RJ, Alford CA. Congenital cytomegalovirus infection. Occurrence in an immune population. N Engl J Med 1977; 296:1254-1258.
5. Ahlfors K, Harris S, Ivarsson S, Svanberg L. Secondary maternal cytomegalovirus infection causing symptomatic congenital infection. N Engl J Med 1981; 305:284.
6. Starr JG, Bart RD, Gold E. Inapparent congenital cytomegalovirus infection. Clinical and epidemiologic characteristics in early infancy. N Engl J Med 1970; 282:1075-1078.
7. Reynolds DW, Stagno S, Hosty TS, Tiller M, Alford CA. Maternal cytomegalovirus excretion and perinatal infection. N Engl J Med 1973; 289:1-5.
8. Weller TH, Hanshaw JB. Virologic and clinical observation on cytomegalic inclusion disease. N Engl J Med 1962; 266:1233-1244.
9. Kumar M, Gold E, Nankervis G. Risk of acquired cytomegalovirus virus(CMV) infection in infants of maternal CMV excretors. Pediatri Res 1975; 9:342.
10. Whitley FJ, Brasfield D, Reynolds DW, Stagno S, Tiller RE, Alford CA. Protracted pneumonitis in young infants associated with perinatally acquired cytomegaloviral infection. J Pediatr 1976; 89:16-22.
11. Dworsky ME, Stagno S. Newer agents causing pneumonitis in early infancy. Pediatr Infect Dis 1982; 1:188-195.

12. Stagno S, Pass RF, Reynolds DW, Moore MA, Nahmias AJ, Alford CA. Comparative study of diagnostic procedures for congenital cytomegalovirus infection. Pediatrics 1980; 65:251-257.
13. Castellano GA, Madden DL, Hazzard GT, Cleghorn CS, Vails DV, Ley AC, Tzan NR, Sever JL. Evaluation of commercially available diagnostic test kits for rubella. J Infect Dis 1981; 143:578-584.
14. Elek SD, Stern H. Development of a vaccine against medical retardation caused by cytomegalovirus infection in utero. Lancet 1974; 1:1-5.
15. Hanshaw JB. Marginal comments. A cytomegalovirus vaccine? Am J Dis Child 1974; 128:141-142.
16. Spector SA, Schmidt K, Ticknor W, Grossman M. Cytomegaloviruria in older infants in intensive care nurseries. J Pediatr 1979; 95:444-446.
17. Yeager AS, Grumet FC, Hafleigh EB, Arvin AM, Bradley JS, Prober CG. Prevention of transfusion-acquired cytomegalovirus infections in newborn infants. J Pediatr 1981; 98:281-287.
18. Nahmias AJ, Alford CA, Korones SB. Infection of the newborn with *Herpesvirus hominis*. Adv Pediatr 1970; 17:185-226.
19. Linnemann CC, Buchman TG, Light TJ, Ballard JL, Roisman B. Transmission of herpes-simplex virus type 1 in a nursery for the newborn identification of viral isolates by D.N.A. "fingerprinting." Lancet 1978; 2:964-966.
20. Kurtz JB, Sykes DW. Herpes-simplex virus (type 1) transmitted to a neonate. Lancet 1974; 2:1580-1581.
21. Nahmias AJ, Josey WE, Naib AM. Neonatal herpes simplex infection. Role of genital infection in mother as the source of virus in the newborn. JAMA 1967; 199:132-136.
22. Whitley FJ, Nahmias AJ, Visintine AM, Fleming CL, Alford CA. The natural history of herpes simplex virus infection of mother and newborn. Pediatrics 1980; 66:489-494.
23. Hanshaw JB. *Herpesvirus hominis* infections in the fetus and the newborn. Am J Dis Child 1973; 126:546-555.
24. Nahmias AJ, Visintine AM. Herpes simplex. In: Remington, Klein, eds. Infectious diseases of the fetus and newborn infant. Philadelphia: Saunders, 1976.
25. Arvin AM, Yeager AS, Bruhn FW, Grossman M. Neonatal herpes simplex infection in the absence of mucocutaneous lesions. J Pediatr 1982; 100:715-721.
26. Kibrick S. Herpes simplex infection at term. What to do with mother, newborn, and nursery personnel. JAMA 1980; 243:157-160.
27. Whitley RJ, Nahmias AJ, Soong SJ, Galasso GG, Fleming CL, Alford CA. Vidarabine therapy of neonatal herpes simplex infection. Pediatrics 1980; 66:495-501.
28. Ch'ien LT, Whitley RJ, Nahmias AJ, Lewin ED, Linnemann CC, Frenkel LD, Bellanti JA, Buchanan RA, Alford CA. Antiviral chemotherapy and neonatal herpes simplex infections: a pilot study—experience with adenine arabinoside (ARA-A). Pediatrics 1975; 55:852-859.
29. Clercq ED, Descamps J, Verhelst G, Walker RT, Jones AS, Torrence PF, Shugar D. Comparative efficacy of antiherpes drugs against different strains of herpes simplex virus. J Infect Dis 1980; 141:563-574.

30. Offit PA, Starr SE, Zolnick P, Plotkin SA. Acyclovir therapy in neonatal herpes simplex virus infection. Pediatr Infect Dis 1982; 1:253-255.
31. Fay O, Tanno H, Roncoroni M, Edwards VM, Mosley JW, Redeker AG. Prognostic implications of the e antigen of hepatitis B virus. JAMA 1977; 238: 2501-2503.
32. Nielsen JO, Dietrichson O, Juhl E. Incidence and meaning of the "e" determinant among hepatitis-B-antigen positive patients with acute and chronic liver diseases. Lancet 1974; 2:913-915.
33. Alter HJ, Seeff LB, Kaplan PM, McAuliffe VJ, Wright EC, Gerin JL, Purcell RH, Holland PV, Zimmerman HJ. Type B hepatitis: the infectivity of blood positive for e antigen and DNA polymerase after accidental needlestick exposure. N Engl J Med 1976; 295:909-913.
34. Okada K, Kamiyama I, Inomata M, Imai M, Miyakawa Y, Mayami M. e Antigen and anti-e in the serum of asymptomatic carrier mothers as indicators of positive and negative transmission of hepatitis B virus to their infants. N Engl J Med 1976; 294:746-749.
35. Schweitzer IL, Dunn EAG, Peters RL, Spears RL. Viral hepatitis B in neonates and infants. Am J Med 1973; 55:762-771.
36. Schweitzer IL, Mosley JW, Ashcavai M, Edwards VM, Overby LB. Factors influencing neonatal infection by hepatitis B virus. Gastroenterology 1973; 65:277-283.
37. Stevens CE, Beasley RP, Tsui J, Lee WC. Vertical transmission of hepatitis B antigen in Taiwan. N Engl J Med 1975; 292:771-774.
38. Okada K, Yamada T, Miyakawa Y, Mayumi M. Hepatitis B surface antigen in the serum of infants after delivery from asymptomatic carrier mothers. J Pediatr 1975; 87:360-363.
39. Shiraki K, Yoshihara N, Kawana T, Yasui H, Sakurai M. Hepatitis B surface antigen and chronic hepatitis in infants born to asymptomatic carrier mothers. Am J Dis Child 1977; 131:644-647.
40. Dupuy JM, Kostewicz E, Alagille D. Hepatitis B in children. Analysis of 80 cases of acute and chronic hepatitis B. J Pediatr 1978; 92:17-20.
41. Dupuy JM, Giraud P, Dupuy C, Drouet J, Hoofnagle J. Hepatitis B in children. Study of children born to chronic HB s Ag carrier mothers. J Pediatr 1978; 92:200-204.
42. Beasley RP, Hwang LY, Lin CC, Stevens CE, Wang KY, Sun TS, Hsieh FJ, Szmuness W. Hepatitis B immune globulin (HBIG) efficacy in the interruption of perinatal transmission of hepatitis B virus carrier state. Lancet 1981; 2:388-393.
43. Barin F, Goudeau A, Denis F, Yvonnet B, Chiron JP, Coursaget P, Mar ID. Immune response in neonates to hepatitis B vaccine. Lancet 1982; 1:251-253.
44. Centers for Disease Control. Inactivated hepatitis B virus vaccine. Morbid Mortal Week Rep 1982; 31:317-328.
45. Howard JB, McCracken Jr. GH. The spectrum of group B streptococcal infections in infancy. Am J Dis Child 1974; 128:815-818.
46. Dworzak DL, Hodges GR, Barnes WG, Rosett W. Group B streptococcal infections in adult males. Am J Med Sci 1979; 277:67-73.

47. Bayer AS, Chow AW, Anthony BF, Guze LB. Serious infections in adults due to group B streptococci. Am J Med 1976; 61:498-503.
48. Grossman J, Tompkins RL. Group B beta-hemolytic streptococcal meningitis in mother and infant. N Engl J Med 1974; 290:387-388.
49. Franciosi RA, Knostman JD, Zimmerman RA. Group B streptococcal neonatal and infant infections. J Pediatr 1973; 82:707-718.
50. Baker CJ, Barrett FF. Transmission of group B streptococci among parturient women and their neonates. J Pediatr 1973; 83:919-925.
51. Aber RC, Allen N, Howell JT, Wilkenson HW, Facklam RR. Nosocomial transmission of group B streptococci. Pediatrics 1976; 58:346-353.
52. Hammerschlag MR, Baker CJ, Alpert S, Kasper DL, Rosner I, Thurston P, Webb BJ, McCormack WM. Colonization with group B streptococci in girls under 16 years of age. Pediatrics 1977; 60:473-476.
53. Mauer M, Thirumoorthi C, Dajani AS. Group B streptococcal colonization in prepubertal children. Pediatrics 1979; 64:65-67.
54. Vollman JH, Smith WL, Ballard ET, Light IJ. Early onset group B streptococcal disease: clinical roentgenographic and pathologic features. J Pediatr 1976; 89:199-203.
55. Ablow RC, Driscoli SG, Effman EL, Gross I, Jolles CJ, Uauy R, Warshaw JB. A comparison of early-onset group B streptococcal neonatal infection and the respiratory-distress syndrome of the newborn. N Engl J Med 1976; 294:65-70.
56. Menke JA, Giacoia GP, Jockin H. Group B beta-hemolytic streptococcal sepsis and the idiopathic respiratory distress syndrome: a comparison. J Pediatr 1979; 94:467-471.
57. Baker CJ, Kasper DL. Correlation of maternal antibody deficiency with susceptibility to neonatal group B streptococcal infection. N Engl J Med 1976; 294:753-756.
58. Baker CJ, Barrett FF. Group B streptococcal infections in infants. The importance of the various serotypes. JAMA 1974; 230:1158-1160.
59. Ingram DL, Suggs DM, Pearson AW. Detection of group B streptococcal antigen in early-onset and late-onset group B streptococcal disease with the Wellcogen Strep B latex agglutination test. J Clin Microbiol 1982; 16:656-658.
60. Edwards MS, Kasper DL, Baker CJ. Rapid diagnosis of type III group B streptococcal meningitis by latex particle agglutination. J Pediatr 1979; 95:202-205.
61. Baker CJ, Rench MA. Commercial latex agglutination for detection of group B streptococcal antigen in body fluids. J Pediatr 1983; 102:393-395.
62. Dorand RD, Adams G. Relapse during penicillin treatment of group B streptococcal infections. J Pediatr 1976; 89:188-190.
63. Kenny JF, Zedd AJ. Recurrent group B streptococcal disease in an infant associated with the ingestion of infected mother's milk. J Pediatr 1977; 91: 158-159.
64. Troug WE, David RF, Ray CG. Recurrence of group B streptococcal infection. J Pediatr 1976; 89:185-186.

65. Broughton DD, Mitchell WG, Grossman M, Hadley WK, Cohen MS. Recurrence of group B streptococcal infection. J Pediatr 1976; 89:183-185.
66. Baker CJ. Group B streptococcal infections in neonates. Pediatr Rev 1979; 1:5-15.
67. McCracken GH, Feldman WE. Group B streptococcal infections: editorial comment. J Pediatr 1976; 89:203-204.
68. Schauf V, Deveikis A, Riff L, Serota A. Antibiotic-killing kinetics of group B streptococci. J Pediatr 1976; 89:194-198.
69. Seighman AJ, Bottone EJ, Hanna BA. Intramuscular penicillin administration at birth: prevention of early onset group B streptococcal disease. Pediatrics 1978; 62:842-843.
70. Lloyd DJ, Belgaumkar TK, Scott KE, Wort AJ, Aterman K, Krause VW. Prevention of group B beta-hemolytic streptococcal septicemia in low birthweight neonates by penicillin administered within two hours of birth. Lancet 1979; 1:713-715.
71. Siegel JD, McCracken GH, Threlkeld N, Milvenan B, Rosenfeld CR. Single dose penicillin prophylaxis against neonatal group B streptococcal infections. N Engl J Med 1980; 303:769-775.
72. Siegel JD, McCracken Jr. GH, Threlkeld N, DePasse BM, Rosenfeld CR. Single-dose penicillin prophylaxis against neonatal group B streptococcal disease. Lancet 1982; 1:1426-1430.
73. Baker CJ. Early onset group B streptococcal disease. J Pediatr 1978;93:124-125.
74. Pyati SP, Pildes RS, Jacobs NM, Ramamurthy RS, Yeh TF, Raval DS, Kilien LD, Amma P, Metziger WI. Penicillin in infants weighing two kilograms or less with early onset group B streptococcal disease. N Engl J Med 1983;308:1383-1389.
75. Thygeson P, Mengert WF. The virus of inclusion conjunctivitis. Arch Ophthalmol 1936; 15:377-410.
76. Heggie AD, Lumicao GG, Stuart LA, Gyves MT. *Chlamydia trachomatis* infections in mothers and infants. Am J Dis Child 1981; 135:507-511.
77. Hammerschlag MR, Anderka M, Semine DZ, McComb D, McCormack WM. Prospective study of maternal and infantile infection with *Chlamydia trachomatis*. Pediatrics 1979; 64:142-147.
78. Schachter J, Grossman M, Hold J, Sweet R, Goodner E, Mills J. Prospective study of chlamydial infection in neonates. Lancet 1979; 2:377-380.
79. Frommel GT, Rothenberg R, Wang S, McIntosh K, Wintersgill C, Allaman J, Orr I. Chlamydial infection of mothers and their infants. J Pediatr 1979; 95:28-32.
80. Komaroff AL, Aronson MD, Schachter J. *Chlamydia trachomatis* infection in adults with community-acquired pneumonia. JAMA 1981;245:1319-1322.
81. Armstrong JH, Zacarias F, Rein MF. Ophthalmia neonatorum: a chart review. Pediatrics 1976; 57:884-892.
82. Forster RK, Dawson CR, Schachter J. Late followup of patients with neonatal inclusion conjunctivitis. Am J Ophthalmol 1970; 69:467-472.
83. Beem MO, Saxon EM. Respiratory-tract colonization and a distinctive pneumonia syndrome in infants infected with *Chlamydia trachomatis*. N Engl J Med 1977; 296:306-310.

84. Schachter J, Grossman M, Holt J, Sweet R, Spector S. Infection with *Chlamydia trachomatis*: involvement of multiple anatomic sites in neonates. J Infect Dis 1979; 139:232-234.
85. Martin DH, Koutsky L, Eschenbach DA, Daling JR, Alexander ER, Benedetti JK, Holmes KK. Prematurity and perinatal mortality in pregnancies complicated by maternal *Chlamydia trachomatis* infections. JAMA 1982; 247:1585-1588.
86. Beem M, Saxon E, Tipple M. Treatment of *Chlamydia trachomatis* conjunctivitis in infants. Presented at the 18th Interscience Conference on Antimicrobial Agents and Chemotherapy, 1978.
87. Barsam PC. Medical Intelligence, current concepts, specific prophylaxis of gonorrheal ophthalmia neonatorum. A review. N Engl J Med 1966; 274: 731-733.
88. Kohen DP. Neonatal gonococcal arthritis: three cases and review of the literature. Pediatrics 1974; 53:436-440.
89. Stark AR, Glode MP. Gonococcal vaginitis in a neonate. J Pediatr 1979; 94:298-299.
90. Thadepelli M, Rambhatia K, Maidman JE, Arce JJ, Davidson Jr. EC. Gonococcal sepsis secondary to fetal monitoring. Am J Obstet Gynecol 1976; 126:510.
91. Reveri M, Krishnamurthy C. Gonococcal scalp abscess. J Pediatr 1979; 94: 819-820.
92. Nishida H, Risemberg HM. Silver nitrate ophthalmic solution and chemical conjunctivitis. Pediatrics 1975; 56:368-373.
93. Thatcher RW, Pettit TH. Gonorrheal conjunctivitis. JAMA 1971;215:1494-1496.
94. Podgore JK, Holmes KK. Ocular gonococcal infection with minimal or no inflammatory response. JAMA 1981; 246:242-243.
95. Nazarian LF. The current prevalence of gonococcal infections in children. Pediatrics 1967; 39:372-377.
96. Branch G, Paxton R. A study of gonococcal infections among infants and children. Public Health Rep 1965; 80:347.
97. Cooperman MB. Gonococcus arthritis in infancy. A clinical study of forty-four cases. Am J Dis Child 1927; 33:932-948.
98. Shore WB, Winkelstein JA. Nonvenereal transmission of gonococcal infections to children. J Pediatr 1971; 79:661-663.
99. Nelson JD, Mohs E, Dajani AS, Plotkin SA. Gonorrhea in preschool and school-aged children. Report of the prepubertal gonorrhea cooperative study group. JAMA 1976; 236:1359-1364.
100. Farrell MK, Billmire E, Shamroy JA, Hammond JG. Prepubertal gonorrhea: a multidisciplinary approach. Pediatrics 1981; 67:151-156.
101. Folland DS, Burke RE, Hinman AR, Schaffner W. Gonorrhea in preadolescent children: an inquiry into source of infection and mode of transmission. Pediatrics 1977; 60:153-156.
102. Litt IF, Edberg SC, Finberg L. Gonorrhea in children and adolescents: a current review. J Pediatr 1974; 85:595-607.
103. Singleton AF. Vaginal discharge in children and adolescents. Evolution and management: a review. Clin Pediatr 1980; 19:799-804.

104. Altcheck A. Pediatric vulvovaginitis. Pediatr Clin North Am 1972; 19:559-580.
105. Auman GL, Waldenberg LM. Gonococcal periappendicitis and salpingitis in a prepubertal girl. Pediatrics 1976; 58:287-288.
106. Northup WP. General gonococcal peritonitis in young girls under puberty: report of 2 cases, 1 simulating appendicitis, operated. Arch Pediatr 1903; 68:388.
107. Murphy TV, Nelson JD. Shigella vaginitis: report of 38 patients and review of the literature. Pediatrics 1979; 63:511-516.
108. Groothuis JR, Bischoff MC, Jauregui LE. Pharyngeal gonorrhea in young children. Pediatr Infect Dis 1983; 2:99-101.
109. Hein K, Marks A, Cohen MI. Asymptomatic gonorrhea: prevalence in a population of urban adolescents. J Pediatr 1977; 90:634-635.
110. Wald ER. Gonorrhea. Diagnosis by gram stain in the female adolescent. Am J Dis Child 1977; 131:1094-1096.
111. Centers for Disease Control. Sexually transmitted diseases treatment guidelines 1982. Morbid Mortal Week Rep Suppl 1982; 31:33S-60S.
112. Rendin RW, Bourgeois AL, Lin FL. Penicillinase-producing *Neisseria gonorrhoea* in a prepubertal female. J Pediatr 1979; 94:431-432.
113. Rettig PJ, Nelson JD, Kusmiesz H. Spectinomycin therapy for gonorrhea in prepubertal children. Am J Dis Child 1980; 134:359-363.

SIXTEEN

Outpatient Approach to Sexually Transmitted Diseases

James Q. Del Rosso
Southeastern College of Osteopathic Medicine
North Miami Beach, Florida

Richard B. Prior
The Ohio State University
College of Medicine
Columbus, Ohio

INTRODUCTION

The major objectives of this chapter are (1) to stimulate the awareness of the primary care practitioner in sexually transmitted diseases (STDs) and (2) to provide fundamental concepts for the clinical and laboratory approach to office diagnosis. Utilization of these concepts coupled with a sound understanding of the involved diseases will provide the clinician with an organized, practical approach to patient evaluation. The development of such an approach should lead to improved physician-patient interaction, diagnostic acumen, therapy, and cost effectiveness.

As with any area of medicine, diagnostic accuracy is based upon the development of a differential diagnosis for each problem encountered. To organize a complete differential and ultimately to obtain a proper diagnosis, the clinician must utilize a series of basic skills in conjunction with his knowledge of disease. The requisite skills include accurate history taking, sound physical diagnostic ability, appropriately collected laboratory specimens, and properly performed laboratory tests. By reviewing considerations for diagnosis and basic clinical and laboratory methods, this chapter intends to facilitate the development of a diagnostician with regard to STDs and related disorders.

Awareness of STDs and Their Sequelae

A major consideration facing the clinician is the broad spectrum of conditions for which the rule of sexual transmission has been confirmed or implicated [1-5]. Etiological agents include bacteria, protozoa, viruses, ectoparasites, and possibly fungi (Table 1). Many of these organisms can also be transmitted by nonsexual means. Most of these pathogens are capable of producing various clinical presentations, including the asymptomatic state (Table 2). Syndromes range from uncomplicated urethritis or vaginitis to more serious conditions such as pelvic inflammatory disease, hepatitis, or neonatal infection. Familiarity with the various clinical syndromes and a high index of suspicion for STDs must be adopted before a diagnostic approach can be established.

Table 1 Pathogens Implicated in STDs

Bacteria	Ectoparasites
Calymmatobacterium granulomatis	*Phthirus pubis*
Campylobacter jejuni	*Sarcoptes scabiei*
Chlamydia trachomatis	
Gardnerella vaginalis	
Streptococcus agalactiae (group B streptococcus)	Protozoa
Haemophilus ducreyi	*Entamoeba histolytica*
Mycoplasma hominis	*Giardia lamblia*
Neisseria gonorrhoeae	*Trichomonas vaginalis*
Salmonella sp.	
Shigella sp.	
Treponema pallidum	Fungi
Ureaplasma urealyticum	*Candida albicans?*
Viruses	Helminths
Cytomegalovirus	*Enterobius vermicularis*
Epstein-Barr virus?	
Hepatitis A virus	
Hepatitis B virus	
Herpes simplex virus	
Human retrovirus?	
Molluscum contagiosum virus	
Papillomavirus	

Source: Refs. 1 and 2 and Chapter 11.

Table 2 Clinical Syndromes and Implicated Sexually Transmitted Pathogens

Syndrome	Pathogen
Acquired Immune Deficiency Syndrome	Cytomegalovirus? Epstein-Barr virus? Human retrovirus?
Arthritis	*Chlamydia trachomatis* (Reiter's syndrome) Hepatitis B virus *Neisseria gonorrhoeae* *Salmonella* sp. *Shigella* sp. *Treponema pallidum*
Asymptomatic cervicitis/ urethritis	*Chlamydia trachomatis* Cytomegalovirus Herpes simplex virus *Neisseria gonorrhoeae* Papillomavirus *Trichomonas vaginalis* *Ureaplasma urealyticum*?
Asymptomatic enteritis	*Campylobacter jejuni* *Entamoeba histolytica* *Giardia lamblia* *Salmonella* sp. *Shigella* sp.
Asymptomatic proctitis	*Chlamydia trachomatis* Herpes simplex virus *Neisseria gonorrhoeae* Papillomavirus *Treponema pallidum*
Cervicitis	Same as asymptomatic group listed above
Dermatoses	*Candida albicans* Hepatitis B virus Herpes simplex virus Molloscum contagiosum virus *Neisseria gonorrhoeae* Papillomavirus *Pediculosis humanus* *Phthirus pubis* *Sarcoptes scabiei* *Treponema pallidum*
Enteritis	Same as asymptomatic group listed above
Epididymitis	*Chlamydia trachomatis* *Neisseria gonorrhoeae*

Table 2 (Continued)

Syndrome	Pathogen
Genital ulcers	*Chlamydia trachomatis* (lymphogranuloma venereum strain) *Calymmatobacterium granulomatis* *Haemophilis ducreyi* Herpes simplex virus *Treponema pallidum*
Hepatitis	Cytomegalovirus Hepatitis A virus Hepatitis B virus *Treponema pallidum*
Pelvic inflammatory disease	*Chlamydia trachomatis* *Neisseria gonorrhoeae* *Mycoplasma hominis*? *Ureaplasma urealyticum*?
Perihepatitis	*Chlamydia trachomatis* *Neisseria gonorrhoeae*
Proctitis	Same as asymptomatic group listed above plus *Enterobius vermicularis*
Urethritis	Same as asymptomatic group listed above
Vaginitis	*Candida albicans* *Gardnerella vaginalis* *Trichomonas vaginalis*
Infections of obstetric significance	*Chlamydia trachomatis* Cytomegalovirus *Streptococcus agalactiae* Hepatitis B virus Herpes simplex virus *Neisseria gonorrhoeae* Papillomavirus *Treponema pallidum*

Source: Refs. 1, 2, and 10 and Chapter 11.

The morbidity associated with many STDs is largely related to sequelae [1, 6]. Pelvic inflammatory disease with resultant infertility, chronic pelvic pain, and increased risk of ectopic pregnancy is a frequent complication of gonococcal and chlamydial infection [2,6]. The estimated yearly financial burden of pelvic inflammatory disease in the mid-1970s, reflecting some 850,000 or more cases, was $1.25 billion [6]. Certain STDs in the pregnant female are associated with fetal wastage, serious neonatal infection, and impaired growth and development

[1,5,7-9]. Male patients may develop such complications as epididymitis, periurethral abscess, prostatitis, and urethral stricture [1,10,11]. Each STD patient should be categorized as having complicated or uncomplicated disease, and possible sequelae should be appreciated by both the patient and the physician.

A growing concern in the United States is the decline in teaching of STDs in medical schools and the lack of clinical experience in many medical residency programs [12,13]. This void in medical education forms the basis for lack of awareness during years of clinical practice. The primary care physician should be continuously updated regarding STDs and their ever-changing clinical spectrum. The application of improved diagnostic and therapeutic measures to patients with STDs depends upon the continuing education of the primary care physician.

INITIAL EVALUATION

Sexual History

The sexual history is probably the most routinely neglected portion of patient evaluation. Most clinicians encounter no difficulty during routine patient interviews, but are uneasy when faced with sexually related diseases. This is unfortunate, as detection of STDs and other sexual problems is facilitated by a thorough sexual history.

Understanding is the key to reducing patient apprehension when obtaining a sexual history. Assurance of confidentiality and a concerned, relaxed, nonjudgmental attitude will comfort most patients. A brief explanation of the importance of a thorough sexual history assures the patient that the physician's goal is to solve his or her problem. Identification of sexual contacts is best deferred until a specific diagnosis is confirmed [15].

Various sexual attitudes and practices should be appreciated and accepted by the physician if an appropriate physician-patient relationship is to be established. The physician intolerant of promiscuous or homosexual behavior is not likely to provide comprehensive patient care. Attention to sexual orientation is critical. Such knowledge directs appropriate questioning, identifies disease risks, and assists in the selection of sampling sites and laboratory tests [16-18].

Specific questions included in the sexual history are somewhat dependent upon the clinical circumstances. However, certain information should always be elicited when evaluating a patient for STDs and should include the following [10,15]:

1. Chief complaint and associated symptomatology.
2. A review of systems, including the presence of dysuria, genital irritation, discharge, rash, pruritus, adenopathy, abdominal pain, dyspareunia, diarrhea, hematochezia, anogenital pain, or malodorous vaginal secretions.
3. Onset and duration of symptoms.
4. Recent dates of sexual intercourse.

5. Sexual orientation (heterosexual, homosexual, or bisexual).
6. Approximate number of recent sexual partners and known STDs among sexual contacts.
7. Previous STDs and therapy utilized.
8. Present and recent medications, especially antibiotics, topicals, and vaginal preparations.
9. Past medical and surgical history.
10. Drug sensitivities.
11. History of genitourinary instrumentation (i.e., cytoscopy, abortion, dilatation and curretage).
12. Time of last urination (might affect presence of discharge).
13. Obstetrical-neonatal history, menstrual history, modes of contraception, and history of douching in the female.
14. History of serological tests for syphilis, including screening tests (hospital admission, employment, military, etc.), prenatal testing, blood donation, and premarital testing [19].
15. Dysuric females should be asked to distinguish whether their dysuria is "internal" (felt inside the body) or "external" (felt as urine passes over inflamed vaginal labia). The former is correlated with cystitis/urethritis, and the latter with vaginitis [20,21].

Evaluation of Signs and Symptoms

As previously stated, most of the pathogens implicated in STDs produce a variety of clinical syndromes as evidenced by different symptoms and physical findings [1-4]. For example, gonococcal urethritis may cause dysuria and a purulent discharge in the male; however, it may also be asymptomatic and barely detectable (or undetectable) on physical examination [10,15,22]. Likewise, the female patient with gonococcal disease may demonstrate mucopurulent cervicitis or no apparent pathology on visual inspection [2,15]. Such elusive features may also be seen with chlamydial infection in both sexes. Sexually transmitted disease-related proctitis and enteritis syndromes, frequently affecting homosexual males, produce similar symptoms (including the asymptomatic state) despite different etiologies [3,23-25]. Thus the absence of signs and/or symptoms does not preclude the presence of a sexually transmitted pathogen. Recognition of this premise is the basis for treating contacts of known STD cases despite an otherwise unremarkable history and physical examination.

Despite classic "textbook descriptions" for specific STDs, overlapping signs and symptoms are commonly encountered with different syndromes. This is frequently the case in cervical, vulvar, vaginal, and female urinary tract infections [1,22,26-28]. For example, dysuria, frequency, and pyuria in a young female should not reflexly implicate cystitis, since vaginitis and anterior urethral syndrome are also likely possibilities. In such cases a pelvic examination should be performed, with appropriate measures taken to rule out the latter two disorders.

In general, an etiological diagnosis of an STD based solely on clinical appearance is best avoided in order to circumvent errors in diagnosis and therapy. Basic laboratory tests are required to make a presumptive diagnosis, prescribe initial rational therapy, and arrange for appropriate follow-up [4]. Notable exceptions are the identification of the crab louse or classic lesions of condyloma acuminata by visual inspection. The presence of one STD should always alert the clinician to the possibility of other STDs in a patient.

Conditions other than STDs must be included in the differential diagnosis of each patient's problem. Genital ulcerations always mandate a search for an STD such as syphilis, herpes genitalis, or chancroid; however, noninfectious causes must be considered [1]. Examples of the latter include carcinoma, extramammary Paget's disease, trauma, Crohn's disease, erythema multiforme, and excoriated dermatoses such as lichen sclerosus or hyperplastic dystrophies.

With these factors in mind, the history and physical examination is performed in order to uncover signs of disease and carefully evaluate the extent of disease. A differential diagnosis is then developed based upon the constellation of signs and symptoms affecting the given patient. Confirmation of a specific diagnosis requires the performance of laboratory tests designed to detect pathogens considered in the differential diagnosis.

Physical Examination

A systematic approach to physical examination is the best means of assuring complete evaluation of patients on a repetitive basis. Since the manifestations of STDs are not limited to the anogenital region, a general physical examination of each patient is the ideal. Physical findings such as scleral icterus, mucosal ulcers, rash, a swollen knee, or right upper quadrant abdominal tenderness may reflect an underlying STD.

In a busy ambulatory practice some physicians may feel that time precludes the performance of a complete general physical examination in every case. Such an attitude may sacrifice diagnostic accuracy in select cases, especially when the patient is a poor historian. Ultimately, the detection of STDs is dependent upon a high index of suspicion, correlation of the physical examination with information elicited in the history, and the clinician's ability to recognize STD pathology. A complete history dictates features of the physical examination which should not be overlooked. A homosexual male, for example, should always undergo visual inspection of the anogenitalia, oropharynx, and skin. Evaluation of the female patient for STDs should include pelvic examination with both abdominopelvic and genitorectal evaluation.

Studies designed to detect errors in physical diagnosis have shown that errors of omission are more common than errors of commission [29,30]. Physical diagnostic ability is a function of patience, concentration, sound fundamental knowledge, and adherence to a logical stepwise approach. All physicians should constantly reassess their capabilities and methods of physical diagnosis and not assume competence because they have performed a specific procedure many times.

The following assumes the clinician's ability to perform a general physical examination and focuses on evaluation of the anogenitalia and oropharynx. Materials needed for specimen collection and adjustable lighting should be readily available in order to expedite the evaluation. Most patients appreciate a cursory description of each step prior to its completion, especially those requiring palpation or instrument insertion.

The Male Patient

The male patient [10,15] is asked to disrobe, allowing exposure of the chest, abdomen, anogenitalia, and lower extremities. Underwear is inspected for staining with discharge. The external genitalia and inguinal skin are examined visually and by palpation with gloved hands. Care should be taken to inspect and palpate the penis, with attention to the urethral canal and scrotal contents for evidence of pain, inflammation, induration, or edema. Hairy regions should be evaluated for the presence of lice, rust-colored excreta, or nits attached to hair shafts. Palpation of inguinal nodes for size, tenderness, induration, and degree of fixation should be routine.

In the uncircumsized male the foreskin should be retracted and the concealed portion of the foreskin and glans examined. The urethral meatus is then visualized for evidence of discharge or other abnormalities. With the penis held firmly at midshaft with one hand, the urethral contents may be "stripped" anteriorly with the free hand in an attempt to elicit discharge.

Genital ulcers, vesicles, and erosions are to be examined closely and carefully palpated. The presence of pain and the location, size, number, and character of lesions should be noted.

Digital rectal, anoscopic, and sigmoidoscopic examination is recommended in homosexual males, especially those with gastrointestinal and rectal symptomatology.

The Female Patient

In 1978 Komaroff et al. published a study designed to develop logical management strategies for urinary and vaginal infections [20]. They concluded that women with "internal" dysuria and urinary frequency without vaginal irritation and discharge do not need a complete pelvic examination. Although this strategy may satisfy a clearly defined subset of patients, its clinical application has serious limitations. The subset of patients described by Komaroff et al. should receive a pelvic examination in order to evaluate for cervical infection with *Neisseria gonorrhoeae* and *Chlamydia trachomatis*, both of which can cause "internal" dysuria and frequency [22,28] (also see Chap. 9). Exclusion of a pelvic examination in females with genitourinary symptomatology is not recommended.

A pelvic examination is a simple and practical test to perform when evaluating a female for the possibility of STDs. It allows the physician to fully assess the etiology of symptoms, test for asymptomatic STDs in sexually active patients, and evaluate for noninfectious disorders such as vulvar lesions, cervical lesions, and structural anomalies.

The following reviews the basic steps involved in the anogenital examination of the female patient when evaluating for STDs [15].

After a brief explanation of the necessity for pelvic examination and the steps involved, the patient should assume the lithotomy position on a table equipped with adjustable stirrups. The examiner, seated at the foot of the table, should have both hands gloved and is encouraged to maintain eye contact with the patient. Both parties should be comfortable before proceeding. Most females are accustomed to draping. Thus the absence of drapes may cause apprehension in some patients. If used, drapes should not preclude visual inspection of the abdomen, anogenitalia, inguinal region, or thighs.

The external genitalia and pubic hair should be carefully inspected and palpated. Stepwise examination of inguinal nodes, vulvar skin, urethral meatus, introitus, Bartholin's ducts, and Skene's ducts is then completed. The examiner should carefully evaluate for erythema, excoriation, inflammation, vaginal discharge, urethral discharge, induration, edema, ulceration, erosion, discoloration, and areas of abnormal-appearing epithelium.

The anal region may be examined visually at this time; however, digital palpation of the anus and rectum should not be undertaken before manual examination of the vagina and pelvic organs unless gloves are changed.

Palpation and "stripping" of the urethra is extremely important. A gloved index finger, lubricated with warm water, is inserted into the vagina. The urethra is then palpated through the anterior vaginal wall for evidence of edema, inflammation, induration, or anomalies such as diverticuli. Since females with urethritis rarely exhibit spontaneous urethral discharge, exudate may be evident by compressing the urethra anteriorly against the pubic symphysis and milking it toward the meatus.

Prior to speculum insertion, the same gloved finger should be pressed gently but firmly against the posterior vaginal wall for several seconds. This allows for perineal relaxation and easier insertion of a speculum, lubricated with warm water. The largest speculum that may be comfortably accommodated by the patient should be used for examination of the vagina and cervix. Proper angling of the speculum on insertion results in ready visualization of the cervix once the blades are opened. In those cases with uterine malposition such as marked anteversion, viewing the cervix may require repositioning of the speculum or prior localization of the cervix by manual examination.

Once visualized, the vagina should be examined for the presence of rugal folds, erythema, malodor, discharge, purulence, ulcerations, and other obvious abnormalities. If discharge is present, the clinician should attempt to evaluate its character and source (physiological versus vaginal versus cervical). In an excellent article on vaginal infections, Eschenbach reviews the character of normal versus abnormal discharge and the rapid laboratory approach suggested on initial evaluation [26]. It is not acceptable to diagnose the etiology of vaginal discharge solely on appearance; however, the physician should attempt to distinguish physiological discharge from an abnormal discharge. Certain characteristics favor a normal vaginal discharge. These include the absence of discharge at the introitus, pooling in the dependent region of the vagina, lack of adherence to the vaginal walls, a white color, high viscosity, floccular consistency, an acidic pH of no more than 4.5, and absence of malodor, especially a fishy amine odor. Candidal vaginitis may mimic a physiological discharge in color, viscosity, consistency, pH, and lack of odor, but frequently consists of a scant discharge with marked vaginal erythema or white, curdlike deposits which adhere to the vaginal walls. Additionally, candidiasis is sometimes associated with an erythematous vulvitis. A low viscosity, grayish, homogeneous exudate that adheres to vaginal walls is associated with both nonspecific vaginitis and trichomoniasis. Cervical pathogens, including *N. gonorrhoeae, C. trachomatis*, and herpes simplex virus, should also be considered in females with vaginal discharge, especially a purulent discharge. Women with cervicitis generally interpret their discharge as vaginal in origin. According to Eschenbach, 25% of women complaining of discharge have cervicitis [26].

The cervix should be visually inspected for discharge, inflammation, erosion, ectropion, ulceration, and friability. Mucus noted at the cervical os is cleared by gently twirling a dry cotton-tipped swab at the cervical portio. If mucopus is present, it generally assumes a green or yellow tinge when compared against the white surface of the cotton swab [2]. The cervix is touched with the cotton swab to test for friability. The blades of the speculum can be used to gently compress the cervix in an attempt to exude endocervical discharge. After specimen collection is completed, the speculum is slowly removed and the entire area of the vaginal mucosa carefully examined.

Bimanual examination, including both abdominopelvic and genitorectal assessment, is an integral part of the pelvic examination. With one hand on the abdomen and the index and middle finger of the other hand inserted in the vaginal orifice, stepwise palpation of the abdomen, vagina, cervix, uterus, and adnexal structures is completed. Uterine size and position should be carefully evaluated and superior displacement of the cervix performed to check for the presence of tenderness ("chandelier sign").

Genitorectal examination allows for evaluation of the rectum and cul-de-sac. Gloves should be changed prior to genitorectal examination to avoid the possibility of iatrogenic rectal inoculation with pathogens such as the gonococcus [31]. Specimen collection for bacteriological testing should be completed prior to digital rectal evaluation if use of lubricants other than water is anticipated.

Anoscopic and sigmoidoscopic examination is suggested for females with proctocolitic symptomatology and those who have engaged in rectal intercourse.

Oropharyngeal Examination

Routine examination of the oropharynx may prove beneficial if such abnormalities as ulceration or pharyngitis are noted. Oral chancres are generally laden with spirochetes; however, with the exception of lip chancres, treponemes present on dark-field microscopy of oral chancres are not diagnostic of syphilis. This is due to the presence of commensal spirochetes such as *Treponema microdentrium* in normal mouth flora [19].

Only 20 to 30% of pharyngeal gonorrhea patients demonstrate signs or symptoms of pharyngitis, so the lack of a "sore throat" and an unremarkable pharyngeal examination do not rule out the possibility of pharyngeal gonorrhea [32-35]. Homosexual males and females who practice fellatio should have a pharyngeal culture for gonorrhea despite the absence of signs and symptoms.

Genital Dermatology

Physicians evaluating patients for STDs will frequently encounter a variety of dermatological disorders affecting the genitalia. Approximately 80% of 877 consecutive patients seen in a cutaneous-vulvar disease clinic suffered from conditions that were primarily dermatological. Generally, such conditions were readily diagnosed by a physician trained in dermatology. Sexually transmitted diseases accounted for 30% of patients seen at the same clinic [36].

Although a complete review of genital dermatology is beyond the scope of this chapter, clinicians should familiarize themselves with genital dermatological disorders and the cutaneous manifestations of STDs (i.e., syphilis, disseminated gonococcemia). Two excellent reference texts are *Practical Dermatology of the Genital Region* by G. W. Korting and *Vulvar Disease* by Edward G. Friedrich [37,38].

Pediatric Patients and STDs

All of the pathogens that cause STDs in adults may also affect children and adolescents [2]. In addition to the passive transfer of pathogens to newborns, STDs may be transmitted to children or adolescents via sexual abuse or by willing sexual participation. In a review of pediatric STDs, Bell alerts the medical community of the need for an increased index of suspicion in the pediatric age group [2]. Ginsburg refers to primary and secondary syphilis as the "stranger to practicing pediatricians" and warns pediatricians about the possibility of acquired syphilis in children with innocuous-appearing lesions and exanthems [39].

Evaluation of children and adolescents for STDs is complicated by legal implications and the need for additional knowledge regarding etiological possibilities. For example, in the prepubertal female, *Enterobius vermicularis* is a cause of vulvovaginitis that must be considered, as is *Shigella* sp. in cases of hemorrhagic vaginal discharge [2]. Childhood epididymitis suggests an underlying structural anomaly and enteric bacterial pathogens, as opposed to a sexually transmitted pathogen in sexually active young adult males [11].

Five basic fundamentals for gynecological examination of neonates, children, and adolescents have been described by Cowell [40]: (1) knowledge of reproductive tract anatomy and physiology from infancy to adolescence, (2) understanding of the normal somatic pubertal process of growth and sexual maturation in girls, (3) a working knowledge of age-specific gynecological disorders for each of the different age categories from infancy to puberty, (4) the ability to communicate, and (5) the technique of gynecological pelvic examination in children and young adolescents. Pediatric gynecological examination should be performed only by physicians who are knowledgable and adequately trained in pediatric gynecology. For interested physicians, pelvic examination workshops are sponsored by the Adolescent Section of the American Academy of Pediatrics. The techniques and materials needed for gynecological examination in children and adolescents have been reviewed in detail by Cowell [40] and Capraro [41].

Specimen Collection

A major factor affecting the diagnostic yield of a laboratory test is proper specimen collection. Most specimens required for the diagnosis of STDs include discharge or scrapings for microscopy and culture. Serological tests are also helpful in select cases such as syphilis and viral hepatitis.

Vaginal Specimens

Approximately 75 to 80% of vaginitis cases are accurately diagnosed when rapid laboratory testing is applied. Such testing does not include Gram staining or culturing and is simple to perform. The remaining 20 to 25% of cases require repeat examination and culturing [26]. Simple, rapid laboratory testing is amenable to the office setting and includes vaginal pH testing, the "sniff" test for amine odor, and microscopy for identification of trichomonads, clue cells, mycelia, lactobacilli, and leukocytes [4,26].

Vaginal pH is determined by simply applying vaginal discharge to pH paper. The normal vaginal pH of not more than 4.5 can be altered by many factors, including microbial pathogens, vaginal medications, and amniotic fluid. Vaginal syndromes associated with *Gardnerella vaginalis* and *Trichomonas vaginalis* generally create a basic vaginal pH [4,26].

Testing for amine odor, the "sniff" test, is often helpful. Application of 10% potassium hydroxide (KOH) to a glass slide containing vaginal secretions often elicits a fishy amine odor characteristic but not specific for nonspecific vaginitis. *Trichomonas vaginalis* infection may also result in a positive "sniff" test [4,26].

In order to microscopically assess vaginal secretions, a dry cotton-tipped swab is placed in vaginal discharge and the specimen is smeared on two glass slides. The first slide, containing a small amount of vaginal discharge, is mixed with a few drops of normal saline. The slide is then examined microscopically for trichomonads, clue cells, lactobacilli and leukocytes. The second slide is coated with a generous sample of vaginal secretion, mixed with 10% KOH, and examined for *Candida* [4,26].

Gram staining of vaginal discharge is generally not helpful in the evaluation of vaginitis [21]. However, Spiegel et al. recently demonstrated the utility of the Gram stain for diagnosing bacterial vaginosis (nonspecific vaginitis) by direct Gram stain of vaginal fluid [42]. These investigators concluded that a microscopically detectable change in vaginal microflora from the *Lactobacillus* morphotype (large gram-positive rods), with or without the *Gardnerella* morphotype (small gram-variable rods), to a mixed flora with few or no *Lactobacillus* morphotypes can be used in the diagnosis of bacterial vaginosis. The use of the vaginal specimen in the diagnosis of gonorrhea is not routinely recommended [15]. In one study approximately 33% of females with gonorrhea would have been undetected if the vagina was the sole site for Gram-stained smears and culture [43]. A notable exception is the prepubertal female, where the alkalinity and epithelial immaturity of the vaginal epithelium make the vagina the optimal sampling site for gonorrhea culturing [44,45].

Urethral and Endocervical Specimens

The urethra and endocervix are sites commonly evaluated for gonococcal and chlamydial infection [22,46], and samples are usually obtained for Gram staining and culture. For the male the urethra is "stripped" and a sterile swab (Calgiswab) or bacteriological loop is inserted approximately 2 to 3 cm into the urethral orifice. Once inserted, the swab or loop is twirled slowly and allowed to remain within the orifice for a few seconds. The collected specimen is evenly smeared onto a clean glass slide. A second swab similarly inserted may be applied to appropriate culture media (see Sec. III). Every effort should be made to avoid contamination of the collected specimens. In the screening for gonococcal urethritis in asymptomatic males, Gram-stained smears alone are not sufficient, and cultures should be obtained [22].

In the female patient the urethra is frequently involved in cases of gonococcal and chlamydial disease, and samples are collected, Gram stained, and cultured as in the male patient. This is especially helpful in the evaluation of women with dysuria and urinary frequency [22,27,28] (see also Chapter 9.) The collection of a urethral specimen should be done in conjunction with an endocervical specimen, as the latter is the most common site of involvement in asymptomatic gonorrhea in females [46]. Also, women who are contacts of known gonorrhea cases and those with genitourinary symptoms (vaginal discharge, dysuria, etc.) should routinely be evaluated with endocervical smears and cultures for *N. gonorrhoeae*.

Specimens from the endocervical canal are obtained by first removing mucoid material from the cervical portio with a dry cotton-tipped swab. A second, dry, sterile cotton-tipped swab is then inserted approximately 2 to 3 cm into the endocervical canal, moved from side to side, and allowed to remain 10 to 30 sec for absorption of organisms to the swab. The specimen is smeared on a glass slide and Gram stained. The same technique is utilized when obtaining specimens for gonococcal cultures. Certain commercial vaginal lubricants have been shown to interfere with growth of the gonococci and should be avoided before specimen collection [47].

When culturing for *C. trachomatis*, adequate specimen collection requires retrieval of cellular material, rather than merely body fluids. Swabs should be rubbed vigorously against the mucosa. The type of swab used is important, with cotton-tipped swabs on aluminum shafts reported to yield higher frequencies of *C. trachomatis* from clinical samples than Calgiswabs or swabs on wooden shafts [48].

Rectal Specimens

The role of the rectal specimen for gonococcal disease in the female was defined in a study by Bhattacharyya and Jephcott [49]. In this review 45% of females with gonorrhea had anorectal involvement. In approximately 5% of females the anorectum was the sole site of gonococcal isolation. The significance of these findings is apparent by the frequency of asymptomatic rectal gonorrhea and the high failure rate of standard gonorrhea treatment regimens when the rectum is involved.

The spectrum of anorectal STDs in homosexual males provides a wide variety of etiological possibilities (see Table 2 and Chap. 10). Unfortunately, no single rapidly performed test is routinely reliable for distinguishing the various causes of proctitis syndromes.

Detection of gonorrhea by rectal Gram stain may allow for more rapid detection of disease, but its relatively poor sensitivity (30 to 50%) enhances the need for culture [3]. Anoscopic directed sampling for Gram staining may increase diagnostic yield in patients with symptomatic gonococcal proctitis and obvious sites of purulence. Samples for rectal Gram staining or culture are collected by inserting a sterile cotton-tipped swab approximately 2 to 3 cm into the anorectal orifice. The swab is then rotated, allowed to remain in the canal for several seconds, and, if not coated by stool, is utilized for specimen collection [3]. Whenever possible, rectal specimens should be obtained prior to digital, anoscopic, or sigmoidoscopic examination, as certain lubricants have been shown to inhibit growth of gonococci [47].

If diarrhea is present, fresh stool can be examined microscopically for leukocytes. Identification of fecal leukocytes by methylene blue stain is rapid and indicates with good reliability the presence of disrupted intestinal mucosa [50].

Fresh stool specimens for direct examination and culture are often necessary for the diagnosis of enteric pathogens. Multiple specimens are frequently required for identification of intestinal parasites such as *Giardia lamblia* and *Entamoeba histolytica*.

Genital Ulcer Specimens

Ulcerations of the genitalia mandate a thorough search for a sexually transmitted pathogen [2] (also see Chap. 6). In the United States herpes and syphilis cause the majority of STD-related genital ulcers. Less common causes include *Haemophilus ducreyi* (chancroid) and lymphogranuloma venereum strains of *C. trachomatis* [1,2].

Vesicular lesions suggest herpetic disease. Vesicles generally provide a greater diagnostic yield of herpes simplex virus than do ulcers, especially when the ulcers have been present for several days [4,51]. This is true for Tzanck smearing and viral culture. Therefore the bases of vesicles or fresh erosions are ideally suited for collecting specimens for smear or culture. When obtaining samples for Tzanck smear, a #15 surgical blade is used to scrape the base of the lesion, and the epithelial debris is thinly smeared onto a dry glass slide, air-dried, and appropriately stained [4,52].

Syphilis must be considered in all cases of genital ulcerations. Chancres may be single or multiple, are generally painless, and are commonly indurated with raised borders [16]. Preparation of a specimen for dark-field microscopy, the best diagnostic test for primary syphilis, requires the collection of serous exudate from the ulcer. This may necessitate the removal of overlying crusted granulation tissue before the sample is obtained [53].

Once herpes genitalis and syphilis have been ruled out, evaluation for less common causes of STD-related genital ulceration may be undertaken.

THE OFFICE-BASED LABORATORY

General Considerations

The office-based laboratory can be a tremendous resource for the clinician, particularly in the evaluation of STDs, where certain simple procedures may provide at least a preliminary diagnosis [4]. While certain tests must be performed in referral laboratories to obtain accurate results, other tests can be performed in the office setting during the patient's initial evaluation. In all cases the proper collection, handling, and processing of specimens are extremely important factors in ensuring accurate results [4,54,55]. Misdiagnosis in the area of STDs leads not only to medical mismanagement, but also can be a traumatic and damaging experience for patients and their sexual contacts. In selecting tests to perform in the office laboratory, the physician should consider utility of the test, turnaround time for results, and cost. Regardless of where the tests are performed, the advantages and limitations of each test employed must be known in order to interpret results effectively.

When performing laboratory procedures on specimens from patients with suspected STDs, it is logical to assume that all clinical specimens are potentially infectious and therefore should be considered biohazards [56]. The STDs are caused by a wide variety of organisms, ranging from viruses and bacteria to protozoa and parasites. Thus prudent handling of specimens by personnel is warranted. The use of disposable gloves is recommended, and all specimens should be discarded in a properly marked biohazard waste container. Office laboratory space should be clearly marked and restricted to personnel performing the tests. Work areas should also be disinfected daily.

Specimens to be cultured in the office laboratory should be processed immediately following collection. If samples are to be transported to a referral laboratory for culturing, they should be placed in the appropriate transport media and delivered as soon as possible. Unnecessary delays will only result in the decreased viability of organisms. Storage of specimens for culturing at a later time is usually not practical in the office setting. Most STD pathogens will not survive the usual freezer temperature of $-20^{\circ}C$ and require temperatures of $-70^{\circ}C$ or lower for storage. Freezers capable of producing these lower temperatures are not normally found in the office laboratory.

In addition to the necessary skills and expertise needed to perform office-based tests, the physician should require some form of quality assurance in the office laboratory. The step-by-step procedures for each test should be written and incorporated into a manual on laboratory procedures. These procedures should be reviewed periodically and updated when necessary. Also, records should be kept of daily recordings of incubators, water baths, refrigerators, and room temperatures. Microscopes should be cleaned and aligned regularly by a competent technician, stain reagents should be checked periodically with known positive and negative smears, and new orders of media should be checked for sterility and support of appropriate growth [4]. Retrospective comparison of presumptive test results with subsequent diagnosis may indicate potential problems. For example, the culture from a male with a "positive" smear for gonococcal urethritis should grow *N. gonorrhoeae* in over 95% of cases. Frequencies under 95% would indicate lack of culture sensitivity or possibly "overreading" (false positives) of the Gram-stained smear by the microscopist. Also, it is recommended that office laboratories participate in some form of survey program [4]. The College of American Pathologists has a program called EXCEL directed at the office laboratory whereby performance of the laboratory is compared with those of other laboratories [57]. There is an annual fee of $60 plus $76 for the Microbiology Module, Series XL-4; however, it is worth the cost to know that office laboratory tests are being performed correctly and are providing accurate results. The Centers for Disease Control also offer short courses on laboratory diagnosis of STDs for both clinicians and laboratory personnel [58].

Once laboratory test results are available, the physician must interpret them. The reliability of tests in determining the presence or absence of disease is often defined by the test's sensitivity and specificity [59]. Sensitivity indicates the frequency of positive test results in patients with the disease and is a measure of the test's ability to detect disease (percent of true positives). On the other hand, specificity indicates the frequency of negative test results in patients without the disease under study and is a measure of the test's ability to exclude disease (percent of true negatives). However, a more important parameter to consider is the predictive value of the test. The positive predictive value of a test is the likelihood that a patient yielding a positive test actually has the disease. The negative predictive value is the likelihood that a patient with a negative test does not have the disease. To compute these predictive values, the prevalence of the disease in the population being tested must be known in addition to the sensitivity and specificity of the test [59,60]. Predictive value tables for various prevalence rates can be found in *Gradwohl's Clinical Laboratory Methods and Diagnosis* [61] or they can be computed for a given prevalence rate using simple mathematics when the sensitivity and specificity of the test are known (Table 3).

The concept of predictive values is not new, since it was first described by Bayes in 1763 [62]. For a test to be useful in predicting disease (positive predictive value), it must have a high specificity. As an example, assume that for gonococcal urethritis Gram stain sensitivity and specificity are 95 and 98%, respectively, when read by an *experienced* microscopist. The positive predictive values of this test for various theoretical prevalence rates of gonococcal urethritis are shown in Table 4. The lower the prevalence of gonorrhea, the less accurate the test in predicting disease. On the other hand, excluding the possibility of a sexually transmitted disease and assuring patients that they are not infected are at least as important as making the proper diagnosis for infected patients [63]. For a test to be useful in excluding disease (negative predictive value), it must have a high sensitivity. The VDRL (Venereal Disease Research Laboratory) test is an excellent screening test to rule out the possibility of secondary syphilis, since during this stage of syphilis the test's sensitivity is 100% [64]. Because predictive values vary according to the test's sensitivity and specificity and the prevalence of the disease under study, it is recommended that clinicians be familiar with these parameters when interpreting test results.

With these general considerations in mind, the following is a brief listing of the microscopic, cultural, and other important laboratory procedures commonly

Table 3 Mathematical Formulas Used for Computing the Positive and Negative Predictive Values of Laboratory Tests

$$\text{PPV} = \frac{(\text{P})(\text{Se})}{(\text{P})(\text{Se}) + (1-\text{P})(1-\text{Sp})}$$

$$\text{NPV} = \frac{(1-\text{P})(\text{Sp})}{(1-\text{P})(\text{Sp}) + (\text{P})(1-\text{Se})}$$

where
PPV = positive predictive value of test
NPV = negative predictive value of test
Se = sensitivity of test
Sp = specificity of test
P = prevalence of the disease

Source: Refs. 59-61.

Table 4 Predictive Values of Positive Gram-Stained Smears Read by Experienced Microscopists for Various Prevalence Rates of Gonococcal Urethritis in Males

Theoretical prevalence (%)	Positive predictive value[a] (%)
5	71
10	84
20	92
30	95
40	97
50	98
60	99

[a]Computed using a Gram stain sensitivity and specificity of 95 and 98%, respectively.

used in evaluating patients for suspected STDs. Also included is a brief discussion of their applicability in the office setting.

Microscopic Tests

Bright-Field Microscopy

Bright-field microscopy is used primarily in venereology to examine unstained specimens such as skin scrapings and vaginal secretions and stained specimens of exudate or infected body fluids. Basic equipment and materials needed include (1) a microscope equipped with low-power objectives (40X and 100X), a "high dry" objective (400X), and an oil immersion objective (1000X); (2) staining reagents; (3) glass slides and cover slips; (4) pipettes; (5) a flame source to fix smears; and (6) accessory materials such as immersion oil, lens paper, and marking pencil. A water source and sink or deep-set pan are also required.

Unstained Specimens. Bright-field microscopic examination of unstained specimens is useful for (1) detecting ectoparasites, (2) examining vaginal secretions for trichomonads, clue cells, lactobacilli, candida, and leukocytes, and (3) examining uncentrifuged and centrifuged urine for leukocytes and bacteria.

Ectoparasites. The most definitive means of diagnosing scabies is identification of the mite, its eggs, or its excrement (scybala) [16]. A hand lens should be used to locate burrows or unscratched papules. Selection of fresh, unexcoriated burrows will make identification most likely. A surgical blade coated with mineral oil is then vigorously scraped against the burrow or papule. The collected material is placed on a glass slide under a cover slip and examined microscopically [16]. Crabs are frequently diagnosed by physical examination alone. Adult lice and nits can easily be identified in infected hair with a hand lens. When noted, however, the hair should be plucked, placed on a glass slide, and examined microscopically to confirm the diagnosis [65] (also see Chap. 13). The microscopic examination of specimens under the low-power objective (40X) for mites, eggs, fecal pellets, or nits is simple, has a high diagnostic value, and is a practical procedure for the office setting.

Vaginal Secretions. Wet mount preparations are useful for evaluating vaginal secretions. The specimen of vaginal discharge is mixed with one or two drops of normal saline on a clean glass slide. The specimen is then covered with a glass cover slip and examined microscopically under the high dry objective (400X) for actively motile flagellates of *T. vaginalis*, clue cells (epithelial cells coated with small bacilli), lactobacilli, and leukocytes [1,26,54] (also see Chap. 5). Care must be taken to examine the specimen before the slide dries. The finding of trichomonads is diagnostic for trichomoniasis. However, although the saline wet mount is an economically and technically feasible procedure, it will only identify 60% of infected patients [66]. A 10% KOH solution is used to demonstrate *Candida* organisms under the 100X objective on a separate slide. The slide is examined for the mycelia (pseudohyphae) form, which is present virtually only when an infection is present [26]. Loffler's methylene blue solution may be used to stain leukocytes, bacteria, and ameba and has been used as a screening test in patients suspected of having bacterial dysentery [54].

Urine Samples. Wet mount preparations are also useful for evaluating urine samples for leukocytes and bacteria. A drop of uncentrifuged urine or sediment from centrifuged urine is placed on a glass slide and covered with a cover slip. The samples are then examined microscopically under the high dry objective (400X) for leukocytes and bacteria. The finding of at least 1 leukocyte per microscopic field of an uncentrifuged midstream urine specimen or at least 20 leukocytes per field of centrifuged urine is indicative of pyuria. The finding of at least 1 bacillus per field in an uncentrifuged midstream specimen of urine is microscopic evidence of bacteriuria [1].

Stained Specimens. The most widely used stain for evaluating patients with STDs is the Gram stain. Another stain which uses Wright or Giemsa stain (Tzanck test) is helpful in certain cases for evaluating herpes lesions.

The Gram Stain. Currently the Gram stain is the only acceptable immediate diagnostic aid for the evaluation of potential gonococcal infection [67]. The basic Gram stain procedure used for smears of exudates or infected body fluids is outlined in Table 5. For males, an immediate and firm diagnosis of gonococcal urethritis can be made with the aid of the Gram stain, provided that the smears are read by experienced microscopists [68]. Gram-stained smears performed on urethral exudates from men with symptomatic urethritis are highly sensitive (93 to 99%) and highly specific (98%), with an overall accuracy of approximately 98%

Table 5 The Gram Stain Procedure

1. Make thin smear of material onto clean slide and allow to air dry.
2. Heat-fix material by passing the slide through a flame three or four times.
3. Overlay smear with crystal violet solution for 1 min.
4. Wash slide with water.
5. Overlay smear with Gram's iodine solution for 1 min.
6. Wash slide with water.
7. Flood slide with decolorizer (acetone-alcohol) until the solvent flows colorlessly from slide (usually about 10 sec or less).
8. Wash slide with water.
9. Overlay smear with safranin counterstain for 1 min.
10. Wash slide with water, then allow slide to air-dry or blot dry with bibulous paper.

Source: Ref. 54.

[68-71]. The finding of typical gram-negative diplococci within the polymorphonuclear leukocytes of urethral exudate is correlated with positive culture results in 98% of cases. Similarly, when the Gram stain is unequivocally negative for the gonococci, the culture is also negative in 98% of cases, and the finding of four or more polymorphonuclear leukocytes per high-power field (1000X) in at least five fields is correlated with nongonococcal urethritis [63]. However, Gram stains of urethral exudates from as many as 15% of males may not be indicative of either gonococcal or nongonococcal urethritis, commonly showing extracellular atypical pleomorphic gram-negative organisms or small numbers of polymorphonuclear leukocytes [72]. The Gram stain is not reliable for asymptomatic urethral infection. For females the Gram stain sensitivity for gonococcal cervicitis is only 55 to 65% in venereal disease clinic laboratories. Gram staining has no place in the diagnosis of pharyngeal infections in either sex, and rectal smears are rarely performed as a routine procedure [67].

For any clinical specimen, reliable use of the Gram stain depends on the experience of the individual reading the smear. Without extensive experience, the accuracy of interpreting Gram-stain smears decreases. In a recent study Gram stain sensitivities and specificities varied from 79 to 96% and 52 to 97%, respectively, for urethral smears and from 15 to 59% and 61 to 100%, respectively, for cervical smears [73]. Results were dependent upon the microscopist reading the smear, with the most accurate results obtained by those microscopists reading more than 200 slides per week for several years [73]. Unfortunately, such expertise is usually restricted to venereal disease clinics. In a survey conducted at the 1981 American Academy of Family Physician's Annual Scientific Assembly, 31% of the private physicians sampled did not do Gram stains in their offices; of those who did, the majority believed the test was less than 80% accurate in their hands [74]. Thus the predictive values of the Gram stain are lower in private practice settings, and the physician must interpret smear results accordingly [75].

The Tzanck Test. The Tzanck test is used for evaluating suspected herpes lesions. A smear of the base of a vesicle is made, air-dried, and fixed with 95% methanol. The slide is then stained with Wright or Giemsa stain and examined for giant multinucleated cells containing intranuclear eosinophilic inclusion bodies. However, the Tzanck test is not very sensitive, and many cytologically negative specimens will eventually be positive by cell culture [4]. In addition, the typical histology seen with herpes simplex virus cannot be distinguished from that of varicella zoster virus [76].

Dark-Field Microscopy

A regular bright-field microscope can be converted into a dark-field microscope by changing the condenser. The dark-field condenser is specially designed to create a hollow cone of light. When no specimen is in the field, light fails to enter the objective lens. When a specimen is present, the light is reflected into the objective lens and the viewer sees a lighted object against a dark background.

The dark-field microscope is useful for evaluating primary syphilis, since the very thin (0.1 to 0.2 μm wide) treponemes can be seen in fluid from the chancre. In many cases a sample of lesion material that is dark-field positive (treponemes visualized) is definitive evidence for treponemal infection [53]. However, the dark-field examination is not usually a routine office procedure. It is also a useless procedure if performed on material obtained and transported to a laboratory. Patients with such lesions must be examined within the vicinity of a dark-field microscope [55]. Most venereal disease clinics or other appropriate laboratories have dark-field microscopes and the experienced personnel needed to identify *Treponema pallidum* in dark-field preparations made from lesions. Therefore patients with genital ulcers should be referred to these facilities for dark-field examinations.

Fluorescence Microscopy

Fluorescence microscopy involves the use of a special microscope equipped with emitter and barrier filters and a light source capable of producing short-wavelength light. It is principally used for detecting antigen-antibody conjugates. In venereology fluorescence microscopy is primarily used for (1) the fluorescent treponemal antibody-absorbed (FTA-ABS) test and (2) the delayed fluorescent antibody confirmation of *Neisseria* from the primary isolation plate. Newer applications include the use of fluorescein-labeled monoclonal antibodies for the culture confirmation of *C. trachomatis*. Direct application of fluorescein-labeled monoclonal antibodies to clinical samples for the rapid (within 30 min) detection of *N. gonorrhoeae, C. trachomatis,* and herpes simplex virus has been reported [77], and these procedures should be available in the near future. However, these tests require the use of a fluorescence microscope and therefore are not likely to be performed in private office settings. Fluorescence microscopes are very expensive, and experienced personnel are required to use them correctly. Such procedures are normally performed in referral laboratories.

Cultures

Neisseria gonorrhoeae

Culturing for *N. gonorrhoeae* is a feasible office procedure, provided that the appropriate quality assurances previously mentioned are performed. The gonococci are fastidious, aerobic bacteria requiring an enriched medium, high humidity, and increased CO_2 tension (5 to 10%) for growth. Enriched media contain heated blood or hemoglobin and nutritional supplements (chocolate agar). The media are made selective for *Neisseria* sp. by the addition of various antibiotics, including vancomycin or lincomycin. Thayer-Martin, New York City, modified New York City, and Martin-Lewis media are routinely used to isolate *N. gonorrhoeae*. These media can be obtained commercially and should be refrigerated (2 to 8°C) until used. Before inoculation, the plates must be warmed to room temperature. For inoculation the swab is rolled directly on the medium in a large Z pattern and cross-streaked immediately with a sterile wire or plastic loop. The cultures should then be placed in an incubator set at 35 to 36°C within 15 min. If a CO_2 incubator is not available, a candle extinction jar can be used and incubated in a regular air incubator. The candle must be relighted each time the jar is reopened. The plates should be examined for visible growth daily for 3 days. Suspicious colonies should be Gram-stained and tested for oxidase production. A presumptive diagnosis of gonorrhea made on the basis of oxidase-positive gram-negative diplococci growing on selective medium is approximately 98% accurate for specimens from a genitourinary site [67]. Further identification is necessary to provide a definitive diagnosis for infection at all sites, but particularly for isolates obtained from the pharynx or rectum. Such identification involves sugar fermentation, fluorescent antibody, or coagglutination tests. Cultures grown in the office laboratory can be confirmed if the laboratory has the materials and expertise, or they can be sent to referral laboratories for confirmatory testing. Screening for penicillinase-producing *N. gonorrhoeae* should also be requested if not routinely done in the office. Descriptions of the methods used for tests which determine β-lactamase production are available through state health department laboratories and are included in commercial kits.

When office cultures are processed correctly, high culture sensitivity for *N. gonorrhoeae* can be expected. For male urethral cultures sensitivity should be greater than 95%. For females, a single cervical culture has been reported to be only about 80 to 93% sensitive [24,78,79]; however, by combining cervical and rectal cultures taken on two separate occasions, sensitivity to detect gonorrhea increases to greater than 95% [24,67,80,81]. The small number of false negative results may be due to vancomycin-susceptible strains. In modified New York City medium, vancomycin is replaced with lincomycin, and Young reported 100% sensitivity using this medium in a limited number of patients [82].

For those office laboratories not wishing to process cultures for *N. gonorrhoeae*, several transport systems are available. Originally, Transgrow medium was promoted as an effective means to transport and grow gonococcal cultures. However, in a recent report, sensitivity of Transgrow medium with off-site evaluation was only 64%, while sensitivities of direct plating on Thayer-Martin medium and modified Stuart's transport system with on-site evaluation were 87 and 85%, respectively [83]. Other commercial transport systems include nonnutrient holding medium (Amies) and selective growth transport medium (JEMBEC, Microcult, Isocult) [69].

Chlamydia trachomatis

Processing cultures for *C. trachomatis* is not an office procedure. In vitro growth of this obligate intracellular parasite requires the use of cell cultures, and clinical samples for culture must be sent to referral laboratories. Cost for these cultures is high and clinicians must exercise informed judgment when deciding the need for chlamydial cultures. Chlamydial cultures are recommended for (1) the pregnant patient, (2) females with gonococcal disease, (3) cervicitis cases, (4) cases of vaginal discharge where other infectious causes have been ruled out by microscopy and culture, (5) cases of pelvic inflammatory disease, (6) unexplained female urethritis, (7) homosexual males with signs and symptoms of proctitis and a negative rectal smear for gonorrhea, (8) sexually active males with epididymitis, and (9) known sexual contacts of patients with chlamydial infection. Sexual partners of patients with chlamydial urethritis, cervicitis, or proctitis should be evaluated and treated.

Following collection, it has been recommended that samples for culture of *C. trachomatis* be kept at 4°C during transportation and that they should be frozen at −20°C or lower if not processed within 24 hr of collection. However, Kallings and Mårdh have shown that chlamydial samples can be stored in 2-SP (a sucrose buffer with additives) transport medium for as long as 2 days at room temperature and for 4 days at 4°C with no appreciable loss of viability of the organism [48].

Viruses

Processing cultures for viral isolation using tissue culture techniques is not an office procedure, and clinical samples must be sent to referral laboratories. The factor having the greatest impact on the success of viral cultures is the collection and handling of the specimens. For herpes simplex virus, vesicles have a higher yield of live virus than ulcers. Time from collection to tissue culture inoculation also affects results, but the use of virus culture transport systems such as Virocult can allow a delay of several days. Samples should be transported at 2 to 8°C and not frozen. Results can be expected in as little as 1 day after the referral laboratory receives the sample.

Other Microorganisms

While many of the microorganisms listed in Table 1 could be cultured in the office laboratory (i.e., *Campylobacter jejuni, G. vaginalis, Streptococcus agalactiae,*

H. ducreyi, Mycoplasma hominis, Salmonella and *Shigella* spp., *Ureaplasma urealyticum, E. histolytica,* and *T. vaginalis*), the need for highly specialized media makes it extremely difficult and impractical. More importantly, special materials and expertise not normally found in the office laboratory are required to identify and confirm isolates. Therefore it is recommended that, with the exception of *N. gonorrhoeae*, samples for culture of these microorganisms be sent to referral laboratories. For microorganisms not previously discussed in this section, it is suggested that the physician consult with the referral laboratory to determine the proper specimen collection method and transport medium.

Other Important Tests

Serology Tests

Blood samples for serological tests (treponemal, chlamydial, herpes, hepatitis, etc.) must be sent to a referral laboratory, since highly specialized materials, equipment, and personnel are required to perform these assays. However, certain nontreponemal tests for syphilis could be performed in the office setting. While the VDRL test requires a microscope to read test results (flocculation), the rapid plasma reagin (RPR) card test does not. The RPR test uses carbon-containing cardiolipin antigen which detects antigen. Flocculation occurs with a coagglutination of the carbon particles, and this coagglutination can be read macroscopically.

The RPR card test can be done during the initial patient visit. The combination of a clinically suspicious lesion and a reactive RPR card test is sufficient to initiate therapy immediately [84]. If RPR testing is not available, the physician must choose between immediate therapy without laboratory confirmation of diagnosis or delay therapy until such confirmation is made. If therapy is delayed, the blood sample must be sent to a referral laboratory for a VDRL or RPR test. Since the sensitivity of these tests increases with the duration of untreated disease, an initially negative test should be repeated after 1 to 2 weeks [84].

For screening purposes, blood samples found to be reactive using a VDRL or RPR test should be repeated. If the repeated test is reactive, the test should be confirmed with a specific treponemal test [FTA-ABS or MHA-TP (microhemagglutination assay for *Treponema pallidum*)] [84].

An excellent article by Jaffe on the laboratory diagnosis of syphilis which includes (1) a description of the nontreponemal and treponemal tests, (2) optimal selection of these tests according to the clinical situation, and (3) interpretation of test results may be found in the *Annals of Internal Medicine* [84].

Two-Glass Urine Test

Occasionally a male patient may present with persistent urethritis symptoms, no objective physical signs, and no identifiable pathogens. A "two-glass" urine test is an office procedure that involves the collection of initial and midstream urine samples. The samples are then examined and compared for appearance (clear or hazy) and for the presence of threads [15]. Microscopic examination of centrifuged samples can also be done [72]. Anterior urethritis is characterized by a predominance of leukocytes in the initial urine sample. An equal number of leukocytes in both specimens may be indicative of posterior urethritis or prostatitis. This test has been more popular in Great Britain than in the United States. In Great Britain the "two-glass" urine test is often used as a "test of cure" in patients without an expressible discharge. However, Munday et al. have shown that use of this test for diagnosis and in the assessment of cure is limited owing to its poor predictive value in both untreated and treated patients [85].

Quantitative Bacterial Cultures

An involved method (amenable only to office laboratories with good microbiology capabilities) which uses quantitative bacterial cultures can be used for determining prostatic inflammation [86,87]. Briefly, sequential urine specimens obtained before and after prostatic massage are cultured semiquantitatively in an effort to localize the disease process. Prostatic inflammation is suggested when colony counts of prostatic samples significantly exceed urethral and bladder samples.

GUIDELINES FOR EVALUATING SEXUALLY TRANSMITTED DISEASES

The best means of developing a diagnostic approach is to understand the pathophysiology, epidemiology, and clinical presentations of each sexually transmitted pathogen. In this manner a logical protocol for diagnosis may be devised and adjusted as needed. Standard approaches to diagnosis and therapy may serve as guidelines, but should not be used in a cookbook fashion. There is no substitute for understanding the pathogens and their various presentations when evaluating patients for STDs.

The previous sections in this chapter have reviewed the essentials in clinical and laboratory diagnosis applicable to the office-based practitioner. The following are general guidelines to consider when evaluating patients for STDs.

1. The presence of one STD signals the possibility of a second pathogen. The second disease may be overt, asymptomatic, or in an incubating phase [16].
2. Every STD patient has at least one sexual partner who is carrying the same pathogen(s). All sexual contacts of an STD patient should be evaluated and treated. Epidemiological treatment of asymptomatic sexual contacts is recommended [88,89].
3. Complications of STDs may be averted by early diagnosis, proper treatment, appropriate follow-up, and detection of the asymptomatic patient.
4. Asymptomatic disease exists in both males and females and is the major impetus to eradication of STDs. Asymptomatic gonococcal and chlamydial urethritis in the male are definite clinical entities [22,23].

5. Site of infection should be specified in the diagnosis. For example, the male with a urethral discharge positive for gonococci on Gram stain and culture does not have "gonorrhea" per se; rather, the diagnosis is gonococcal urethritis, and his chart should be so labeled. Site of involvement affects choice of therapy. For example, gonococcal treatment regimens utilizing ampicillin fail to eradicate 20% of male rectal gonorrhea and 50% of pharyngeal gonorrhea, prompting a need for alternative therapy [5,89]. Sequelae also vary with site of infection.

6. Knowledge of a patient's sexual orientation, frequency of activity, approximate number of sex partners, and routes of contact (i.e., vaginal, coitus, anal coitus, fellatio, analingus) assist in assessing disease risk and type.

7. Evaluation for pregnancy by history, physical examination, and laboratory tests is essential. A serum pregnancy test should be performed in all suspected cases even when urine testing is negative. Pregnancy introduces the potential for obstetric and neonatal complications of STDs and affects therapeutic choices. All pregnant women should be screened at regular intervals for STDs. The presence of ectopic pregnancy must be ruled out in all cases of suspected pelvic inflammatory disease.

8. Initial examination of rape victims should include (1) cultures for *N. gonorrhoeae* from any potentially infected sites; (2) if possible, cultures for *C. trachomatis* from any potentially infected sites; (3) examination of vaginal specimens for *T. vaginalis* by wet mount and, if available, by culture; (4) a bimanual pelvic examination for women; (5) a serological test for syphilis; and (6) a sample of serum that is frozen and saved for future testing [89]. Regardless of initial test results, a complete re-evaluation should be performed 1 month later. The complex problems faced by physicians during the forensic evaluation of sexual assault victims are discussed by Woodling et al. [90].

9. Sexually transmitted diseases must be considered in all cases of child abuse. Conversely, an STD in a child should be considered as evidence of sexual abuse until proven otherwise [89]. Physicians experienced in pediatric gynecology should evaluate such cases. These children should be evaluated for STD pathogens as described under the guidelines for management of rape victims, but with particular sensitivity to clinical procedures that may be traumatic [89]. Pharyngeal cultures in abused children and their siblings have been shown to be helpful in detecting cases of sexual abuse [91].

10. Geographic location and patient population determine the prevalence of a specific disease and affect the predictive values of laboratory tests. The sensitivity and specificity of a test also determine the predictive values.

11. Laboratory diagnosis is dependent on proper acquisition of samples from appropriate sampling sites. Sampling sites should be chosen based on the probability of greatest yield, routes of contact, patient sex, age, sexual preference, and the suspected pathogen.

12. Antimicrobial susceptibility patterns are subject to change owing to a variety of factors. The gonococcus, by virtue of penicillinase production, is an

excellent example [92]. Physicians are encouraged to review *Morbidity and Mortality Weekly Report*, a Centers for Disease Control publication, and communicate with local health department officials regarding STD patterns in their area.

13. A single, nonreactive nontreponemal serological test for syphilis (VDRL, RPR) does not exclude syphilis. Conversely, a positive test does not confirm the presence of syphilis. The VDRL and RPR tests are approximately 70% sensitive during the primary stage, but are virtually 100% sensitive during the secondary stage [16,64,84]. Repeat serological testing in 4 to 6 weeks is required in suspected cases of syphilis. A reactive VDRL or RPR test should be titered, and the diagnosis of syphilis confirmed by specific treponemal serological testing (FTA-ABS or MHA-TP). False reactive VDRL or RPR tests do occur, especially in cases of low titer positivity.

14. Although herpes genitalis is frequently associated with visible lesions on the external genitalia, herpetic cervicitis may be the sole manifestation of primary herpes simplex infection. Such patients may be symptomatic or asymptomatic [93]. Virus shedding has been shown to occur in women without signs or symptoms of active herpetic disease [94].

15. Although the Papanicolaou smear has been valuable in screening for neoplastic disease, its value in the diagnosis of STDs such as trichomoniasis and herpes is limited. The collective error rate (false positive and false negative results) in such STDs is high [95-98].

16. Appropriate patient follow-up and documentation of cure are critical. Poor response to therapy may indicate noncompliance, organism resistance, reinfection, improper treatment, incorrect diagnosis, or complicated disease.

These guidelines for the diagnosis and treatment of STDs are by no means inclusive. The practicing physician is encouraged to formulate additional ones by combining clinical experience with the material presented in *Sexually Transmitted Diseases: A Clinical Syndrome Approach.*

REFERENCES

1. Holmes KK, Handsfield HH. Sexually transmitted diseases. In: Petersdorf RG, et al., eds. Principles of internal medicine. Vol. 1. New York: McGraw-Hill, 1983:889-902.
2. Bell TA. Major sexually transmitted diseases of children and adolescents. Pediatr Infect Dis 1983; 2:153-161.
3. Baker RW, Peppercorn MA. Gastrointestinal ailments of homosexual men. Medicine 1982; 61:390-405.
4. Murphy MD. Office laboratory diagnosis of sexually transmitted diseases. Pediatr Infect Dis 1983; 2:146-152.
5. Handsfield HH. Sexually transmitted diseases. Hosp Pract 1982; 17:99-116.
6. Holmes KK. Pelvic inflammatory disease. In: Petersdorf RG, et al., eds. Principles of internal medicine. Vol. 1. New York: McGraw-Hill, 1983:902-908.

7. Knox GE. Cytomegalovirus: import of sexual transmission. Clin Obstet Gynecol 1983; 26:173-177.
8. Minkoff H. Hepatitis. Clin Obstet Gynecol 1983; 26:178-185.
9. Stevens CE, Krugman S, Szmuness W, Beasley RP. Viral hepatitis in pregnancy: problems for the clinician dealing with the infant. Pediatr Infect Rev 1980; 2:121-125.
10. Hook EW, Stamm WE. Sexually transmitted diseases in men. Med Clin North Am 1983; 67:235-251.
11. Sufrin G. Acute epididymitis. Sex Transm Dis 1981; 8:132-139.
12. Brandt EN. Physicians and sexually transmitted disease: a call to action. JAMA 1982; 16:2032.
13. Stamm WE, Kaetz S, Holmes KK. Clinical training in venereology in the United States and Canada. JAMA 1982; 248:2020-2024.
14. Alexander B. Taking the sexual history. Am Fam Physician 1981; 23:147-151.
15. Morton RS. Gonorrhoea. London: Saunders, 1977:62-122.
16. Noble RC. Sexually transmitted diseases—guide to diagnosis and therapy. New York: Medical Examination Publishing, 1979:9-18, 68-72.
17. Felman YM, Morrison JM. Examining the homosexual male for sexually transmitted diseases. JAMA 1977; 238:2046-2047.
18. Council on Scientific Affairs. Health care needs of a homosexual population. JAMA 1982; 248:736-739.
19. Fuimara NJ. Infectious syphilis. Dermatol Clin 1983; 1:3-22.
20. Komaroff AL, Pass TM, McCue JD, Cohen AB, Hendricks TM, Friedland GF. Management strategies for urinary and vaginal infections. Arch Intern Med 1978; 138:1069-1073.
21. McCue JD, Komaroff AL, Pass TM, Cohen AB, Friedland G. Strategies for diagnosing vaginitis. J Fam Pract 1979; 9:395-402.
22. Wong ES, Stamm WE. Urethral infections in men and women. Annu Rev Med 1983; 34:337-358.
23. Handsfield HH, Lipman TO, Harnisch JP, Tronca E, Holmes KK. Asymptomatic gonorrhea in men. N Engl J Med 1974; 290:117-123.
24. Dans PE. Gonococcal anogenital infections. Clin Obstet Gynecol 1975; 18:103-119.
25. Dritz SK. Medical aspects of homosexuality. N Engl J Med 1980; 302:463-464.
26. Eschenbach DA. Vaginal infection. Clin Obstet Gynecol 1983; 26:186-202.
27. Stamm WE, Wagner KF, Amsel R, Alexander ER, Turck M, Counts GW, Holmes KK. Causes of acute urethral syndrome in women. N Engl J Med 1980; 303:409-415.
28. Stamm WE. Management of the acute urethral syndrome. Drug Ther 1982; 12:155-164.
29. Wray NP, Friedland JA. Detection and correction of house staff error in physical diagnosis. JAMA 1983; 249:1035-1037.
30. Wiener S, Nathanson M. Physical examination—frequently observed errors. JAMA 1976; 236:852-855.
31. Bertholf ME, Stafford MJ. Colonization of *Candida albicans* in vagina, rectum and mouth. J Fam Pract 1983; 16:919-924.

32. Wiesner PJ, Tronca E, Bonin P, Pedersen AHB, Holmes KK. Clinical spectrum of pharyngeal gonococcal infection. N Engl J Med 1973; 288:181-185.
33. Harrison WO. Pharyngeal gonorrhea. JAMA 1981; 246:2726-2727.
34. Tice AW, Rodriguiz VL. Pharyngeal gonorrhea. JAMA 1981; 246:2717-2719.
35. Weisner PJ. Gonococcal pharyngeal infection. Clin Obstet Gynecol 1975; 18:121-129.
36. Tovell HMM, Young AW. Classification of vulvar diseases. Clin Obstet Gynecol 1978; 21:955-961.
37. Korting GW. Practical dermatology of the genital region. Philadelphia: Saunders, 1981.
38. Friedrich EG. Vulvar disease. 2nd ed. Philadelphia: Saunders, 1983.
39. Ginsburg CM. Acquired syphilis in prepubertal children. Pediatr Infect Dis 1983; 2:232-234.
40. Cowell CA. The gynecologic examination of infants, children, and young adolescents. Pediatr Clin North Am 1981; 28:247-266.
41. Capraro VJ. Gynecologic examination in children and adolescents. Pediatr Clin North Am 1972; 19:511-528.
42. Spiegel CA, Amsel R, Holmes KK. Diagnosis of bacterial vaginosis by direct Gram stain of vaginal fluid. J Clin Microbiol 1983; 18:170-177.
43. Bhattacharyya MN, Jephcott AE, Morton RS. Diagnosis of gonorrhea in women: comparison of sampling sites. Br Med J 1973; 2:748-750.
44. Rubinow A. Gonococcal arthritis in a 4-year old girl. Postgrad Med 1981; 69:53-57.
45. Barsett-Connor E. Gonorrhea and the pediatrician. Am J Dis Child 1973; 125:233-238.
46. Holmes KK. Gonococcal infections. In: Petersdorf RG, et al., eds. Principles of internal medicine. Vol. 1. New York: McGraw-Hill, 1983:939-945.
47. Singh B, Cutler JC. The effect of vaginal lubricants on *Neisseria gonorrhoeae*. Am J Obstet Gynecol 1976; 126:365-369.
48. Kallings I, Mårdh PA. Sampling and specimen handling in diagnosis of genital *Chlamydia trachomatis* infections. Scand J Infect Dis Suppl 1982; 32: 21-24.
49. Bhattacharyya MN, Jephcott AE. Diagnosis of gonorrhoea in women–role of the rectal sample. Br J Vener Dis 1974; 50:109-112.
50. Harris JC, Dupont HL, Hornick RB. Fecal leukocytes in diarrheal illness. Ann Intern Med 1972; 76:697-703.
51. Jarratt M. Genital herpes infection. Dermatol Clin 1983; 1:85-92.
52. Lerner AM. Infections–with herpes simplex virus. In: Petersdorf, et al., eds. Principles of internal medicine. Vol. 1. New York: McGraw-Hill, 1983:1162-1167.
53. Fitzgerald TJ. *Treponema*. In: Lennette EH, et al., eds. Manual of clinical microbiology. 3rd ed. Washington, DC: American Society for Microbiology, 1980:389-393.
54. Gulick P, Hall G, McHenry MC. Office microbiology. Med Clin North Am 1983; 67:39-55.
55. Isenberg HD, Washington JA, Balows A, Sonnenwirth AC. Collection, handling, and processing of specimens. In: Lennette EH, et al., eds. Manual of

clinical microbiology. 3rd ed. Washington, DC: American Society for Microbiology, 1980:52-82.
56. Richardson JN, Huffaker, RH. Biological safety in the clinical laboratory. In: Lennette EH, et al., eds. Manual of clinical microbiology. 3rd ed. Washington, DC: American Society for Microbiology, 1980:960-964.
57. College of American Pathologists. EXCEL (External Comparative Evaluation for Laboratories) Program, Microbiology Series XL-4, 1984. Skokie, Ill. 60077.
58. Centers for Disease Control. Laboratory Improvement Program Office, Laboratory Training and Consultation Division. Building 3, Room B12, Atlanta, Ga. 30333.
59. Vecchio TJ. Predictive value of a single diagnostic test in unselected populations. N Engl J Med 1966; 274:1171-1173.
60. Wiegert HT, Wiegert O. The impact of disease prevalence on the predictive value of laboratory tests in primary care. J Fam Pract 1979; 8:1199-1203.
61. Galen RS. Statistics. In: Sonnenwirth AC and Jarett L, eds. Gradwohl's clinical laboratory methods and diagnosis. Vol. 1. St. Louis: Mosby, 1980:41-68.
62. Bayes T. An essay toward solving a problem in the doctrine of chance. Philos Trans R Soc 1763; 53:370.
63. Kraus SJ. Semiquantitation of urethral polymorphonuclear leukocytes as objective evidence of nongonococcal urethritis. Sex Transm Dis 1982; 9:52-55.
64. Syphilis, a synopsis. Public Health Service Publication No. 1660, January 1968. Washington, DC: U.S. Government Printing Office, 1967:96-108.
65. Orkin M, Maibach HI. Scabies and pediculosis pubis. Dermatol Clin 1:111-121.
66. Spence MP, Hollander DH, Smith J, McCaig L, Sewell D, Brockman M. The clinical and laboratory diagnosis of *Trichomonas vaginalis* infection. Sex Transm Dis 1980; 7:168-171.
67. Young H. Advances in routine laboratory procedures for the diagnosis of gonorrhoea. In: Harris JRW, ed. Recent advances in sexually transmitted diseases. Edinburgh: Churchill Livingstone, 1981:59-71.
68. Jacobs NF, Kraus SJ. Gonococcal and nongonococcal urethritis in men: clinical and laboratory differentiation. Ann Intern Med 1975; 82:7-12.
69. Riccardi NB, Felman YM. Laboratory diagnosis in the problem of suspected gonococcal infection. JAMA 1979; 242:2703-2705.
70. Rothenberg RB, Simon R, Chipperfield E, Catterall RD. Efficacy of selected diagnostic tests for sexually transmitted diseases. JAMA 1976; 235:49-51.
71. Prior RB, Spagna VA. Application of a *Limulus* test device in rapid evaluation of gonococcal and nongonococcal urethritis in males. J Clin Microbiol 1981; 14:256-260.
72. Swartz SL. Diagnosis of nongonococcal urethritis. In: Hobson D, Holmes KK, eds. Nongonococcal urethritis and related infections. Washington, DC: American Society for Microbiology, 1977:15-18.
73. Goodhart ME, Ogden A, Zaidi A, Kraus SJ. Factors affecting the performance of smear and culture tests for the detection of *Neisseria gonorrhoeae*. Sex Transm Dis 1982; 9:63-69.
74. Spagna VA, Prior RB. *Limulus* lysate assay for gonorrhea. Am Fam Physician 1983; 27:227-231.

75. Kleris GS, Arnold AJ. Differential diagnosis of urethritis: predictive value and therapeutic implications of the urethral smear. Sex Transm Dis 1981; 8:110-116.
76. Moffet HL. Clinical microbiology. 2nd ed. Philadelphia: Lippincott, 1980: 164.
77. Nowinski RC, Tam MR, Goldstein LC, Stong L, Kuo CC, Corey L, Stamm WE, Handsfield HH, Knapp JS, Holmes KK. Diagnosis of sexually transmitted diseases with monoclonal antibodies. In Program and abstracts of the International Society for STD Research, 5th international meeting, Seattle, Washington, 1983 (Abstract 88).
78. Caldwell JG, Price EV, Pazin GJ, Cornelius CE. Sensitivity and reproducibility of Thayer-Martin culture medium in diagnosing gonorrhea in women. Am J Obstet Gynecol 1971; 109:463-468.
79. Holmes KK. The *Chlamydia* epidemic. JAMA 1981; 245:1718-1723.
80. Barlow D, Nayyar K, Phillips I, Barrow J. Diagnosis of gonorrhoea in women. Br J Vener Dis 1976; 52:326-328.
81. Chipperfield EJ, Catterall RD. Reappraisal of Gram-staining and culture techniques for the diagnosis of gonorrhoea in women. Br J Vener Dis 1976; 52: 36-39.
82. Young H. Cultural diagnosis of gonorrhoea with modified New York City (MNYC) medium. Br J Vener Dis 1978; 54:36-40.
83. Spence MR, Guzick DS, Katta RA. The isolation of *Neisseria gonorrhoeae*: a comparison of three culture transport systems. Sex Transm Dis 1983; 10: 138-140.
84. Jaffe HW. The laboratory diagnosis of syphilis—new concepts. Ann Intern Med 1975; 83:846-850.
85. Munday PE, Altman DG, Taylor-Robinson D. Urinary abnormalities in nongonococcal urethritis. Br J Vener Dis 1981; 57:387-390.
86. Meares EM. Prostatitis and related diseases. DM. 1980; 26:1-39.
87. Meares EM. Prostatitis syndromes: new perspectives about old woes. J Urol 1980; 123:141-147.
88. Johnson RE. Epidemiologic and prophylactic treatment of gonorrhea: a decision analysis review. Sex Transm Dis 1979; 6:159-167.
89. Centers for Disease Control. Sexually transmitted diseases treatment guidelines 1982. Morbid Mortal Week Rep Suppl 1982; 31:33S-60S.
90. Woodling BA, Evans JR, Bradbury MD. Sexual assault: rape and molestation. Clin Obstet Gynecol 1977; 20:509-530.
91. Groothius JR, Bischoff MC, Jauregui LE. Pharyngeal gonorrhea in young children. Pediatr Infect Dis 1983; 2:99-101.
92. Handsfield HH. PPNG infections: current status and guidelines for therapy. Drug Ther 1982; 12:118-124.
93. Corey L, Adams HG, Brown ZA, Holmes KK. Genital herpes simplex virus infections: clinical manifestations, course, and complications. Ann Intern Med 1983; 98:958-972.
94. Adam E, Kaufman RH, Mirkovic RR, Melnick JL. Persistence of virus shedding in asymptomatic women after recovery from herpes genitalis. Obstet Gynecol 1979; 54:171-173.

95. Hume J. Trichomoniasis, candidiasis and *Gardnerella vaginalis*—vaginitis as sexually transmitted diseases. Dermatol Clin 1983; 1:137-152.
96. McLennan MT, Smith JM, McLennan CE. Diagnosis of vaginal mycosis and trichomoniasis—reliability of cytologic smear, wet smear, and culture. Obstet Gynecol 1972; 40:231-234.
97. Perl G. Errors in the diagnosis of trichomonas vaginalis infection—as observed among 1199 patients. Obstet Gynecol 1972; 39:7-9.
98. Guinan ME, MacCalman J, Kern ER, Overall JC, Spruance SL. The course of untreated recurrent genital herpes simplex infection in 27 women. N Engl J Med 1981; 304:759-763.

SEVENTEEN

The Patient's Perspective

Carol A. Kitchen
Merry B. Krempasky
Courtland Storck
Venereal Disease Clinic
Columbus Health Department
Columbus, Ohio

INTRODUCTION

Why? How long? How did I? What is it? These are a few questions patients are asking today concerning their health status. With increased public awareness concerning sexually transmitted diseases, clinicians must be prepared to address their questions with direct and concise answers. This chapter reviews the most frequently asked questions in a leading sexually transmitted disease clinic.

GENERAL QUESTIONS

1. *What is venereal disease?*
   Venereal disease refers to any sexually transmitted disease and includes over twenty common disorders other than gonorrhea or syphilis.

2. *How many sexually transmitted diseases are there?*

   At least 22 different etiologies (agents) have been identified as having the potential to be spread through sexual contact. The most common sexually transmitted diseases are nongonococcal urethritis, gonorrhea, trichomoniasis, genital herpes, venereal warts, syphilis, and chlamydial infections.

3. *Is there any way to prevent getting a sexually transmitted disease?*

   The best way is to avoid sex, but since this is not a reasonable approach, other measures may be taken. Condoms, if used properly by the male, will prevent the transmission of most sexually transmitted diseases. Also, avoid multiple and casual sexual contacts.

4. *How long does it usually take to obtain test results for various sexually transmitted diseases?*

Gonorrhea culture	2 to 4 days
Syphilis serology	1 to 3 days
Herpes culture	2 to 10 days
Trichomoniasis wet prep	Same day to 3 days
Chlamydia culture	3 to 7 days

5. *Can one determine how long a person has had a sexually transmitted disease?*

   No. The different stages of syphilis correspond to duration of disease, but are only rough estimates. A knowledge of incubation periods in conjunction with the dates of sexual contact probably provides the best estimate of disease duration.

6. *Can sexually transmitted diseases recur spontaneously following treatment?*

   Yes. Genital herpes can recur at various intervals for life. Venereal warts can recur following treatment at intervals over approximately 2 years. All other sexually transmitted diseases do not recur unless re-exposure to the infection has taken place.

7. *Can I have a sexually transmitted disease and not have symptoms?*

   Yes. Many sexually transmitted diseases can be asymptomatic. The presence of disease does not always produce symptoms.

8. *What sexually transmitted diseases are associated with swelling of the penis or scrotum?*

   Any of the sexually transmitted diseases characterized by a break in the skin of the penis can produce swelling. Herpes and syphilis are the most common diseases. The bites of crabs and scabies can also result in swelling. Swelling in the absence of penile sores can be the result of prolonged mechanical rubbing of the penis (masturbation, continuous intercourse). Scrotal enlargement, with tenderness, usually implies inflammation of the epididymis by extension of gonococcal or nongonococcal urethritis.

9. *What sexually transmitted diseases cause a discharge from the penis?*
The most common are gonorrhea and nongonococcal urethritis.

10. *Could sexually transmitted diseases cause swelling of the vagina (vulva)?*
This area is very sensitive and swelling could be due to irritation, trauma, or an infection. *Trichomonas* or *Candida* vaginal infections and genital herpes can be associated with vulvar or vaginal swelling.

11. *What sexually transmitted diseases are associated with vaginal itching?*
Vaginal itching may or may not indicate a sexually transmitted disease. When vaginal itching is accompanied with symptoms of excessive discharge or unpleasant odor, it could indicate any of the sexually transmitted diseases which infect the cervix or vagina.

12. *What sexually transmitted disease could cause abnormal vaginal bleeding?*
Irregular vaginal bleeding could indicate a wide range of problems. The sexually transmitted diseases that can cause irregular vaginal bleeding are those which involve the cervix and upper genital tract.

13. *Why does my partner not have any symptoms?*
It is possible to possess and transmit a sexually transmitted disease without demonstrating symptoms. This is referred to as an asymptomatic infection or asymptomatic carrier state.

14. *Why do sex partners need to be checked? Can I not give them the same medication prescribed for me?*
Your partner needs a complete evaluation. Other infections could be present that require additional therapy. A complete medical history is necessary before medication can be safely prescribed under any circumstances.

15. *If I have a sexually transmitted disease, is it necessary to have my partners treated?*
Treatment for sex partners depends upon the specific sexually transmitted disease and the time period since the last contact. Therefore it is necessary to give a brief history of your sexual activity.

16. *Do I have to have my parents' consent to be treated for a sexually transmitted disease?*
No. Health providers do not require consent from parents to treat minors for sexually transmitted diseases.

17. *How is my privacy assured?*
All material pertaining to the evaluation of sexually transmitted diseases is strictly confidential and that right is protected by law. If it is necessary to notify sex partners, you have the option of doing this yourself or the agency where you are treated will do it.

18. *Can you get venereal disease from someone because they are dirty?*
You can only if they are infected with a sexually transmitted disease. The cleanliness of the individual has nothing to do with the transmission of disease.

19. *Do condoms protect against venereal disease?*
    Condoms are one of the best methods of protection against most sexually transmitted diseases if used correctly. Today many individuals are choosing alternate methods of birth control that are effective against pregnancy but totally uneffective in preventing the transmission of sexually transmitted diseases.

20. *Should family members take any precautions if I have a sexually transmitted disease?*
    Generally not. If scabies or pubic lice are present, family members should avoid using towels, bedding, or other personal objects that may harbor the pubic louse or scabies mite. Scabies patients should avoid close bodily contact until they are cured, and some authorities recommend that all family members of scabies patients be treated. Other sexually transmitted diseases are rarely, if ever, transmitted among family members except via sexual contact.

21. *Why do I have to come back after I finish all of the medication?*
    There is a possibility that the particular disease may persist despite adequate therapy or another disease may become apparent on a repeat exam. Re-exposure to an untreated sex partner may also result in reinfection. You must remember that the absence of symptoms does not guarantee cure.

22. *Can I drink alcohol while taking tetracycline?*
    There are no definite contraindications to ingesting alcohol and tetracycline simultaneously. Moderation is advisable so as not to forget the reason you are taking the tetracycline.

23. *I was told that I should not take tetracycline while on birth control pills. Is this true?*
    Some authorities recommend that some alternate method of birth control be utilized while taking tetracycline. The possibility exists that tetracycline may interfere with the actions of oral contraceptives.

GONORRHEA

1. *Can gonorrhea recur spontaneously following proper treatment?*
   No, if a negative test of cure is established following treatment, the infection cannot spontaneously recur. It is possible to be reinfected if a new exposure to gonorrhea occurs.

2. *Can areas other than the cervix and urethra be infected?*
   Yes, gonorrhea can infect the throat and rectum of males or females. Infrequently it can be transported via the bloodstream and infect the joints and cause skin lesions. A newborn can develop infection of the eyes during vaginal delivery from an infected cervix.

3. *How common is gonorrhea?*
Gonorrhea is the most common reported communicable disease in the United States. Over 1 million reported cases occur in the United States each year.

4. *Can I get gonorrhea if I am re-exposed, or can I develop an immunity to it?*
Yes, you can become infected with gonorrhea on re-exposure. However, you do not become immune to gonorrhea or any of the other diseases transmitted through sexual contact.

5. *Can you tell how long I have had gonorrhea?*
The tests that are done only show the presence of the organism, not the duration of the infection. The incubation period, the time from exposure to established disease, is usually 2 to 10 days. The incubation period plus the duration of symptoms may help determine the length of time you have been infected.

6. *I cannot tell my sex partners they could have gonorrhea. What can I do?*
Most health departments throughout the United States have programs to handle this situation. Sexual contacts can be notified confidentially and your name will remain anonymous.

7. *What are the symptoms of gonorrhea in women?*
Approximately 80% of women have no specific symptoms. Some women may complain of a yellow vaginal discharge, burning when they urinate, abnormal menstrual bleeding, or lower abdominal pain.

8. *What are the symptoms of gonorrhea in men?*
The most common symptom is profuse urethral discharge with or without burning on urination. It is possible to be asymptomatic and still be infectious. Gay men may notice white or yellow mucus in the stool, rectal or anal irritation, or a sore throat.

9. *If I am allergic to penicillin, are there other medications that will cure gonorrhea?*
Yes, there are numerous medications that can be used to treat gonorrhea.

10. *If I have gonorrhea, should my partner or partners be treated?*
Yes, your sex partners in the past 30 days should be examined and given preventive treatment.

11. *If I have gonococcal pelvic inflammatory disease (PID), will I be sterile?*
Pelvic inflammatory disease can result in the scarring and occlusion of the fallopian tubes. Studies conducted upon women who have experienced a single episode of PID have suggested that approximately 15 to 20% may become sterile. Subsequent episodes increase the likelihood of sterility.

12. *Can gonorrhea during pregnancy harm a developing fetus?*
Gonorrhea will not harm a developing fetus; however, an infant delivered vaginally through an infected cervix can develop gonococcal infection of the eyes.

13. *If I have not had rectal intercourse, how could I become infected there?*
The close proximity of the rectum and vagina allows infected vaginal secretions to directly involve the rectal area.

14. *Can any sexually transmitted disease cause joint pain?*
A rare complication of gonorrhea is known as disseminated gonorrhea. The organism spreads via the bloodstream and settles in certain joints, especially the wrist, knees, and small joints of the hands.

15. *How long can women have gonorrhea without having symptoms?*
The infection can remain asymptomatic for several months.

16. *Can I have gonorrhea and not have symptoms?*
Many people who have gonorrhea do not have symptoms. Estimates suggest approximately 80% of women and 10% of men are infectious and have no symptoms.

17. *Do I need to be examined at any time following treatment?*
Yes, a 1-week follow-up exam is recommended in order to repeat gonorrhea cultures. If the cultures are negative, confirmation of a cure is established.

18. *Can I be examined for gonorrhea while I am menstruating?*
Yes, menstruation does not hamper gonorrhea detection and may aid in the isolation of the organism by serving as a nutrient.

19. *Does gonococcal PID result from having the infection a long time?*
The length of time a woman has an infection does not influence the risk of PID. Previous tubal infections and the presence of an intrauterine device increase the risk of PID infection.

20. *Is gonorrhea the only infection that causes PID?*
No, *Chlamydia trachomatis* and other bacteria can cause PID.

NONGONOCOCCAL URETHRITIS

1. *Is nongonococcal urethritis (NGU) a sexually transmitted disease in every case?*
There are cases of NGU resulting from urethral strictures or trauma which are not sexually transmitted, but these account for only a small percentage of cases. With *C. trachomatis* accounting for approximately 60% of the cases and the rare occurrence of NGU in celibate individuals, NGU is most often a sexually transmitted disease.

2. *Is NGU very common?*
It is estimated that approximately twice the number of men become infected with NGU than gonorrhea. Each year there are about 2 million cases of NGU in the United States.

3. *If I have NGU, do I need to inform my sex partner?*
Yes, your sex partner should be examined and treated to (1) further identify the causative organism and other sexually transmitted diseases and (2) prevent reinfection when sexual intercourse is resumed.

4. *Can I be cured of NGU?*
The present cure rate for NGU is about 85% with proper treatment, follow-up, and treatment of sex contacts. Treatment failures may require subsequent antibiotic therapy and other diagnostic tests.

5. *How long does it take for the symptoms of NGU to occur?*
The incubation period for NGU is usually 7 to 28 days. There is significant overlap with the incubation period of gonorrhea so that a diagnosis cannot be made based solely on this information.

6. *Could I have gotten NGU from physical or emotional strain?*
No, NGU is caused by organisms that are transmitted via sexual contact. Lifting heavy objects or psychological stress does not cause an infection. This fact emphasizes the need to have sexual contacts evaluated and treated.

7. *I am pregnant. What can I take if I am an NGU contact?*
You will be treated with erythromycin, which can safely be taken during pregnancy. This medication is effective treatment for *C. trachomatis*, which can cause infection of the newborn if left untreated.

8. *I took medicine last week for gonorrhea. Why do I still have an infection?*
It is possible to have a recurrent urethritis following treatment for gonorrhea. Approximately 20% of gonorrhea patients have concurrent NGU and the medication given for gonorrhea does not always eradicate the NGU infection. The possibility also exists that the original gonococcal infection was not cured or reinfection has occurred. Further tests need to be done with the possibility of receiving a different treatment.

SYPHILIS

1. *What is syphilis?*
Syphilis is an infectious disease caused by a spirochete (*Treponema pallidum*) which penetrates the skin and enters the bloodstream.It is usually transmitted by direct contact during sexual activity. Infected pregnant women can infect the unborn child via the bloodstream. Incubation period is between 10 to 90 days.

2. *Can syphilis recur?*
A person is able to obtain the disease again with exposure to an infected sexual contact. The initial episode does not confer immunity to the disease.

3. *How is syphilis diagnosed?*
Syphilis is diagnosed by a combination of clinical and laboratory findings or incidentally by routine serological blood testing. In the primary stage patients have a painless hardened sore called a chancre. In the secondary stage patients may have a skin rash involving the chest, back, palms, and soles. In the latent stage patients are free of signs and symptoms. The signs and symptoms of syphilis frequently mimic other diseases. A clinician must be alert to the possibility of syphilis to ensure a correct diagnosis.

4. *If I am allergic to penicillin, can syphilis be treated?*
   Yes. The course of treatment usually involves tetracycline or erythromycin therapy over a period of 10 to 15 days.
5. *Why is my blood test positive following treatment of syphilis?*
   During the course of disease your body produces antibodies to fight the infection. Even though treatment is given and the disease is cured, antibodies within the body are still produced and form the basis of a positive blood test. These antibodies, however, do not provide immunity against future infection.
6. *Are all rashes on the hands and feet results of syphilis?*
   No. Syphilis should be ruled out in these situations; however, a wide variety of unrelated skin conditions can be present in that fashion.
7. *Why is syphilis more common in the gay population?*
   Syphilis is more common in the gay community for several reasons. A substantial minority of gay males have casual sexual relationships with multiple partners. Anal intercourse provides a potential, asymptomatic means of disease transmission. Premarital and prenatal screening for syphilis is a routine procedure in the heterosexual population which has no equivalent in the gay population. Prejudice in certain medical communities has restricted the availability of qualified care for gay patients.
8. *What are my complications of having syphilis?*
   A tragic complication of syphilis occurs when a child is infected in utero and develops congenital syphilis. Routine screening for syphilis during pregnancy has made this a rare event. An untreated syphilis victim may also develop serious diseases of the heart and nervous system.

HERPES

1. *What is herpes genitalis?*
   Herpes genitalis is a noncurable sexually transmitted disease caused by the herpesvirus. An eruption of painful blisters and ulcers occurs in the genital area which resolves over a period of days without scar formation. The disease can recur at any time without sexual contact, since it can persist for life in the infected person.
2. *How long am I going to have these herpes sores?*
   Initial outbreaks of herpes sores usually persist for 2 to 5 weeks, but symptoms such as fever, itching, and burning resolve by the second week. Recurrences of the herpes lesions persist usually for only 5 to 7 days.
3. *Can I have herpes without knowing it?*
   Females may shed the virus from the cervix and recurrences of genital herpes can also be so mild that the disease goes unnoticed. It is probable that most

disease transmission occurs via sexual contact with asymptomatically infected individuals.

4. *Should I be rechecked every time I have herpes lesions?*
No. Recurrences are part of the natural history of herpes infection and do not indicate a new infection. However, do not hesitate to seek medical attention if doubt exists or troublesome symptoms restrict daily activities.

5. *Is herpes curable?*
No. There are several treatment modalities which can modify the course of an outbreak of genital herpes, but at this time there is still no cure for herpes.

6. *Will I have signs or symptoms before an recurrent episode?*
Possibly. Some patients with recurrent genital herpes will experience certain symptoms prior to the appearance of sores. Itching and burning in the genital area have been the most commonly reported events before the actual outbreak of the lesions.

7. *How is herpes transmitted?*
Herpes is usually transmitted via direct contact with an oral or genital source where there is active shedding of the virus.

8. *Can I spread herpes to other parts of my body?*
Yes. A person can inoculate other parts of the body with infected secretions. It is important for a person with herpes to practice good personal hygiene. Always wash your hands after contact with the lesions and avoid rubbing your eyes.

9. *Do I have herpes if I have a "cold sore" on my lip?*
The possibility of herpesvirus infection is suggested by a history of recurrent lip sores. Herpes type I is the virus that most commonly causes recurrent oral lesions and can be transmitted to the genital area via oral-genital contact.

10. *What are the complications of having herpes?*
An infected pregnant female can infect the newborn if she has active herpes at the time of vaginal delivery. Cesarean section should be performed if documented or suspected active genital herpes exists at the time of delivery. Herpes infection of the cervix has been associated with an increased risk of cancer of the cervix. A Pap smear should be obtained yearly to allow the early diagnosis of this possible complication.

11. *Can I have sex when I have herpes?*
A genital herpes patient should abstain from sexual activity when showing signs and symptoms of disease. In case of doubt, a condom can provide relative protection against disease transmission.

12. *If my partner and I both have herpes, can we have sexual relations?*
Despite the fact that reinfection with the herpesvirus is a rare event, sexual contact is best avoided during an active herpesvirus infection. This advice

applies to all individuals with oral or genital lesions, regardless of the disposition of sexual contacts.

13. *Does a condom protect me from getting herpes?*
There have been laboratory studies that demonstrated the use of condoms reduced the risk of transmitting herpes.

14. *Is there any medication that is effective in the treatment of genital herpes?*
Despite the numerous remedies that have been proposed, acylovir (Zovirax) is the only approved treatment for genital herpes, and this applies only to the initial (primary) episodes. Acylovir has been shown to significantly accelerate the healing process and decrease viral shedding. The application of other creams and ointments to the lesions may prolong the healing process and increase the risk of secondary infection. Symptomatic relief can be obtained with warm sitz baths and analgesics.

15. *Is acylovir effective in the treatment of recurrent herpes?*
Topical acylovir has been shown to have the most beneficial effect for the initial episode of herpes. Some individuals have found it to be of some benefit on recurrent lesions. Recurrent lesions should be kept clean and dry to prevent secondary infections and promote healing.

TRICHOMONIASIS

1. *Does trichomoniasis recur following proper treatment?*
No. Recurrent trichomoniasis is most commonly a reinfection via sexual contact with an asymptomatically infected person.

2. *Why can I not take metronidazole while I am pregnant?*
Metronidazole should not be administered during the first trimester of pregnancy because of the possibility of promoting birth defects. Metronidazole has also promoted tumors in laboratory animals and should be used during pregnancy and breast feeding only when vaginal symptoms are especially troublesome.

3. *Why can I not drink alcohol when I take metronidazole?*
Alcohol and metronidazole taken together produce abdominal cramping, nausea, vomiting, and headaches.

4. *Why are yeast (Candida) infections so common? Are they sexually transmitted?*
Candida vaginitis or vulvitis is not a sexually transmitted disease. Certain conditions (antibiotic treatment, weight change, birth control pills, pregnancy) allow the overgrowth of these organisms which are otherwise normal body inhabitants.

VENEREAL WARTS

1. *What causes venereal warts?*
Venereal warts are the manifestations of infection by the wart virus (papillomavirus). Their growth may be enhanced by abnormal vaginal discharge, heavy

perspiration, poor personal hygiene, and certain medical disorders (i.e., diabetes). Pregnancy may also cause venereal warts to proliferate.

2. *Are venereal warts contagious?*
   Yes. You can transmit the wart virus during sexual contact. The susceptibility of becoming infected varies between individuals but is generally transmitted in three out of four cases.
3. *What is the incubation period for venereal warts?*
   In most cases 2 to 4 months, but 8- to 9-month incubation periods have been recognized.
4. *How often will I need to return for podophyllin treatment?*
   Podophyllin is left on treated sites 4 to 6 hr and washed off with soap and water. Weekly applications for a period of 1 month are usually sufficient for most cases.
5. *Is it possible for venereal warts to recur without being reexposed to them?*
   Yes. Recurrences can take place without reinfection and are most common in women during pregnancy or following childbirth.
6. *Can I have venereal warts and not know it?*
   Yes. Warts may occur in the vagina and/or cervix in women and inside the urinary passage or rectum of both sexes.
7. *What do venereal warts look like?*
   People often confuse skin tags and warts. Warts are round, flat, or sponge-like in appearance (pink or dark in color) 1 mm to 2 cm in diameter, and usually multiple in number.
8. *How can my warts be treated?*
   There are several ways to treat warts. Medication can be applied locally to the warts. They can be cauterized, frozen, or surgically removed. Specific treatment depends upon location of the warts and their severity. These procedures are only cosmetic, and the warts may reappear following any therapeutic approach.
9. *Can regular skin warts be present on the genitals?*
   Rarely. While genital warts can be transferred to nongenital sites, the transfer of the skin wart virus to the genitals has been an unusual event. Sexual transmission is the rule in genital warts.
10. *How can I tell the difference between skin warts and genital warts?*
    There may be differences in appearance that separate skin warts and genital warts. Skin warts are small, flat, hard, and white to pale pink. Genital warts may grow considerably in size, are soft, may be darkly pigmented, and may have a slightly pointed appearance.
11. *Are venereal warts associated with any complication?*
    Rarely. There are cases where newborn have venereal warts in their throats following contact during vaginal delivery. There are a few occasions where warts have developed into cancers. Recent evidence suggests that cervical

warts are associated with cancer of the cervix, and annual Pap smears are recommended.

MOLLUSCUM CONTAGIOSUM

1. *Which areas of the body does molluscum contagiosum most affect?*
   Molluscum contagiosum is usually found on thighs, buttocks, lower abdomen, and external genitalia.
2. *Is molluscum contagiosum treatable?*
   Yes. Depending on location and severity, they can be treated by injecting medication into the lesion or surgical removal. The majority of cases will resolve without therapy.
3. *If I have molluscum contagiosum, is there a chance I have other sexually transmitted diseases?*
   Yes. Since molluscum contagiosum can be acquired via sexual contact, a routine sexually transmitted disease evaluation is recommended.
4. *Are molluscum lesions potentially dangerous?*
   No. Despite the fact that a virus causes molluscum lesions, there are no complications associated with this disorder.
5. *Is molluscum contagiosum always transmitted via sexual contact?*
   No. Transmission can occur through close personal contact of any kind. Saunas, hot tubs, and swimming pools are places where the virus may also be acquired.

PUBIC LICE

1. *Are pubic lice always sexually transmitted?*
   Usually, but pubic lice can survive away from the human body for up to 24 hr; therefore bedding, clothing, or towels used by an infected person can occasionally be the cause of spread to another person. Other modes of transmission (toilet seat, animals) are strictly myths.
2. *How are pubic lice treated?*
   Recommended therapy is 1% gamma benzene hexachloride in cream or lotion form. A thin layer is applied to the thighs, trunk, and axillary regions, left on from 8 to 12 hr, and washed off with soap and water. Pregnant or breast-feeding women should use crotamiton (Eurax), and not gamma benzene hexachloride.
3. *What are the white things that stick to the pubic hair?*
   These are the nits, or eggs, of the pubic louse. Female lice lay about three eggs per day. These look like small pieces of glue stuck to the base of the pubic hair.

4. *Do pubic lice jump from place to place?*
   No. They move very little in the course of a day: 6 in. maximum.
5. *What are the small brownish red specks I have found in my underwear?*
   This is the fecal material passed by lice after they have fed upon the blood of the host.
6. *Can my pets have pubic lice?*
   No. Pubic lice cannot live on animals. A human host is necessary for the louse to survive.
7. *Do pubic lice carry other diseases?*
   No. Pubic lice have not been found to carry any diseases harmful to humans.
8. *Should I have an exterminator spray my house or apartment since I have pubic lice?*
   Definitely not! The pubic louse is not able to survive longer than 24 hr off the human body.
9. *Will the medication used to treat pubic lice kill the lice inside nits or eggs?*
   Yes. One application of gamma benzene hexachloride will normally kill adult lice as well as the developing larva inside the egg. Nits do remain attached to the hair shaft though, and a fine-toothed comb may be needed to remove them.

SCABIES

1. *What is needed to treat scabies?*
   Gamma benzene hexachloride is used to treat older children and adults. Young children and pregnant or breast-feeding women should use crotamiton (Eurax).
2. *How long will the itching continue after I have been treated for scabies?*
   This varies among individuals, depending upon how sensitive they are to the scabies infestation and the degree of involvement. The itching is due to an allergic reaction to the scabies mite. Normally the itching will subside within 2 weeks.
3. *Can scabies live off the human body?*
   The scabies mite can survive only a few days when not in contact with the human body. Articles of clothing and bed linen used 2 to 3 days prior to treatment should be washed in the hot cycle of the washer and dryer.
4. *Do animals carry scabies?*
   Animals carry scabies mites that result in mange. Humans are rarely infected and have a mild condition when compared to true scabies.
5. *Are scabies transmitted only through sexual contact?*
   No. Mites may be transmitted via close body contact, often incidental to sexual intercourse, and can be spread via infected bedding or clothing.

Index

About the Editors

VINCENT A. SPAGNA is a Clinical Assistant Professor of Medicine at The Ohio State University College of Medicine, Columbus, and a staff member at Riverside Methodist Hospital, Columbus, Ohio. He received his M.D. degree in 1974 from New York Medical College, New York City, and took his residency at The Ohio State University College of Medicine, where he completed a fellowship in infectious diseases and also received the M.S. degree in medical microbiology. Dr. Spagna has served as Assistant Clinical Director of the Venereal Disease Clinic of the Columbus Health Department, and has conducted (with Dr. Prior) extensive research in the clinical and laboratory aspects of sexually transmitted diseases, resulting in several publications and a patented test for the office evaluation of urethritis/cervicitis syndromes. Dr. Spagna is board certified in Internal Medicine, a member of Alpha Omega Alpha (Medical Honorary) Society, and holds memberships in numerous medical and microbiological societies.

RICHARD B. PRIOR is an Associate Professor in the Department of Medicine, and Associate Professor in the Department of Microbiology at The Ohio State University, Columbus, where he has been a faculty member since receiving the Ph.D. degree in 1972. Dr. Prior has contributed to the medical literature and lectured extensively in the areas of clinical microbiology and infectious diseases. He has conducted research in these fields with emphasis on venereal diseases, and developed and patented (with Dr. Spagna) a simple test for office evaluation of urethritis/cervicitis syndromes which uses the *Limulus* (horseshoe crab) lysate assay. Dr. Prior is a member of numerous societies including the American Society for Microbiology and the American Venereal Disease Association.